CHILDHOOD and ADOLESCENCE

A Psychology of the Growing Person

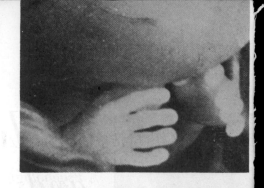

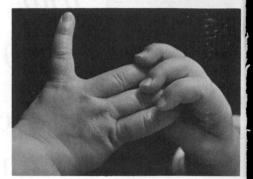

Random House
NEW YORK

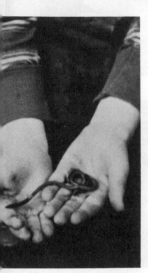

Childhood and Adolescence

A Psychology of the Growing Person

SECOND EDITION

L. Joseph Stone
VASSAR COLLEGE

Joseph Church
BROOKLYN COLLEGE OF THE CITY UNIVERSITY OF NEW YORK

Photo Credits / Title Page

(Top left) Edith L. Potter, *Fundamentals of Human Reproduction*
(Below left) Wayne Miller
(Right) *Children in Community*

Foreword to the First Edition

By Otto Klineberg

Columbia University

This book really needs no introduction by me, or by anyone else. The authors speak for themselves—and for children—clearly, soundly, constructively. They are men of recognized competence in the field of child study; I am just a little embarrassed at being asked to present to the reading public the work of two specialists who know much more about this subject than I do. By contrast, however, I can perform a pleasant function which would have been just a little embarrassing for them. I can tell everyone else that this is an excellent book.

It is rare in my experience to encounter a book which satisfies the scientific canons of sound and rigorous scholarship and at the same time makes such good reading. The subject matter may be responsible in part, since there are few of us who are not interested in children, but I have read too many dull books about them to feel that this is an adequate explanation. I think that what has happened in this case is that the authors not only know children but are genuinely fond of them, and that their warmth and enthusiasm somehow become clothed in clear and readable prose that delights the reader even as it instructs him.

On the theoretical side, the authors are frankly and explicitly eclectic. They are neither Freudian nor anti-Freudian, for example; they apply Freudian principles of explanation when appropriate, but not otherwise. They deal with learning theory, but they do not force all the data into that or any other psychological system. They obtain their material from many sources—from observation and experimentation with children, of course, but also from animal psychology (with reference to the effects of isolation on development), from sociology (in the excellent discussion of the part played by peer cultures), from cultural anthropology (for the purpose of cross-cultural comparisons). They are not extremist; in the long-standing quarrel between traditional and so-called progressive schools, they take their stand in favor of a "liberal" school which builds on the contributions and avoids the excesses of both. I for one find this general standpoint very palatable, since in my judgment truth is not the exclusive property of any one system or viewpoint, and a constructive eclecticism gives us a sounder and more complete picture of the complex reality of child behavior.

There are many different groups of readers to whom this book should bring both pleasure and profit. I think first of teachers and students of child psychology (or child study) who should find this a suitable and attractive textbook. It seems to me to be appropriate also as a text or at least as required reading in courses on educational psychology, in which knowledge of the child must surely be a major preoccupation. It should be helpful to others who deal professionally with children, for example, teachers and school administrators, social workers, pediatricians. Cultural anthropologists and other social scientists who do field work outside our society will find in it a clear picture of what is known about American children, which should serve as a sound basis for comparisons with child development under different social conditions.

Finally, but far from least important, the book has much to offer the reader who is sometimes identified as the "intelligent layman," and more particularly the fathers and mothers who are looking for guidance in understanding their own children. It has been suggested that Americans are so insecure in this respect that they become eager disciples of the so-called experts, and our comic magazines are filled with unflattering references to the "techniques" of the child psychologist. It is true that in the fairly recent past many people followed rather slavishly the rules which such experts laid down, only to discover a little later that new experts had developed new rules. This book helps us all to put those rules in proper perspective. It sees the parent not as a slave to the child, or to the expert, but as a partner in the process of adaptation and socialization. It offers no blueprint for child-rearing, but it does provide something more important, a clear and readable and sound guide to child understanding.

It gives me great satisfaction to write this word of introduction to a book which I have enjoyed so much.

Preface to the Second Edition

This is a revised edition of a book that first went to press just a decade ago. These ten years have been lively ones in the field of child development, and this revision seeks to incorporate the new advances in knowledge about psychological development, in ways of conceptualizing development, and in techniques for studying children and the developmental process. At the same time, the authors have tried to retain those features of the earlier edition that gave it its special character.

For many adults, children are a relatively little understood subspecies of humanity, sometimes enchanting, sometimes exasperating, but in either case baffling. It is our aim to convey a more accurate understanding of children by describing—like a naturalist reporting on a new species—the shape, size, nature, haunts, habits, and activities of the breed, from conception to the point at maturity when it loses its special identity and becomes part of mankind at large.

Our description seeks to be a systematic, integrated, and interpretive one, rather than a simple compilation or summary of facts. We have tried to include all the facts that we judge to be important for an understanding of childhood and development, but subordinated to the child as a person in a world. Our outlook is in part ecological, with strong emphasis on the material and social context of behavior and development; in part it is phenomenological, in an attempt to convey how things appear to the child himself. Our facts are drawn not only from psychology but also from anthropology, sociology, psychiatry, and zoology. We have profited likewise from the insights of poets, novelists, and just plain people with a sharp eye for the doings of children.

Before we tell the prospective reader about what is new in the present edition, we want to stress what has been conserved from the first one. Our concern is still with all aspects of childhood: as something worthy of study in its own right, as the period on which adulthood is founded, and as the embodiment of general principles of behavior and development. We are concerned both with child psychology and with developmental psychology. Our focus is on the child as a person. It is still our contention that it is impossible to understand child development apart from the material, personal, and cultural context in which the child develops. Our general scheme of organization, as in the first edition, is chronological, in terms of age periods, and follows the young person through the major phases of growth. Topics such as emotion, perception, social relations, self-awareness, physical and motor development, and schooling are discussed in the context of the particular age period. We have felt free, however, to depart from this general scheme of age divisions whenever it seemed necessary to stress either the continuities or discontinuities of functioning across ages.

We have tried once again to keep in mind various kinds of readers and their diverse needs: psychology students and their instructors, teachers and prospective teachers, parents and prospective parents, clinicians, researchers, medical students and practicing pediatricians and psychiatrists, nurses, home economists, and others. While our primary emphasis has been on depicting the child, we have also been concerned with the application of knowledge about children to practical problems of child-rearing, education, and social action. Although we have been concerned at every point with the practical implications of facts and concepts, we have not tried to spell them all out in detail. This is because we believe that the most effective applications derive from a general understanding of how a child functions rather than from a set of prescriptions, no matter how well founded these may be. Obviously, each reader will approach this book in a way in keeping with his or her own interests. But this does not mean that thus-and-such sections are addressed only to certain kinds of readers, or that readers looking only for a particular kind of information should read only the immediately relevant sections. The more practice-oriented passages are rooted in theoretical ones and cannot properly be understood in isolation from them. Moreover, the practice-oriented sections carry much of the factual and theoretical material of the book.

This revised edition attempts to take account of the new facts and new ways of thinking about development that have emerged in the past decade. Among the general changes that have taken place in the past ten years is a recognition of developmental psychology as a major field of psychology at large. Not only has there been an increased interest in studying children as children, but also in a developmental approach to understanding phenomena which have not traditionally been thought of as developmental. Thus, the experimental psychologist of perception has become increasingly involved in studying what newborn babies see, hear, smell, or otherwise react to, and how perceptual capacities are elaborated early in life. The decade has seen renewed interest in all aspects of cognition and cognitive development, including perception, the acquisition of knowledge, thinking, imagination and creativity, and symbolic functioning. There has been wider awareness of the destructive effects on cognition of early material and psychological privation, and of the need to find ways of offsetting such consequences, as in special programs of "enrichment." We have rediscovered important analogies between human development in infrahuman species, and the past ten years have seen an outpouring of research dealing with the effects of early experience on the later psychological functioning of sundry beasts, including monkeys, fowl, rodents, turtles, and even insects. We have become newly sensitive to the influence of context not only on postnatal behavior and development but also on anatomical and physiological development before birth. The concept of "critical periods" in development has undergone considerable elaboration in the time between editions. There has been a revival of interest in values and the moral and ethical dimensions of human action, and in the ways codes of values are imparted to children. Above all, we have come to comprehend the extreme plasticity of young human beings, with all that this implies about both the danger of damaging them and the opportunity and obligation to rear them to humane adulthood.

More specifically, the present volume is almost half again bigger than its predecessor. The bulk of the new research shows up in the early chapters, dealing with the neonate, prenatal development, and infancy. We have also brought together in a new chapter scattered sections from the first edition on developmental principles and approaches and added further treatments of theories and research methods. In later chapters, we have revised our accounts of language learning and concept formation and proposed a new conception of intellectual development and intellectual differences. As the child moves out into the world of school and society, we have become concerned with the impact of the technological and social revolution and its effect on the very character of childhood and youth and on the processes of identity formation. In general, throughout this edition, we have included more reports of specific studies and discussion of research techniques, without, we trust, losing sight of the child and the flow of his development. In trying to knit together the knowledge and insights of the past and present, we have also tried to anticipate the future. For it seems clear that it will be a long time before we can have a final human psychology, if only because culture keeps evolving and human behavior changes with it.

In the preface to the first edition, we made acknowledgments to the teachers and colleagues who had contributed to our thinking, and ten years later we still find ourselves in the debt of Heinz Werner, Gardner and Lois Murphy, Otto Klineberg, L. K. Frank, K. M. Dallenbach, R. B. MacLeod, Max Wertheimer, Bruno Klopfer, Margaret Mead, Benjamin Spock, Mary Essex, Eveline Omwake, Barbara Biber, and Eugene Lerner. Our erstwhile editor, Charles D. Lieber, has continued to give us sage counsel over the years. We think it does no injustice to our teachers and associates to say that we have learned most from the children we have known, in nursery schools and elsewhere, including our own. Each of us owes his own children special gratitude for the bits of their lives that we have watched and enjoyed and which they have allowed us to smuggle into these pages. Each at his or her own level of sophistication has contributed information on the inner workings of childhood. The later influences are too numerous to list, which in no way diminishes our obligation to the students and thoughtful readers whose comments have helped shape this revision. In the pages that follow we pay tribute and express our debt to the many researchers who have made it necessary to revise this book and who, in doing so, make the authors proud to be a part of the enterprise of developmental psychology.

L.J.S.   J.C.

Contents

CHILDHOOD and ADOLESCENCE

A Psychology of the Growing Person

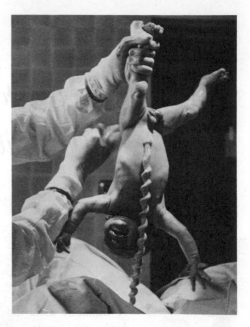

In our society, where almost all babies are born in hospitals, the birth process may be a secret veiled from all but the professional workers who officiate. Even the mother, if she has been heavily anesthetized, may not get a good look at her baby for a day or more.

Eve Arnold

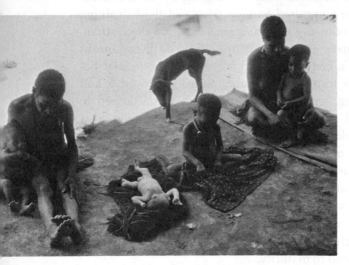

In many societies, childbirth is a public event: Everybody knows what a newborn baby looks like. Here, in New Guinea, Iatmul children—and animals—welcome a new arrival to the village, twenty minutes old.

Gregory Bateson and Margaret Mead, FIRST DAYS IN THE LIFE OF A NEW GUINEA BABY/N.Y.U. Film

1 *The Birth of the Baby*

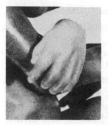

A moment after he has emerged from his mother's body, the newborn baby is dangling by his feet from the doctor's upraised hand, a trickle of fluid draining from his nose and mouth. A smart slap on the bottom, and he gives a thin, reedy wail. The birth cry marks the baby's first breath and serves as a boundary between his former waterborne, parasitic existence and his status as an air-breathing, separate organism. He is still attached to his mother by his umbilical cord, but this has ceased functioning as a life line and will shortly be clamped off and severed—a painless operation. In another fifteen or twenty minutes, the placenta in which the umbilical cord terminates, having separated from the lining of the mother's womb, will be delivered, with its attached membranes, as the afterbirth. The neonate immediately has drops of silver nitrate solution (or penicillin ointment) put into his eyes as insurance against infection, he is labeled with his family's name and given a brief physical examination, and a new human being is on the long road to maturity.

One of the odd by-products of our urban-suburban civilization is that many Americans never see a newborn baby until confronted with their own. Many new parents, whose expectations are based on the idealized "newborn" babies shown in advertisements (usually babies two or three months old), are taken aback at their first sight of their tiny, wet, sticky, possibly red and wizened baby. It is because so many people are unfamiliar with neonates that we must begin with a description of the baby's physical appearance. Later on, we shall talk a good deal about the

3

biological and psychological individuality that exists from birth—and, indeed, from conception—but let us first describe newborn-ness in general, the still somewhat fetal character that neonates have in common. Note that we speak of the baby as a neonate not only as he is within the first few minutes after birth but also during the first few weeks of postnatal life.

Physical Appearance of the Neonate

The newborn baby seems incredibly small: average weight 7 pounds (3+ kg.) (although we have a newspaper clipping announcing the birth of a baby weighing 17 pounds [7.7 kg.]), average length 20 inches (51cm.); since he* keeps his legs drawn up, he is likely to look even smaller. His proportions are very different from those of later life: His head makes up a quarter of his overall length (try to picture an adult with these proportions) and seems to rest directly on his puny shoulders, his neck being all but invisible; his almost useless legs are about a third of his total length. When he is held vertical under the arms, his head lolls and his bowed legs hang helplessly. His feet, which seem disproportionately long, are bent inward at the ankles, so that the soles are almost parallel. His facial proportions, too, will undergo many changes; his cranial vault is well developed, but his features are small and unarticulated, and he seems virtually chinless. His nose may have been flattened and his head squeezed out of shape (*molded*) in his passage through the birth canal. This molding disappears within a week or two. The neonate may still be wearing his fetal hair, dark and coarse, not only on his crown but sometimes elsewhere: low across his brows or far down his back, for instance. This hair, if present, will eventually be replaced by a regular crop, either gradually or after an intervening period of baldness. The baby at birth is still wet with the *amniotic fluid* in which he was immersed before birth and his skin is coated with a cheeselike protective substance, the *vernix caseosa*, which, when it dries, gives his skin a chalky cast. Depending on his maturity, his coloring may range from pale livid to rosy pink, perhaps tinged with the so-called *normal physiological jaundice of the newborn* (see below). Both eye and skin pigments are slow to develop, so that virtually all babies are born with smoky blue eyes and even Negro neonates may have light skins for the first few days. The

---

* Except where sex differences are an issue, we shall refer throughout to the child as "he." This is to avoid the awkwardness of "he or she" and the feelingless neutrality of "it."

neonate's skull has six soft spots, or *fontanels,* openings covered with a tough, resilient membrane; the most conspicuous of these is at the very top of the head and may not close over until age one and a half.

The genitals of the newborn are at first surprisingly large and prominent. Neonates—both boys and girls—in many cases have enlarged breasts which may secrete a milklike substance called "witch's milk," and girls may have a brief "menstrual" flow shortly after birth. These phenomena are caused by hormones absorbed from the mother's bloodstream and subside rapidly.

The neonate is likely to look scrawny because he has not yet fully developed his layers of body fat, except for the fat pads that fill out his cheeks. The fat pads play an important part in sucking and, incidentally, keep the baby's toothless mouth from having the withered look of an old person's. Premature babies (defined not by age since conception but by a birth weight of less than 5 pounds [2¼ kg.; the European cutoff point, however, is 2½ kg.]) have underdeveloped fat pads and look remarkably senile. At the other extreme, very mature neonates may be well plumped out with body fat and so resemble the pink pudginess shown in advertisements.

We should not be misled by the unprepossessing, almost larval look of the average neonate. All his body structures are present, some ready for full functioning, others only in rudimentary form. He is a real human being, down to the last eyelash and the miniature nails on fingers and toes. All the nerve cells are present at birth, but in immature form—the brain more than doubles in size, from 350 cc. to 750 cc., between birth and age one, and doubles again by age six. In the neonate's jaws are buds for two sets of teeth. The newborn girl's ovaries contain what is thought by some to be a lifetime supply of rudimentary ova, although mature sperm cells do not form in the testes of the boy until middle childhood.

The "feel" of a neonate is something to be experienced. A skilled adult can hold him in one hand, fingertips bracing the back of his skull, the heel of the palm holding his shoulders, the forearm supporting his almost nonexistent buttocks. But not all newborn babies feel alike to hold. Some remain compactly and comfortably curled, like kittens, others sprawl like bundles of loosely joined sticks, some are tense and stiff, still others squirm and writhe or flail. Even at this age, we see the beginnings of marked individual differences in behavior.

Basic Life Processes in the Neonate

If the neonate is to grow and flourish, his first order of business is to stay alive. Although our concern in this book is not primarily with the physiological processes that maintain life, these are so central in the existence of the newborn baby that we must see how they settle down to dependable operation before we go on to examine the rudiments of behavior in the neonate.

The complete transition from fetal to postnatal ways of living takes between two weeks and a month. It is the end of this transition that marks the end of the neonatal period and the beginning of infancy. The transition begins, however, with the birth cry; and when we consider the drastic change of environment involved in being born, from the dark, waterborne passivity of the womb to autonomous life in the light and air, the neonate does a remarkable job of adapting. His various body mechanisms may work unevenly and inharmoniously, but they do work, and the baby is a lot more durable than he seems to anxious parents.

Prior to birth, as we have said, the baby lived in total darkness, suspended in a fluid bath (*the amniotic fluid*) at a constant temperature, and cushioned against mechanical buffetings. He received oxygen, water, nutrients, and other substances (some perhaps beneficial and others demonstrably harmful) directly into his bloodstream through the umbilical cord that joined him by his navel to the placenta and so to his mother's bloodstream (see page 23), and discharged body wastes and other bloodborne materials into the blood flowing to the placenta. Although most prenatal metabolic wastes are disposed of in this way, once the fetus's kidneys are working he excretes small amounts of urine directly into the amniotic fluid. In addition, he swallows mucus and amniotic fluid containing shed skin and hair, and solid wastes are formed in the bowel as *meconium*, a greenish-black, tarry substance which also contains bile from the liver. (Meconium is not ordinarily excreted before birth.) Once he is born, the baby's body must shift to new patterns of circulation and must do for itself the jobs of respiration, digestion, and temperature control.

RESPIRATION

Breathing is a new activity for the neonate, although there is some evidence that he may "practice" in the uterus. The baby's first breath may be stimulated simply by his being exposed to air, it may be set off by a sneeze or a yawn, or it may be stimulated by the traditional (in our society) slap on the bottom, producing the birth cry which sets in chain the whole complicated reflex pattern of lifelong inhalation and exhalation. Almost any sort of stimulation can be used to start the baby breathing, as by massage; by dipping him into warm water, or cold water, or an alternation of both; by mouth-to-mouth breathing; or by various more drastic measures that are sometimes called for. The neonate's lungs are at first congested with mucus and amniotic fluid, and he may have to spend a few days with his head lower than his feet to facilitate drainage. The muscle groups active in breathing are poorly coordinated for some weeks after birth, and the neonate's respiration tends to be noisy, shallow, and irregular. Because the soft palate has not yet been integrated into respiration, the neonate's breath may rattle in his throat in an alarming but innocuous way.

CIRCULATION

The shift from fetal to postnatal circulation begins with the first breath. The abdominal muscles surrounding the umbilical vessels contract, and circulation through the cord slows down immediately and ceases within a few minutes, making it possible to clamp off and sever the cord. The navel opening heals over within five days, and the dried, atrophied stump of umbilical cord drops off in a week or two. Increased pressure in the left atrium of the heart closes a flap over the *foramen ovale*, the opening between the left and right ventricles, and the foramen grows permanently closed within ten days. The shutting off of the umbilical arteries forces blood to the lungs, which now take over the job of aeration previously done by the pools of maternal blood surrounding the capillaries from the infant's side of the circulatory system of the placenta. The oxygen level of the blood reaches 90 per cent of normal within three hours after birth. The acid-alkaline balance (pH) of the blood is normal in a week or so, and blood pressure is normal within ten days.

A day or so after birth, a number of babies develop what has been called normal physiological jaundice of the newborn (or, more technically, *icterus neonatorum*). The jaundice is caused by the presence in the blood of a substance called bilirubin, produced when red blood cells break down and perhaps involving liver function. The authorities differ on the cause of the breaking down of the red corpuscles, some holding that the baby is born with a surplus which has to be eliminated, others suspecting that it is due to incompatibilities of ABO blood types between

7

mother and child, which sometimes, it now appears, lead to disorders comparable to those produced by the Rh incompatibilities to be discussed later (see page 33). In any case, moderate icterus of brief duration seems to be self-limiting and with no serious consequences for the baby, but requires close observation to differentiate it from much rarer severe jaundice and kernicterus which can have serious consequences of brain damage. There is growing evidence of specific genetic factors in the latter, related to enzyme production and to triggering effects of certain foods and chemicals, such as the fumes of common moth balls.[1] Notice the analogy here to the condition known as phenylketonuria, discussed on page 42.

DIGESTION

The baby, unlike the fetus, must take in sustenance through his mouth, digest it in his alimentary tract, and eliminate wastes by urination and defecation. (We leave out of account the elimination of wastes through sweating, the shedding of dead skin and hair, and the necessity of cropping off dead or superfluous tissue as in nail and hair trimming.)

From birth the baby's digestive tract is equipped with enzymes to handle all the basic foods except some starches, and in a short time the neonate takes in from his surroundings the beneficent bacteria necessary to digestion. (Since vitamin K, which is important for blood clotting, is produced by the intestinal bacteria, any lesion in the first few days holds the threat of serious hemorrhage.) It is usually assumed in American hospitals that babies cannot eat for a day or two after they are born. Certainly the mother's milk does not "come in" until eighteen or twenty-four hours after the birth, although her breasts may secrete a milklike substance called *colostrum*, thought by some to have nutritional value. However, observations of babies born into some "primitive" societies, such as Iatmul, where they are breast-fed by wet nurses immediately after birth, would suggest that neonates are indeed capable of managing food almost at once. Whenever he begins, the newborn's eating is likely to be unskilled. At first, he takes fluids in 1- or 2-ounce doses, of which a good part may be promptly regurgitated, and more often than not the infant, in the American hospital regime at least, loses weight for the first few days of life. The excretion of meconium and the elimination of mucus and other wastes furthers this weight loss. A fair number of babies, from the age of two or three weeks, suffer badly from colic, marked by severe gastric pain. The cause of colic is unknown, and it usually clears up spontaneously by age three months.

TEMPERATURE REGULATION

Mechanisms for internal temperature control develop slowly, so that the newborn is at the mercy of fluctuations in environmental temperature and may easily become chilled or overheated. His sweat glands begin operating only when he is about a month old, the absence of sweating meanwhile making it easier for him to conserve heat and body fluids. Parents, in adjusting the environment to the baby's needs, often err on the side of keeping him too warm and may incidentally interfere with the normal development of temperature-regulating mechanisms.

IMMUNITY AND SUSCEPTIBILITY

Among the substances absorbed by the fetus from his mother's bloodstream are antibodies which give him several months of immunity to various infections. Indeed, the sicknesses traditionally associated with "teething" from age six months onward probably represent simply the coincidental wearing off of earlier immunities acquired from the mother. In spite of his borrowed antibodies, the newborn baby is very susceptible to infections of the gastrointestinal tract, respiratory system, and skin. (A goodly number of babies also develop early such allergic reactions as hay fever and eczema.) It will take the baby some years to build up his own system of resistances, and parents in the interim have to protect him against infection. Some parents, of course, are overprotective, to the point where they may severely restrict the baby's experience. Moreover, over-protection retards the necessary formation of the baby's own immunities, and may have the paradoxical result of making the baby more vulnerable rather than less.

Behavioral Capacities of the Neonate

The past decade has seen a revolution in the study and understanding of the psychological capacities of the newborn. When we consider that people have been having and rearing babies for as long as there have been people, it is amazing how little was securely known about neonatal behavior. In the past several years, there has been an outpouring of research by such investigators as Bartoshuk, Blauvelt, Bridger, Caldwell, Crowell, Fantz, Graham, Lipsitt, Lipton, Richmond, Steinschneider, Stechler, White, and Wolff[2] (to mention just a few) which has completely changed our thinking about the neonate and given us a new respect for his abilities. This revolution has been the product of several things: of a new awareness that one cannot understand development without knowing its origins; of improved observations and ingenious test devices; of the shrewd use of "index" or "indicator" responses, physical reactions to sensory stimulation, such as changes in heart rate, brain waves, or skin conductance; of an awareness that the baby's *state*— whether he is awake or sleeping or somewhere in between, whether he is calm or distressed, hungry or sated—is an important consideration in evaluating his behavior. An important consideration has been our re-discovery that human development has a number of infrahuman analogs, and that work with animal species permits a number of experimental manipulations impossible with human subjects. We have also learned that human neonates *habituate* rather quickly, that they will stop re-sponding to a stimulus as the novelty wears off, so that our measurements have to take account of whether a response comes early in a series or late.

The newborn spends much of his time sleeping, perhaps twenty hours a day. During the first few weeks, sleeping and waking are only a matter of degree, and the neonate rarely appears fully awake except when hungry, startled, or otherwise distressed. When he is crying and an adult picks him up, he ordinarily quiets immediately—if only temporarily —indicating his responsiveness to the sensations that go with being held, cuddled, and rocked. When awake and in reasonable physiological balance, as just after a feeding (or the elimination that is likely to follow a feeding), he may stare fixedly but somewhat blankly at a face or a spot of light that happens to fall within his field of view. Asleep or awake, he is subject to fits and starts and tremors reflecting the spread of stimula-tion in his still immature nervous system. A still unexplained recent finding is that the sleeping newborn shows the brain wave pattern and the rapid eye movements (REM) that in adults signal the occurrence of dreaming—it is as though the physiological mechanisms of dreaming are present from the beginning, anticipating the arrival of something to dream about.[3] In fact, the proportion of REM sleep is distinctly higher in the infant than it will be later.

POSTURE AND MOVEMENT

Most babies quite early have a "preference" for lying either on their backs or on their bellies, as shown by agitated movements or crying when the baby is put down in the less favored position and by relaxation when placed in the favored one—the mother's becoming sensitive to such cues is an important part of learning to communicate with her baby. On back or belly, the baby keeps his arms and legs flexed, his fingers curled more or less tightly into fists, and his head turned to one, favored side. Babies who regularly lie on their backs are likely to develop a bald spot and some flattening of the skull at the place where it meets the mattress. This flattening is harmless and disappears, although not always completely, as the baby begins to vary his sleeping position, somewhere around age six months. When in distress, the newborn squirms, twists his head from side to side, and flails his limbs—not randomly, but, as high-speed cinematography shows, in a highly stereotyped pattern.

Lying alone on a table or in a bassinet, the neonate is virtually helpless, but he becomes a different creature when in contact with a responding human adult. That is, his *state* changes, and with it his capabilities, according to his behavioral context. We have already mentioned the way his crying stops when he is picked up and held close. When he is hungry, he engages in complex *rooting* behavior: Like newborn infrahuman mammals, he "searches" the adult body with his mouth as though for a nipple; he clutches firmly at whatever handholds he finds—clothing, hair, folds of skin—and propels himself, if not restrained, with trunk, arms, and legs, so actively that the adult may wonder if, like the Duchess's baby in *Alice in Wonderland*, he isn't changing into a small pig. Most first-time mothers (in our society) who are breast-feeding their babies have to be shown how to get themselves and the neonate into position for nursing, and how to put the breast into the baby's mouth; but as long as the mother plays her part properly, the neonate adapts reciprocally. Sometimes, according to Gunther,[4] the mother's breast blocks the baby's nostrils and produces partial suffocation. Films made by Helen Blauvelt show that when the neonate is picked up to be carried against an adult shoulder, he presses his cheek against the adult's. The usual adult response is to press back, which only pushes the baby's head over to the other side. If, instead, the adult tilts her (or his) head away from the baby's, the baby's head slides down to the base of the adult's neck, and when the adult straightens up her head, the two are perfectly interlocked. Blauvelt[5] has described a number of patterns of mother-child adaptations and compared them to those she observed in sheep and goats; in these infrahuman species, such reciprocal adaptations, which are so uniform as to seem like ritual, play an important part in establishing right after birth the mother-child relationships essential to the young animal's survival. Thus, Spitz[6] has spoken of the "intricate ballet" constituting early mutual adaptations in the mother and infant dyad.

The newborn baby has only a limited command of his hands, which, when not in use, he is likely to keep fisted. As we know, people learn to use their hands in a variety of ways—to feed themselves, to draw and write, to pick their noses and to pick pockets, to make love, to mold clay, to handle tools—but it is possible to specify quite briefly the newborn baby's total repertory. He may, in waving his arms, score his face with his fingernails, for which reason his shirt sleeves may have to be folded or sewn closed over his hands; but it will be at least a month before he can scratch at an insect bite or a patch of eczema. He does grasp when his hand is properly stimulated, but he does not as yet reach out to grasp things that he merely sees.[7] He clings when rooting, and when nursing he soon begins to clasp the breast or bottle, but he does not yet cling to the adult who holds him upright against the adult's body. He may be able to suck his thumb at birth—it appears that some fetuses suck their thumbs prenatally—but many newborn babies cannot find their mouths with their hands, try as they may, while others, when hungry, hook the whole hand into the mouth.

EMOTIONS

The newborn baby's emotional expression is often intense, but it lacks variety. Distress, whether from hunger, pain, heat, cold, or whatever, comes out as tearless crying, thrashing, and turning red all over. (Although the tear glands play no part in most neonates' crying, they act continuously to bathe the eyeballs and will step up their activity to wash away irritants.) Crowell and associates[8] and others have recently demonstrated that newborn babies show a galvanic skin response, which is one autonomic index of emotionality in older subjects. When the baby is contented, as after a feeding, he may, awake or asleep, smile.[9] This early "pleasure smile" must be distinguished both from the *social smile*, which appears during the second month in response to the human face or voice, and from the "gas smile," the twisted precursor of a burp. For the most part, however, the neonate is blankly unemotional.

Nearly a half century ago, the famous behaviorist John B. Watson[10] postulated three basic emotions present at birth and linked to reliable, unconditioned stimuli: fear, produced by loss of support; rage, produced by restraint; and love, elicited by fondling. These emotions later, by associative conditioning, became attached to new stimuli. Subsequent observations have failed to support Watson's hypothesis. Although loss of support (or a loud noise or a flash of bright light) will provoke a Moro response (to be described on page 16), careful observation by the

Shermans and by Bridges and others[11] indicates that one cannot differentiate among kinds of unpleasant emotion in the newborn. Second, while vigorous crying and kicking can be produced by partial immobilization of the neonate, snug swaddling arrests crying and struggling and soothes the baby.[12] Last, there is no indication that the neonate feels affection toward anybody or anything, although such affection develops quickly in the first few months. We might mention here the early beginnings of an important form of social behavior, imitation of the behavior of others; the earliest recorded imitation appears at ten to twenty days of age, when the baby imitates the adult's sticking out his tongue.[13]

SENSORY CAPACITIES AND PERCEPTION

The neonate's sense organs are in good working order, but they bring him only a limited amount of information. We must bear in mind that there are decided individual differences in sensitivities of various kinds and in strengths of reaction to stimulation. There is some evidence to suggest that some newborns, within a few minutes after birth, turn to look in the direction of sounds that catch their attention.[14] Within a day or two, the neonate can, somewhat unreliably, track a moving object with his eyes. A few babies right after birth can turn their heads to follow a moving object, and most can do so within a few weeks. Fantz[15] has shown that the newborn baby discriminates patterns; thus, he spends more time looking at black and white figures than at unfigured colored areas, and a crude approximation of the human face is looked at significantly more than is a nonsensical arrangement of the same features. Fantz's technique for determining the direction of the baby's gaze is an interesting one: By peering through a hole in the screen on which the stimulus materials are mounted, he can see which of two forms is reflected on the baby's eye in the region of the pupil. There is evidence, however, that the neonate's eye has a fixed focus for objects at a distance of about 7½ inches (19 cm.), which may mean that more distant objects are seen as blurred.[16]

Tactual cues are important in guiding the baby's rooting behavior, and it seems likely that olfactory cues play a part. The neonate reacts with distress to unpleasant olfactory stimuli, such as ammonia or asafetida,[17] and to unpleasant gustatory ones such as quinine.[18] Although the neonate seems indifferent to whether he is held head up or head down, the vestibular apparatus of his inner ear is working, as shown by the eye movements—like those of adults—that occur after he has been spun on a turntable.[19] He is relatively insensitive to painful stimulation at birth, but his sensitivity, as measured by his reactions to pin pricks or mild electric shock, increases rapidly in the first few days.[20] Nevertheless, circumcision in the first week requires no more anesthetic than the distracting effect of a sugar ball in the baby's mouth. His reactions to internal pain, as of colic or hunger cramps, are much more pronounced. It is not clear whether the newborn tries to turn away from or to push away noxious stimuli. If he does, it is weakly and ineffectually: Observation shows that he cannot rid himself of a cleaning tissue spread over his face, which means that accidental suffocation is a real danger for very young babies, when simple head-turning is insufficient to remove an obstruction. There is some reason to believe that it is the strong intensity of a stimulus that makes it noxious to the newborn, rather than its more specific qualities as perceived by adults. Well into infancy the child reacts aversively to strong light, and in later infancy to loud noises and strongly flavored foods, though marked individual differences in responsiveness are noted. We must point out, however, that babies are often impervious to stimuli that are very prominent for adults and older children. The young baby may not react at all, for instance, to thunder, fire sirens, or the clatter of trash cans. The smells that older children and adults find disgusting, such as the odors of body wastes, affect the neonate not at all. On the other hand, the baby may react very negatively to stimulation that seems innocuous to adults, such as the crackling of stiff paper.

The use of such index responses as change in heartbeat or respiration has made it possible to study hearing in the newborn baby. Bartoshuk[21] has shown that increase in heartbeat varies directly (obviously, there is a ceiling) with increases in the intensity of sound, yielding a curve of auditory response virtually identical with that of the adult, provided that the sound is turned on when the baby's heartbeat is at a given rate. For any one level of sound intensity, there seems to be a more or less fixed level of corresponding heart rate, which means that the amount of change in heartbeat depends upon the rate at the moment of stimulation. Thus, if the baby's heart is beating at a relatively slow rate at the moment of stimulation, there will be a large increase to the level of heart rate corresponding to the particular intensity of the stimulus. If the heart is beating faster, less of an increase in rate is necessary to reach the same response level. If the baby's heart is beating at a rate faster than that associated with the stimulus, it will slow down to the appropriate level. It is not clear whether the observed decrease in heartbeat in response to sound means that the baby is in a state of agitation when stimulated and that the stimulation serves to focus his attention and so to calm him, but this seems to be the case in some circumstances.[22] The general relationship between the magnitude of change and the level of activity just prior to stimulation is called the *law of initial values* (LIV). Such psychophysical studies of vision and hearing in the neonate promise to make possible the early diagnosis of blindness and deafness.

LEARNING

Until recently, studies of whether newborn babies learn were limited for the most part to the method of classical conditioning. Attempts to associate such stimuli as a flash of light or the sound of a buzzer with such responses as sucking or autonomic reactions to electric shock yielded equivocal results. Now, studies by Papoušek and by Siqueland and Lipsitt show that head-turning can be conditioned to particular sounds during the first few days after birth, provided the baby is given immediate reinforcement in the form of milk or dextrose squirted into his mouth.[23] We know, too, that goslings and ducklings and lambs and kids learn to know their mothers within a few hours after hatching or birth. We also know that by the end of the neonatal period human babies have learned where milk comes from, as seen by their turning toward the breast or opening their mouths and straining toward the bottle.

REFLEXES

There is a wide array of reactions which can be rather dependably elicited in the newborn and which are often called *reflexes*. Some of these have little behavioral significance but may be very useful to the physician for diagnostic purposes, like the familiar knee-jerk (patellar) reflex. One of these, the plantar response, is interesting because it undergoes a change with development. If one strokes the sole of the neonate's foot, his toes fan up and outward in the *Babinski response*. Later in infancy, and for the rest of life except in conditions of brain damage and stupor, stroking the sole of the foot causes the toes to do the opposite, to curl downward. Other reflexes have practical adaptive significance but are primarily vegetative, that is, they do not involve the voluntary muscles. Such are the pupil's contraction to an increase in light, and salivation when something is placed in the mouth. Then there are "reflexes" involving complex motor behavior, such as the grasping and rooting responses, which probably should not be called reflexes since they can be varied adaptively instead of following a rigid pattern, since they cannot be elicited unless the baby is in the proper motivational state, and since

15

later on they will be superseded by new and more mature forms of action.

Of considerable importance to the neonate's survival is the sucking response, present at or shortly after birth. Tactile stimulation of the lips or cheek causes the baby to turn his head toward the source of stimulation (a nipple is the usual stimulus, but an experimenter's finger will work as well), try to take it into his mouth, and begin to suck. If the stimulus is indeed a milk-producing nipple, sucking and swallowing occur in fairly well-coordinated alternation. The sucking response may not appear unless the baby is hungry, but this is not a hard condition to meet. Newborn babies, according to Kron's observations,[24] show striking and consistently maintained individual differences in rate and intensity of sucking. Kron has also shown a distinct change and stabilization of the sucking response in the first few days. As mentioned before, if one wants to turn a young infant's face in a given direction, as for nursing, it does no good to push against his cheek—he turns his head in the direction that the push comes from. One should, it follows, touch the cheek on the side toward which one wants him to turn. If restraining a baby's head causes him distress, as Watson suggested, conceivably it is because he is being stimulated to turn his head in two directions at once.

We have already mentioned the *Moro response*, or infantile startle pattern. The Moro response can be set off by any sudden, intense stimulation, such as a loud noise. The neonate reacts by stretching wide his arms and legs, often crying at the same time, and then hugging himself together again. The tension subsides visibly within a few seconds. There is then usually a refractory phase, as with many other responses, during which the response cannot be elicited. Successive stimulations lead to a decrease in response, as though the baby were becoming habituated.

Apart from the scant "voluntary" use of hands mentioned above, the neonate, as stated, shows a *grasping reflex* when his palm or fingers are stimulated. He reacts by taking a firm grip on the rod or finger used to stimulate him—so firm in some babies that they can hang by their hands for as long as a minute.[25] Voluntary grasping supplants reflex grasping at about age four months, but even then, once the baby has something in his hand, the still-persistent grasp reflex makes it impossible for him to let go. One can also elicit a vestigial grasp reflex of the toes by stimulating the sole of the neonate's foot just at the base of the toes (note that the Babinski response is stimulated by stroking the middle of the sole, where the arch will be).

If the baby is supported horizontal on his belly, he may perform swimming movements (*swimming reflex*). If he is held vertical with his feet lightly touching a firm surface, he may move his legs as though walking (*stepping reflex*). These two responses disappear shortly after birth, to reappear later in more mature form. When the neonate lies prone, if the bottoms of his feet touch a surface he pushes against it, in some cases with sufficient force to move his body; this response accounts for reports of newborn babies' "crawling." Slightly later, he pushes back with his feet when lying supine.

Within the first hour after birth, given the right stimulating conditions, the baby shows such important vegetative reflexes as vomiting, sneezing, hiccoughing, yawning, and blinking. Boy babies can have a reflexive erection of the penis, and usually do just prior to urination. Wolff has reported rather frequent erections in neonates, apparently like those recently found to occur regularly during sleep in adult males of all ages, just before each REM sleep period. Attempts to identify analogous cycles of clitoral excitation in females are still inconclusive.[26]

LIMITATIONS OF THE NEONATE

Our description might lead the reader to conclude that any handling of the baby would produce great outbursts of reflex activity. Such is not the case. In fact, during routine care such as dressing and undressing, bathing, and medical examination, the baby for the first several months is remarkably passive, placid, and malleable. Most of the newborn's actual response capabilities may go unnoticed by parents, who may, however, at the same time anthropomorphically (or "adultomorphically") credit him with qualities of mind, morality, and purpose that the scientific observer is unable to verify.

For all his rudimentary humanity, it is as well to stress what the neonate cannot yet do. The only vocal sounds he makes are crying and the noises that accompany digestive processes. He cannot yet (with some rare exceptions) raise his head, or roll over (except by accident), or move his thumb and fingers separately. His hands do not reach out to things at a distance. He cannot control elimination. Although he begins almost immediately to pay attention to human faces, he cannot tell one face from another. He does not know that he has feet. He has nothing to remember and remembers nothing. His life is governed largely by the rhythms of his digestive tract and other physiological processes, and the rise and ebb of wakefulness, the triggers that set off reflex discharges, and the kind mercies of those who take care of him.

INDIVIDUAL DIFFERENCES AND INDIVIDUALITY

Right from the beginning, as we have said, the neonate manifests an individual uniqueness that is the product both of his special genetic make-up and of conditions in the uterine environment. Newborn babies are decidedly different one from another in the tonus of their bodies, the forcefulness or sluggishness with which they react, the speed at which they move their limbs, the zeal and vigor with which they attack the nipple and the patterning of bursts of sucking, their sensitivity to light or sound or touch, their irritability, their alertness; they differ in size and shape, in the absolute and relative size of body organs, in blood chemistry, and in hormonal balance.[27] Within a short time, the very proteins of the child's body become so individualized that they reject tissues transplanted from other individuals.[28] These, of course, are differences along single "dimensions," the scales defined by opposites such as fast-slow on which people can be assigned to various positions. In addition, however, each baby has a cluster of characteristics which adds up to an overall pattern of unique individuality which, unlike his positions on single scales, he shares with no one else in the world.

Let us stress an obvious but often neglected fact. People change as they grow, but they still retain their individuality. We know very little as yet about what the anatomical, physiological, and temperamental differences observable at birth mean for later development. Predictions made from early behavior to later functioning work out at better than chance expectations, but there are too many exceptions, including some very dramatic reversals, for us to have much confidence in the prognostic value of neonatal characteristics.[29] Nevertheless, it seems probable that the differences between any two individuals would mean that they would respond to and assimilate and integrate even very similar life experiences in different ways. We shall set forth as we go along some of the evidence for the radical role of the psychological environment in determining the course of postnatal development, but while experience may transform the individual it in no way diminishes his individuality. Even such an event as oxygen deficiency at birth, which is significantly associated with later intellectual impairment, has a differential effect on different individuals; as Graham and her associates[30] have pointed out, too many individuals escape the expected consequences of traumatic birth for us to make predictions in the particular case.

Prenatal Development

Now the baby is safely born, and the reader has some acquaintance with his lineaments, but before we follow the neonate toward adulthood, we must turn back and see where he has come from. For the baby at birth is already nine months old, and is considered a year old in the reckoning of several Oriental cultures. In addition, he has a genetic history linking him with a multitude of ancestors back to the dawn of life. (Our practice of drawing a family tree as spreading out from a single pair of founders is somewhat misleading; not only can a single couple have a throng of descendants, but the child has many progenitors, doubling in number each generation back—two parents, four grand-parents, eight great-grandparents, and so on.) We shall first follow the child's development from conception to birth, and then go still further back for a brief look at some principles of genetic inheritance.

CONCEPTION

The child begins life as a single cell, or *zygote*, formed by the union of two germ cells, or *gametes*, one contributed by the mother and one by the father. The paternal germ cell is called a *sperm* or *spermatozoon*, a microscopic free-swimming cell with a whiplike tail. Spermatozoa are produced in the *testes* (testicles), bodies which are also endocrine glands producing the male sex hormone *testosterone* and perhaps others. The two testes are contained in a pouch of skin, the scrotum, which is a part of the external male genitalia. The maternal germ cell is called an *ovum*, a tiny speck barely visible to the naked eye, but still some 85,000 times greater in volume than the sperm. Ova are formed in the *ovaries*, two bodies corresponding to the testes in the production of both germ cells and hormones but situated in the abdomen above and to each side of the uterus (as endocrine glands, the ovaries and testes are called *gonads*).

Sperm are continuously and copiously manufactured in the mature testes, so that the man is almost always fertile, that is, capable of siring a child. The woman, by contrast, usually produces only one mature ovum (that is, she *ovulates*) each lunar month of four weeks. Ovulation occurs as a part of the intricate, recurring pattern of fertility known as the *menstrual* or *estral* cycle, marked externally by the flow of blood from the vagina, that appears every twenty-eight days, on the average, in healthy adult human females. (In some other mammalian species, such as the cat and rabbit, ovulation is a response to coitus.) Ovulation takes place sometime between the end of menstruation and the midpoint of the menstrual cycle, the entire cycle being measured from the beginning of one menstrual flow to the beginning of the next. At ovulation, a blisterlike swelling on the surface of the ovary ruptures, releasing the ovum into the abdominal cavity, at the mouth of the Fallopian tube, which leads into the uterus. (There are two Fallopian tubes, one per ovary, but usually only one ovary produces an egg in any given month.) The ovum is drawn into the Fallopian tube and is carried down it (a distance of about three inches [7.5 cm.]) for the next three or four days. However, it is only during the six or seven hours immediately following ovulation that the ovum remains fertile; after that time, it begins to deteriorate. This does not mean, though, that sexual intercourse has to coincide with these few hours of fertility for conception to take place. Since sperm can live as long as two or three days within the woman's body, intercourse as much as seventy-two hours prior to ovulation can lead to pregnancy.

If the ovum is not fertilized, the ensuing chemical changes play their part in the sequence whereby the lining of the uterus (the *endometrium*), ready to receive and nourish a zygote, instead breaks down and is shed as menstrual blood. Immediately after menstruation, the uterine lining begins once more to build up, to thicken and become engorged with blood, until it is again ready for pregnancy.

In sexual intercourse, the male ejaculates about a teaspoonful of male fluid, or *semen,* containing upward of 350 million spermatozoa, into the vagina, near the *cervix,* the neck-like projection that surrounds the opening to the uterus. Unlike the ovum, which drifts passively downstream in the Fallopian currents, the spermatozoa can swim by lashing their tails. Some succeed in working their way through the cervical opening, through the uterus, and upstream into the Fallopian tube. The journey takes one or two hours. The casualties among the sperm cells are enormous, but, even so, a goodly number enter the tube that contains that month's ovum and there lie in wait. When the ovum arrives, the host of spermatozoa is drawn toward it and surrounds it. However, only a single sperm can unite with the ovum. The structures of the joined sperm and ovum break down and recombine to form a single cell, and a new individual has begun life.

STAGES OF PRENATAL DEVELOPMENT

Our newly formed person will go by several names, corresponding to important stages in his development, before he emerges as a neonate. The first stage lasts about two weeks, until the time menstruation would be expected, and is called the *germinal period* of gestation. During this time the zygote, which becomes a hollow sphere, is successively transformed into a *blastocyst,* marked by the formation of an inner cell mass at one side of the egg; a *gastrula,* marked by the appearance of a rudimentary gut; and a *neurula,* which shows the formation of primitive nerve tissue. During the ensuing six weeks, when all the organ systems are taking shape, our creature is called an *embryo.* Thereafter, from age eight weeks until birth, the developing child is called a *fetus.* The total gestation period is estimated at 266 days on the average. However, since it is usually impossible to date conception exactly, pregnancy is reckoned from the beginning of the last menstruation, and the normal term is set at 280 days, or ten lunar months. It is standard practice to describe prenatal development in lunar rather than calendar months, so the accompanying scale is provided to help the reader translate lunar months into the more familiar scheme. It will be noted that ten lunar months is approximately equal to the nine calendar months popularly allotted to pregnancy.

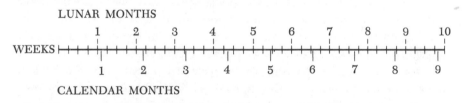

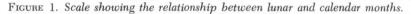

FIGURE 1. *Scale showing the relationship between lunar and calendar months.*

The Germinal Period. During the first two weeks of pregnancy, the mother has no awareness of the events going on inside her, nor can they be reliably detected by laboratory tests. Immediately after fertilization, the zygote in its slow passage down the Fallopian tube begins the process of cell division which will ultimately produce a human body consisting of some 26 billion cells. To see how successive cell divisions can produce this huge total, the reader has only to try carrying out successive multiplications by two: 1, 2, 4, 8, 16, 32, 64, 128, 256, 512, 1024, 2048, 4096, 8192, 16,384, and so on. The reader should not suppose, however, that the cells divide and subdivide all at once according to this neat numerical scheme. For instance, in a two-celled structure, if one cell divides, the total number becomes three; if another cell divides, the total becomes four. Cell division goes on in spurts, with resting interludes of several hours. We must stress the obvious point that the two cells formed by a cell division do not go their own ways like the two halves of an amoeba, each of which is a separate organism. Rather, they remain together in an organized way, with the growth and operation of the individual cell subordinated to the "master plan" of the total organic structure. It is interesting that early division is accomplished with no increase of total bulk: The cells increase in number but the resulting cells are smaller. Here we must signal an ambiguity. In some infrahuman species, the cells are at first all alike in composition; they are *equipotential* and in experiments can be transplanted from place to place without disturbing the total design. Thus, tissue from the eye region becomes limb tissue if transplanted to the region of a future limb. Later, cell tissues become *specialized* and *self-determining*, so that, if transplanted, they grow according to the design of their original location. Now, specialized eye tissue, even though an eye has not yet begun to form, will, if transplanted, grow into a misplaced eye. In other infrahuman species, however, it appears that even in the unfertilized egg the cytoplasm has already differentiated in composition and determines which kinds of cells will develop out of the various regions. We do not yet know which of these principles applies to human development.[31]

By the time it is seven days old and has come to rest within the uterus, the blastocyst is a hollow sphere of cells except for the inner cell mass at one side. Most of the blastocyst will be devoted to the housing for the developing organism. The cells surrounding the cavity make up the *trophoblast*, which will become the *placenta* and the *chorion*, or outer sac (see page 23). From the inner cell mass will develop the *amnion*, or inner sac; the yolk sac, which is thought to be nonfunctional in human embryonic development; the *body stalk*, which becomes the umbilical cord; and, finally, the *germinal disk*, from which the embryo itself will later emerge. The new organism sets about planting itself, almost literally sinking its roots into a portion of the surrounding uterine tissues. Secretions from the trophoblast eat a recess in the uterine lining and the blastocyst embeds itself in this recess, sending out tendrils which take root in the bloodfilled lakes in the endometrium. These tendrils take shape as capillaries, called the *chorionic villi*, which are linked with the developing umbilical vein and arteries. The villi, together with some surrounding maternal endometrial tissues, are elaborated into the *placenta*. Nutrients—oxygen, water, sugars, fats, amino acids, minerals, and so forth—and other substances such as hormones, antibodies, viruses, and blood fractions, which we shall discuss later, are absorbed from the mother's blood via the placenta; and waste products, such as carbon dioxide, are discharged into it. While the mother's blood supplies all the nutritive raw materials for the baby's growth, synthesis of complex amino acids and carbohydrates may begin at implantation. The placenta serves not only as a filter through which materials pass back and forth between the mother's and baby's blood, but also as an endocrine gland, secreting hormones which become an integral part of the mother's physiology and presumably help regulate the baby's own growth.

When fully developed, the human placenta is a disk-shaped fleshy slab, 6 to 8 inches (15 to 20 cm.) across, slightly more than an inch (25 mm.) thick, and weighing about a pound (slightly under one-half kilogram). It is a somewhat spongy-surfaced mass of blood vessels on the side attached to the uterine lining, and smooth on the side to which the baby is connected by the umbilical cord, a rubbery tube containing a vein that carries fresh blood from the placenta to the baby and two arteries carrying waste-laden blood to the placenta (reversing the functions of veins and arteries in nonfetal circulation but duplicating the relations between the adult's heart and lungs). The baby is enclosed within a double-walled (chorion and amnion) membrane extending out of the placenta in the form of a balloonlike sac filled with the amniotic fluid (at full term, about 2 quarts or liters) in which the child floats.

The Embryo. It should be made explicit that the stages into which prenatal development is divided are not always clearcut. Many things are going on simultaneously, so that one cannot always say with assurance precisely when any one system begins to take shape. It should also be clear that human embryology, unlike infrahuman embryology, cannot be studied experimentally, and knowledge of the subject is based partly on the study of embryos removed surgically and partly on extrapolations from infrahuman embryonic development. It is possible that liberalization of the laws governing abortion will greatly increase the accuracy of our knowledge, as will some new developments in techniques for lighting and photography within the body.

It is during the period of the embryo that the baby's organ systems are emerging and he is most vulnerable to environmental insults of the kind we shall talk about later. Some idea of the appearance of the embryo and fetus can be gained from the accompanying photographs.

Between ages two and three weeks the embryo starts to take animal shape and reaches a length of 1/12 inch (2 mm.). All its body axes and poles are determined. A neural plate has formed and folded into a tube, the upper end of which will be the brain, and somites, indicative of the spinal vertebrae, have begun to appear. The heart, at first a single tube, is growing by a process of looping and infolding and soon begins to beat, apparently even before there is any blood for it to circulate. A beginning digestive tract can be distinguished. By three weeks of age, the embryo's tissues have clearly specialized into *ectoderm*, which will become skin and nerve tissue; *mesoderm*, which will become bone, muscle, and supportive tissue; and *endoderm*, from which the alimentary tract and digestive organs emerge. Circulation through the body stalk and yolk sac is in operation, and placental nutrition has begun. Earlier, there was direct diffusion from the mother's blood through the surface of the blastocyst. By age four weeks, or one lunar month, the embryo has grown to about $\frac{1}{7}$ inch (3+ mm.) in length, has a clearly visible (but not recognizably human) head and spinal cord, and buds for arms, legs, and tail. The lenses are forming in the primordial eyes, the location of the ears has been marked off, some isolated nerves have appeared, blood is flowing through the microscopic veins and arteries, and various glands and organs are taking rudimentary shape.

By this time, the mother herself is probably aware of pregnancy. Most obviously, menstruation will be two weeks overdue. In addition, the woman may feel a heaviness and fullness of the breasts and see an enlargement and darkening of the nipples and surrounding areolas. She

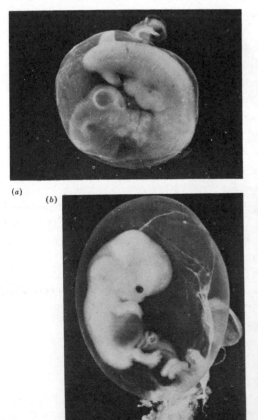

Some stages in prenatal development. (a) Embryo at about five weeks. (b) Embryo at about nine weeks. (c) Fetus at about fifteen weeks. This photograph shows the normal relationship of the umbilical cord and placenta. (d) Fetus and placenta at about sixteen weeks. (e) Fetus at about twenty-two weeks.

Edith L. Potter, *Fundamentals of Human Reproduction*

(c)

(a)

(b)

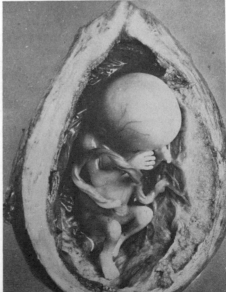

may have to urinate more often than usual. She may have morning sickness, the nausea that afflicts some two-thirds of women in the early weeks or months of pregnancy. There are a number of possible emotional attitudes toward pregnancy, which, coupled with somatic symptoms and perhaps generating further psychosomatic reactions, can make pregnancy a very different experience for different women. Most women, though, find pregnancy a mixture of discomfort and rewards, hopes and anxieties, pain and elation. Many women report that later pregnancy is a time of unparalleled physical well-being.

During the second lunar month, the embryo reaches a length of about 1¼ inches (3 cm.). At five weeks, rudimentary gill pouches appear, the forerunners of throat, esophagus, jaws, and external ears. The embryo's tail reaches its maximum length at about six weeks and thereafter ordinarily regresses. The head becomes clearly distinct from the body, accounting for about half the embryo's total size. The eyes migrate forward from the side of the head, lids begin to form, and humanlike facial features emerge. The limb buds grow and become paddle-shaped, and digits appear, first as ridges and then as separate members, the fingers being more advanced than the toes. The endocrine system has taken shape, the adrenal medulla secretes adrenalin, and the testes (in

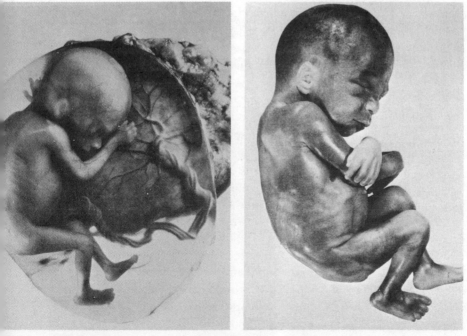

(d)   (e)

male embryos) have begun to produce androgens. At this point, though, there is still no visible difference between the sexes. Isolated reflex movements can be elicited, indicating that there is at least rudimentary neural transmission. In sum, by the end of the embryonic period, the baby has become clearly human, with all his human anatomy present, if only in primitive form.

The Fetus. The fetal period of development, from eight weeks to birth, is given over to the elaboration and growth of structures laid down in the embryonic stage. During the third lunar month, the fetus reaches a length of about 3 inches (7½ cm.) and a weight of about ⅔ ounce (20 g.). The humanizing of the face continues as the lips take shape and the nose comes to stand out. The eyelids are fused shut. The fingers are well developed and fingernails and toenails are forming. An expert can distinguish the sexes by their very slightly different external genitalia, although the boy's testes do not descend from the abdominal cavity into the scrotum until prenatal age seven months or later. The primitive kidney begins secreting small amounts of urine, although, as we have said, most waste disposal is handled via the placenta. By age ten weeks, the fetus, tiny though it is, makes breathing movements if removed from the mother's body. Reflex movements of the lips, resembling sucking, may occur. The feet will show the Babinski response.

During the fourth lunar month, the fetus doubles in length to almost 6 inches (15 cm.) and increases sixfold in weight to about 4 ounces (115 g.). Most of the bones have been formed by four months, although ossification, the replacement of cartilage by true bone, will not be complete for many years. Some spontaneous movements of the fetus can be detected by stethoscope by fourteen weeks, although the "quickening," the first movements of which the mother is aware, does not come until about seventeen weeks. During the fourth month, reflexive swallowing occurs, and the fetus ingests small amounts of amniotic fluid. In fact, if too much amniotic fluid is present, the treatment is to inject saccharine into the amnion, stimulating the fetus to swallow additional fluid and discharge the excess through the placenta.[32] Not only is this an ingenious medical technique, but it indicates differential taste sensitivity even in the fetus. Hormone secretion becomes ever more complicated, and the digestive system is beginning to function. The liver secretes bile which collects in the intestine.

Growth in length continues rapid throughout prenatal life, but the rate drops off in the later months. The unborn baby gains weight very slowly until the beginning of the seventh month, when he begins filling

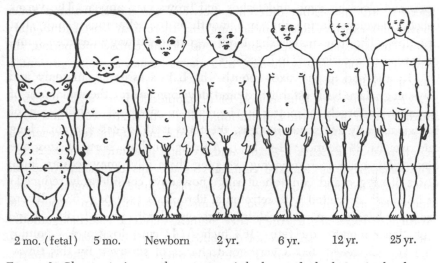

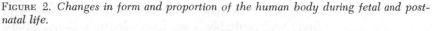

2 mo. (fetal) 5 mo.   Newborn   2 yr.   6 yr.   12 yr.   25 yr.

FIGURE 2. *Changes in form and proportion of the human body during fetal and post-natal life.*
SOURCE: Robbins, W. J., et al., *Growth*. New Haven: Yale University Press, 1928.

out rapidly, going from 20 ounces (580 g.) to 7 pounds (3+ kg.) in four months. In the fifth lunar month, the body hair begins to appear, and by the seventh month the fetus is densely covered with down. This down is shed, although not always completely, shortly before birth. By age five months, although the fetus weighs only 11 ounces (320 g.), his metabolic equipment is working well enough so that he can produce insulin in sufficient quantities to take care of some of his mother's carbohydrate regulation. During the fifth lunar month the fetus's heartbeat can be heard with the help of a stethoscope. The quickening, as we have said, comes early in the fifth month. It is felt first as a mild fluttering, but later in pregnancy as good solid kicks. (It is not until the sixth month that an observer can feel, with his hand against the mother's belly, the baby's movements.) Age five months (four and a half calendar months) is the midpoint of pregnancy, and the mother's condition will usually be obvious to other people. Any morning sickness will probably be past, and she will be in the most comfortable period of pregnancy. A fetus born at this time will inevitably succumb, although babies weighing as little as 12 ounces, indicating an age of just over five months, have been known to survive.

In the sixth month, the baby grows to a foot (30 cm.) in length and a weight of 20 ounces (580 g.). His lids separate, so that he can now open and close his eyes, and lashes and brows may appear. The vernix caseosa develops during the sixth month as the sebaceous glands start operating. The fetus makes slight but regular breathing movements, and he is reputed occasionally to hiccough.

By the end of the sixth month, the baby's essential anatomy and physiology have been established, and development for the remainder of gestation is largely a matter of increase in size and stabilization of functioning. By age seven months, the fetus is 15 inches (38 cm.) long and weighs 2½ pounds (1+ kg.). Although babies born at this age have a fair chance of surviving, keeping them alive may require large doses of oxygen and consequent risk (nowadays considerably reduced) of blindness associated with retrolental fibroplasia (see page 530). There are other hazards and vulnerabilities associated with prematurity. At age eight lunar months, the fetus, 16½ inches (42 cm.) long and 4 pounds (1.8 kg.) in weight, has a very good chance of survival. By this time— although in some cases not until years later—one or both of the male testes (the left one first) will probably have descended into the scrotum. The baby fills out rapidly during the ninth and tenth lunar months, gaining an average of close to half a pound a week. He sheds his prenatal body hair. He loses much of his red, wizened, fetal look and becomes more babyish in appearance. Since he is filling out so quickly, a difference of only a few days in maturity at birth can make a considerable difference in the neonate's looks, just as it does in his behavioral capabilities.

During the final months of pregnancy, the mother will probably feel healthy, but she is likely to suffer some discomforts of a mechanical sort. Her inner organs are becoming crowded by the expanding fetus. She must make postural adjustments to a new distribution of weight—note the swaybacked posture of many women in late pregnancy. By the tenth lunar month, many women experience their bodies as awkward and cumbersome and look forward to childbirth as a welcome liberation.

Prenatal Environmental Influences

The normal process of prenatal development that we have described is so usual that we may fail to see that the transformation of a single cell into a human baby is an altogether remarkable event. The zygote, after all, does not contain a miniature model of the creature it is to become, which has only to grow bigger, but instead a wealth of information, coded in molecular form, which regulates successive steps in the evolution of the organism. Note that the genetic code does not stop operating at birth. The entire business of growing up and growing old constitutes, together with prenatal development, a single, continuing process. We shall discuss a little later some details of genetics, but here we must mention two aspects of the way genetic constitution is expressed in development. We must remember, first, that every cell of an organism contains exactly the same genetic information as every other cell of that organism, but this information is used in different ways by different cells at different periods of development. Second, the units in the genetic code, like the words in a sentence, change meaning according to their context. Both these statements can be reduced to one by saying that genetic mechanisms operate in various ways according to their environments. We must stress that there are many different levels of relevant environments, some inside the organism and some outside it. The gene does its work in the context of its position on the chromosome. The chromosome operates in the context of other chromosomes. The cell nucleus operates in the context of the surrounding cell matter. The single cell acts according to its position in the cell cluster. Events in the cell cluster as a whole (even as a zygote in the Fallopian tube), and later in the embryo, are governed by environing conditions of temperature, electrical potential, chemical balance, orientation with respect to the uterine wall, gravity, atmospheric pressure, and, at successive stages of development, various other specific factors, including in due time, personal-social-affective influences.

It is fortunate that the intrauterine environment is usually quite stable and varies only within very narrow limits, since experimental manipulation of the prenatal environment of animal embryos indicates that even minor alterations can produce serious deformities. (The study of developmental anomalies is called *teratology*.) In addition to the general conditions mentioned above, the following agents are some that have been shown to alter embryonic development in one species or another: poisons; drugs; viruses; x-rays and other forms of ionizing radiation; abnormal blood conditions of the mother, such as hormone imbalance, anemia, or anomalous proteins; excess or deficiency of certain vitamins; oxygen lack; and iodine deficiency.[33] Among the deformities produced by environmental factors are anencephaly (lack of a brain), harelip, phocomelia (the "seal flippers" recently found to have been caused by the drug thalidomide), cleft palate, syndactyly (failure of the digits to separate), extra members or missing members, sex reversal or ambiguity of sex, and a host of other conditions, some minor and some so severe as to lead to spontaneous abortion. While only a relatively few pregnancies eventuate in such developmental disasters, recent teratological research is of great interest for the light it throws on general principles of growth. Moreover, such research promises to bring many of the newly understood factors under control, and to eliminate vague fears of "hereditary taints." What we do not yet know very much about is ways of manipulating the prenatal environment to produce superior forms of somatic development; for the time being it seems safest to say that the normal environment is the ideal one. However, there is now evidence from the study of rats that injection of pituitary growth hormone into the pregnant mother has favorable effects on the development of the brain in the offspring.[34] Notice, too, the inescapable reciprocity of influences; not only does the mother affect the development of the baby, but the zygote, embryo, and fetus are a part of the mother's environment and modify her physiology from the moment of conception.

Whether teratogenic agents have an effect, and what the effect is likely to be, varies with certain conditions: the time of development at which the agent is introduced, the part of the organism that is affected, how large a dose is present, and both strain and individual differences among organisms. Note, too, that teratogens can act on the embryo in two different ways: directly, as in the case of rubella (German measles) virus or x-rays, or indirectly, by altering the mother's physiological state in

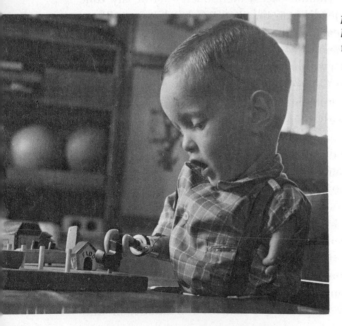

Phocomelia of the kind produced by thalidomide.
Esther Bubley

ways that will have an effect on the developing baby. Now let us look more closely at the governing variables of prenatal environmental influences.

TIMING

It is a principle of embryonic development that organs and organ systems emerge in a fixed sequence, with just so much time allowed for each—though the times, of course, overlap. That is, in the total timetable of growth, each organ system has its own *critical period*. During its critical period, the organ system is both highly responsive to growth-stimulating influences and highly vulnerable to disruptive ones. Put another way, it is the part of the organism that is growing most rapidly that is most sensitive to deleterious agents. If the organ system does not develop normally during its critical period, it does not have a second chance—the focus of growth shifts to successive systems.

The importance of timing is illustrated by the differential effects of grossly excessive amounts of vitamin A given to pregnant white rats at different stages of gestation: Between eight and 10 days, the most likely consequence is anencephaly; between 11 and 17 days, cleft palate; between 18 and 20 days, cataract.[35] Some teratogens, such as thalidomide, seem to act only at one stage of development, and are innocuous at other times. Others (like the vitamin excess mentioned) act at any time but have different effects depending on the stage of development. Thus, maternal rubella during the embryonic period may cause brain damage, blindness, deafness, or peripheral deformities in the offspring, depending on the time of infection. It is estimated that 30,000 defects and 20,000 fetal deaths resulted from the German measles epidemic of 1963–1965 in the United States. (Because rubella is a mild, inconsequential disease except for its effects in the early months of pregnancy, many physicians recommend that girls be given every opportunity to contract it in childhood. Reports in 1966 indicate that a safe and effective vaccine has been developed by the National Institutes of Health.)[36] It further follows from what we have said that the same anomaly can be produced by a variety of teratogens.

Let us emphasize that the effects we are speaking of, which alter the design of the organism (its *morphology*), occur only during the germinal and embryonic periods when the baby's organ systems are first emerging. During the fetal period, various illnesses and toxins can produce permanent damage, but they no longer alter the basic structural design. The fetus apparently reacts, too, to prolonged maternal malnutrition and fatigue, which find chemical expression in the bloodstream, to nicotine, and to alcohol. The baby born to a morphine-addicted mother is likely to show signs of morphine addiction; the New York City Commissioner of Health estimated that some 600 such babies were born in New York alone in 1965.

LOCUS OF EFFECTS, SIZE OF DOSE, AND ORGANISM DIFFERENCES

Some portions of the organism are structurally more central to total functioning than others; if these central systems are deformed, other, secondary, often widespread deformities follow in their wake. If, on the other hand, it is one of the peripheral systems that is affected, the damage may be quite circumscribed. We may, of course, be misled by the most striking feature of an anomalous condition and fail to see that it is only a part of a syndrome. For instance, the stunted limbs of phocomelia are only one of the effects produced by thalidomide. Other features of the "thalidomide syndrome" are a temporary strawberry mark extending from the forehead down the nose and across the upper lip, and, with varying incidence, a saddle-shaped or flattened nose, a missing external ear and a downward displacement of the internal auditory canal (hearing, however, is normal), paralysis of one side of the face, and malformations of the alimentary tract and of the heart and circulatory system.[37]

Some teratogens have no effect unless they surpass a certain minimum dose. On the other hand, the threshold may be a dual one: Vitamin A deficiency can be as serious for the baby as a surplus. Sternglass[38] concludes, from a survey of available cases, that prenatal ionizing radiation as a cause of childhood cancer does not show a threshold effect, that is, there is no safe range of exposure. Reasoning that radiation induces cancer by acting on a gene, he concludes that the main effect of increasing exposure to radiation is to increase the probability of changing the gene structure.

The same teratogen may have different effects or no effects depending on the species involved. Even closely related strains may show differential reactions to the same teratogen, and individual members of the same strain—including litter mates—may respond differently.

Although we have been talking about environmentally induced abnormalities of physical development, the very same principles of environmental regulation apply to normal development. The hereditary make-up of the organism is not a single fixed entity which simply unfolds on schedule. It contains many possible modes of expression, varying with environmental circumstances. For instance, worker bees and queen bees are both genetic females, but only the queens, fed on an exclusive diet of royal jelly, become fertile adult females. The workers, fed on pollen and nectar, become sexless adults.

OLD AND NEW CONCEPTIONS OF PRENATAL INFLUENCES

The kind of prenatal environmental influences we are talking about is, of course, quite different from that which has always figured in old wives' tales: The pregnant woman who saw a tree struck by lightning gives birth to a child who will have a blaze of white in his hair; the mother who listens to good music throughout pregnancy will produce a musically talented child; by thinking pleasant thoughts, one guarantees a child of cheerful disposition. Unlike these magical influences, the ones we are discussing require direct physical action on the tissues of the embryo, as by x-rays, by the transmission of biochemical agents from the mother's bloodstream to the child's, or by privation of materials needed for normal growth. Nevertheless, there is firm evidence from animal experimentation[39] and suggestive evidence from the study of human beings[40] that the mother's emotional state can have a bearing on her unborn child's development. As we know, emotional arousal is accompanied by physiological changes, and the endocrine and neurohumoral products of arousal can be transmitted from the mother's bloodstream to that of the child. The exact relationships are still unclear, but it is evident—through research at the level of the rat and mouse—that severe or prolonged stress to the mother, such as that engendered by electric shock, sudden exposure to cold, or crowded living conditions, can affect infantile body size, viability, adrenal size and activity, anxiety level, and learning ability.

RH INCOMPATIBILITY

One important form of prenatal influence, illustrating reciprocal action between genetic and environmental factors, is that of blood incompatibility between a mother whose blood does not contain Rh factor (that is, is Rh negative) and a baby whose blood is Rh positive. Rh factor is a genetically determined blood component found in all rhesus monkeys ("Rh") and 85 per cent of white people (as against nearly 100 per cent of other racial groups). When Rh factor is introduced into Rh negative blood, as sometimes used to happen in transfusions before the Rh factor had been recognized, antibodies that combat the Rh factor are produced. When an Rh negative woman marries an Rh positive man (the

only potentially dangerous combination), she may conceive an Rh positive child (if the father carries two Rh positive genes, the child is certain
to be Rh positive; if he carries one Rh positive and one Rh negative gene,
then the chances are half-and-half). If the unborn child is Rh positive,
and even a small rupture of the placental capillary structure allows some
of his blood to mingle with his mother's, this may lead, as in the case of
transfusion, to the production of Rh antibodies in the mother. However,
the antibodies are usually produced too slowly to affect a first Rh positive
fetus. If, however, the mother carries subsequent Rh positive children
and receives additional Rh positive blood, her now-sensitized blood steps
up production of antibodies which may enter the fetal bloodstream and
cause destruction of its Rh positive red blood cells. The damage caused
by Rh antibodies to the baby's Rh positive blood can sometimes lead to
miscarriage or, at or shortly after birth, to death or brain defects.
Fortunately, total transfusion techniques for the newborn have been
developed which can prevent damage from Rh incompatibility. Indeed,
techniques have been worked out for transfusing the fetus's blood before
birth. For reasons unknown, Rh reactions appear somewhat less frequently than purely statistical considerations would lead one to expect.

In spite of all the variety of possible environmental influences on
prenatal development, most embryos develop in essentially normal environments and are born sound of body. The interest of prenatal influences for the purposes of this book is the important lesson, first formulated in these terms by Hebb,[41] that all aspects of development and
behavior are determined 100 per cent by heredity and 100 per cent by
environment in that neither can operate except in interaction with the
other—a sometimes neglected consideration. This point becomes especially vital when we get on to the chief business of our book, psychological development, where we shall pay particular attention to the role of
the affective-personal-social-symbolic environment. From this point of
view it makes no sense to speak of the "relative contributions" of heredity
and environment or to seek for pseudo-quantifications of the relationship.
    If, in this chapter, we dwell on patterns of physical development, it
is because psychological development emerges from a context of biological conditions. We are not in a position to make precise correlations
between anatomical or physiological variables and psychological ones,
but we do know that certain gross relationships exist. We know that there
are some ways of behaving that are peculiarly human. We know, too, that
there are variations in human behavior corresponding to the state of the

nervous system, to endocrine functioning, to physique, to strength and mobility; and we know that some of these variations do not follow as direct consequences of constitution but are socially mediated in diverse and often subtle ways.

Biological Inheritance

A complete account of modern genetics, the science of how biological characteristics are transmitted from one generation to the next, would be far beyond the scope of this work.[42] This is particularly true because new findings in molecular biology require that we rethink some of the established concepts of earlier genetics. We shall begin with a brief presentation of some standard genetic notions and then go on to discuss some of the more recent phenomena in this field and some principles that the reader may find helpful in thinking about how hereditary traits find expression. Genetics has several useful applications. To begin with, knowing something about the traits of two individuals (and perhaps of their parents), the geneticist can make certain limited predictions about some of their children's characteristics. Note that he cannot usually make predictions for a particular child; for most traits he can forecast only the probability that the trait will appear in a given proportion of offspring. The geneticist may also be able to apply hindsight: Given an individual with such and such characteristics, he may be able to reconstruct something of his genealogical history, a partial pedigree.

EUGENICS AND EUTHENICS

Perhaps the most important application of genetics is in *eugenics,* the improvement of a species—human, animal, or plant—by selective breeding, by matching parents to produce certain desired traits in their progeny and by preventing unions likely to produce unfavorable traits. Eugenic procedures are standard practice in animal husbandry and agriculture, although most of the selective breeding techniques used by farmers were devised long centuries before Gregor Mendel enunciated the principles of genetics.

At the human level, we find crude eugenic measures in the practice, at various times and places, of infanticide, by which unwanted or unfit members were eliminated from the species; in Hitler's lunatic campaign of racial purification (with some uncomfortable parallels in the racial segregation practiced in the United States and South Africa, and more subtly elsewhere); and in the scattered and rarely invoked laws for the sterilization of criminals, mental defectives, psychotics, epileptics, or other people considered substandard. In a modern eugenic view, inadequate members of society might well be discouraged from having children, not because of flawed heredity but because of the unpropitious environments for development that they are likely to provide. The real barrier to human eugenics (apart from strong human preferences for unprogrammed matings, somewhat modified currently by a fad for computer-matching of couples) is that we know too little about the mode of inheritance of complex characteristics (assuming that they are hereditary) to know how to proceed in eliminating the genes from the population. Instead of restrictive eugenic measures, most geneticists recommend matings across as many geographical and social barriers as possible with a view to increasing human heterogeneity. Some combinations would work out badly and others well; but the odds in favor of superior combinations would be increased over what they are now, and selective factors should work to control the propagation of the unsuccessful combinations.

Eugenics is often contrasted with *euthenics,* ways of improving the species by manipulating the environment. Proponents of eugenics and euthenics have often been at odds with each other, although it should be obvious that measures of both sorts can go hand in hand. It is also lamentably clear that attempts to change the environment so as to provide a benign climate for development—as by eliminating racial discrimination—are likely to run up against powerful resistance.

SOURCES OF GENETIC KNOWLEDGE

The reader should understand that our knowledge of genetic mechanisms, like our knowledge of prenatal development, is based largely on studies of infrahuman species. Unlike fruit flies and mice, human beings cannot be bred under controlled laboratory conditions. This means not only that we have no way of regulating matings and rate of reproduction, but also that we have no satisfactory way of keeping environments standard, which we would have to do to be confident that the variations we observed were of genetic origin. A favored technique in human genetics, the study of identical twins reared in different environments, has several limitations. First, such twins are far from numerous. Second, we have no systematic way of specifying and contrasting significant aspects of the environment. Third, unless twins are followed longitudinally, through life, we are forced to reconstruct their early histories from questionable evidence. There is the further practical difficulty in human genetics that people live too long, and have to wait too long to reproduce, to make good subjects for even nonlaboratory research. The human geneticist is often less an experimental scientist than an archivist, tracing traits back through historical and family documents and hospital records.

HEREDITARY MECHANISMS

The trait-carrying elements of heredity are thought to be *genes,* giant molecules in the *chromosomes,* which are rodlike bodies in the cell nucleus, visible under the microscope during periods of cell division. All organisms produced by a sexual mating have two sets of chromosomes, arranged in pairs, one set—half of each pair—inherited from each parent. Human beings normally have 23 pairs, or 46 chromosomes. Ordinarily, when a cell divides, the chromosomes split lengthwise in two, so that there are 92, which are then divided equally between the two resulting cells. Germ cells, spermatozoa and ova, however, have a peculiarity. At one stage of development (*meiosis,* or *reduction division*), instead of the individual chromosomes splitting, the chromosome pairs simply separate, with one set going to one new cell and the other to the other. That is, the mature human germ cell contains only 23 chromosomes rather than 46. When a sperm and ovum combine, each contributes 23 chromosomes so that the zygote has the usual 46. Since some people still entertain the notion that it is either the father or the mother who is exclusively responsible for the child's heredity, it is important to note that the child gets half his chromosomes from each parent. Which parent the child "takes after," whether in appearance or behavior, is a complicated matter that cannot be resolved by references to "your side of the family." Even where certain trait resemblances are clear, the child may take after the other parent in other respects. In meiosis, the chromosomes do not divide themselves neatly according to their (grand) maternal and (grand) paternal origins. In other words, the set of 23 chromosomes that one parent passes on to his or her offspring may include some chromosomes inherited from that parent's father and some from the mother. Furthermore, although the genes that make up a single chromosome generally stay together as a unit, there is evidence that corresponding genes sometimes trade places with each other between members of a chromosome pair, so that the chromosomes themselves may change in character. Hence, a given parent has not two kinds but a great variety of germ cells, each sperm or ovum representing a different sorting and shuffling of potentialities. These facts help explain how members of the same family resemble each other, since each child has 46 chromosomes drawn from a pool of only 92, and how at the same time they can be quite dissimilar, since their chromosomal inheritance can be any one of a vast number of possible combinations of genes.

We still do not understand the subtle differences in composition among the genes that control different structures or that determine the different forms that a given structure can take: Noses can be straight or hooked or retroussé, hair can be blond or brown or red or black, or straight or wavy or kinky, and so forth for all the varieties of human constitution. The fact is, nevertheless, that many physical characteristics do have a stable pattern of inheritance. With an exception to be noted in a moment, there are two genes for every trait. Certain traits occur given the presence of a single gene without regard to the contribution of the second, counterpart gene. Such traits are called *dominant*. Among dominant human traits are brown or hazel eyes, short stature, blood types A, B, and AB, high blood pressure, Rh factor, and allergy. Other characteristics occur only when two like genes are present; these are called *recessive* traits: blue eyes, adherent ear lobes, normal vision, and so forth. When a dominant gene is paired with a recessive gene, only the dominant trait is expressed. In such cases, we must distinguish between *phenotype*, the phenomenal or observable characteristic, and *genotype*, the underlying genetic make-up which does not necessarily correspond to the phenotype. Thus, a phenotypically brown-eyed person who genotypically has a pairing of brown-eye and blue-eye genes will look just like an individual who has two genes for brown eye color. It follows that two phenotypically brown-eyed parents each of whom carries a recessive blue-eye gene can have blue-eyed children. The same genotype-phenotype terminology can be applied to environmentally caused modifications; thus, the queen and worker bee are genotypically the same but phenotypically very different. A number of traits are partially dominant, so that a single gene produces an intermediate effect, for example, medium skin pigmentation or wavy hair. Some genes may be dominant in one biological context but not in another. For instance, baldness is dominant in men but recessive in women (although there are more bald women—that is, women with two genes for baldness—than the reader may realize).

The example of baldness should remind us that not all of our genetic make-up has found full expression at birth—remember such genetically influenced characteristics as growth rate, adult stature, age of onset of puberty, and the different ways in which men's beards grow. The serious degenerative condition of the nervous system called Huntington's chorea, which is hereditary, is usually not manifested until adulthood; by the time it is recognized, the sufferer may already have children of his own.

Genetic Sex Determination. The two members of any pair of chromosomes are very much like each other, with one important exception. In males, one chromosome, arbitrarily designated X, is paired with an undersized one called Y. It is the Y-chromosome that determines maleness at the human level. The sperm, then, are of two kinds: half carry an X-chromosome and half carry a Y. Women, on the other hand, have two X-chromosomes, and every ovum therefore carries an X. When a sperm carrying an X-chromosome (and its constituent genes) joins with an ovum, the result is obviously XX, and a daughter is conceived. When a Y-carrying sperm joins with an ovum, producing XY, a male zygote is formed. (Although this is the normal pattern, we should point out that, because of errors in chromosome replication, other combinations occur: XXY, XXX, XXXX, XXXXY, or a single X without the second gene. This last case produces an underdeveloped female. See page 42.) Any combination containing a Y produces a male. The Y-chromosome acts by differentiating the primordial gonads as testes rather than ovaries, and the testicular hormones govern the further elaboration of the male's primary and secondary sex characteristics.[43]

The Y-chromosome carries fewer genes than the X, which means that some genes on the X have no matching counterparts on the Y. Some of these X-chromosome genes produce what is known as *sex-linked recessive traits*. Sex-linked recessive traits are produced by gene forms which are recessive when paired with a normal gene but which find full expression in the male, who lacks a corresponding gene on the Y-chromosome which would suppress its effect. Perhaps the best-known of the sex-linked recessives are red-green color-blindness (other forms are only partially sex-linked) and bleeder's disease, or hemophilia, a condition in which the blood does not clot, so that even a minor wound can cause a fatal hemorrhage. Although these conditions can appear in women, provided both X-chromosomes carry the genes for them, they are far more common in men. Thus, red-green color-blindness is found in some 8 per cent of men, but only 0.4 per cent of women. Although sex-linked recessive traits appear most often in males, they are always transmitted to the son by the mother, who supplies his X-chromosome.

We said earlier that half the sperm cells are X and half Y. This assertion runs up against the fact that in many species, including man, more males are conceived than females. The *sex ratio,* the number of males per 100 females, varies in human populations from 103 to 107 at birth (because of higher mortality among males, the sex ratio shifts in the opposite direction at later ages). Either more Y sperm than X are produced, or Y sperm have an advantage of some sort in fertilization.*

MUTATIONS AND EVOLUTION

It is clear that when a cell divides there is duplication of the nucleus, so that each daughter cell will have a full complement of chromosomes and genes. The subject of how the gene duplicates itself has recently become an active and fascinating field of study. Ordinarily the gene reproduces itself with absolute fidelity, so that a child's genes are exact copies of parental genes. Occasionally, however, there occurs a change in gene structure, a *mutation*, which produces a minor or major change in physical constitution. (We mention only in passing that synthetic or natural genelike structures can sometimes be substituted for a real gene in the course of cell metabolism and thereafter function as a gene; it is suspected that viruses act in this way, particularly viruses responsible for cancer.[46])

The occurrence of mutations is thought to provide the raw materials on which natural selection operates in the process of evolution; mutations constantly appear as though to be tried out, with the maladaptive mutants perishing and the fitter ones (in terms of the given conditions) surviving, sometimes at the expense of the parental strains. Of course, physiological and behavioral mechanisms that serve a species well may prove ill-suited if the ecological context changes too drastically. The environment may be so altered, as by flood, drought, fire, glaciers, housing developments, highway construction, man-made pollution, and mass spraying with pesticides, as to dislocate or destroy some of its inhabitants. Rachel Carson was only a more eloquent spokesman than most for the standard biological view that the balance of nature is an intricately interconnected system, and that trifling with it is likely to produce unforeseen and possibly disastrous consequences.[47]

As viable mutations accumulate over generations, new species emerge. It used to be thought that mutations occurred spontaneously or

---

* We might note that in certain species, such as some birds and fishes, males are XX and females XY. In many species, fathers are more or less redundant. Queen and worker bees are genetic females with fathers, but the male drones are a product of parthenogenesis, or virgin birth, and have only one set of chromosomes, including an X. (The females are XX.) Some strains of fish are exclusively female; some such are entirely parthenogenetic, while some have their eggs fertilized, but without union of the cell nuclei, by the males of related strains.[44] The evidence for experimental parthenogenesis in mammals is still questionable, but the phenomenon may have been demonstrated in rabbits.[45]

perhaps even in response to a mystical evolutionary driving force, or *élan vital,* toward improvement of the species. Nowadays, and with good evidence, mutations are believed to be the product of natural radiation from terrestrial and cosmic sources. We should remind the reader that human beings are currently raising the level of background radiation through the explosion of nuclear bombs and the manufacture of radioactive materials, and may incidentally be conducting a mammoth but unplanned experiment in evolution. So far, there is no direct evidence of genetic effects from the large-scale release of ionizing radiation and free radioactive substances, but our knowledge from laboratory studies of the effects of radiation on living tissues should make us profoundly skeptical of experts who find no menace in increased exposure. This is especially so if we consider also the possible effects on infrahuman animals and plants which play an important part in human ecology.

SHORTCOMINGS OF THE TRADITIONAL GENETIC MODEL

The simple gene-chromosome model we have sketched works reasonably well as far as we have gone. It needs some supplementary concepts, however, to account for the whole range of genetic phenomena. For instance, we ordinarily categorize people in two rigidly exclusive classes as male or female, when in fact one can recognize at least seven genetic gradations of sex, from supermale at one extreme through various degrees of intersex to superfemale at the other extreme, plus some subvarieties. It appears that males and females do not have different genes for primary and secondary sex characteristics, but that their sex organs take shape in keeping with different endocrine patterns. In any event, geneticists now believe that sex differentiation is determined by genes in addition to those on the X- and Y-chromosomes. In general, we must assume a principle of *gene interaction,* in two different senses. First, some traits, such as height, are governed not by one but by a constellation of genes; second, even where one gene may control the trait, the action of other genes is necessary to its expression.

The principle of gene interaction has a reciprocal in the principle of *pleiotropy,* that a single gene may regulate a number of traits. Pleiotropic action may be of two kinds. Either a number of structures take shape in keeping with the character of the gene, or, more commonly, the gene affects only a single trait which then has repercussions on other functions. (Notice that this is the genetic equivalent of the ramification of early environmental effects mentioned on page 30.) For example, the hereditary condition *phenylketonuria* consists primarily of a defect in the enzyme which metabolizes phenylalanine. If this defect goes uncorrected, the metabolic disorder has as a secondary consequence brain damage and serious mental deficiency. Fortunately, phenylketonuria is easily diagnosed in early infancy by the presence of abnormal metabolites in the blood or urine, and if proper dietetic measures are taken, the individual can develop normally. Some geneticists hold that all genes are pleiotropic and have multiple influences.

We should also mention the fact of *expressivity,* that the same gene may lead to different forms of the same trait in different individuals. To the extent to which allergy, for instance, is a hereditary condition, it may be variously expressed as hay fever in one individual and eczema in the next; the presence of the gene may mean that this person is sensitive to ragweed pollen and that one to Brazil nuts.

One further phenomenon, mentioned in connection with sex determination, should be recalled. An error in cell division can result in the formation of one or more extra chromosomes or the loss of a chromosome. An abnormal complement of chromosomes has been associated with Down's syndrome (mongolism),[48] leukemia, and with certain anomalies of sex mentioned earlier. The interesting point about these conditions is that, like mutations, they are genetic without necessarily being inherited. It appears that these chromosomal anomalies are generally produced in ova by the action of viruses or radiation. If we remember that the woman carries her lifetime supply of ova from an early age, then we can see that the longer she lives, the greater the probability that one or more ova may be affected. Since the male sperm supply is constantly replenished, the odds are against the father's acquiring and passing on an anomaly. It used to be thought that depletion of the maternal tissues accounted for the greater number of mongoloid babies born to women past forty than to younger mothers. It now appears likelier that older mothers simply have had more exposures to anomaly-producing agents. In areas having a high level of natural radiation, all sorts of anomalies are more common than in low-radiation regions. Whenever a new virus is introduced into a community, the number of birth defects rises temporarily until the women of the community have developed antibodies.

In all this discussion we have sidestepped a logical problem that arises in talking about genetics. This is the difficulty of saying what we mean by "trait." Sometimes the term designates a distinct anatomical component, such as an eye or a finger, which can take different forms; it may refer to the particular form that a feature may take, such as the curliness of hair; it may mean the presence or absence of some component, such as eye pigment or an enzyme or a sixth toe; it may denote a pattern of related traits, as in mongolism, which involves many physical anomalies; or it may refer to some anatomically unlocalized characteristic of the way the total organism functions, such as intelligence or temperament or schizophrenia.

If we cannot specify what we mean by a trait, it becomes very difficult to specify a gene-trait relationship. Part of the difficulty is that genetics has been studied and taught largely in terms of discontinuous, all-or-none traits such as blood types or eye color, which show a single gene pattern of inheritance but are a numerically small part of the individual's make-up, and less in terms of traits showing continuous variation, such as stature or strength, which are determined by a multiplicity of genes and are numerically more significant.[49] It is clear that we cannot think of development as an additive process by which the gene contributes its particle to an organic mosaic. Instead, we must think of the genes as key links in the biochemical sequence by which the organism undergoes successive metamorphoses. In other words, we do not know where the organism's total morphology is encoded in the zygote nucleus, or the successive morphologies through which the organism passes en route to maturity. There is some evidence, as we said earlier (page 29), that the morphology of the germinal period, before implantation, is encoded in the differential structure of the cytoplasm of the ovum, but this obviously cannot tell the whole story. It will become evident that we have retained the image of metamorphosis in speaking of postnatal psychological development, although we do not know of any corresponding biological transformations.

BIOLOGY AND PSYCHOLOGY

If our later chapters seem to slight genetic factors, it is not because we think them insignificant but because relatively little firm knowledge is available about the genetic components of normal individual variations in development. Somewhat more is known of the social-environmental influences that shape the individual as a person. Where the individual's constitution enters significantly into his personal relationships, as in extremes of beauty or ugliness, responsiveness and unresponsiveness, in cases of deformity or impaired mobility, in sensory handicaps which limit reception of environmental information, and in organic impediments to learning, understanding, and thinking, we shall take due account of it. Here two points should be borne in mind. First, these constitutional conditions, even when *congenital* (present at birth), are not necessarily hereditary. Second, our knowledge of biological correlates of human psychological functioning is largely restricted to pathological states. There are no human counterparts for the studies of the interacting effects in dogs of early experience and selective breeding.[50] On the other hand, we know a great deal—although not nearly enough or in enough detail—about environmental correlates of group and individual differences in the development of attitudes, values, morality, intelligence, temperament, and emotional reactivity. We are even coming to know something about the way the psychological environment shapes the individual's somatic development.[51]

Moreover, we know now that in the first few decades of this century psychology fell into a fatalistic use of hereditary concepts which actually retarded our coming to grips with important issues. Social-class differences in intelligence, for instance, were interpreted as a sort of social survival-of-the-fittest; and a recognition and effective analysis of the effects of psychological privations, and of the nature of optimal environments, is only now getting under way. Thus redressing the balance and taking account of current research strategy, we are inclined to focus more of our attention on the way psychological processes develop under the influence of environmental conditions, though we have emphasized that such processes are determined 100 per cent by heredity and 100 per cent by environment.

Hence, the authors' environmental stress in the ensuing chapters is not to be taken as antibiologism. We wish rather to insist that genetic constitution is not a set of fixed givens of behavior but is subject to variation in interaction with physical and personal environmental conditions. As yet, the standard concepts of the several biological sciences are inadequate to describe behavior and psychological development. We have only the rudiments of an organismic-ecological biology—particularly a physiology—of the total, functioning person or animal. A complete biology will be a biology not only of isolated physiological subsystems (digestive, respiratory, reproductive, and so on), but of their interrelationships and of how they work in the service of the organism's commerce with its behavioral surroundings. We need a means for the biological phrasing not only of the functions common to all organisms (such as growth, metabolism, and homeostasis) but also of such higher-order activities as manipulation, language, play, empathy, learning, knowledge, and imagination.[52]

44

The Birth Process

Having introduced the reader to the newborn baby and then turned back successively to the baby's prenatal incarnations and to his ancestry, we must now bring the child once more into the world. Toward the end of pregnancy, the fetus turns head down and comes to rest with his head in the lower part of the uterus, now well down in the mother's pelvic basin. The baby is then in position for the usually headfirst passage into the light and air. As he turns head down, the mother's high-prowed profile sags; pressure against her upper abdomen is eased and she breathes more freely. It is from this relief from pressure that the baby's change of position is called the *lightening*. The lightening may come as early as four weeks before birth, or it may wait until the onset of *labor*, the process by which the baby is expelled from the mother's body. The specific trigger (or triggers) for the start of labor is unknown, though some of the hormonal components are understood. Once begun, labor consists of spontaneous rhythmic contractions of the involuntary longitudinal uterine muscles, aided by the voluntary abdominal musculature, and the relaxation of the circular muscles of the cervix. The muscular contractions gradually squeeze the baby out of the uterus and through the vagina into the open.

The mother may be made aware of the onset of labor by any of three signs. One sign is labor pains, produced by the recurrent uterine contractions, initially of mild intensity and spaced fifteen or twenty minutes apart, and then of steadily increasing duration, frequency, and sharpness. Labor pains may begin in the back, but migrate forward as they continue. (False labor pains, which cannot always be distinguished from genuine ones, have sent many a woman on a futile trip to the hospital.) Another first sign may be a "showing," the appearance from the vagina of a small spot of mucus brightly spotted with blood—this is a plug that had formed in the cervix and now is released as the cervix begins to relax and dilate. Yet another sign may be a gush of clear fluid from the vagina; this follows what is called the "bursting of the bag of waters," the rupturing of the amniotic sac that has enclosed the fetus, releasing the amniotic fluid.

Obstetricians recognize three stages of labor. The first and longest part is the period when the cervix is being dilated to permit passage of the baby's head. (The pelvic girdle has already enlarged during pregnancy, facilitating birth.) The mother is usually encouraged to remain active during the first stage, since there is nothing she can do to help the process, which at first involves only involuntary musculature, and since activity may reduce her discomfort. The first stage lasts an average of fourteen hours for first babies, but with great individual variation, and considerably less for subsequent deliveries, as policemen and taxi-drivers well know.

The second stage of labor includes the baby's passage through the vagina and his delivery into the outside world. This stage may last from under twenty minutes to an hour and a half. The mother can actively speed the birth process during the second stage by "bearing down," tightening her (voluntary) abdominal muscles in concert with the uterine contractions. This participation by the mother seems also to help reduce pain. The baby's head turns so that the back of his skull appears first. The vaginal and surrounding tissues have softened during pregnancy and can be stretched considerably; if it appears that the tissues are in danger of tearing, the doctor makes a small lateral nick (*episiotomy*) to enlarge the opening. Such a cut heals neatly, as a tear might not. Once the occiput has been forced out, the rest of the baby's head comes quickly free, face down and draining. The doctor (or midwife) supports the head with one hand and draws gently on the baby. The rest of him, with the shoulders oriented vertically, in line with the long axis of the vulva, rapidly and easily slips out. The doctor holds the baby aloft by the ankles and, if breathing has not begun spontaneously, slaps him on the buttocks to get him started. As soon as the blood vessels of the umbilical cord stop pulsating, the cord is clamped and cut. Drops of silver nitrate—now, more often, penicillin ointment—are put into the baby's eyes as insurance against gonococcal infection. An identifying band is fastened around the baby's wrist or ankle and, in most hospitals, his footprint is taken on an identification card bearing the mother's thumbprint. These measures, of course, are a precaution against giving mothers the wrong babies. Then, if his muscle tone, color, and breathing indicate that he is functioning normally, the baby is put aside while the doctor and nurse attend to the mother. This first evaluation of the baby has been systematized in the Apgar Score (named for Dr. Virginia Apgar), the sum of ratings on five three-point scales: breathing effort, muscle tone, heart rate, reflex irritability, and color (from grayish to rosy). Preliminary findings from large-scale research show the scores to be good gross predictors of the baby's chances for healthy survival and a useful means of identifying neonates who need special care.[53]

The third and final stage of labor consists of the delivery of the *afterbirth,* the placenta with its attached amniotic and chorionic membranes and remainder of the cord. The third stage takes less than twenty minutes and is virtually painless. The doctor carefully examines the afterbirth to make sure that all of it has been delivered and that there are no abnormalities. The mother is given hormone injections which hasten shrinkage of the uterus, pressing shut any broken blood vessels, and, if she is planning to nurse her baby, which stimulate milk production. Note that these hormone injections are the human equivalent of behavior found in other mammals—even herbivorous mothers, such as sheep and goats, become carnivorous and eat the hormone-rich placenta. The licking of newborn animals in which their mothers engage, and which is so essential both to the infant's survival and to the formation of a bond between mother and young, is probably stimulated by hormones in the amniotic fluid that coats the infant. To return to the human mother, the doctor or nurse will, if necessary, knead her abdomen to restore tone to the uterine muscles. The mother loses a pint of blood or less in giving birth—about what she would donate to a blood bank. For the next ten to fourteen days, the uterine lining disintegrates and is shed in a process (the *lochia*) resembling menstruation.

We have described the usual birth sequence, in which the baby emerges headfirst, in what is called a *vertex presentation.* An occasional baby does not turn head downward in the womb, and is born buttocks first, with somewhat more difficulty, in what is called a *breech presentation.* Some babies, because of the mother's physical condition or because the baby is disproportionately large, or to forestall the consequences of Rh incompatibility, are delivered surgically, by Caesarian section. If the uterine contractions weaken or stop during labor, the baby may have to be delivered by forceps, tongs that fit around the baby's head and enable the doctor to draw him from the mother's body. The use of forceps during the first stage of labor or early in the second is referred to as high-forceps delivery and is a dangerous procedure, since inaccurate placement of the forceps and the greater force needed to pull out the baby may disfigure him or cause brain damage. For a time, high-forceps deliveries were popular because they shortened both the mother's and the doctor's labors, but recognition of the dangers involved has now led most physicians to consider the use of high forceps an emergency procedure. Low forceps, as one might expect, refers to the use of forceps at the stage of actual delivery, and involves less risk since the forceps can be placed quite accurately. The use of forceps is virtually routine in some hospitals and is almost completely shunned in others, the frequency of use in the United States varying from one per cent to 84.5 per cent.[54]

"NATURAL" CHILDBIRTH

Attitudes toward the birth process have varied widely from era to era and from place to place. For many years it was thought proper that women should suffer in giving birth as punishment for original sin. The first use of anesthetics in delivery was condemned from the pulpit as flying in the face of the Divine Will. Eventually, as we know, the entire process of birth was turned over to the physician and his instruments, the mother being anesthetized unconscious, partly in an attempt to avoid all pain. More recently mothers and doctors have come to a more balanced view.

If the mother chooses to have no anesthetics during the labor or to take them only sparingly at the final, most painful point of delivery, the process is called "natural childbirth." The mother may also have had a course of exercises during pregnancy, designed to limber her body, and lessons in how to cooperate in the birth process. There can be distinct satisfactions for the mother in "being there" when her baby is born and in participating in the act of birth. We suspect, too, that minimal use of anesthetics reduces the chance of birth complications for the baby. There is a good deal of evidence that most anesthetics adversely affect the baby's activity, alertness, and general functioning for hours and days after birth. How "natural" a childbirth a mother has must be decided in terms of her individual temperament. And if natural childbirth is to include the father's presence in the delivery room, his temperament must be considered, too.

The advantages of natural childbirth have sometimes been obscured by its more fanatical advocates, who proclaim dogmatically that childbirth is inherently painless and is made painful only through fears instilled by a cultural mythology. It seems safer to say that taking part in the act of birth reduces the mother's pain, to point out that the pain of childbirth limits itself by numbing the mother's tissues, and to say that memory of the pain of childbirth evaporates quickly. Because, as we shall emphasize repeatedly, sound development can take place only in a social milieu, it makes no sense to speak of "natural" as opposed to "artificial" human practices, on the analogy of the animal "in the wild." The Noble Savage is a mythical creature; people all over the world, even in the most "primitive" preliterate societies, are as various and "artificial" in their childbirth practices as in the conduct of all the other affairs of life. And those who would wholly emulate the happy primitive should first consider the figures on health, longevity, and infant and maternal mortality in technical and nontechnical civilizations. We must remember, of course, that the folklore of childbirth, including the notion that the bed of pain is punishment for original sin, is still rampant and may produce exaggerated and groundless fears in many women. These fears may be further reinforced by the surgical atmosphere of hospitals.

CHILDBIRTH IN THE HOSPITAL

Our description of the birth process assumes that the baby is born in a hospital, as is nowadays true of almost all American infants. The trend to having babies in the hospital with a physician in attendance has contributed, along with improved community and individual hygiene and better diets, to a sharp drop in infant and maternal death rates over the past half century. For instance, in 1900, 162.4 of every 1000 American babies surviving birth and the neonatal period died in the first year of life. This figure had dropped to 99.9 per 1000 in 1915 and to 25.2 per 1000 in 1961. But note that while the infant mortality rate among white babies dropped from 98.6 per 1000 in 1915 to 22.4 in 1960, the rate for nonwhite babies dropped only from 181.2 to 42.6 in the same period, reflecting the systematic exclusion of Negroes, Indians, and other nonwhites from the material benefits of citizenship. In the period 1915–1935 the maternal mortality rate per 10,000 live births fluctuated between 58.2 and 79.9; in 1961 it was 3.2 (But nonwhite maternal deaths are four times as frequent as white.) The United States' 1961 infant mortality rate of 25.2 per 1000 may be compared to rates of 15.5 in Sweden, 15.4 in the Netherlands, 13.3 in Iceland, and, rather surprisingly, 13.6 in Lebanon.[55]

However, the services of a doctor and the facilities of a hospital are essential only in those unusual instances when something goes wrong. That a normal birth does not require any particular setting or assistance is shown by the many successful births that occur in taxicabs, with driver, policeman, or fireman acting as midwife, or even at home when the mother is alone. As other countries become more Americanized, there is a movement toward hospital births. But in the United Kingdom and on the Continent, the professional midwife still officiates at a large proportion of births, calling in medical help or arranging for hospitalization in the event of complications. In this country, physicians have come to prefer their familiar, dependable, centralized resources provided by a hospital, and mothers the sense of specialized techniques always in reserve.

As is so often the case, the very real advantages of a hospital setting are bought at the cost of certain disadvantages. In this instance, the price is a psychological one. First and foremost, hospital personnel are oriented to the treatment of serious pathology and sometimes forget that mothers and their babies are normal, healthy people. In their well-founded zeal for medical sterility, hospitals have brought about a certain emotional sterility as well. Fathers and other children in the family are regarded as hotbeds of contagion and are rigorously kept away from the baby until he has left the hospital. The mother cannot be wholly excluded, but she too is suspect and is kept apart from the baby as much as possible, all the babies being together in a nursery except at feeding times. A few years ago, just as many hospitals became aware of the psychological need for relaxing their hygienic regulations, antibiotic-resistant strains of staphylococcus became a serious—for neonates, deadly—menace, and new and still more stringent sanitary measures had to be instituted. The hierarchical organization of the hospital, with authority concentrated in the physician and transmitted through nurses and attendants, favors the establishment of rigid procedures and routines which may be at odds with the psychological needs of individual mothers and their babies and may further intimidate patients already awed by an atmosphere of medical omniscience and omnipotence. Since doctors and nurses are in short supply, they cannot easily vary their procedures and may be forced into time-saving routines. The obstetrician may be tempted to dose the mother heavily with anesthetics or to use medications and forceps to hasten delivery. The mother may be discouraged, overtly or more subtly, from breast-feeding her baby, since successful breast-feeding requires that the baby be brought to the mother for all his feedings around the clock and that a first-time mother be instructed in the techniques of breast-feeding. Cumulatively, the ways of hospitals may convey to parents an uneasy feeling that their baby belongs not to them but to the hospital. Let us note, however, that the hospital nowadays has less time—usually four or five days—to work its effect than in the era of the two-week hospital stay when mothers were kept immobilized for a ten-day lying-in period and then allowed to sit on the edge of their beds and "dangle" briefly.

Rooming-In. One arrangement that combines the benefits of hospital delivery with a close mother-child relationship is found in programs of *rooming-in.* Here the baby lives in his mother's hospital room, and she begins early to take care of him. The father, subject to reasonable sanitary restrictions, can visit his wife and child. As it turns out, mothers, fathers, and babies thrive under rooming-in. For one thing, a generally healthy mother need no longer be kept in enforced idleness, wondering if the baby she hears crying in the nursery is hers. The mother gets some practice in caring for her baby before she suddenly has to take him home and be wholly responsible for him with no expert to turn to. Mother and child can get an early start on the business of coming to know each other and to adapt to each other's rhythms. Most important, the parents can feel that the baby is really theirs.

Interestingly enough, rooming-in simplifies hospital administration and cuts costs. When we stop to think about it, keeping babies in a centrally located nursery is efficient only if they receive all their care there, assembly-line fashion. If babies have to be distributed to their mothers for feeding and then collected again after meals, the coming and going is highly inefficient, especially if some of the babies happen not to be hungry on the hospital's schedule and in the not too rare event that the wrong baby gets deposited with the wrong mother, with consequent fireworks (since the babies are all clearly labeled, mismatchings are quickly set straight but can nevertheless occasion some emotionality). Another welcome by-product is that the chances of nursery epidemics are reduced when neonates are kept apart from each other in their mothers' rooms.

Like natural childbirth, rooming-in does not have to be an all-or-none matter. Just as maternal and paternal (and the obstetrician's) temperament have to govern just how "natural" a childbirth will be, so can degrees of rooming-in be provided to suit varying individual tastes. Experienced mothers may look upon the lying-in period as a rare opportunity for luxurious living uncluttered by workaday responsibilities. Similarly, the lying-in period has been shortened, in keeping with the principle of "early ambulation" followed in modern surgery, but many such mothers would like to indulge themselves with a few extra days of bed rest and, quite legitimately, resist being hurried onto their feet and out of the hospital.

REFERENCES / Chapter 1

[1] Doxiadis, S., Valaes, T., Karaklis, A., and Stavrakakis, D. Risk of severe jaundice in glucose-6-phosphate-dehydrogenase deficiency of the newborn. *The Lancet*, Dec. 5, 1964, pp. 1210–1212.
[2] Bartoshuk, A. K. Human neonatal cardiac responses to sound: a power function. *Psychonomic Science*, 1964, 1, 151–152; Blauvelt, H., and McKenna, J. Mother-neonate interaction: Capacity of the human newborn

for orientation. In Foss, B. M. (ed.) *Determinants of Infant Behavior*. New York: Wiley, 1961, pp. 3–29; Birns, B., Blank, M., Bridger, W. H., and Escalona, S. B. Behavioral inhibition in neonates produced by auditory stimuli. *Child Development*, 1965, 36, 639–645; Crowell, D. H., Davis, C. M., Chun, B. J., and Spellacy, F. J. Galvanic skin reflex in newborn humans. *Science*, 1965, 148, 1108–1111; Fantz, R. L. Visual perception from birth as shown by pattern sensitivity. In Caldwell, B. M., Fantz, R. L., Greenberg, N. H., Stone, L. J., and Wolff, P. H. New issues in infant development. *Annals of the New York Academy of Science*, 1965, 118, 783–866; Graham, F. K. Behavioral differences between normal and traumatized new borns. I. The test procedures. *Psychological Monographs*, 1956, 70, no. 20; Graham, F. K., Matarazzo, R. G., and Caldwell, B. M. II. Standardization, reliability, and validity. *Psychological Monographs*, 1956, 70, no. 21; Lipsitt, L. P., and Levy, N. Electrotactual thresholds in the neonate. *Child Development*, 1959, 30, 547–554; Engen, T., Lipsitt, L. P., and Kaye, H. Olfactory responses and adaptation in the human neonate. *Journal of Comparative and Physiological Psychology*, 1963, 56, 73–77; Lipsitt, L. P., Engen, T., and Kaye, H. Developmental changes in the olfactory threshold of the neonate. *Child Development*, 1963, 34, 371–376; Richmond, J. B., Lipton, E., and Steinschneider, A. Observations on differences in autonomic nervous system function between and within individuals during early infancy. *Journal of the American Academy of Child Psychiatry*, 1962, 1, 83; Stechler, G. Newborn attention as affected by medication during labor. *Science*, 1964, 144, 315–317; White, B. L. The development of perception during the first six months of life. Paper given at meetings of the American Association for the Advancement of Science, 1963; Haynes, H., White, B. L., and Held, R. Visual accommodation in human infants. *Science*, 1965, 148, 528–530; Wolff, P. H. Observations on newborn infants. *Psychosomatic Medicine*, 1959, 21, 110–118.

[3] Roffwarg, H. P., Muzio, J. N., and Dement, W. C. Ontogenetic development of the human sleep-dream cycle. *Science*, 1966, 152, 604–619.

[4] Gunther, M. Infant behavior at the breast. In Foss, B. M. (ed.) *Determinants of Infant Behavior*. New York: Wiley, 1961, pp. 37–44.

[5] Blauvelt and McKenna, *op. cit.*

[6] Spitz, R. A. Paper read at meeting of the New York Psychoanalytic Society, March 1, 1966.

[7] White, *op. cit.*

[8] Crowell *et al.*, *op. cit.*

[9] Wolff, *op. cit.*; see also Chastaing, M. Premiers sourires enfantins. In *Rencontre/Encounter/Begegnung*. Utrecht and Antwerp: Spectrum, 1957, pp. 80–87.

[10] Watson, J. B. *Psychology from the Standpoint of a Behaviorist*. Philadelphia: Lippincott, 1919, pp. 199–201.

[11] Sherman, M. The differentiation of emotional responses. *Journal of Comparative Psychology*, 1927, 7, 265–284; Bridges, K. M. B. Emotional development in early infancy. *Child Development*, 1932, 3, 324–341.

[12] Wolff, *op. cit.*; Lipton, E. L., Steinschneider, A. and Richmond, J. B. Swaddling, a child care practice. *Pediatrics*, 1965, 35, 521–567.

[13] Zazzo, R. Le problème de l'imitation chez le nouveau-né. *Enfance*, 1957, 2, 135–142.

[14] Wertheimer, M. Psychomotor coordination of auditory and visual space at birth. *Science*, 1961, 134, 1692.

[15] Fantz, R. L. Pattern vision in newborn infants. *Science*, 1963, 140, 296–297.

[16] Haynes *et al., op. cit.*

[17] Engen, Lipsitt, and Kaye, *op. cit.;* Lipsitt, Engen, and Kaye, *op. cit.*

[18] Pratt, K. C. The neonate. In Carmichael, L. (ed.) *Manual of Child Psychology.* New York: Wiley, 1954, pp. 215–291.

[19] *Ibid.;* Tauber, E. S., and Koffler, S. Optomotor response in human infants to apparent motion: Evidence of innateness. *Science*, 1966, 152, 382–383.

[20] Lipsitt and Levy, *op. cit.*

[21] Bartoshuk, *op. cit.*

[22] Birns *et al., op. cit.*

[23] Papoušek, H. Conditioning during early postnatal development. In Brackbill, Y., and Thompson, G. G. (eds.), *Behavior in Infancy and Early Childhood.* New York: Free Press, 1967; Siqueland, E. R., and Lipsitt, L. P. Conditioned head-turning in human newborns. *Journal of Experimental Child Psychology*, 1966, 3, 356–376.

[24] Kron, R. E., Stein, M., and Goddard, K. E. A method of measuring sucking behavior of newborn infants. *Psychosomatic Medicine*, 1963, 25, 181–191.

[25] Pratt, *op. cit.*

[26] Fisher, C., Gross, J., and Zuch, J. A cycle of penile erections synchronous with dreaming (REM) sleep. *Archives of General Psychiatry*, 1965, 12, 29–45.

[27] Williams, R. J. The biological approach to the study of personality. Paper given at the Berkeley Conference on Personality Development in Childhood, 1960.

[28] Burnet, F. M. Immunological recognition of self. *Science*, 1961, 133, 307–311.

[29] Escalona, S., and Heider, G. M. *Prediction and Outcome.* New York: Basic Books, 1959; Kagan, J., and Moss, H. A. *Birth to Maturity.* New York: Wiley, 1962; Thomas, A. S., Birch, J. G., Hertzog, M. E., and Korn, S. *Behavioral Individuality in Early Childhood.* New York: New York University, 1963.

[30] Graham, F. K., Ernhart, C. B., Thurston, D., and Craft, M. Development three years after perinatal anoxia and other potentially damaging newborn experiences. *Psychological Monographs*, 1962, 76, no. 3; see also Yacorzynski, G. K., and Tucker, B. E. What price intelligence? *American Psychologist*, 1960, 15, 201–203; Windle, W. F. Neuropathology of certain forms of mental retardation. *Science*, 1963, 140, 1186–1191.

[31] Fischberg, M., and Blackler, A. W. How cells specialize. *Scientific American*, September, 1961, 121–140.

[32] Barth, L. G. *Embryology.* New York: Holt, Rinehart, & Winston, 1953, p. 195.

[33] Mintz, B. (ed.) *Environmental Influences on Prenatal Development.* Chicago: University of Chicago, 1958; Montagu, M. F. A. *Prenatal Influences.* Springfield, Ill.: Thomas, 1962.

[34] Zamenhof, S., Mosley, J., and Schuller, E. Stimulation of the proliferation of cortical neurons by prenatal treatment with growth hormone. *Science,* 1966, 152, 1396–1397.

[35] Mintz, *op. cit.*

[36] Meyer, H. M., and Parkman, A. D. Paper read at meetings of the American Pediatrics Society, April 27, 1966.

[37] Taussig, H. B. The thalidomide syndrome. *Scientific American,* August, 1962, pp. 29–35.

[38] Sternglass, E. J. Cancer: Relation of prenatal radiation to development of the disease in childhood. *Science,* 1963, 140, 1102–1104.

[39] Montagu, *op. cit.,* Chapter 8.

[40] *Ibid.*

[41] Hebb, D. O. Heredity and environment in mammalian behaviour. *British Journal of Animal Behaviour,* 1953, 1, 43–47; see also Anastasi, A. Heredity, environment, and the question "How?" *Psychological Review,* 1958, 65, 197–208.

[42] For a more detailed treatment, the reader is referred to standard textbooks of genetics, e.g., Gardner, E. J. *Principles of Genetics.* New York: Wiley, 1960. A sensitive philosophical analysis of genetics is given in Dobzhansky, T. *Mankind Evolving.* New Haven: Yale, 1962. The reader who wishes to keep abreast of current developments can follow them in the pages of *Scientific American.* A brief but informative introduction is given by Lennox, B. Chromosomes for beginners. *The Lancet,* 1961, i, no. 7185, 1046–1051.

[43] Mittwoch, U. Sex differences in cells. *Scientific American,* July, 1963, pp. 54–62.

[44] Miller, R. R., and Schultz, R. J. All-female strains of the teleost fishes of the genus Poeciliopsis. *Science,* 1959, 130, 1656–1657.

[45] Pincus, G. The breeding of some rabbits produced by artificially activated ova. *Proceedings of the National Academy of Sciences,* 1939, 25, 557–559.

[46] Sloan-Kettering Institute for Cancer Research. Progress report/Viruses and cancer. New York: 1963.

[47] Carson, R. *The Silent Spring.* Boston: Houghton Mifflin, 1962.

[48] Warkany, J. Etiology of mongolism. *Journal of Pediatrics,* 1960, 56, 412–419.

[49] Medawar, P. H. *The Future of Man.* New York: Basic Books, 1959. Medawar calls these two kinds of traits the "segregative" and the "polygenic."

[50] Freedman, D. G. Constitutional and environmental interactions in rearing of four breeds of dogs. *Science,* 1958, 127, 585–586; Scott, J. P., and Fuller, J. L. *Genetics and the Social Behavior of the Dog.* Chicago: University of Chicago, 1965.

[51] Levine, S. The psychophysiological effects of early stimulation. In Bliss, E. L. (ed.) *Roots of Behavior.* New York: Harper, 1962, Chapter 17; Smith, C. J. Mass action and early environment in the rat. *Journal of Comparative and Physiological Psychology,* 1959, 52, 154–156; Rosenzweig, M. R., Krech, D., Bennett, E. L., and Zolman, J. F. Variation in environmental complexity and brain measures. *Journal of Comparative and Physiological Psychology,* 1962, 55, 1092–1095; Thiessen, D. D., Zolman, J. F., and Rodgers, D. A. Relation between adrenal rate, brain cholinesterase activity, and hole-in-wall

behavior of mice under different living conditions. *Journal of Comparative and Physiological Psychology,* 1962, 55, 186–190; Ader, R. F. Social factors affecting emotionality and resistance to disease in animals: III. Early weaning and susceptibility to gastric ulcers in the rat. A control for nutritional factors. *Journal of Comparative and Physiological Psychology,* 1962, 55, 600–602.

[52] G. G. Simpson (*Science,* 1963, 139, 81–88) has proposed that biology be considered the unifying science since it subsumes all of physics and chemistry. It seems to us that the same argument could be adduced in support of psychology, as a still higher-order, more inclusive science. We leave it to the sociologists to argue their case.

[53] Apgar, V. Perinatal problems and the central nervous system. In U. S. Dept. of Health, Education, and Welfare, Welfare Administration, Children's Bureau. *The Child with Central Nervous System Deficit.* Washington: U. S. Government Printing Office, 1965, pp. 75–76.

[54] Testing system gauges infants' survival chances. *The New York Times,* June 23, 1963, p. 54.

[55] All figures are from *Statistical Abstract of the United States.* Washington: U. S. Government Printing Office, 1957 and 1962.

2   *The Infant: 1*

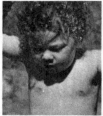Development during infancy—from the age of a few weeks until the baby is walking securely and beginning to talk—is a dramatic thing to watch. Striking and radical changes take place within this relatively brief period. During these first fifteen months or so outside the womb, the baby changes from a helpless—if sometimes noisy—neonate unable to change position, to a high-powered, willful pedestrian investigating and exploiting everything within reach in the most active way possible, tasting, chewing, fondling, probing, tugging, pushing, pounding, and tearing. As a child's activity increases, his sleeping time decreases. Some newborn babies spend all their time sleeping except at mealtimes or when in distress; by the end of infancy, the child may sleep as little as ten hours at night, with one or two naps during the day—there are great individual differences (as we shall keep emphasizing) in this respect as in all the others. In the first year, the baby adds almost 8 inches (20+ cm.) to his length and gains about 15 pounds (6+ kg.), trebling his birth weight. He acquires half a dozen temporary teeth and a full head of hair. Early in infancy his face loses its neonatal look and becomes the smooth, chubby face of a baby.

Socially, the infant progresses from blank, unblinking staring at faces to smiling at people, to demanding company, to laughing, to active participation in social games. After midyear, he will know that some people are strangers and may hide his face or shriek with dismay when they come near. The term "infancy" comes from the Latin *infans,* which means "not speaking"—and no matter how much he vocalizes, or how much his vocalizations change during this period, his babblings stop short of true speech. By the time he is a year old, however, he can understand a great many words and phrases, listens attentively to those he does not understand, and may (there are great individual differences) use a few words of his own. The limited emotional repertory with which he began life differentiates into half a dozen recognizable kinds of feeling states: pain-distress, aversion, anger, fear, affection, elation, and perhaps others.

From being a neonate whose existence is dominated by his own volatile inner processes with only a rudimentary awareness of the world around him, the baby moves on in infancy to a quite elaborate knowledge of his surroundings, of people and objects and their attributes, of space and spatial relations, of causal sequences, of his own body and its workings, and of countless possibilities for action. But the world becomes a place in which to learn and live and act only by virtue of the emotional attachments and meanings that are formed in this crucial period for the development of basic attitudes of optimism or pessimism, of trust or mistrust.

In this chapter, we shall begin the detailed description of infancy with an account of developmental landmarks, the conspicuous transformations of behavior (along with what they tell us about what the baby is perceiving, feeling, and thinking) that appear in a fairly stable sequence in the first year or so. We could arrange these landmarks under such headings as posture and locomotion, emotions and their differentiation, social relations, perception and cognition, tastes and preferences, and learning. To do so, however, would give us a logical but artificial set of parallel strands. Instead, we prefer to examine the baby's total development chronologically, describing diverse sorts of behavior that first occur at about the same time. This is in hopes of conveying some sense of the baby's integrated functioning. Even so, we shall not be describing the whole baby, but only certain abstractions from the totality. We hope that these will be relevant and meaningful abstractions that reflect the organization of behavior and development in real babies, but meanwhile it must be the reader's task to keep in mind the baby as a flesh-and-blood creature living at home with his doting but no doubt harried parents and, in various families, brothers and sisters and uncles and aunts and grandparents.

Landmarks in the Infant's Behavioral Development

A word of warning is in order. The ages we give for the appearance of items of behavior are approximate. The so-called developmental scales from which many of the items are drawn have some serious defects as guidelines to the normal course of infant development. They take little account of the wide but perfectly normal range of ages at which a given kind of behavior may emerge. They assume that behavioral development during infancy is for the most part *autogenous,* that is, a product simply of growth and maturation, whereas we have come to know a great deal about the effects of social and cultural influences on development, even in early infancy and even on growth and maturation. In fact, it seems that infancy itself has changed in the last twenty-five years, so that today's babies—at least the measured and observed ones in American research centers—are decidedly different creatures from yesterday's.

The changes that we think we have seen can be related in part to improved medical care, sanitation, and diet, so that babies are healthier and stronger than they used to be. Equally important, parental attitudes and practices have changed, thanks in large measure (in the United States) to Dr. Benjamin Spock, whose widely read book on child care has been a powerful influence in the last twenty years, so that parents are better able to relax and enjoy babies. There is greater faith in the competence of babies, and they are given increased freedom to explore and manipulate. Affluence, of course, plays a part in all this, and babies are given more playthings and exposed to ever greater varieties of stimulation.

In general, infants seem to be more advanced in their functioning than in times past, and though the authors are not always happy about the fosterings of precocity that can be observed, it seems to be true that the older scales of baby development underestimate the abilities of infants brought up under favorable conditions. Another difficulty with baby scales is that they tend to focus on the easily measurable physical side of development, with minimal attention to cognition, which makes their occasional use as infant intelligence tests doubly illogical. The use of such tests may reveal gross impairments, and they have considerable utility in comparisons of groups, but they do a poor job of predicting later intelligence in the individual case. Both the scales and the authors are guilty of the error of ethnocentrism, of assuming that development in a broadly Western setting is representative of development everywhere.

We know in fact that development follows quite different patterns and proceeds at different rates in other social settings. But we do not know enough to permit a coherent account of development around the world. We shall allude to known cultural differences, and to their possible origins in the baby's life circumstances, but our description will be mainly of so-called Western development, with no implication intended that this is the one right way to grow up.

Our knowledge of infancy, like our knowledge of the neonatal period, has been revolutionized in the last decade. Our former ignorance is easily explained by the fact that the child goes underground into the bosom of his family from the time he leaves the hospital at a few days of age until he resurfaces several years later in the nursery school. Our new knowledge is a result of willingness on the part of psychologists to go where the babies are—their homes, well-baby clinics, and pediatricians' offices. It also reflects a new attitude on the part of pediatricians, public health workers, and psychiatrists, a new interest in research, and in research on normal and healthy babies as well as on sick or disturbed ones. Parents, too, deserve credit for the willingness and even enthusiasm with which they cooperate in research. But just because so much of our knowledge is new, it must be regarded as provisional, and many of the generalizations we make will almost certainly have to be revised as our knowledge becomes more detailed and secure in the years ahead.

ONE TO THREE MONTHS

In the first chapter, we described the behavioral capabilities of the neonate as he exists for about a month after birth and the reader may wish to go back and review the behavioral repertory the baby brings with him into the world. Our present description begins at the end of the neonatal period, or approximately one month of age. Now, during his second month, the baby is awake more than he was as a neonate and shows more sustained response to an increasing variety of sights and sounds. By the age of one month many babies, when prone, can raise their heads slightly to look at something (some specially mature babies do so at birth) or, held in the feeding position, to strain for the nipple, although a number of perfectly healthy babies cannot raise their heads until age two months or later. Notice that raising the head and opening the mouth as the nipple comes into view implies that the baby now recognizes the bottle visually, at a distance, instead of having to wait until the nipple actually touches the region of his mouth. At the age of a month, however, when he is in the feeding position, he may react to almost anything held before his eyes—a gray or white cube, a sphere, a cylinder, a cone, or even a loosely bunched cleaning tissue—as though it were a bottle. Here we have an example of the baby's *physiognomic* perceiving, reacting to the global properties of things rather than to specific attributes. We expect the range of equivalence to be narrowed until the baby reacts only to a close copy of an actual bottle, with the nipple aimed at his mouth, as he learns to discriminate the essential features of the bottle and to rule out irrelevant ones.

In his second month, the baby's crying will stop at the sight of his mother, or when other people caress him. Many babies, before they are two months old, stop crying at the approaching footsteps of the mother. By about age six or eight weeks most babies respond with a smile to a moving human face seen in front view—or, for that matter, to a crude approximation of a face.[1] By this age, the baby sheds tears when he cries; his earlier crying was real and vociferous but usually tearless. He now, in addition to his crying and the sounds that go with digestion, produces vocalizations described by Gesell[2] as "small throaty sounds." He still cannot really change position, but he may arch his back and flail from side to side when in distress. He sometimes kicks his legs in the air, but he ordinarily keeps them flexed, knees wide apart, as though squatting. He eats at frequent intervals and still takes two or more night feedings. If he is howling with hunger, he now calms down as soon as he is held in the nursing position, even before the bottle comes into view. He can track a moving person or a trinket through an arc of 100 degrees or more (some babies swivel their heads around to look over their shoulders), but if he loses sight of a moving object he does not search for it. At age two months, babies begin to blink when something approaches their eyes at a fast clip.[3]

By about age two months, when an adult leans over and talks to him—it matters little what is said, and gibberish works as well as speech—the baby writhes about and works his mouth as though struggling to answer back. Some babies actually squeeze out a few strangled sounds. Later, this kind of response gets elaborated into babbled conversations between adult and child.

Early in the third month, the baby begins to reach out and bat at dangling objects, but he does not yet open his fingers to try to grasp things. This first reaching out to things may signal the start of the gradual transition from an inert, passive orientation to an active, manipulative, exploratory one. Interestingly enough, reaching toward objects is one form of behavior very much subject to environmental, experiential influences. Burton White and his associates have shown that babies living in the barren, unstimulating conditions provided by some institutions do not reach out to grasp until almost five months. But when such babies were given extra stimulation in the form of interesting stabiles (like a mobile in structure but stationary) to look at, additional handling, play, cuddling, and talking, they too reached out to grasp at just past age three months, a phenomenal advance.[4] Accommodation of the lens of the eye is essentially complete by age three months, and the eyes converge on an object as it approaches the baby's nose.

The baby becomes more social, even to the point of enjoying mild roughhousing. Vocalizations change to gurgles and coos, which the baby utters both spontaneously and in response to people. By this age, the baby smiles in delight when the adult pretends to be angry, whereas genuine anger provokes shrieks of dismay. Some babies, in the vicinity of age three months, begin to croon or hum to music. Those babies who have suffered colic in early life are likely to be free of it by age three months, to the benefit of their and their parents' dispositions.

THREE TO SIX MONTHS

In many ways, age three months is a transition point. The change in the baby is often summarized by saying that he is "becoming human." It is hard to define the subtle ways in which "becoming human" expresses itself, but the baby has lost his neonatal look and is physically a highly individualized infant. He seems to be newly alert and responsive and gives the impression of having a beginning inner life. In part, the baby's new status may have to do with his differential reaction to familiar and unfamiliar people. He greets members of his household with smiles and wriggles and gurgles, whereas strangers may be met with a solemn, reserved, watchful stare. Whatever the manifestations, parents seem to have no difficulty recognizing the change when it occurs.[5]

By age three months—and sometimes earlier—many babies "sleep through" the night, from an evening feeding to five or six or seven in the morning. The age at which a baby sleeps through seems to be a matter both of the baby's physical maturity and also of parental experience, since, according to a study by Moore and Ucko,[6] second and subsequent babies sleep through at younger ages than firstborn ones. The baby's readiness to sleep through is usually shown by his taking sizable amounts at daytime feedings, by the diminishing fervor of his crying when he wakes up during the night, and by his relative indifference to the bottle when he is given a nighttime feeding. Some babies wake up during the night not so much because they are hungry as because they are ready for a period of play and sociability; such episodes are usually transitory. The baby's ability to sleep is related to a general stabilization of physiological rhythms that goes on during infancy.

Roughly coincidental with his beginning to sleep through, the baby's evening bedtime behavior may show an interesting change. Previously, when sleepy and put to bed, he was likely to fuss or whimper briefly and then drift off to sleep. Now, as though recognizing that bedtime means the end of companionship and activity, many babies begin to react with cries of woe and anger. This bedtime screaming may be the first use of the voice in something resembling voluntary communication. For the baby who acts this way does not merely scream and go on screaming. Instead, he yells briefly and then stops, as though listening for a reaction. Indeed, in our experience, if a parent starts toward the baby's sleeping place, the baby will stay quiet as long as the parent keeps moving in the right direction. If the parent, heartened by silence and hopeful that the baby has gone to sleep, stops to listen, there will be a series of howls, punctuated by silences, each howl more forceful and prolonged than the one before, apparently as a way of insisting that the parent keep coming.

The baby's resistance to going to sleep means several days of torment for parents, humanely responsive to the baby's distress and the possibility that he may suffer some lasting harm without their intervention, but frazzled and fatigued by the demands of child care—piled on top of everything else—and desperate for repose. However, even the most indulgent of parents will find that they have to draw a line between social times and sleeping times, and the baby may simply have to be allowed to scream himself to sleep. According to Spock,[7] and experience supports him, once the parents steel themselves not to respond to the baby's bedtime crying, the baby will cry for some twenty minutes (which feels like an eternity to the anxious parents) the first night, less the next two or three nights, and thereafter not at all. (C. D. Williams[8] reports on the extinction of crying in a twenty-one-month-old by withholding all reinforcement for six nights, with the child crying for forty-five minutes the first night; obviously, behavior at two such different ages is not altogether comparable.) To the surprise and relief of guilt-ridden parents, the baby awakes the next morning refreshed and with no trace of rancor or resentment. We might mention that the process may be eased by leaving a soft light on in the baby's room, or even by allowing the baby to fall asleep in a bassinet or cradle right in the midst of family activity.

We stress this matter of bedtime and sleeping through because it reveals a new level of awareness on the baby's part, because it marks the time when parents can have some time to themselves and can themselves sleep through, thus enjoying parenthood and each other more, and also because it exemplifies a very important general phenomenon, the establishment of semi-autonomous internal "biological clocks." That is, the baby's cyclic daily (*circadian*) rhythms of activity and repose, of hunger, ingestion, and elimination, and of accompanying physiological changes such as regular fluctuations in body temperature, seem to be set initially by recurring events in the environment, particularly by the family's schedules and routines. Over a period of several months, they become self-sustaining (although obviously not immutable) and relatively insensitive to random departures from the usual round.

At the risk of digression, we might point out that biological clocks are common to virtually all species, including man, bees, oysters, and flowering peas.[9] Furthermore, the environmental programming of cycles seems to be produced not only by such obvious regularities as feeding schedules and the alternation of daylight and darkness, but also by such unlikely-seeming forces as the gravitational pull of the moon. For instance, oysters along the east coast open and close with the rise and fall of the tides. When moved to the Middle West and kept in a pan of shallow water, oysters for a time continue to open and close in concert with the tidal ebb and flow of their home waters. Gradually, however, they shift to the nonexistent tidal pattern of their new location, indicating that their cycles are not a response to the tides as such but directly to the geodetic forces that produce tides. It seems to follow that much of what we have been inclined to dismiss as superstition, such as the farmer's wanting to plant his crops by the dark of the moon, or the supposed relation between phases of the moon and women's menstrual cycles, may turn out to have some basis in fact.

Our society's great concern with time and schedules is often absurd to behold. Nevertheless, there seem to be some advantages to the stabilization of the baby's physiological rhythms, for the parent because it simplifies child care and for the baby because it appears to liberate him for play, exploration, and learning and to provide a foundation for his eventual mastery of time.

By age three or four months the baby may enjoy the playful fright that comes when a parent says "Boo!" and then smiles and tickles him. It may give him hiccoughs, but as often as not he enjoys these, too. It is toward four months that many babies laugh (rather than merely smile or

gurgle) for the first time, in the form of a hearty chuckle, perhaps in response to having the belly nuzzled or nudged by an adult. By this time, if
not earlier, the baby takes active pleasure in his bath. From about three
months on, when the baby is awake and on his back, he no longer keeps
his head turned to the favored side but holds it in the midline, his gaze
aimed straight up, although he turns head and eyes freely to see where a
voice is coming from. As we said in Chapter 1, some neonates may search
for the source of a sound, but the general rule seems to be that the baby
will turn his head and eyes toward a familiar voice at two or three
months, and to other sounds at four or five months—he hears the sounds
at earlier ages, as indicated by his change of state, but he doesn't necessarily turn to the source.

The four-month-old baby can be propped in a sitting position for
short periods, and can half-recline indefinitely in the baby carriers that
have come into widespread use in the United States. He may begin to eat
solid foods—more accurately, strained, mushy solids. At first, eating
entails a fair amount of spluttering, choking, coughing, and spitting—and
even gagging and vomiting—but it is usually easy to tell, each time that
one tries, whether the baby is agreeably disposed toward food in this new
form. (In a number of cultures this does not seem to matter and masses
of mush are relentlessly crammed into the infant's mouth.) An incidental
observation is that adults, spooning solids into young babies, cannot
resist making empathic feeding movements with their own mouths, as
though magically but unconsciously inducing the baby to do the same.

As we have said, the baby growing up in a normally stimulating
situation reaches out to take hold of things given visually by the time he
is three or four months old. The baby spreads his fingers to grasp, but his
thumb is not yet opposed to his fingers (a few babies show thumb
opposition almost from the beginning), and his hand bends backward at
the wrist in a strained, spastic manner that parents may find alarming.
When picking up things from the floor or a table top, the baby does best
by corralling them with his forearm and sweeping them against his body.
Although the baby can pick something up in his hand, he cannot yet
intentionally let go. Either the thing he is holding gets knocked out of his
hand when he moves it, or drops unnoticed from his relaxing fingers as
his attention strays to something new. If he really wants to get rid of
something he is holding, he rubs it against his body until it is worked
loose from his grip. A development of this period, seemingly associated
both with the baby's newfound skill in grasping and with his growing self-
awareness, is his ability to reach up and remove a cleaning tissue spread

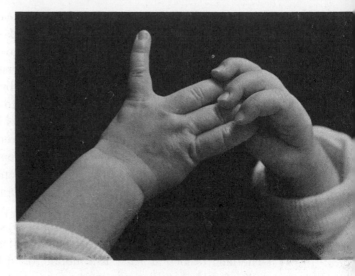

The hands of a baby.
Wayne Miller

over his face. At three months, the baby waves his arms ineffectually in the vicinity of his head, which he wags from side to side, by four months he can wipe the tissue away with his hand or arm, and before five months he simply reaches up, grasps it, and pulls it away—although there may be a delay of several seconds during which the baby seems to be considering the proper course of action. By age five months, quite a few babies will remove the tissue and then put it back again as though playing peek-a-boo.

By age four months, if one holds the baby during preparations for a meal, he will wait, another clear sign that he anticipates things to come. It is a tense kind of waiting, marked by escaping bleats and whimpers and by straining toward the warming bottle or the room where he is customarily fed. Sometime in this period, instead of howling the moment he wakes up in the morning, the baby begins to lie in his crib softly crooning and crowing and babbling a while before yelling to be picked up. Parents often become aware of this change almost as of something wrong. Instead of being dragged awake by the baby's screams, they come to of their own accord into a somewhat uncanny stillness hardly broken by the unprecedented sounds of good cheer from the infant.

As the baby approaches age five months, he can go four or five hours between feedings (longer, of course, during the night) and consumes generous amounts of milk and solids at each meal. He settles down to a pattern of two or three well-defined naps during the day, quite different from his earlier drifting in and out of sleep. He studies and plays with his fingers, one hand carrying the other to his eyes for visual inspection and to his mouth for tasting. Whatever he picks up goes to his mouth for sampling—and this will probably continue to be true for another year or more. If he cannot pick something up, he may pull his mouth to it. He still has to be braced in a sitting position, but he can stay this way for ever-longer periods before his head begins to loll and his body to slump. Notice how his horizons broaden as he shifts from recumbent to upright. The provisions made for babies in different households or different cultures may make a vast difference in perceptual scope. Prone, the four- to five-month-old baby can push his chest and shoulders clear and hold his head erect, as in the classic family album photograph of the nude baby on the fur rug. During his waking periods, the baby can stay contentedly alone at least long enough to let his mother finish a few household tasks uninterrupted. It helps to keep him content to give him something to look at, such as a mobile, or to finger, such as a suspended doll or rattle, or to listen to, such as music or a family conversation. The five-month-old baby given patches of different colors to look at begins to show clear preferences, with "warm" colors (red, orange, yellow) being looked at more than "cool" ones (green, blue, violet), and intense and fully saturated colors being preferred to weak and dull hues.[10] By this time, the baby's ankles have begun to straighten so that the soles of his feet no longer stare each other in the face.

Between five and six months of age, the baby becomes able not only to grasp but also to hold on, manipulate, and let go of rings and rattles and rags. He uses both hands in a coordinated way to handle things, to stretch out a piece of cloth while he inspects its intricacies, and he can transfer things from one hand to the other. It seems to be the case that the baby turns any new object around so as to examine the far side, indicating, as does the baby's reaching out to grasp things, that objects never exist for him as flat projections but instead are perceived as continuing on around out of view, like proper solid things.[11] This applies equally to really two-dimensional patterns, like designs on his playpen pad, which the baby tries to pick up. At a somewhat older age, having failed to pick up a design or picture, the baby may lower his eyes to the surface as though to peer at the hidden side. This phenomenon of implicit perception, of being aware of the presence of things or parts of things that are not directly perceived, is an important part of adult perception, but we shall talk later about differences in what is perceptually given for the baby as compared with the adult. There seem to be two different reasons that the baby may examine an object from several angles. The first, and more primitive, seems to be that the baby is looking for the best orientation to get the object into his mouth. The second, more sophisticated one, seems to be curiosity about what the far side is like, about what surprises may lie around the bend. Now, when the baby puts things into his mouth, it may be with a view to chewing on them rather than simple mouthing or tasting or sucking; his baby teeth are beginning to push through the gums, and chewing relieves the discomfort. This is the time when many breast-fed babies are weaned to bottle or cup, sometimes to protect the mother against the baby's new urge to bite.

SIX TO NINE MONTHS

It is around the age of six months that the baby is likely to discover his feet (for some babies, this discovery comes as early as age four months). He does not at first experience them as part of himself, but as strange objects which occasionally swim into view above the horizon of his belly (most six-month-olds are pretty chubby) and which his hands clutch at and capture and bring to his eyes for viewing and, within a month or so, to his mouth for tasting and chewing. To get ahead of our story for a moment, the baby's pained surprise when he bites down on his foot, as though he hadn't expected it to hurt (or at least to hurt *him*) is one among many indications that knowledge of his own body is not given to the baby at birth, simply by virtue of its being an operating biological entity, but that the body, its extent and its capacities for feeling and action, is learned through a series of discoveries during a long apprenticeship. The baby's knowledge of his body can be at several levels, however, since he can make use of different parts of his body before he explicitly discovers them. Thus, he could not grasp and handle his kicking feet if his feet did not cooperate at least to the extent of stopping kicking. Somewhat later, his feet raise themselves to be caught. At a still later age, but before they assume their main function of walking, the feet act as prehensile tools, assistant hands that fetch things out of reach of the hands or that support an object while the hands play with it.

At six months, the baby may be able to roll completely over (most babies can turn from back to belly before they can turn from belly to back), although there are wide individual variations in the age at which rolling over becomes possible. The stepping reflex—set off by supporting the baby upright with his feet lightly touching a firm surface—returns about now, having disappeared shortly after birth. Indeed, many babies of this age—or even younger—can lock their knees and stand on an adult lap with the adult's encircling arm for support. Most babies in our three-meals-a-day society settle down at about this time to a schedule of three meals a day plus occasional juice, snacks, and, if there is an interval between supper and bedtime, a bottle just before going to sleep. The bedtime bottle staves off hunger pangs as a threat to sleep and, just as important, provides a final period of social contact, cuddling, and sooth-ing before the end of the day's activities.

Somewhere between five and eight months of age, and characteristi-cally at six months, about half of all babies show a decided fear of strangers, or *stranger anxiety*. We have already mentioned the reserve that the three-month-old shows toward strangers; now he is likely to scream, clutch at the parent, and strain to put as much distance as possible between himself and the stranger. Stranger anxiety is important in practical terms, since it affects leaving the baby with new caretakers while the mother goes outside the home, and because many a visiting grandparent or aunt or uncle has suffered wounded feelings at the hands of a rejecting baby who has been rushed through the process of getting acquainted or reacquainted. The wise stranger keeps his distance, know-ing that the baby's reaction to a novel stimulus has components of both fear and curiosity. With a bit of patience on the visitor's part, the baby's curiosity dominates his fear, and aversion soon changes to friendliness. Stranger anxiety is also an important consideration for the scientist doing research with infants. One cannot test a baby in a tearful panic. In addition, one must remember that stranger anxiety applies both to people and to strange things and places, and the research setting and test materials may at first be just as threatening to the baby as the unfamiliar researcher.

Stranger anxiety is interesting also in terms of developmental prin-ciples. It indicates that the baby has acquired during this first six-month period of his life a scheme of the familiar (and ordinarily has formed powerful emotional attachments to it) so that a contrast of the strange becomes possible. The attachments that the baby forms for his own family (and house and yard and crib and playthings) has its infrahuman counterparts. Notice, however, that stranger anxiety is the culmination of a process that goes on over a span of five or six months, whereas the infrahuman baby generally forms a stable attachment within a few hours after birth (or, in the case of fowl such as geese or chickens, hatching). That is, there seems to be a *critical period* for the formation of primary attachments, analogous to the critical periods of embryonic development (see page 31).

The emotional bond to the mother formed by the hatchling goose or duck or chicken is called *imprinting*, a term which some authors would like to generalize to all mother-child attachments, including the human. Shortly after hatching, the gosling (which we may take as the prototype, although there are some species and strain differences) will follow the first moving object which comes within its field of view (the mother's calling and answering calls from the hatchlings probably also play a part)[12] and thereafter is attached to that particular object. Ordinarily, the first moving object is the mother goose, but in her absence, a football or tin can dangling from a conveyor belt, or the renowned ethologist Dr. Konrad Lorenz (who has been a pioneer in the study of imprinting) waddling, honking, and flapping his arms, will serve almost as well. We know that the gosling or baby turkey imprinted to a human being grows up to court human beings as though seeking to make them sexual partners.[13] We are not aware of what effect imprinting to such inanimate objects as a tin can or a football has on the behavior of these birds as adults—it is possible that such birds end up on the experimenter's dinner table somewhat short of full maturity. The authors have wondered about the role siblings play for each other in the imprinting process, since the duck or chicken may hatch out a half-dozen young at a time, and, in theory at least, the young might be expected to imprint on one another.

The case is somewhat different with higher mammals such as sheep and goats. Immediately after birth, the mother goat, presumably stimulated by her own tissue needs and the hormones present in the placenta and in the amniotic fluid coating the kid, eats the placenta and begins licking the baby. Her licking stimulates the kid into wakefulness and he staggers to his feet. Then begins a reciprocal stimulus-response sequence that has all the earmarks of a ritualized dance. The mother licks the kid from nose to tail, edging her body alongside his so that as her tongue moves down his body, he is in a position to nose along the underside of hers, ready to take hold of the nipple. However, just as he is about to nurse, the mother reaches his tail, turns around so that they are once again head to head, and the process is repeated. This goes on for two hours or more, until the mother stands still and allows the kid to nurse. Out of this stimulus-response ritual comes a stable bond between nanny and kid. If the mother and young are kept apart for as long as four hours after birth, the ritual does not take place and the attachment fails to occur. Or, if the ritual is prematurely interrupted, an odd thing happens: The kid nurses and, sated, wanders away. The next time he is hungry, however, he approaches mother goats at random, as though he did not know which was his mother, and is butted away. Even if he approaches his own mother, *she* does not recognize *him* and will not permit him to nurse. Failure to form the usual bond dooms the kid to death by starvation, or if human beings intervene and feed him, abnormal development is likely.[14] If he is left with the flock, various neurotic symptoms appear. If he is raised in a human setting, he is permanently alienated from goat society.

The effect of human rearing is especially visible in the sheep, which develops such unsheeplike traits as solitary independence.[15] Sackett,[16] in a summary of studies of early influences on the development of monkeys, finds much the same story. Harlow,[17] in his studies of rhesus monkeys reared by terrycloth dummies (with built-in nursing bottles), found that such monkeys were socially inadequate, showed bizarre mannerisms reminiscent of human psychotics, were unable to mate, and, in the case of females artificially inseminated, were unloving and even abusive mothers with firstborn babies (apparently they could act normally with later-born babies). However, recent findings by Meier[18] contradict Harlow's. The chief difference between Meier's and Harlow's rearing conditions seems to be that Meier's young animals could see each other, although kept separate, while Harlow's were kept out of each other's sight, and it is just possible that this difference accounts for the contrary findings.

One further point should be made about imprinting and stranger anxiety. Some authors, such as Freedman,[19] hold that the critical period for imprinting is brought to an end by the appearance of the "flight response," the tendency of the young bird to avoid unfamiliar objects after a few days of age, making impossible the proximity needed for imprinting. These experts view the flight response as the infrahuman equivalent of stranger anxiety. This position assumes that the flight response appears autogenously, as a product of maturation, as the next developmental step after an approach period. It is our view that the flight response, like all fear, is a response to strangeness, and that strangeness can only be perceived against a framework of the familiar. Thus, in our view, the young fowl who avoids normal imprinting objects does so because he has already formed a deviant attachment, as to his pen, and everything else appears strange and frightening. Indeed, Moltz and Stettner[20] have shown that the critical period for imprinting can be considerably extended if the animal is kept in an almost structureless environment after hatching. There is also experimental evidence to show that some supposedly automatic fear reactions need not appear at all. For instance, young fowl flee panic-stricken if a hawklike form is "flown" across the barnyard, which may seem like an instinctive fear. However,

Melzack and associates[21] have shown that if young chickens are exposed to the hawk shape from the time they are hatched, this fear does not develop. Kuo,[22] likewise, has completely and permanently altered dog-cat and cat-rat relationships by manipulating early experience.

To return to the human baby, whether stranger anxiety appears, and how strongly, seems to depend on how varied the baby's caretakers have been. Those babies who have known only a few adults are likely to display marked stranger anxiety. Those who have been taken care of by many adults, as in the kibbutzim of Israel, tend not to.[23] No one, to our knowledge, has seriously investigated whether children raised from early infancy by a nursemaid form a primary bond to the nurse rather than the parents, but casual observations lead us to suspect that this may sometimes be the case. There is the further question whether stranger anxiety is good or bad. It is our hunch that it is good insofar as it reflects a strong emotional attachment which should facilitate cultural learning and may foretell a later generalized capacity for strong affections. It seems to be good, too, in that it shows clear perceptual discrimination among people. On the negative side, stranger anxiety may represent an attachment so strong as to interfere with the normal weanings from infantile ways. In general, development entails relinquishing old attachments and forming new ones—at later stages, of different kinds, such as friendship, erotic love, parental love, commitment to a field of endeavor, loyalties to institutions and principles, feelings for art objects and keepsakes—a sometimes painful fact celebrated in Philip Roth's novel *Letting Go*.[24]

Furthermore, if we take it as a normal part of development that the child will grow away from identification with his family toward identification with humanity at large, too thorough an identification with the family can obstruct independence of thinking and the assumption of new and different systems of values. Here we are talking about the phenomenon of *ethnocentrism*, an unquestioning acceptance of one's own culture's outlook on and evaluation of things, so pervasive that it seems inconceivable (or deranged or depraved) that anyone could possibly think differently. One common outcome of ethnocentrism is that people of alien cultural backgrounds (including people from other regions or strata of our own society) may strike us as so peculiar as to seem subhuman. Such prejudice appears not only as hostility or fear of the kind found between Negroes and whites in the United States, but also in a patronizing attitude which sees representatives of "exotic" cultures as "quaint." Fortunately, as we shall see later, in complex societies there are some inherent mechanisms that help to some degree to counteract ethnocentrism.

Although the strange is often threatening, it is important to see that novelty is also sometimes an attractive quality as a departure from the humdrum habitual. Novelty produces fear reactions, as in stranger anxiety or even when the baby sees his father partly disguised with shaving-cream lather. But it can often produce fascination or amusement, and in the case of the human baby we have no system for predicting which novel objects or situations will produce which kind of reaction. At the infrahuman level, we have Helen Bruce's finding[25] that exposing freshly impregnated female mice to strange males tends to block pregnancy. However, a further analysis, by Eleftheriou, Bronson, and Zarrow,[26] indicates that a great variety of unfamiliar stimuli will produce the same effect, so that it is novelty as such that is the disruptive stimulus.

It is in the six- to nine-month age period that some babies begin to hold out their arms to be picked up, although others do not do so until a year of age, and a few perfectly normal babies never do at all. By age six months, the baby is highly responsive to his parents' moods and emotions and may even, according to Lewis,[27] show distress in response to words indicative of displeasure but enunciated matter-of-factly. He enjoys hiding his face with a corner of a blanket, peering out from time to time as though to see if anything has changed. His vocalizations are becoming more mature and differentiated, with consonants emerging between the vowel sounds; cooing sounds give way to gurgles, gurgling to babbling, where the child tries out a great variety of speech sounds—apparently the same all over the world. The conversationlike exchanges of nonsense sounds between parent and baby that began at age two or three months by now are a stable pattern of play—and one of central importance in the infant's emotional and linguistic development.

The baby's first teeth, ordinarily the two center lowers, are likely to erupt during the seventh month. Teething may be preceded by some discomfort, and usually is marked by a compelling urge to chew on things. Once his teeth have appeared, the baby begins to chew—even milk and baby foods. Salivation increases, and since the baby has not yet learned to keep his mouth closed and swallow his saliva, he is likely to drool copiously from now until age two or later, when his set of "milk teeth" is complete. We have already said that the immunities given by antibodies absorbed prenatally from the mother's blood wear off at about this time, so that teething coincides with—but does not, as old wives' tales would have it, cause—a new vulnerability to illness. Moreover, as the baby gets older he is exposed to more people and places, and so has more opportunity to pick up infections. Sicknesses during infancy and toddlerhood may produce raging fevers, as high as 104° or 105° (41° C.), which may be accompanied by convulsions, delirium, or even hallucinations. Alarming as such symptoms may be, generally healthy babies with good medical care usually recover rapidly with no discernible ill effects.

During his seventh month, the baby will probably begin to be able to stay sitting up without support, but he still has to be helped into a sitting position. He also assumes the Buddha-like pose characteristic of infancy, and as he plays with something on the floor in front of him, he may droop forward until he is helplessly nose against floor. He will be content to play in his playpen, provided he is not left there too long and particularly if his mother is within sight or hearing. We should note that the early self-reliance expected of babies in European-style cultures is seen as inhuman in societies where babies and young children are carried almost constantly during the daytime hours. Furthermore, in some societies it is considered animal-like and degrading for the child to play or creep on the ground.

In his feeding table or high chair, the baby amuses himself by banging objects together or on the table top or tray. He may even discover the delightful game of dropping things overboard. At some point this becomes an even more delightful social game in which parents play the role of retrievers, but at first, accidental dropping aside, it seems to be a way of exploring spatial relations in which the baby watches or listens for the impact of the dropped object. Later, this ability to release things into space and the knowledge of what becomes of them is assimilated to the all-important social exchange of the game of drop-and-retrieve.

This is an early manifestation of the child's fascination with repetitive playing with new discoveries until they are fully mastered. The adult is likely to find such repetition boring and foolish and perverse, unless he can see the analogy to his own involvement with some new gadget. It is hard for the adult, who takes so much for granted, to realize how new and fresh the world is for the baby, how many things there are to discover and experiment with and assimilate. It may help if the adult can remember discovering the way raindrops trickle down a window pane, fusing and sticking and accumulating and branching, and how the better part of a rainy day during his childhood could go to tracing the movements of the raindrops, or discovering how one can fog a window pane or mirror by breathing on it, and then trace designs in the mist.

Parents who quickly get their fill of the drop-and-fetch game have tried various escapes. It does no good to fasten the plaything to the table with a length of string. In the first place, this spoils the point of the game, which is social interaction which the baby himself can control. Second, the baby cannot yet perceive the spatial relation by which the string is an instrument for hauling in the plaything. At a slightly later age, he may discover, in playing with the string, that moving the string causes the attached plaything to move, and then that pulling on the string brings the toy closer. At first, however, he can utilize this knowledge only to the extent of making a single wide sweep of his arm, which may bring the plaything within reach but which can also send it flying. It is later still before the baby can shift his grip to a point on the string nearer the lure, and later again before he is able to reel it in hand over hand.

Another by-product of the baby's new skill in the use of his hands is that he may have to be given a spoon to hold while he is being fed solids, or else, once his first ravenous hunger has been appeased, he will be more interested in the spoon his mother is holding than in the food it contains. By this age, many babies have decided food preferences, especially if they are given a variegated diet, and will clamp their lips and jaws tight when an unfavored food is offered. Some babies approach unfamiliar foodstuffs with their nose, as though the odor is the deciding factor in whether the food should be given a try. Most babies seem insensitive to routine smells of cooking, people, body wastes, and so forth, but take delight in sniffing at flowers and other sources of novel odors.

The baby at this age enjoys a passive form of peek-a-boo in which the adult drapes a piece of cloth over the baby's head and face and then at the proper moment snatches it away and exclaims, "Boo!" Note that the suspense of being shut off from the world for more than a few seconds at a time becomes unbearable for the baby, and he may frantically claw away the cloth. There are two general principles hidden in this simple observation. The first is that when the baby is shut off from the world, he is also shut off from himself. We all need sensory stimulation from the outside world to maintain our sense of identity, as has been demonstrated by experiments in sensory deprivation.[28] Witkin and his associates[29] have shown that the younger the person, the more important visual information is for staying oriented. The second principle concerns affective arousal and comes from Dumas' theory of emotion.[30] This principle says that all mild emotional arousal is pleasant. It is obvious that we get pleasure from being petted or fondled or from their verbal equivalents, such as words of endearment or compliments, but we also enjoy the mock-fright of a ghost story or the safe terror of a roller-coaster ride. As emotions become more intense, they differentiate more sharply into pleasant and unpleasant. At a still more intense level of arousal, all emotions become disagreeable, so that what was pleasant at an intermediate level becomes painful. At the final level of arousal described by Dumas, just to complete the picture, functioning either disintegrates or is paralyzed. The baby's feelings of mock-dissolution in a game of peek-a-boo can shift very rapidly to panic—a sense that he and the world are actually on their way out of existence, and the baby needs a good deal of time and testing of the world's durability before he can feel comfortable shut off from it.

Although one can elicit a few sorts of imitation beginning shortly after birth, it is from age six months on that imitation, provoked and unprovoked, flowers most abundantly. The baby imitates such gestures as those involved in breaking an egg into a bowl or in brushing away a fly. Within a short time he will imitate such functional acts as using a sponge or cleaning tissue to wipe up spilled fluids. Social games with the parents evolve out of the baby's imitating what they do and also from the parents' imitating the baby, particularly the sounds he makes in babbling. The baby quickly learns the behavior needed to cue parental participation in social games: slapping the high-chair tray, sham-coughing, sniffing, puffing out the cheeks to have the air squeezed out, puckering the lips as though to whistle (many babies enjoy using a forefinger to plug up and so turn off parental whistling). From somewhere around six months, the baby joins in heartily when he hears his parents laughing, even though he has no idea what the joke is about, and at a slightly later age he tries to start new rounds of merriment by making a strained laughing sound. Notice that long before he can talk, the baby is inventing ways of communicating his wants to other people, and that his wants far transcend mere satisfaction of physical needs.

As the baby approaches seven months, he makes crawling movements when on his belly. Although these are mostly abortive, he may succeed in propelling himself for short distances—forward, sideways, or backward, more as chance dictates than from any intention of his. By this age, quite a few babies travel short distances by rolling over and over. Somewhere between ages six and eight months, the baby becomes able to hold on to an adult's fingers and half pull himself, half let himself be pulled into a sitting position. A little later, he can sit up by himself, different babies accomplishing this in different ways. Some babies, from a prone position, walk their hands under the chest until the trunk is almost erect, simultaneously swinging their legs forward and around. Another style of sitting up is to lie on one side with knees drawn up and to half-push, half-rock the body sidewise into the vertical, with the buttocks as the pivot and the head traveling in a 90 degree arc—the reader must bear in mind how different a baby's proportions are from a grownup's. As we have said, infants sit with their feet together close to the body, sometimes with ankles crossed. Toddlers, by contrast, will squat, kneel, or sit with legs jutting straight forward. The preschool child sits with knees slightly spread and forelegs folded back like wings, his heels by his hips.

As the baby approaches eight months, he will probably become able to crawl. (Crawling differs from creeping in that one crawls on one's belly, whereas one creeps with the torso clear of the ground.) Typically, the baby crawls by dragging himself along with his forearms and pushing with legs and feet (plus whatever other wriggling and writhing may be involved), but there are many possible individual styles. Some babies crawl feet first, some use only their arms, some travel by swiveling on their arched bellies, some, as we have said, by rolling from place to place; we shall presently describe some varieties of creeping as well. Some babies enjoy rocking on their bellies, an activity which may incidentally pump out gobbets of vomit. (In general, infants do a good bit of mechanical vomiting unrelated to gastrointestinal infections or motion sickness.) We should note here that some babies neither creep nor crawl, but stay where they are put, until they are able to walk.

At about this age, the baby begins to try to feed himself with a spoon, making a splendid mess of food, himself, and surroundings. The problem is partly one of poor muscular control, but partly also of not knowing too precisely where his mouth is. Here we must point to a distinction: Even though the baby at this age has no difficulty popping a thumb into his mouth, this is a different task from inserting a spoon, where one must take account of the size and position of the object intervening between hand and mouth. Even with the simpler task of eating a piece of toast or a slice of apple, one can observe that the baby has to poke around to find his mouth. Moreover, when eating a cracker, he may try to put it in at right angles to his mouth, and be at a loss to know why it won't go in. A spoon presents the additional complication that it has to be aimed right and, besides, must be kept right side up lest gravity rob it of its cargo. One can reproduce the baby's movements in trying to use a spoon by holding one's thumbnail up, and then making a scooping movement away from the body, up and around and back toward the mouth, with the thumbnail turned down, like an airplane at the top of a loop. The reader who finds it hard to imagine how the baby's body regions can be so imprecisely localized might remember the standard test for drunkenness of having to touch a fingertip to the nose with eyes closed, or the neurological test of having to close the eyes and bring the tips of the index fingers together, or the game of having to wriggle a particular finger with them interlaced and the arms crossed.

By age eight months, the baby will have acquired one or two additional teeth, and each remaining month of infancy will bring him another pair. Between eight and nine months, the baby's thumb becomes fully opposed, and he can grasp pincers-fashion with great accuracy. This means that he can feed himself pellets of food, such as green peas or bits of meat, as well as lick his fingers dipped into soft foods, gnaw at larger chunks grasped in his whole hand, and cram food into his mouth with his palm. As we have noted, the baby practices new skills tirelessly until they have been thoroughly incorporated into his repertory; thus with pincers grasping: With thumb and forefinger he practices picking up bits of fluff, snippets of cloth or thread, crumbs, specks of dust, grains of sand or dirt—the tinier the better, it would seem. He uses his whole hand to try to grasp shadows, sunbeams, and tobacco smoke. Indeed, later in the first year he may practice picking up wholly imaginary granules, which he carefully deposits in his other, cupped hand or sets down on a shelf or gives to a cooperative adult. By age eight or nine months, the baby will have outgrown his bathinette or dishpan or kitchen sink and will move to the family tub. This means endless opportunities for exploration and experimentation, especially if the baby has a supply of washcloths, plastic cups, floating toys, and so forth. The water must be kept shallow, however, or the baby, whose buoyancy works against his balance, will topple, and more than one baby left untended in a tub has drowned there.

On dry ground, the baby can get onto hands and knees, either by pushing up from prone or by tilting forward from a sitting position. At first, the infant can only rock back and forth on hands and knees; a short while later, he learns how to shift his weight so as to free one limb after the other in creeping. Notice that creeping seems to require a certain amount of conscious deliberation—the baby has to figure out where he is and what to do next. Once he has found the combination, of course, creeping quickly becomes smooth and automatic and often incredibly rapid. As we have said, there are numerous individual styles of creeping. Some babies leapfrog forward, moving both hands together and both legs. Bearwalking, with legs held straight, is sometimes the first form of creeping, while for some babies it is an advanced form midway between creeping and walking. One little girl we know used one leg simply for support and poled herself along with the other, like a gondolier. Some infants move sitting, either by hitching themselves along or by pulling or pushing with the hands. One baby used her feet oar-fashion, placing them forward and then sliding them outwards to the sides, which propelled her rump along the floor. At a more advanced stage of creeping, a baby may push himself along with his feet, sliding his hands on a sheet of paper or a rag. The creeping baby may take any one of a number of approaches to carrying something with him. He may simply drag it along in one hand, he may hold it off the floor and travel three-legged, or he may carry it in his mouth, dog-fashion.

Once the baby can move about easily, one can demonstrate the "visual cliff" effect, the fact that he will stop short at the edge of a precipice, even when in fact there is a sheet of heavy plate glass covering the void to prevent him from falling.[31] The visual cliff reaction is important because it shows that perception of depth is innate or develops very early. (But we can just as well infer depth perception from the baby's first reaching out to swat at a dangling toy.) The visual cliff response has been observed in newly hatched chicks and in white rats whose eyes have just opened, as well as in various other species, attesting to its wide distribution in animals for which it is a meaningful form of behavior. One should not conclude, however, that it is safe to leave an infant unguarded on a bed or table. The baby has to see the cliff to take account of it, and he is liable to play his well-liked game of flopping backward onto the bed when sitting with his back at the brink. Or, if he is rolling toward the brink, he may not see it until too late. In addition, some babies react to the drop-off as inviting rather than menacing and have to be restrained from flinging themselves into space (we propose the name of "Geronimo response" for this reaction). Some babies (and some puppies we have observed) want so badly to get down on the floor that they seem oblivious to the danger of falling as they try frantically to get down. The creeping baby learns very readily to go up a flight of stairs, but coming down remains beyond his powers for some time. The visual cliff effect usually restrains him from trying to go downstairs headfirst, and his body awareness has not reached the point where he can figure out the process of going down backward, feetfirst. It is only at about age eleven months that one can teach the baby to creep backward downstairs or to slide feetfirst off a bed or couch. The basis of the baby's perception of the visual cliff is thought to be motion parallax, the fact that objects at different distances from the observer have a differential displacement on the retina. The importance of motion parallax for the baby's depth perception has received further confirmation in a study by Bower.[32]

The baby's creeping further reveals his ability to detour around obstacles to get to something he wants. The ability to detour requires a more sophisticated perception of spatial relations than may be obvious. For instance, if the baby is given the task of getting a doll that is separated from him by a transparent screen, it is not usually before age one year that he can reach around the screen instead of persistently trying to penetrate it to get at the doll. A chicken separated from corn by a short length of wire fence may starve to death without ever discovering that she has only to walk around the fence to get at the food. Not long after he begins creeping, the baby wends his way snakelike through the rungs of chairs, beneath coffee tables, and in general through and around whatever passageways space offers him for exploration.

We have already mentioned some of the social games that babies begin to enjoy at this age. Others include give-and-take, passing a toy back and forth with an adult. Here parents may get another inkling of the baby's devotion to repetitive activities, the baby's interest continuing long after the adult has grown bored. Although the infant gladly hands things to an adult in a game of give-and-take, he now for the first time shows frustration and even resentment when something is taken away from him. Earlier, his reaction, if any, probably did not go beyond a mild and momentary perplexity. An important ingredient in the baby's frustration seems to be that now objects are *conserved,* that is, they continue to exist for him when they pass out of his perceptual ken, whereas at earlier ages the baby acted as though objects that went out of view went right out of existence. Conservation also makes possible the game of finding things that his parents have hidden. Although he can find a toy hidden under a box while he was watching, if there are two similar boxes he will not know which one to look under. He can learn with repeated trials, but no one, to our knowledge, has so far systematically investigated what cues the baby can learn to respond to—position (whether to the left or the right), color differences, size differences, different designs on the box, or whatever. If one hides a small object consistently in the same hand, the baby will learn after a few trials to reach for the correct hand; if one then changes hands, he will continue indefinitely to try the previously correct hand, eventually in the form of a ritualistic vestigial touching, before going on to the now correct hand. We shall return to the matter of conservation later.

The baby takes gleeful pleasure in this-little-piggy and allied games, in just being talked to or sung to, in being swung by his armpits (one must be careful about picking the baby up by his upper arms lest one dislocate his shoulders) between an adult's legs or being jiggled high in the air, in being tumbled about on a bed, including being shoved over from a sitting position. Late in this period, and even more so in late infancy, the creeping baby enjoys being chased by a mock-ferocious adult, and will initiate the game by paddling away, looking over his shoulder for the adult to follow and perhaps even making cries in imitation of those the adult utters in chasing him. While it is important that the baby not be caught too quickly, it is also the case, as with peek-a-boo, that the catching not be too long delayed and the suspense too prolonged. In much the same way, the baby may now begin a favorite pastime of late infancy, that of running away or hiding from his parents when they try to get him for a bath or bedtime or whatever. Even if the infant is not yet mobile and so is unable to take refuge in a closet or behind a door, he may begin to feign total preoccupation with what he is doing whenever his parents want his attention. Along the same lines, he takes great delight in his parents' simulated inability to see him as they search in all sorts of unlikely hiding places, calling out, "Where's Baby?" Again the tension cannot be too long maintained or the delicious excitement turns into frustration and panic.

It is worth pausing to mention that not much before age three does the child have any notion that successful concealment also requires silence; when hiding, he squeals and giggles with great abandon, apparently not realizing that he is betraying his whereabouts. By age nine months, many babies resent extended confinement in a playpen. The now-mobile baby wants to be out exploring the wonders of the house or yard or park, and parents have to impose their first taboos on dangerous or damageable objects and locations.

It is characteristic of United States middle-class babyhood that the infant has monthly medical checkups in the course of which he receives a number of immunizing injections or vaccinations. As David Levy[33] has pointed out, this practice makes for a natural experiment by which to study the acquisition of a particular fear. What we would expect is a steadily expanding gradient of anticipation of pain: at first the baby reacts only when the needle goes in; then, when the doctor or nurse approaches; then when being undressed for the examination; then when entering the examining room; then in the waiting room; and ultimately, by whatever intuition the baby senses it, when leaving home to go to the doctor's—as one mother put it, "We always take a taxi to come to the doctor's. Now, whenever he sees the taxi pull up to the house [note that this one-year-old could differentiate between taxicabs and cars in general, presumably on the basis of distinctive markings] he starts to howl." It is only at about age two, when the inoculations are much more widely spaced, that many babies can make friends with doctors and nurses. The sequence we have described can indeed be observed in many babies, but other babies seem not to find injections particularly bothersome, others seem not to anticipate the injection and react only after the fact, and others seem to develop a stolid stoicism that endures medical procedures without flinching. We are at a loss to account for these widely varied individual styles. We should also point out that there are other features of medical examinations besides injections that babies find distressing—the handling, the having things done to oneself, are also disagreeable to a number of babies.

NINE TO TWELVE MONTHS

During the final quarter of his first year the baby continues the transition, by stages we shall describe in a moment, from a horizontal to a vertical organism. He becomes less passive and no longer lies quietly while being changed or cleaned or dressed. Instead, he wriggles and twists and has to be given a plaything to keep him occupied and tractable—he may even get his first angry smack on the bottom from a parent who finds it impossible to cope with a flailing baby and a soiled diaper at the same time. On the other hand, he begins to cooperate in getting dressed, holding out an arm to go through the sleeve, raising head and shoulders to allow the shirt to pass behind his back, and so forth, so that dressing the child becomes much less a matter of stuffing him into his clothes. Even so, it may be as late as age three before one no longer has to remind the child to "push" his arm or leg through. If, as is often the case, the baby's customary plaything while being changed is his diaper pins (closed, we hope it is superfluous to add), one may see his first primitive awareness of number: If he is given or can find only one safety pin, he looks around for its mate.

His self-awareness reaches a new stage at about ten months when he recognizes himself in the mirror. (There is some evidence that culturally deprived children as old as age four years do not recognize their own reflection or photograph.[34]) He was earlier able to recognize the person holding him, as shown by his comparing person and reflection, but his reaction to his own image develops more slowly, from simple interest to playfulness to affection to clear recognition, manifested by his reaching up to touch the hat he sees mirrored in the glass or comparing his overalls with their reflection. It is only later that one sees the child posing and posturing before the mirror, or draping himself with odd garments and admiring the effect. As early as nine months the baby begins to shriek or shout as a way of letting people know that he wants something, like his dinner. When shrieking, he may for the first time discover the sound of his own voice and then make vocal sounds just so that he can listen to them.

Late in the first year, the baby becomes able to play advanced games like pat-a-cake. At first he claps his fists together, then his palms, but he is not likely to produce a clapping sound for a long time to come. If he sees people clapping on television, he may join in this mass game of pat-a-cake. The infant imitates such actions as picking up a sheet of paper and holding it above his head; blowing out a match and kissing movements of the lips; prominent inanimate sounds like the backfire of a car; and babble sounds such as ba-ba and da-da. He can throw things, but with very little control. He comes to understand a great many things that are said to him, mostly in the form of simple commands and requests but also cue words and phrases for familiar games and routine activities like bathing and eating. For instance, here is a mother's account of the behavior of her daughter at age ten months, one week:

> Debbie surprised us today by bringing "Red Fox" on request from her room to the dining room (a distance of 40 feet [13 m.] through several rooms—and a major feat for her to creep the distance both ways, dragging this 12-inch-high animal with her on the return trip). We had not realized she knew its "name" or that she could distinguish between it and "Bear" and "Heffalump," but she demonstrated to us then that she knew each of these equally well by bringing them, too.[35]

In his understanding of words that refer to events that are part of his regular schedule, the infant is probably helped by his biological clock, which signals when things are due to happen.

At about ten months of age the baby becomes able to solve such deceptively easy-seeming problems as how to remove a bead from a transparent wide-mouth jar: At first the baby tries to grasp the bead (or whatever lure is used) directly, through the glass; at a later age—typically between ten and twelve months—he can see that the way to reach the lure is to put his hand through the opening; still later, he knows that he can up-end the container and pour the bead out. It should not be supposed that the transparent container is invisible to the baby; he may steady the jar by grasping its rim as he tries to penetrate its wall. With opaque containers, where visibility correlates perfectly with accessibility, the baby has no trouble, and enjoys putting things into and taking them out of receptacles. He explores apertures and crevices with a probing forefinger. Indeed, many a baby goes through a period where his fore-finger seems to lead the way through the world. With palm and forefinger he palpates textures, quite literally getting the feel of surfaces such as fur and fabric and brick and glass and wire screening. If not restrained, the all-inquisitive infant tries to eat dirt, leaves, bottle caps, cigar and cigarette butts, dead insects—the potential list is endless. He learns to unscrew the caps from bottles and toothpaste tubes, sometimes with lamentable results. He can turn an electric light on and off by pulling a string, although at first he does not control the direction of his pull, and it takes him a while to learn to relax the string so that the switch can reset itself at the end of each yank. He can work simple cupboard latches and he tugs at knobs to open doors and drawers. He can switch on a radio or television set and twist the knob to regulate the volume. Some babies we have observed use the right hand to turn a knob clockwise and the left to turn it counterclockwise. Babies learn that there may be a delay between turning on a TV set and the appearance of picture and sound, although a baby can obviously have no understanding of the set's warming up. The

The teaching of taboos begins in late infancy.
Wayne Miller

The baby makes a plaything of his own reflection.
ABBY'S FIRST TWO YEARS/Vassar Film

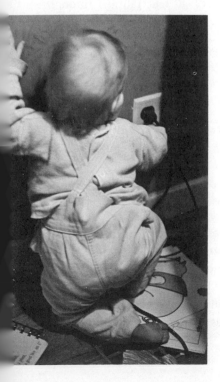

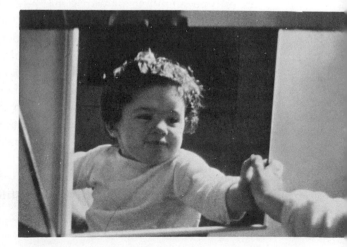

baby may seek to accelerate the emergence of sound by turning the volume to its highest setting, and then be so frightened by the ensuing blast of sound that he cannot go near the set.

The infant learns that toy cars roll forward and back but not sideways. He learns to distinguish among free-rolling, friction-motor, and wind-up cars. He cannot yet work the key on a wind-up car or other mechanical toy and hands it to the adult for winding. He likes to empty pots and pans from their cabinets, to bang them together and to mouth the handles, and to disassemble complicated pieces like double boilers and percolators. At this age, he takes such things apart, but it will be some months before he has either the inclination or ability to put them back together. Late in the first year, though, he may be able to place pierced blocks on a peg. He also practices putting things in things and setting things on other things. He is sensitive only to gross differences in size and seems baffled that he cannot put a large object into a small container. He has to learn by trial and error that he cannot rest a plaything on a vertical or steeply sloping surface, but this learning does not teach him that he can roll a car down an incline, a discovery he makes at about a year and a half. It sometimes seems that babies have a hard time perceiving extended plane surfaces, since we have observed babies doing things like trying to pass a spoon from one hand to the other through a feeding table top and creeping head on into a wall as though unaware that it existed, like the trapped wasp which seems to be trying to fly through the ceiling. It is possible that such surfaces seen close up have for the baby something of the character of a Ganzfeld, a homogeneous surface that fills the field of view and gives the impression of a space-filling fog.[36]

Late in the first year, the baby becomes aware that some things have a "correct" up-down spatial orientation and goes around almost compulsively righting overturned objects. This awareness extends even to such unfamiliar abstract forms as a wooden cone or graduated disks stacked on a central spindle to make a tower. In the same way, he soon learns to turn books and magazines right side up before looking at them and to read them from front to back—although he will probably turn the pages a handful at a time. He shows his recognition of pictured objects by rocking when he sees a picture of a rocking horse; even before he can speak, he may meow at the picture of a cat or make motorlike sounds at the picture of a car. Some such behavior is clearly in imitation of adults, but a great deal of it seems spontaneous. He does not at first distinguish clearly between printed forms and solid three-dimensional objects, as shown by his attempts to pick up the designs on his playpen pad, or letters, designs, and pictures in books.

In his progress from quadruped to biped, the baby goes through a fairly stable sequence of stages. The ages we give should not be taken too seriously—we hear of so many babies nowadays walking at between seven and ten months of age that we suspect that the published norms (approximately thirteen months) are obsolete, assuming they were correct earlier.[37] In any event, the range of normal individual differences is so wide (perhaps eight to twenty months)—and we do not even know much about such development in other societies—that it is probably meaningless to speak of an "average" age for walking. The authors were recently fascinated to watch a motorically precocious six-month-old creep to a large doll cradle, climb in, stand up, and examine his reflection in a mirror, bracing himself by gripping the mirror's frame and shifting his weight as the cradle rocked slightly under him. We shall describe progress toward walking as it is described in textbooks, regardless of when this occurs for any given baby, since the sequence seems to be a stable one.

By age ten months the textbook baby can support his weight when standing, although an adult must give him balance. By eleven months he can be pulled to standing and then, if his grip is transferred to a piece of furniture, he can balance himself. He may even take a few steps holding on with both hands to an adult's fingers. By age one, he can pull himself to his feet. The first few times he does so, he does not know how to get down again and may cry in alarm until someone comes and lowers him. He soon learns, however, to let go and thud onto his seat—a distance, after all, of only 9 or 10 inches, besides which his backside is well padded with fat and diapers. He is able to "cruise," sidestepping while he supports himself on furniture or on playpen railing. Then he stands without holding on; he bounces in place, either to music or, apparently, just for the fun of it. And then, one day—parents usually sense its coming and wait tensely—he gathers himself together and, with hands held high and to the side for balance, he toddles. His first few ventures on foot may last no more than three or four steps, but the baby has clearly made a transition. He almost immediately learns to stand up without holding on to anything—seated, he may draw his feet under him and simply push up; on hands and knees, he shifts his weight backward from knees to feet and then straightens up at the hips and waist. For another month or more, the baby may still prefer to creep when he has a definite destination, but meanwhile he assiduously practices walking until the time

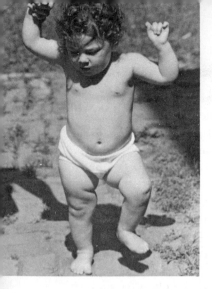

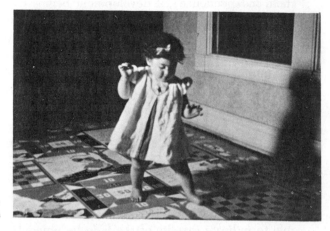

Many babies can walk holding on to an adult's hand.
L. Joseph Stone

A baby's first steps.
ABBY'S FIRST TWO YEARS/Vassar Film

The baby creeps feetfirst down staircases.
ABBY'S FIRST TWO YEARS/Vassar Film

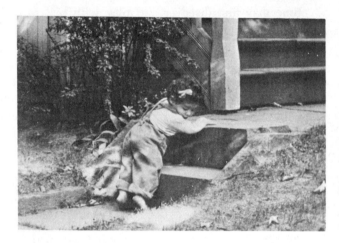

comes when he creeps only as a joke. This joke, incidentally, tells us something about the baby's self-awareness, since he seems able to draw a distinction between the walking baby he now is and the creeping baby he used just now to be.

The reader should bear in mind that the newly walking baby is some 29 inches (74 cm.) tall, which means in Western households that the top of his head will be just below the level of an ordinary table top; by stretching, he can just barely see what is on the table. He will not be able to grasp a doorknob, some 38 inches (97 cm.) from the floor, until almost age two. To return to Witkin's studies of reliance on visual cues for

86

orientation in space (field dependence) as compared to internal cues (field independence), if development begins with field dependence, one would predict that the baby who can stand up in a normal environment would be unable to do so if clues to verticality were abolished, as by placing him in a spherical chamber or one whose walls were greatly out of plumb.

One can observe the baby's growing knowledge of his own body late in the first year as he explores the adult's facial features and then feels his own corresponding ones. If he plays with one adult ear, he then turns the adult's head to find the second ear; if he feels his own ear, he feels both. He may even be able to comply with the request, "Show me your ear" (or nose or eye or mouth or teeth or tongue), but, as we said before, these are not clearly localized and he may have to grope a bit to find them. Also, if he suffers an insect bite or is otherwise injured, he may not be able to indicate the site of the pain he obviously feels. The baby at this time may first discover and play with his own genitals. This discovery seems to come earlier in boys than in girls, presumably because the boy's penis is visible to him in a way that the girl's vulva is not to her. The boy's discovery of his penis comes not out of some inner motivational state but out of his noticing something down there and grabbing it. A diapered society, of course, tends to delay such discovery. Most normal babies by the age of a year masturbate occasionally, especially at bedtime, but babies given adequate attention and playthings do not

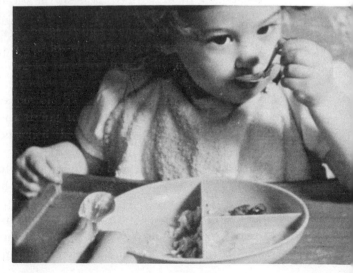

Late in infancy, the child likes to have a spoon to hold while being fed and may try feeding himself in concert with his mother.

ABBY'S FIRST TWO YEARS/Vassar Film

87

concentrate on this source of pleasure. Genital stimulation early in infancy seems to have a soothing effect, as suggested by its use in some cultures to quiet a crying baby. By late infancy, however, genital play seems to produce actual pleasure, but with nothing like the intensity of adult sexual experience.

Around one year of age, the infant waves bye-bye, usually by closing and opening his fist. He can pile one small wooden cube, somewhat precariously, atop another. As we have said, he can fit pierced blocks on a peg, but if they are graduated in size, he cannot yet arrange them in order. Nor can he pile or fit together a set of nesting boxes. He can sometimes get a spoonful of food into his mouth, but the spoon is still likely to reach his mouth upside down. He can drink from a glass, but he has to hold it with both hands. Similarly, he can hold his own bedtime bottle, if he has one, although many babies enjoy the social contact involved in a parent's holding the bottle or holding him while he holds the bottle. He not only enjoys receiving affection but is able to return it with warm hugs and very wet, open-mouth kisses. He tries to sing and enjoys listening to songs, rhymes, and jingles, and being danced around to music in an adult's arms. He may be able to hide a plaything under or behind a couch or in a closet and then retrieve it a day or so later. This is a real-life equivalent of the delayed-reaction experiment, which tests the child's (or animal's) ability to remember the location of a concealed object, except that here it is the baby who hides the lure and not the experimenter.[38] In general, babies perform much better on tasks they set themselves than on those devised by adults. The one-year-old may be able to draw a few strokes with a crayon—often on floor or walls. An occasional bright one-year-old can figure out, apparently without prior demonstration, that he can use a stick to reach and retrieve some desired object lying beyond his grasp, and most one-year-olds can be taught, by demonstration, how to do this.

During the first few months of the second year, as the baby is making the shift from infancy to toddlerhood, he achieves a stable bipedal stance and locomotion, he perfects and integrates his already-acquired manipulatory skills, and begins to say a few words or almost-words. He anticipates his interests as a toddler when he combines walking with grasping to lug, shove, and haul outsized objects. Now he enjoys his herculean efforts for their own sake; later on, they will be subordinated to higher-order activities such as block-building. When the child begins carrying things while walking, his first preference seems to be for large things hugged to his body with both arms, failing which he will carry two smaller things, one for each arm. Apparently, the urge to carry is great, for we have many times observed a baby pick up a bit of thread or lint or dust, hug it against his chest, and walk.

How the Infant Perceives the World

Now that we have surveyed some key features of development during infancy, it is time to examine in more detail a recurring theme of this book, self-world relations. We must begin by understanding that the same physical reality can be perceived very differently by different people. Some of these perceptual differences have to do with differences in individual outlooks, while some are related to differences among groups. Anthropologists are interested in the perceptual differences between cultural groups. Men and women debate, and sometimes quarrel about, sex differences in perceiving. And the developmental psychologist is concerned with age differences. What we perceive is only partly a product of the sensory information that impinges on our sense receptors both from outside and from deep within our bodies. We attend to only a limited portion of the sensory information available to us, and what we attend to can be organized in a multiplicity of ways. How the world looks to us is influenced by our knowledge of how things work, especially when it comes to taking account of governing forces that lie beyond perception, such as x-rays, ultrasounds, magnetism, infrared and ultraviolet light, bacteria, viruses, and the principles of growth. What we perceive is not always clearly distinguished from what we feel, think, believe, crave, and fear. In sum, the world is organized for us as a sphere of meanings and relationships, and not merely as a collection of things. We can draw a distinction between sophisticated modes of perceiving, in which the forces that actuate events are those that are derived from science, and primitive modes, in which the world is held together and animated by demons, spirit forces, and magic.

As nearly as we can reconstruct the perceptual experience of the very young baby from his behavior, the world at first is only a diffuse field in which objects come and go but without a stable framework. Objects seem to come into the baby's awareness at first in terms of immediate threat or gratification to him. Soon after, there may be connections between things, but the connection is always personal, through the infant. His mother's presence may portend changing, soothing, and pleasure, but he has little comprehension of the operations involved. Orange juice may signify that a bath will follow, but these are related for him as a familiar sequence of sensations, not as events in a world that includes his mother's schedule, too. Similarly, he has no idea of the geographical framework relating the kitchen where he gets his juice and the bathroom where he is bathed. The difficult thing for most adults to grasp is that, although everything is related to "my" wants and feelings, there is at first no *me*. There simply are states of hunger or wetness, of orange-flavored-fluid-followed-by-warm-immersion, all in a context of familiar person and place. But there is no *I am* hungry or *I feel* tired or *I taste* orange juice. The baby's experience is personal, because it is only his feelings of which he is aware, but he has not yet defined himself as an entity, just as he at first has no knowledge of a world that exists apart from his own feelings. This state of affairs in which the child's universe is centered upon himself, without his being aware of himself at the center, has been named *egocentrism* by Piaget.[39] We shall return repeatedly to the theme of egocentrism.

We have already seen many aspects of perceptual development during infancy. In the visual sphere, we have seen the newborn baby's preference for moderately complex forms over simple ones, and for facelike forms over nonsense patterns. We have seen him learn to recognize his nursing bottle at a distance, to distinguish between familiar faces and strange ones, and even to fear strange faces. We have seen him become able to reach out and grasp a dangling plaything. He learns to inspect objects visually and to manipulate them in various ways. At first he lacks conservation, so that vanished objects seem to have gone out of existence for him, and he fails to recognize his unfamiliarly accoutred father or mother. Then, when he begins to hunt for objects that have disappeared, we know that conservation is becoming the rule. We have seen him react to two-dimensional designs as though they were three-dimensional solids. Late in infancy, he becomes sensitive to the up-down dimension of objects. As he becomes able to creep, we see him adapting to spatial arrangements, as when he detours around an obstacle. He learns about transparent barriers and the need to go around them, too. Visually given textures invite his fingers to reach out and palpate them. The baby's first rooting behavior reveals a sensitivity to tactile information, and we have seen how he uses his mouth as a sense organ by which to know objects. From an early age, contact with adults comforts him and gives him pleasure.

In the auditory sphere, we have seen how highly selective the baby's hearing is at first. We have noted his early sensitivity to the human voice and the way he strains, as early as age two months, to try to answer back when talked to. From the age of a few months, he turns to see where a voice is coming from; at later ages, he searches for the sources of other kinds of sounds. He reacts to approaching footsteps, and by late infancy he recognizes the sound of his father's approaching car. He becomes responsive to music and may even show decided musical preferences. He becomes able to imitate sounds, and by the end of infancy understands a certain amount of language. We know less about the development of the sense of smell, but it is apparent that the baby's olfactory apparatus operates from birth on. Similarly, the baby develops food preferences, and he comes to recognize visually those foods he likes and dislikes.

In the realm of self-perception, we have seen the baby discover his own hands and feet and become able to use them. He learns to localize certain sensations, so that he can scratch at an itchy place or rub his eyes when sleepy. He learns where his eyes are, and his mouth, and his ears, and so forth. He becomes able to feed himself. He learns to recognize himself in the mirror. He discovers his navel and genitalia, and learns about the sensations caressing of the genitalia brings. He learns control of his body in manipulation and locomotion. He acquires a certain degree of self-control, as in waiting and in observing taboos. He becomes playful, and may even begin to play with his own identity. He becomes self-assertive and obstinate. In general, his burgeoning emotions tell us about his broadening awareness of things, of their characteristics and possibilities. Let us go on now to look at these aspects of perception more carefully.

There is some indirect evidence that the baby's active manipulation and his movements through space play a vital role in organizing his world. Held and Hein,[40] for instance, have shown that kittens whose visual experience is all gained from being passively moved through space (specifically, in a cart propelled by another, actively moving kitten), show defective spatial vision, as in the visual-cliff situation. The Austrian psychologist Ivo Kohler[41] has demonstrated that the effects of wearing distorting lenses gradually disappear as the adult subject moves about in the world, at first gropingly and then, as he becomes reoriented, easily. Once perception has stabilized, on the other hand, movement seems to be less important, since adult subjects who have taken curarelike drugs, which produce a total, temporary, flaccid paralysis, report that perceptual experience is even intensified under the influence of the drug.[42] The importance of active movement may help us understand some of the cognitive deficits that go with "cultural deprivation," which often has as one of its features that children are discouraged from moving about; in institutions where babies are kept immobilized in cribs, even walking may be long delayed.[43]

Another interesting feature of the baby's perception is the things he does not attend to. Loud and conspicuous noises that the adult finds it hard to ignore, such as thunderstorms, sirens, the racket of garbage cans being emptied and thrown back onto the sidewalk, the shrilling of the telephone bell, seem to go unnoticed. By contrast, the baby may scream in dismay at a sneeze or cough, he alerts to his mother's tiptoed approach, and, once he has learned to recognize the noise of airplanes, he detects them flying in the far distance. It is also important to recognize that the baby may be focused on something besides what we take for granted. When we find him staring out the window, at least some of the time he seems to be looking at the glass and the reflections thereon rather than through it. Similarly, the baby discovers reflections, especially his own, on the shiny surfaces of toasters, hub caps, or whatever, including very tiny ones. When the baby examines the draperies, he may be looking at the design or even at the weave of the cloth.

At all ages, we accept the world as given to our senses as real and complete—typically, the color-blind person does not discover his impairment until somebody points it out to him. However, the adult, unlike the

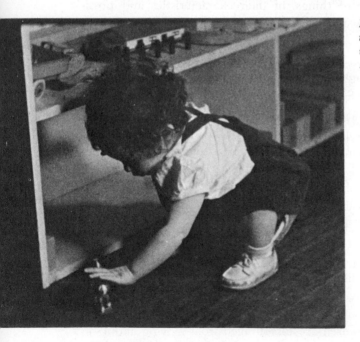

Perceptual realism: The child treats the toy animal as though it were a real one.
ABBY'S FIRST TWO YEARS/Vassar Film

baby, recognizes that the world contains several kinds of reality (what philosophers call *orders* or *levels* of reality). Dreams and pain and other such subjective events are real enough, but they are real in a different sense from cabbages and auto accidents and oxygen and photographs and sentences. Insofar as these realities exist for the young child, they seem to be fused into a common realm where dreams occupy everyday space, thoughts influence objects, feelings take incarnate shape, material objects dissolve into nothingness or change identity without warning, and where the common denominator of causation is magic. This tendency to accept everything as real and real in the same way as everything else has been given the name of *realism.*

We must distinguish between perceptual realism of the kind we are talking about and "realism" in the ordinary sense of realistic, either as hard-headed practicality or fidelity to nature. Realism also comes in such special versions as picture realism, as seen in the child's petting a pictured animal, trying to pick up a pictured string bean, or trying to listen to the ticking of a pictured watch (as did the Hayes' home-reared chimpanzee, Viki[44]); word realism, whereby a statement is treated as though it were a fact; and moral realism, whereby moral and ethical rules are assumed to be absolute, timeless, and built into the natural order of things. We see a suspension of realism in social games where the baby adopts a playful orientation to things, as in peek-a-boo, and a reassertion

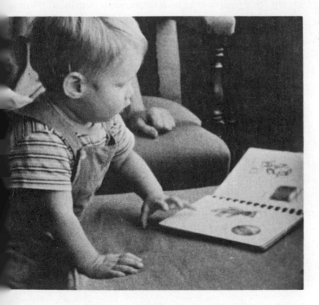

Early exposure to books and pictures facilitates learning to read.

INCITEMENT TO READING/Vassar Film

of realism when the game goes on too long and the baby acts as though he had indeed come to the end of the line. Schiff[45] has demonstrated that infant monkeys can be thrown into terror by the looming effect, produced by rapidly enlarging a shadow on a wall, which gives the impression of a rapidly approaching large object. The chimpanzee shows as much fear of a motion picture of a snake as of a real snake. The three-year-old can lose himself in his play to the extent of trying to eat his sand cake, and we as adults can be so absorbed in a movie or a story as to cry at the death of the hero or gloat at the downfall of the villain, to the point of forgetting where we really are. As we shall see later, preschool age children assume that the television dramas they watch are real events enacted by real characters enclosed within the set. It is a long, slow developmental process learning to sort out the many orders of reality and of reality-like fantasy.

A complicating effect of realism is that we all tend to assume that the reality we perceive is everybody's reality, as though everyone had the same knowledge, understanding, interests, values, moral standards, and vantage point in space. This assumption produces the attitude called *egocentrism* (which we have already discussed in terms of infancy), the failure to realize that one's outlook is peculiarly one's own, with a corresponding inability to take account of other, differing perspectives on a given state of affairs. Egocentrism provides the foundation for *ethnocentrism*, taking for granted the ways of behaving, the values and ideas of the people among whom one grows up. Ethnocentrism is a shared blindness masquerading as knowledge; it is akin to the shared geocentrism that made people think for millennia that the earth was the center around which the universe revolved, and which resisted so bitterly the radical notion put forward by Galileo, Copernicus, and others that the earth was merely one satellite of one star among countless other stars.

Note that egocentrism, as used in the description of immature behavior, does not mean egotistic; it does not mean either selfishness or preoccupation with self. It is perfectly possible to be quite generous in an egocentric way, as when someone gives a present, in all love and benevolence, that is more suited to the donor than to the recipient. We can see this in the way a young child affectionately and self-sacrificingly bestows his sodden toast upon his mother or father. Egocentric behavior occurs not because the child is full of his own importance or preoccupied with thoughts of self but precisely because he is insufficiently aware of himself and the personal nature of his experience, his biased, idiosyncratic outlook on things. Ideally, with maturity, one moves away from ego-centrism and ethnocentrism toward *relativism,* the ability to take account of how things look to other people and in other cultural perspectives, but even adults give abundant evidence of egocentrism—a mother may weep because her children didn't like some foodstuff she had prepared as a special treat. Relativism, it might be added, does not mean a relinquishing of values, but it often enables us to think critically about the values that we do hold.

In most experimental and philosophical accounts of perception, it is assumed that the person contemplates and analyzes the features of the objects around him, and then reconstitutes objects and their spatial and causal relationships from elements of sensation, by a kind of unconscious cerebration. Analytical, contemplative perceiving does occur, but the more usual procedure is to take things in and react to them at a glance. Instead of attending to the detailed properties of things, we apprehend them *physiognomically,* in terms of their overall, expressive qualities, so named on the analogy of the way we perceive the human physiognomy and the play of facial expression. Physiognomic perceiving lasts through life, so that even after we have scrutinized something analytically, and so perhaps changed its physiognomy, we continue to react to it globally, as when we identify a particular make of car. Learning to read requires analysis of the letter forms (although many children can read well before they can reproduce the shapes of letters), but once reading has been mastered, we read physiognomically. This is why we easily miss typographical errors, misread unfamiliar words as familiar ones, and seldom notice the typeface in which a book is printed. We grasp the general sense (correctly or incorrectly) of what we read, ignoring or only half-noticing the physical characteristics of the little black squiggles that are the stimulus for reading. In fact, if color names are printed in inks of a color different from the name, the expert reader has to make a special effort to see the color of the ink.[46]

The physiognomies of things contain what Koffka calls their *demand qualities,* which elicit particular feelings and behavior, often without prior learning. For the baby, knobs have the demand quality of graspability and pullability, crevices that of forefinger-pokeability, textures of palpability, funny faces that of risibility, just as for the adult wet paint demands to be touched and a baby's cheek to be pinched.

Demand quality points to another neglected fact of perception, which is that we react to objects somatically and emotionally in a single sweep of behavior, and not in stages where we first perceive something, then identify it, and then have feelings about it. The general term here is perceptual *participation,* that is, we participate directly in happenings in our surroundings, as though they and we were all segments of the same organism. One of the most striking forms of participation is *empathy,* where we become so involved in some external action that we do it, too, as when we help the pole-vaulter over the bar, restrain the comedian from falling over the precipice, apply "body English" to a billiard or golf ball, yawn in concert with another, clear our throat to remove the frog in somebody else's, writhe and grunt with the wrestlers on television, or open our mouth as we feed the baby. Empathy seems to be the basis of early imitation, such as the neonate's imitation of sticking out the tongue. The way one baby cries in response to another baby's crying is another example of empathy. With age and experience, we come to perceive more objectively and to interpose judgment between perception and action (although it is obvious, from the misunderstandings of everyday life and from students' answers on examinations, that we misperceive much of what we hear) and the somatic components of perceiving become more subdued. Nevertheless, with the proper recording instruments, such as those linked to a polygraph or "lie detector," we can show that even in adults the very simplest stimuli, such as the click of a telegraph key, produce reverberations throughout the body.[47]

An important feature of immature perception is *synesthesia,* the fact that stimulation in one sense modality produces effects in other modalities. The almost universal adult synesthesia is the way odor contributes to flavor, as we become aware when we get a cold and foods lose their familiar "taste." A small number of adults have color-hearing, so that various sound patterns produce characteristic color sensations. It is reported that color-hearing is a common effect of the so-called psychedelic or hallucinogenic drugs such as mescaline, LSD–25, and psilocybin, so that hearing music is accompanied by shifting colors of objects, prismatic effects along edges, and sometimes patterns of color flowing through the air. While the undrugged adult knows that sounds have a visible source, he does not think of the sounds themselves as visible entities. The baby, by contrast, often acts as though he expects to be able to see sounds, as when he quickly pulls an adult's hands apart as though looking for the handclap they have just made, or looks about the room as though seeking the chord that has just been struck on the piano. We even have an instance of a little girl trying to hear the ticking of a watch by holding it to her eyes.[48] For just as sensations are not clearly catalogued for the baby, his awareness of the functioning of his sense receptors is vague and poorly localized. There also seems to be an anticipatory synesthesia, whereby we sense from the visual appearance of something whether it will be rough or smooth to the touch, or wet or sticky or slimy, or hard or elastic or brittle, or warm or cool, or heavy or light. In the same vein, many sounds seem to carry faint visual or kinesthetic images of the things that produce them, as when we hear "a person walking." Even so diffuse a sense as smell may evoke an image of the object that produces the odor, as when we smell an orange (not merely the odor of orange), and this tells us its location in space.

Some of the associations and anticipatory synesthesias seem to be learned rather than organically built in, and these are called *intersensory effects*.[49] Whereas true synesthesias diminish with age, so that we become less likely to confuse taste and smell, sight and sound, temperature and texture, we expect an increase, at least to some maximum, in intersensory effects. We learn to judge food flavors from appearances, and it is only when we sample an alien cuisine that we are taken by surprise by flavors we had not expected. The baby apparently sees sandpaper as rough to the touch, but, to judge by his surprise when the soap bubble bursts, he did not see the latter as fragile. As far as he is concerned, there would be nothing incongruous about striking two wooden sticks together and getting a tinkling sound, or dropping a glass on a cement floor and having it land with a whoosh. He has to learn over a period of years how experience in one modality is correlated with experience in others. He has to learn, for instance, that in general size is positively correlated with weight, but he also has to learn the exceptions, that there are big lightweight things like balloons and foam plastic rafts and eiderdown pillows, and small heavy ones like chunks of gold and lead. Transfer of knowledge between modalities is a complicated matter, still incompletely mapped. For instance, a child of preschool age may be able to recognize by touch alone things that he has previously known only visually, but not the reverse: He may not recognize visually things he has previously known only by touch.

We have already mentioned another important perceptual principle, what Piaget calls the *conservation* of objects. The adult takes it for granted that a material object can go on existing even when not present to the senses. The young infant, by contrast, acts as though an object that has disappeared has evaporated. If one simply places a piece of cloth over a toy the infant is looking at, or lowers behind a screen a toy that the baby is following with his eyes, the infant immediately loses interest, with no sign of surprise or regret or any attempt to look for the vanished object. In other words, objects are not conserved for babies younger than six to eight months.

However, the case of conservation and nonconservation is not a simple one. In the first place, it appears that certain privileged objects, such as parents, may be conserved from almost the beginning of infancy. The baby's howling at evening bedtime, at age two or three months, may imply awareness of being separated from a stable object. Some of the nonconservation shown by babies in experimental tasks may be because the baby is not in actual contact with the lures; objects which are presented only visually may be less stable than those the baby handles. We must also note that conservation is not always the rule in the real world. In the strict physical sense, the law of conservation says that matter or energy can be transformed or dissipated but not destroyed. But as far as the evidence of the senses goes, lots of material substantial things (without mention of dreams and sensations and smoke and mist and light and sounds) do change—milk disappears from the bottle and food from the plate, fat cools and congeals, ice melts, balloons shrink and shrivel, flowers grow and wither, wastes are flushed down the toilet, water dries up or disappears down the drain. What the baby has to do is sort out the stable and the unstable, and when one considers the variety of things he encounters and the poverty of precedent he has to draw on, he does an altogether remarkable job.

So far, we have been talking about the conservation of whole objects. But one can also talk about the conservation of attributes of objects, which is more commonly labeled perceptual *constancy*. It is a fundamental and amazing fact that a given object looks to be the same size, shape, and color, and indeed to retain its identity as itself, under a great variety of viewing conditions. (There are also auditory, tactual, and so forth, constancies, but the phenomenon is most easily illustrated in the realm of vision.) In actuality, as an object moves toward or away from us, the image it projects on the retina changes size, but the object itself continues to seem the same size. Its color looks constant even when the illumination changes, and we see it as having the same shape even though the retinal projection undergoes all sorts of transformations. For instance, we see table tops as having square corners, even though, seen in the customary perspectives, the corners are not projected to the retina as right angles.

From time to time, there has been controversy about whether constancy develops in the life history of the individual or is present from the start. The controversy is still unresolved, but there seem to be a few

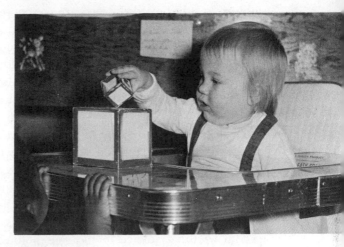

Exploring size relations.
Louis Georgianna

Object conservation.
Bettye Caldwell

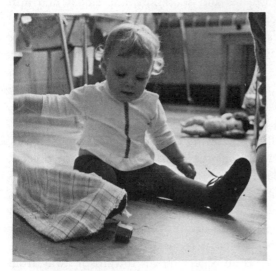

safe generalizations. First of all, we must distinguish between how objects exist for the baby as something to interact with and how they exist as objects to be contemplated. Apparently, as in the experiments mentioned above, unhandled objects are less stable than handled ones. A second distinction is between the baby's orientation to things relative to himself and to things relative to each other. For instance, in creeping or toddling through space, the baby avoids steeply pitched surfaces, seemingly in the knowledge (however ill-defined) that they will send him tumbling. (But he is as likely to try to cross a bridge made of cardboard as one made of wood.) On the other hand, as we have said, it seems to come as a surprise to him that a plaything set down on an incline will also slide or roll or tumble. When it comes to grasping things and putting them in his mouth, the baby handles them appropriately with respect to size. When it comes to fitting two things together, though, or putting one thing inside another, he seems incredibly insensitive to size relations. Furthermore, size constancy seems to break down for the baby beyond a certain distance, so that the two-year-old, seeing people at the far end of the block, can point with surprise to the "little people." All of us, babies and adults alike, have trouble with size and distance in the up-down dimension of space. All of us are subject to the moon illusion, the fact that the moon looks much larger at the horizon than high in the sky, and most of us know the sensation of watching an airplane come in to land and seeing it jump from toy size to airplane size as it approaches. Similarly, we know that people and cars lose their reality viewed from a tall building. The baby reaches up to embrace his mother as she leans out of a third-story window, or he tries to grasp the moon. As far as we know, nobody has ever tried to study color constancy in babies, but it could be done with a discrimination learning task.

In general, the baby's constancy is more easily tricked than the older child's or adult's, as when he fails to recognize a partially disguised parent. His judgments improve with age and experience, his coordination of objects in space becomes more accurate, and his perceptions become more objective and less affect- and action-dominated; but there is every reason to suppose that the baby begins life with a rudimentary perception of objects as constant.[50]

Two further characteristics of the world as perceived by immature human organisms deserve mention, even though we are not sure how they apply in babyhood. These are called *phenomenalism* and *dynamism*. Phenomenalism refers to the fact that babies (and many adults) seem to accept the surface appearances of things without wondering about their deeper structure. This applies particularly to learning about causal chains. The baby learns, pragmatically, a great many causal sequences. He knows how to turn a light on and off, he knows how to pour from a cup (although he may not know how to stop pouring), he knows how to turn on a radio, he knows that if he pulls the cat's tail, he is liable to get scratched, and so on. At the same time, he is not curious about their hidden mechanics. Indeed, a great many adults have no notion about what intervenes between flicking a wall switch and the shining forth of light, of why water comes out of a faucet, of how airplanes fly, how a car works, or even of the workings of their own bodies. One can demonstrate an interesting specimen of adult phenomenalism by asking a group of subjects to draw an island, not as it is represented on a map but as it would be seen from the side, in profile, including what is under the water as well as what is above; they are to start their drawings with a horizontal line representing the surface of the water. It turns out that almost all school-age children and a great many adults (especially females)—even well-educated adults—conceive of islands as floating, not as the peaks of mountains thrusting up from the ocean floor. A large number of subjects reveal their phenomenalism by evading the task, letting the lines showing the flanks of the island peter out or run off the side of the page without coming to any resolution. We have tried this task with residents of the island of Oahu, in Hawaii, and get about the same proportion of floating and indefinite islands as with mainland dwellers.

In place of the many specific causal factors that the scientist is concerned with, the baby—or the naïve adult—seems to get along with a generalized *dynamism*, as though the world were pregnant with some magical force that supplies the motive power for particular events. Many causal doctrines of bygone days, such as animism, animal magnetism, mesmerism, mind over matter, spiritualism, and the like, can be seen as dynamism made concrete and explicit.

SELF-PERCEPTION

Implicit in everything we have said so far is that perception of the world is always simultaneously perception of oneself. We perceive ourselves in several ways. Some parts of our bodies are available to visual inspection, while other parts can be seen only with a mirror or an arrangement of mirrors, and most of what lies beneath the skin can ordinarily not be seen at all. Most of our inner anatomy has no clearcut perceptual representation for us. When we are in good equilibrium, our physiological functioning is a blend of sensations, although we can make some functions stand out, as when we attend to our breathing or our heartbeat. Various physiological imbalances have their own perceptual qualities, as in pain, aches, illness, hunger, fever, thirst, fatigue, sexual arousal, and the physiological components of emotion, such as sweating or the "butterflies in the stomach" that accompany anxiety. We experience our own behavior in terms of the spatial displacements we make and in terms of the feedback we receive from our surroundings. (We are not explicitly aware, except on difficult terrain, of the way the ground feeds back information to our feet in walking, but when that feedback is shut off, as in certain neurological conditions, walking becomes a very difficult matter.) We also experience our own behavior in terms of motivation, emotion, and esthetic and moral considerations.

In general, these self-awarenesses are blended into a total self-awareness, but we can sort out most of the constituents if we try. Somewhere in the course of development, we come to have a sense of identity, of who we are and what we believe in, what we want out of life, what our virtues and failings and competences and inadequacies are. We develop a certain amount of perspective on ourselves so that we can judge our own acts in terms both of how they look to others and of how they measure up to abstract, ideal standards; when we fail to measure up to abstract moral standards, we feel guilt, and when we fail to meet abstract standards of competence, we feel shame.[51] We become able, within limits, to shape our own characters and destinies, and we come to have a conscience and to be concerned for other people.

To return to the baby's self-awareness, his implicit knowledge of his own body is fairly well advanced by the end of infancy, as indicated by his ability to deal adaptively with objects. His active exploration of hands, feet, genitals, navel, and facial features seems to suggest that he has brought some parts of his body into explicit consciousness and so made them his own. He still seems peculiarly insensitive to some body states. He may, for example, carry on normally even though he has a fever or is badly chilled. When he does know that something is wrong, it may be expressed as a general malaise or a being out of sorts, as though the discomfort were not clearly represented to him. He rubs or scratches accurately at itchy patches or places where one tickles his skin with a cleaning tissue, but he may not be able to locate sharp pain such as that caused by an insect bite—he feels the pain, as we have said, but he does not seem to know where it is. By the end of infancy, he will probably respond to his own name, which is most likely the beginning of a verbal definition of self, an important ingredient in the formation of identity. We shall have a good deal more to say about the evolution of self-awareness in later chapters.

Let us look now at the conditions, personal, social, and physical, which shape development and make it possible.

REFERENCES / Chapter 2

[1] Spitz, R. A. The smiling response: A contribution to the ontogenesis of social relations. *Genetic Psychology Monographs*, 1946, 34, 57–125. For a more recent account, see Wolff, P. Observations on the early development

of smiling. In Foss, B. M. (ed.) *Determinants of Infant Behavior II.* New York: Wiley, 1963, pp. 113–138.

2 Gesell, A., Thompson, H., and Amatruda, C. S. *The Psychology of Early Growth.* New York: Macmillan, 1938.

3 White, B. L. The development of perception during the first six months of life. Paper read at meetings of the American Association for the Advancement of Science, 1963.

4 White, B. L., and Held, R. Plasticity of sensori-motor development in the human infant. In Rosenblith, J. F., and Allinsmith, W. (eds.) *The Causes of Behavior.* Boston: Allyn & Bacon, second edition, 1966, Chapter 9

5 Church, J. (ed.) *Three Babies.* New York: Random House, 1966, pp. 13, 180–181.

6 Moore, T., and Ucko, L. E. Night waking in early infancy. *Archives of Disease in Childhood,* 1957, 32, 333–342.

7 Spock, B. *Baby and Child Care.* New York: Pocket Books, 1957.

8 Williams, C. D. The elimination of tantrum behavior by extinction procedures. *Journal of Abnormal and Social Psychology,* 1959, 59, 269.

9 Brown, F. A. Living clocks. *Science,* 1959, 130, 1535–1544.

10 Spears, W. C. Assessment of visual preference and discrimination in the four-month-old infant. *Journal of Comparative and Physiological Psychology,* 1964, 57, 381–386; Staples, R. The responses of infants to color. *Journal of Experimental Psychology,* 1932, 15, 119–141; Valentine, C. W. The colour perception and colour preferences of an infant during its fourth and eighth months. *British Journal of Psychology,* 1913–14, 6, 363–386.

11 Piaget, J. Das Umdrehen des Gegenstandes beim Kind unter einem Jahr. *Psychologishe Rundschau,* 1932, 4, 110–115.

12 Hess, E. H. Imprinting in birds. *Science,* 1964, 146, 1128–1139.

13 Lorenz, K. Z. *King Solomon's Ring.* New York: Crowell, 1952; Schein, M. W., and Hale, E. B. The effect of early social experience on male sexual behavior of androgen-injected turkeys. *Animal Behaviour,* 1959, 7, 189–200.

14 Blauvelt, H. Dynamics of the mother-newborn relationship in goats. In Schaffner, B. (ed.) *Group Processes: Transactions of the First Conference.* New York: Macy Foundation, 1955, pp. 221–258; Moore, A. U. Studies on the formation of the mother-neonate bond in sheep and goat. Paper read at meetings of the American Psychological Association, 1960.

15 Scott, J. P. *Animal Behavior.* Chicago: University of Chicago, 1958.

16 Sackett, G. P. Effects of rearing conditions upon the behavior of rhesus monkeys. *Child Development,* 1965, 36, 855–868.

17 Harlow, H. F., and Harlow, M. K. Social deprivation in monkeys. *Scientific American,* 1962, 207, 136–146.

18 Meier, G. W. Other data on the effects of social isolation during rearing upon adult reproductive behaviour in the rhesus monkey (Macaca-Mulatta). *Animal Behaviour,* 1965, 13, 228–231.

19 Freedman, D. G. The differentiation of identical and fraternal infant twins on the basis of filmed behavior. Paper read at Second International Congress of Human Genetics, 1961.

20 Moltz, H., and Stettner, L. J. The influence of patterned-light deprivation

on the critical period for imprinting. *Journal of Comparative and Physiological Psychology*, 1961, 54, 279–283.

[21] Melzack, R., Penick, E., and Beckett, A. The problem of "innate fear" of the hawk shape. *Journal of Comparative and Physiological Psychology*, 1959, 52, 694–698.

[22] Kuo, Z.-Y. *The Dynamics of Behavior Development: An Epigenetic View.* New York: Random House, 1967, PP 34.

[23] Spiro, M. E. *Children of the Kibbutz.* Cambridge: Harvard, 1958; Caldwell, B. M. Mother-infant interaction in monomatric and polymatric families. *American Journal of Orthopsychiatry*, 1963, 33, 653–664.

[24] Roth, P. *Letting Go.* New York: Random House, 1962.

[25] Bruce, H. M. A block to pregnancy in the mouse caused by the proximity of strange males. *Journal of Reproductive Fertility*, 1960, 1, 96.

[26] Eleftheriou, B., Bronson, F. H., and Zarrow, M. X. Interaction of olfactory and other environmental stimuli on implantation in the deer mouse. *Science*, 1962, 137, 764.

[27] Lewis, M. M. *How Children Learn to Speak.* New York: Basic Books, 1959.

[28] Bexton, W. H., Heron, W., and Scott, T. H. Effects of decreased variation in the sensory environment. *Canadian Journal of Psychology*, 1954, 8, 70–76.

[29] Witkin, H. A., and associates. *Personality through Perception.* New York: Harper, 1954.

[30] Dumas, G. *Traité de Psychologie.* Paris: Alcan, 1923.

[31] Walk, R. D., and Gibson, E. J. A comparative and analytical study of visual depth perception. *Psychological Monographs*, 1961, 75, no. 15.

[32] Bower, T. G. R. Stimulus variables determining space perception in infants. *Science*, 1965, 149, 88–89.

[33] Levy, D. M. The infant's earliest memory of inoculation: A contribution to public health procedures. *Journal of Genetic Psychology*, 1960, 96, 3–46.

[34] Baltimore City Public Schools. *An Early School Admission Project: Progress Report 1963–64.* Baltimore: Baltimore City Public Schools, 1964.

[35] Church, *op. cit.*, pp. 42–43.

[36] Cohen, W. Spatial and textural characteristics of the *Ganzfeld*. *American Journal of Psychology*, 1957, 70, 403–410.

[37] Stolz, L. M. Youth: The Gesell Institute and its latest study. *Contemporary Psychology*, 1958, 3, 10–15.

[38] Hunter, W. S. The delayed reaction in animals and children. *Behavior Monographs*, 1913, 2, no. 1.

[39] Piaget, J. *The Construction of Reality in the Child.* New York: Basic Books, 1954, p. 352. One of the most careful studies of the development of perception in infancy.

[40] Held, R., and Hein, A. Movement-produced stimulation in the development of visually-guided behavior. *Journal of Comparative and Physiological Psychology*, 1963, 56, 872–876.

[41] Kohler, I. *On the Structuring and Transformation of the Perceptual World.* New York: International Universities, 1964.

[42] Smith, S. M., Brown, H. O., Toman, J. E. P., and Goodman, L. S. The lack of cerebral effects of D–Tubocurarine. *Anesthesiology*, 1947, 8, 1–14.

References

[43] Dennis, W., and Najarian, P. Infant development under environmental handicap. *Psychological Monographs,* 1957, 71, no. 7.

[44] Hayes, C. *The Ape in Our House.* New York: Harper, 1951.

[45] Schiff, W. Perception of impending collision. *Psychological Monographs,* 1965, 79, no. 11.

[46] Comalli, P. E., Wapner, S. and Werner, H. Interference effects of Stroop color-word test in children, adults, and aged. Paper read at meetings of Eastern Psychological Association, 1960.

[47] Davis, R. C., Buchwald, A. M., and Frankman, R. W. Autonomic and muscular responses, and their relation to simple stimuli. *Psychological Monographs,* 1955, 69, no. 405; Davis, R. C., Garafalo, L., and Kveim, K. Conditions associated with gastrointestinal activity. *Journal of Comparative and Physiological Psychology,* 1959, 52, 466–475; Lacey, J. I. The evaluation of autonomic responses: Toward a general solution. *Annals of the New York Academy of Sciences,* 1956, 67, art. 5, 123–164.

[48] Church, *op. cit.,* p. 213.

[49] Birch, H. G., and Lefford, A. Intersensory development in children. *Monographs of the Society for Research in Child Development,* 1963, 28, no. 5; Blank, M., and Bridger, W. H. Cross-modal transfer in nursery-school children. *Journal of Comparative and Physiological Psychology,* 1964, 58, 277–282; Caviness, J. A., and Gibson, J. J. The equivalence of visual and tactual stimulation for the perception of solid forms. Paper read at meetings of Eastern Psychological Association, 1962; Lobb, H. Vision *versus* touch in form discrimination. *Canadian Journal of Psychology,* 1965, 19, 175–187.

[50] Bower, T. G. R. Slant perception and shape constancy in infants. *Science,* 1966, 151, 832–834.

[51] Lynd, H. M. Some questions raised by experiences of shame. Paper read at meetings of the American Psychological Association, 1966.

3 *The Infant: 2*

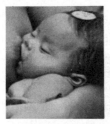

So far, we have talked about the infant's development almost as though it took place in a vacuum. In this chapter, we shall shift our focus from the baby himself to the environmental context in which he develops and in which we shall also see him after infancy. For it must be remembered that the baby is always potentially a great many different people, and which of these he becomes depends on the context in which he develops.

As in prenatal development, there are many levels of relevant context. There is the natural world of earth and vegetation and atmosphere and animal life, all linked together in cyclical exchanges of water, oxygen, nitrogen, carbon dioxide, and so forth, which make life possible. The baby, as a living organism, is part of the symbiotic whole, just as he is subject to the law of gravity and can survive only within a narrow range of atmospheric pressures. Within the natural environment there is the man-made environment of rush-mat huts and perpetual smoky fires of dung-cakes and of farms and cities and highways and vehicles and cribs and plumbing and television sets, and also institutions and ideas and knowledge and works of art, and all the more or less codified personal, economic, and political arrangements which tie societies together—often, to be sure, in antihuman ways.

The larger society does not at first act on the baby directly, but insofar as it affects his parents, it can, through them, influence his development. For we must stress that parents, much as they would like to, cannot wholly regulate their baby's development. Even if we knew all the answers to how to proceed in every individual instance, and even if parents could always act according to plan and not on impulse and emotion, there would still exist the incalculables of natural disasters, epidemics, wars, economic crises, accidents, bereavements, whatever can shape a family and thus its children. For the most conspicuous level of environment for the baby is that of the persons in his family and the interactions that go on among them. At first, exchanges between parents and baby are more the doing of the parents than the baby, although he can be a potent stimulus to parental action and can provide a good deal of feedback through his cries or his smiles of contentment or gurgles of active enjoyment. It is out of these developing exchanges that the baby's general emotional orientation to the world begins to emerge.

The Foundations of Basic Trust

Erikson, whose thinking derives from Freud but who has modified the psychoanalytic scheme of psychosexual development (see pages 165–167) along cognitive lines, has proposed that infancy is the time in which the child learns—obviously, in some as yet unformulated way— whether the world is a good and satisfying place to live in or a source of pain, misery, frustration, and uncertainty. These contrasting orientations are designated as *basic trust* and *basic mistrust,* corresponding closely to everyday notions of optimism and pessimism. The baby has physical needs, for nourishment, cleansing, sleep, warmth, and so forth. Equally important, he has psychological needs, for response, for contact, cuddling, rocking, talk, play and playthings, and the various ways affection shows itself. It is the satisfaction of his needs that gives the baby a sense of the world as a good, stable, pleasant, and, ultimately, manageable place to be—in sum, basic trust. When his needs are not met, or are incompletely met, the world takes on, to various degrees, a dominant cast of threat and frustration—in other words, he develops basic mistrust. Observe that the way parents meet needs can produce either a benign or vicious circle. The baby whose needs are met becomes a satisfying baby who calls forth an ever-growing abundance of love and attention; the baby whose needs are not met becomes irritable, demanding, and ever less lovable. An attitude of basic trust permits the development of variegated emotional responding across a full range from pleasant to unpleasant, whereas serious basic mistrust keeps emotional response in the limited range from distress to dull apathy. And out of variegated emotional functioning we would expect the growth of openness to experience and of the ability to master reality.

Note that meeting needs, especially as the baby grows older, does not always mean giving the baby what he wants. A reasonable amount of delay in giving the baby a feeding or in picking him up after sleep is not going to damage him, even if he acts as though the world were coming to an end. It is when gratification is too long and too consistently delayed that panic sets in. The baby has no time perspective, the crisis seems to him to drag on interminably, he is helpless to do anything about it, and a tiny seed of distrust has been planted.

Eventually, of course, he is attended to. His panic subsides, but it leaves a residue of fear and distrust. It is not only the factual meeting of needs that counts, but the quality of the attention given to the baby. If parents are grudging, if they are hostile or impatient, their movements may be rough and jerky and abrupt. If they feel anxious, their movements may be hesitant, fumbling, and erratic. Handling which lacks the definite, tenderly firm quality of a self-assured, loving parent seems to disorient and frighten a baby. The baby needs handling that expresses love and confidence. With it, he can tolerate a fair amount of normal hardship. Obviously, new parents need some practice before they can operate smoothly with their infant, and what we have said should not be interpreted to mean that there is no room for mistakes. There is bound to be some clumsiness, but within a total context of love and good will and sensitivity, initial clumsiness is of no great consequence.

Some of the things that are good for the baby hurt, like immunizing injections, and self-confident parents have to be ready to hold a squalling baby immobile while the needle goes in. Since the baby is not always a good judge of what is safe or unsafe, parents have to impose limits on his behavior. They have to help the baby sleep through the night and—gradually—to eat on a schedule approximating their own. Since an attitude of absolute trust toward a sometimes treacherous world would probably not be desirable, even if it were attainable, it may be just as well that life contains some built-in irritations and frustrations to temper a baby's basic trust, even in a benign, nurturing setting. A favorable emotional climate is not bland but temperate, with storms and seasons and rain and sunshine, mirroring family circumstances.

We should also make clear that there is no one way to love a baby. Babies are individuals and need different amounts and kinds of affection. Parents, too, are individuals and have different ways of expressing their affection. Some parents are lavish with physical demonstrations of their feelings; others are not, but still manage to convey them. Some parents are soft and tender, some are bluff and hearty, some are sober, some ironic. Furthermore, nobody can love his baby equally at all times and in all circumstances. Babies are sometimes cranky and sometimes exasperating. They can destroy the parents' sleep or a favorite treasure. What is important in terms of the baby's sense of trust is the reliability of his parents' love, the clarity with which it shows through transitory vicissitudes, through the inevitable strains and anxieties.

The evidence for the importance of early parent-child relations for basic trust as a secure foundation for later development comes from several kinds of sources. One fairly ancient tradition, drawn forcefully to our attention by such modern-day workers as Bowlby, Goldfarb, Ribble, and Spitz,[1] and well exemplified by a recent study by Provence and Lipton,[2] compares babies reared in institutions with babies raised normally in their families. In general, rearing in institutions seems to have serious consequences for later emotional and intellectual development. Here we must pause to specify that we mean institutionlike institutions, not those few that seek to approximate family living conditions. Among the consequences pointed to by various observers are inconsolable distress which finally fades into blunted responsiveness, perceptual retardation, as in White's studies[3] of visually-guided grasping, motor retardation and linguistic impairment, as in Dennis's studies,[4] increased susceptibility to infection, repetitive rocking and more bizarre and ritualistic mannerisms, impaired learning ability, and general apathy. Notice that the people who work in institutions are often not aware that anything is wrong: their charges are seen as "good" babies, quiet and undemanding and, at later ages, polite and easily managed. Salimbene gives an account of a thirteenth-century experiment by Frederick II, in which babies were deliberately subjected to institutionlike experiences, and its unforeseen results:

> . . . He wanted to find out what kind of speech and what manner of speech children would have when they grew up if they spoke to no one beforehand. So he bade foster mothers and nurses to suckle the children, to bathe and wash them, but in no way to prattle with them, or to speak to them, for he wanted to learn whether they would speak the Hebrew language, which was the oldest, or Greek, or Latin, or Arabic, or perhaps the language of their parents, of whom they had been born. But he laboured in vain because the children all died. For they could not live without the petting and joyful faces and loving words of their foster mothers. And so the songs are called

"swaddling songs" which a woman sings while she is rocking the cradle, to put a child to sleep, and without them a child sleeps badly and has no rest.[5]

Now it is obvious that not all institution children die, though they are more likely to than family-reared ones, and we do not even know what proportion of them find their way into mental hospitals, but it is clear that, on the average, children raised in the barren, unstimulating setting of an orphanage are in various degrees psychologically stunted and deformed.

Some of our evidence comes from studies of infrahuman species, where actual experiments can be conducted so that we are not limited, as in the study of human babies, to capitalizing on social accidents for knowledge. We have already mentioned Harlow's experiments[6] in which baby rhesus monkeys were "reared" by either a roughly monkey-sized and -shaped dummy covered with soft, cuddlesome terrycloth and warmed from within by a light bulb, or by a similar surrogate whose wire mesh frame was left uncovered. Those monkeys who had a choice of surrogates formed much stronger attachments to the terrycloth one which provided "contact comfort," even when it was always the bare wire frame mother which provided milk. This finding indicates that the baby's attachment to the mother is not based solely on her satisfying his hunger needs (although Igel and Calvin,[7] in a similar study with puppies, found that both contact comfort and nursing were important). Monkeys reared with terrycloth surrogates, as compared to those reared with wire mothers, showed much greater emotional security and curiosity. After a year's separation from the terrycloth mother, the young monkey reintroduced to her bolts to her, embraces her, and clings passionately. Unfortunately, as we have said, the love and security gained from the terrycloth surrogate are not a sufficient condition for normal monkey development, and Harlow's animals grew up neurotic and sexually inadequate.

A whole series of papers out of Denenberg's Purdue laboratory[8] bears on the importance of early mother-child relations in animal development, including the fascinating finding that male mice reared by white-rat mothers with white-rat peers never fought with other male mice, whereas all of those reared by mouse mothers but without age-mates fought when paired with another male.

We cannot mention all the illuminating findings from the field of animal development, but they all seem to point to the fact that manipulations of early experience can have profound effects on physiology, temperament, sexuality, intelligence, and just about every other kind of function that has been investigated. A classic study by Forgays and Forgays[9] shows that rats brought up in an enriched environment of other young rats, mazes, ramps, exercise wheels, swings—the best analogy is a white-rat nursery school—are brighter than rats reared in ordinary bare laboratory cages. This kind of study has been extended by C. J. Smith,[10] who found that rats raised in an enriched environment showed specialized functioning of brain tissue, while rats reared in an unstimulating

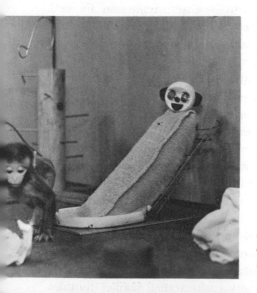

(Left) A Rhesus infant explores a strange environment secure in the presence of his surrogate "mother."
Harry F. Harlow

(Bottom left) Separated from his "mother" in a strange setting the infant Rhesus huddles in fear.
Harry F. Harlow

(Bottom right) Typical "choo-choo" position assumed by Rhesus monkeys reared in a group without a mother figure.
Harry F. Harlow

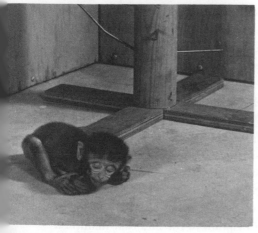

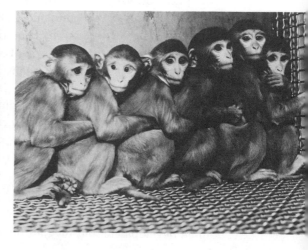

cage environment did not, and by Bennett, Diamond, Krech, and Rosenzweig,[11] who find differences in brain biochemistry associated with rearing conditions. Thompson[12] was among the first to show that "gentling," daily human handling by the human experimenter, affected the animal's emotional development—the age of the animal and the character of the gentling seem to determine whether the animal is made more or less fearful. Levine[13] has shown that stress to the mother during pregnancy (as by electric shock or immersion in cold water), or to the young animal, increases adrenal size and activity and can affect body weight. Schneirla and associates[14] have demonstrated estrangement in young kittens removed temporarily from the litter, Scott and Fuller[15] have shown impaired social relations (to human beings as well as other dogs) in dogs reared in isolation, and Ader[16] has shown that rats weaned early are more susceptible to gastric ulcers than rats weaned later.

Sometimes the significant manipulations are unintentional, and such investigators as Denenberg and Whimbey,[17] and Hatch, Balazs, Wiberg, and Grice[18] have shown that extra-experimental animal husbandry practices, including such seemingly innocuous things as how often one changes the shavings in the cage, can affect development. An important implication of these findings is that rats raised in typical laboratory conditions are in many cases sick or feeble-minded animals, which has a bearing on how we interpret medical and psychological research done with such animals.

On the borderline between animal and human development, let us say only in passing that accounts of so-called feral children, described as having identified with wild animal foster parents, seem all to be either fraudulent or erroneous, so the reader is warned to treat skeptically tales about "wolf boys" and "antelope girls."[19] On the other hand, there have been a number of well-authenticated cases of "closet children," brought up with virtually no contact with the world outside the space in which they were confined, and the severe physical and psychological deficits they showed.[20]

A third set of findings on the importance of early parent-child relations, with implications for the formation of basic trust, comes from studies which seek to relate specific child care practices, such as ways of managing feeding or toilet training or discipline, to particular personality traits at later ages. As a recent review by Caldwell[21] shows, our faith in this approach to studying later development has been largely disappointed and it should probably be abandoned. This is not to say that such practices have no effect. We know from animal studies that maternal temperament has a powerful impact on the young, but we know nothing of the significant specifics of child care. It may be the total quality of parental behavior, expressed, as we have said, in such things as smooth and assured or nervous and erratic or angry and impatient handling, in tones of voice, in amount of talking and play, that makes the most difference.[22] In general, it is very hard to study antecedent-consequent relations in human development simply because so many things impinge on the total process, even if we could be sure we were getting accurate information about child-rearing attitudes and practices, which some studies suggest we cannot.[23]

Schaefer,[24] among others, has tried to capture some of the global aspects of child-rearing in what is called a "circumplex model." In Schaefer's scheme, the mother's behavior toward the child is scored along the two intersecting dimensions of control-autonomy and love-hostility. The crossing of these two dimensions at their midpoints forms four quadrants in which are located such general orientations as "democratic" and "cooperative" in the high autonomy-high love sector; "overindulgent" in the high love-medium control region; "dictatorial" and "demanding" in the high control-high hostility zone; and "neglectful" and "indifferent" in the high hostility-high autonomy quadrant.

This is an ingenious and useful scheme, but it does not go far enough. It leaves out of account such other dimensions and considerations as cognitive stimulation, opportunities and encouragements to explore space, objects and their qualities of taste and texture and pliability and weight and shape, and the relations among objects, the way they come apart and fit together and move and act on each other, and the sensations that arise inside the baby's own body. It omits the way parents convey values to babies, telling by their own behavior what is wicked or virtuous, beautiful or ugly, important or unimportant, nasty or nice, and all the other qualities that give meaning to life. Perhaps the chief lack, though, is that it puts the full onus of responsibility on the mother. This is in line with most people's thinking, as though the mother deserves all the credit when her children turn out well, and all the blame when they come to a bad end. This view leaves out of account the role of the father, both directly, in his dealings with the child, and indirectly, in his sharing of the common family enterprise, in the support—or lack of support—that he gives the mother. It ignores family circumstances that may affect maternal behavior, such things as financial problems, illness, competing demands from other children, or the fact that nobody has ever told the father and mother anything about how to take care of babies, or the

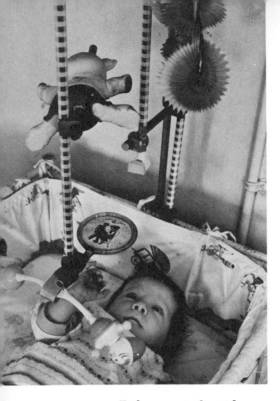

Early perceptual enrichment.
Leonard McCombe, LIFE Magazine © Time Inc.

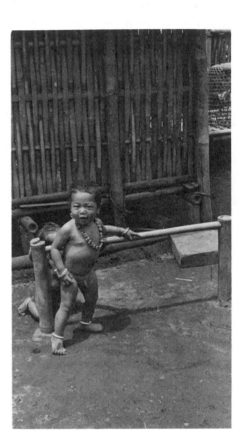

A Balinese walking-rail, which orients the baby away from the world at large.
Gregory Bateson and Margaret Mead, *Balinese Character*

presence or absence of in-laws who may be helpful or harassing. Finally, it leaves the baby a cipher in the family equation.

We cannot safely forget the ways babies vary in tempo and temperament, in activity level and responsiveness, and how such variations affect the way they are perceived by parents. Just whether the baby is a girl or a boy can affect parental attitudes. Babies vary in physical attractiveness, too. It is not enough to say that there are some babies only a mother could love. There are some babies who, for whatever reason, do not call forth love in their own particular mothers. Apart from characteristics of the baby, the mother herself may have reasons of her own for not responding. She may be so immersed in other concerns that she is insensitive to whatever charms the baby may have. The baby may remind

114

her too vividly of her own carnal nature, he may have come at the wrong time in her marriage, he may look like a hated adult of her childhood, or he may symbolize the end of carefree youth and of beauty. And such influences may be powerful without ever coming clearly into awareness.

The lack of conditions necessary to basic trust and normal affective and intellectual development has been summed up in the term "maternal deprivation." In fact, as we can see, a great many kinds of deprivation may be involved besides those that go with normal, loving maternal care and stimulation. The baby may be deprived of sensory stimulation in general, like adult subjects who are experimentally shut off from the customary—if unnoticed—barrage of sights, sounds, kinesthetic and skin stimulation, and the information these bring. Most adult subjects in conditions of extreme sensory deprivation disintegrate psychologically. We would assume that deprived babies, whether in institutions or simply neglected at home, would also lack the necessary shower of stimulation and so would have no opportunity to develop those awarenesses and competences that we take for granted as part of babyhood. But even those babies who are given abundant social and emotional stimulation may be denied opportunities to explore the material world and to acquire ways of symbolizing experience. These children suffer what we might call cognitive deprivation. We shall return to this topic throughout the book, since it seems crucial to fully human development.

Some authors draw a distinction between what we may label deprivation and privation. The latter refers to the absence from the beginning of a relevant kind of stimulation, the former to taking away from the baby something that was previously present, as when he is separated from his family after several months during which he formed an attachment. We would expect that privation would result in retarded development and deprivation in disturbed, pathological development, as seems to be indicated by studies of babies separated from their mothers.[25] The English language makes it hard to maintain this distinction, since we have a verb form, *deprive,* corresponding to deprivation, but none for privation.

We have been talking about things that might be missing from the lives of babies who could belong to parents of great good will, but we must also mention that some parents at some times are not parents of good will, and pediatricians and emergency ward doctors know the syndrome of the "battered child."[26] Statistics are hard to keep and compare, but it is clear that a lot of brutality gets practiced on children, including neonates and infants. The known cases of such brutality in the

United States are increasing, perhaps because many states have recently adopted legislation requiring doctors to report them and freeing them of legal liability in doing so. It seems reasonable to assume that most people who practice brutality on children are seriously disturbed or are persons under unbearable pressures and tensions, for whom the cries of a hungry or sick or lonely baby are the last nerve-shattering turn of the screw, and the chances are that such people didn't really want the baby in the first place. In some cases, however, child-beating expresses a stark and cold-blooded moralism which seeks to purify the baby of its supposed selfishness and perversity. It is also clear that many people who beat babies to the point of injury or death could, in more favorable circumstances, cherish and care for those same babies most adequately. Such extremes, however, should not be allowed to distract us from the fact that most parents convey, and most babies learn, an orientation of basic trust.

Trends in Child Care

People have been giving and receiving advice on how to rear children at least from Biblical times, as witness the injunction to "Spare the rod and spoil the child." Until relatively recently, though, people have simply known and taken for granted, on the basis of tradition, what should be done to and for children. Let us make clear that these givens of folk-wisdom were by no means the same from one society to the next, or even in different segments of complex societies, but each group had its own tradition-sanctioned ways. Obviously, these ways had enough validity to keep the species going, but the historical record of human folly, depravity, pettiness, and cruelty gives us reason to think that improvements can be made.

In stable societies, where relatives are likely to live close together and to act collaboratively as an extended family, there are abundant opportunities to observe and absorb the accustomed practices of the society. In modern European societies, and most particularly in the United States since the end of World War I, where there is a great deal of economic and geographical mobility, and where each generation is supposed to outgrow the stupidities of the one before, families fragment and there is limited occasion to transmit and acquire (or even to find consensus on) the culturally accepted ways of dealing with children—or of doing many other things besides. Increasingly, it is assumed that one learns personal and social functions and skills and values from schools and books and newspaper columns and magazines addressed to special groups—women or teen-agers—in sum, from the Expert. This despite the fact that American anti-intellectualism simultaneously contains a strand of contempt for the expert—the farmer once sneered at the agronomist, the office worker at the efficiency expert and, more recently, the automation expert, the business man at the economist or organizations theorist, and, above all, the parent and grandparent at the child psychologist or psychiatrist. In the folklore, it was assumed that the child care expert was a bachelor or old maid who would disintegrate if saddled with the actual responsibilities of looking after a child. Nevertheless, advice to parents has long been a readily marketable commodity and is supplied in never-abating plenty—along with the latest gadgets—to an insatiably avid public.

The apparent conflict between disdain for the expert and a servile seeking for his counsel may perhaps be reconciled by noting two things. First, parents are truly uncertain of themselves and badly want guidance. Second, they seem to seek out and listen to those experts, or those parts of a given expert's preachments, that best suit their own opinions. That is, they are looking for confirmation for what they already do, rather than for new ways of doing things. David Levy[27] has discussed how mothers both fail to comprehend pediatricians' recommendations and, in addition, act only on so much of what they comprehend as suits their own ideas. Even when they try, people are likely to grasp unfamiliar notions in a distorted way, and the authors, when cast in the roles of experts and teachers, have seen their own ideas come back to them in some very strange guises indeed.

Mothers were told in a 1912 treatise[28] that babies should not be breast-fed if the mother has hysteria or epilepsy, that worry, anxiety, and nervous excitement poison the mother's milk (they may indeed interfere with lactation), that constipation in the nursing mother produced constipation in the baby, that breast milk was exhausted after about seven months (apparently this expert had never heard of the societies in which children are nursed up to age three or four years), that pacifiers produced "great harm" as well as disease, that if one started toilet training at age six weeks one might reasonably hope that the job would be completed, with "much patience and perseverance," by age eighteen months (it apparently didn't occur to anyone then, despite what actual experience might have taught them, that one might start toilet training at age seventeen months and finish the job thirty days later). Between ages one and two years the baby's diet was to consist of fruit, fluids, toast, soup, and gruel. No meat could be given before age two, after which, up to age three, the child might have some scraped beef or white meat of chicken.

If these prescriptions sound slightly unreal today, when babies are given synthetic formula at below room temperature from a disposable bottle, when baby foods are given from early infancy and by age ten months the American baby is gnawing beef from a bone or eating chicken livers and rice or chunks of cheddar cheese, probably some of our current beliefs will seem fully as antiquated in another few years. For this reason, the reader is asked always to exercise a proper skepticism. It is also worth emphasizing that in 1912 only about 80 per cent of babies born alive lived to see their first birthday; that there were not at that time techniques and widespread centers for immunization against whooping cough, diphtheria, poliomyelitis, measles, and the like; there were no antibiotics; and sanitary conditions were far more primitive than they are today, all of which justified a preoccupation with physical health.

One can follow the shifting currents of expert advice on child care, along with changes in underlying values, in successive editions of the United States Government manual *Infant Care*,[29] first published in 1914. (Martha Wolfenstein,[30] who has traced these changes, has summarized them as the "emergence of fun morality," whereby it is—or was in the 1950's—not only all right to have a good time, but morally obligatory.) The early editions are in keeping with the spirit of John B. Watson, the father of behaviorist psychology in the United States. Behaviorism sought to place psychology on a secure scientific footing by eliminating from consideration all such elusive subjective states as motives, will, urges, cravings, ideas, intentions, aspirations, and the like, and by confining study to the directly observable and measurable behavior of the organism. In this view, all behavior is externally determined (or at least triggered) by unconditioned and conditioned stimuli, and stable, recurring behavior patterns are seen as habits. Thus, the main goal in this framework of child-rearing is to instill the proper habits and to avoid teaching undesirable ones. The flavor of Watson's thinking is given in the following widely quoted passage:

> There is a sensible way of treating children. Treat them as though they were young adults. Dress them, bathe them with care and circumspection. Let your behavior always be objective and kindly firm. Never hug and kiss them, never let them sit in your lap. If you must, kiss them once on the forehead when they say good night. Shake hands with them in the morning. Give them a pat on the head if they have made an extraordinarily good job of a difficult task. Try it out.

In a week's time you will find how easy it is to be perfectly objective with your child and at the same time kindly. You will be utterly ashamed of the mawkish, sentimental way you have been handling it.[31]

Oddly enough, though, this streamlined mechanistic view managed to incorporate a Victorian or even medieval moralism according to which the baby was a greedy, scheming, power-mad creature in whom filthy, bestial habits could and would crop up without warning if the parent did not Nip it in the Bud and turned maudlin and indulgent. Something of the rigor of the habit-training way of thinking is given in this quotation from the 1938 edition of *Infant Care*, by which time the habits approach was already coming to be regarded by many people as obsolete:

> . . . Immediately after birth he will begin to form habits, which if they are the right kind will be useful to him all his life. Regularity from birth on is of first importance.
> Through training in regularity of feeding, sleeping, and elimination . . . the tiny baby will receive his first lessons in character building. He should learn that hunger will be satisfied only so often, that when he is put into his bed he must go to sleep, that crying will not result in his being picked up or played with whenever he likes. He will begin to learn that he is part of a world bigger than that of his own desires.[32]

It is not simply that love and affection were left unemphasized, they were regarded by Watson and like-minded thinkers as downright insidious, as Watson indicates:

> In conclusion won't you then remember when you are tempted to pet your child that mother love is a dangerous instrument? An instrument which may inflict a never healing wound, a wound which may make infancy unhappy, adolescence a nightmare, an instrument which may wreck your adult son or daughter's vocational future and their chances for marital happiness.[33]

While Watson was properly modest in his claims for the efficacy of his procedures, he saw as the outcome ". . . a child as free as possible of sensitivities to people and one who, almost from birth, is relatively independent of the family situation."[34] One is tempted to infer that Watson himself had been deeply hurt in his interpersonal relations and proposed this almost psychopathic style of life as a defense against pain.

In the next chapter, we shall describe in some detail various theoretical orientations to behavior and development. Here we must mention them insofar as they played a part in the advice on child-rearing given to parents. Sigmund Freud was an influential figure who, although he came into prominence in avant-garde psychiatric and literary circles before Watson, became a competing force in American child psychology only in the 1920's. Freudian doctrines underwent a subtle sea change in traveling from Europe to the United States. Freud had a pessimistic, Victorian, moralistic outlook and saw man fated by his animal nature to live in lust and violence until the slow process of social evolution would remake him into a truly human being. Americans misinterpreted Freud's emphasis on animality (perhaps in the context of Darwinian doctrine) as an endorsement, and libertarians rallied round the Freudian banner in opposition to the supposed puritanism of Watson's behaviorism. In the American version of Freud's teachings, man is made neurotic by the arbitrary, artificial restraints imposed by society on the free expression of impulse, and the secret of successful child-rearing as popularized in the 1930's and 1940's was to avoid frustrating and inhibiting the child. Aggression was seen as the product of frustration, and not, as in Freud's own later version, as internally motivated by a death-wish or drive to destruction. What seems to have happened is that Freudian psychology thrived in the United States when grafted onto the thinking of anthropologists like Ruth Benedict and Margaret Mead, who stressed the crucial role of the social and cultural environment for the formation of character. The merger of anthropology and psychoanalysis is most clearly seen in the writings of such authors as Erik H. Erikson, Erich Fromm, and Karen Horney, who have been much more sociological and environmentalistic in their views than traditional Freudians. Sometimes, though, the anthropological view of human nature has been anticultural and has taken the form of Romantic Naturalism, first set forth by Jean-Jacques Rousseau and happily embraced by some of the less discriminating progressive educators, which says that the ideal condition for man is that of the happy, noble savage living in a state of nature. This view is strongly implicit in some of the writings of Ashley Montagu and also in the nonanthropological works of Arnold Gesell and his collaborators. The Romantic-Naturalist child contains in himself the seeds of successful development, and to impose the outworn moralities and ideologies of a decadent society is to threaten the child's well-being at its very core. Notice that Gesell and Montagu owe much less to Freud than do the anthropologically oriented psychoanalysts and the psychoanalytically oriented anthropologists, but their prescriptions for child-rearing are very similar.

One other strand that should be mentioned is John Dewey's pragmatism, which merely said that much of what we teach children is obsolete and of no earthly use to them, but which got interpreted by some people to mean that we should teach children only practical skills, as in Life Adjustment courses or in vocational education. Dewey was not particularly concerned with infancy, but his teachings were very much in the air in the 1920's and 1930's.

B. F. Skinner,[35] about whose thinking we shall have more to say in the next chapter and who describes himself as a radical neo-behaviorist, proposes in his Utopian novel *Walden Two* another ideal system of child-rearing based on several assumptions. First of all, human behavior is thought of as shaped by forces lying outside the organism, either in stimuli present at the time of behavior or else in its past history. Notions of self-control, self-determination, will, and purpose are delusions with which people needlessly torment themselves. One behaves as one does because initially random acts set off by need states are selectively reinforced (rewarded) in terms of whether they serve to reduce the need. Eventually, the organism learns which instrumental acts (called by Skinner *operants*) work in which circumstances, and behavior becomes orderly, effective, and to all appearances sensible. To find happiness, one should surrender control to a scientifically engineered society in which child-rearing according to the principles of operant conditioning will insure cooperative, industrious, conflict-free, and ideology-free individuals who will while away their leisure hours with art and music and suchlike creative endeavors. Children are taught by being rewarded for socially useful behavior, whereas aberrant behavior receives no response of any kind and so withers away for lack of external reinforcement. (Internal reinforcement or token reinforcement works only after learning has taken place with real reinforcers.) Punishment should not be used, because it inhibits only the overt act, not the tendency to perform that act, which tendency is perpetuated by the reinforcing effect of punishment. Children are taught to work for delayed reinforcement, and thus to tolerate inevitable frustrations and delays, by gradually stretching out the interval between operant act and reward. Like many Utopia-makers, Skinner paints a coolly rational or rationalistic world without guts, without strong passions, without illness or grief or jealousy, without responsibility or the need to make decisions. One would gather that sexuality in the Walden Two colony is a bloodless coupling for purposes (in Skinner's system, societies are allowed to have purposes, even if individuals are not) of carefully programmed reproduction, and such humor as is practiced is of a dry, cerebral, pedantic sort.

More than a few people find Skinner's vision appealing, to the point of wanting to found Walden Twos of their own (one obscure news item seems to imply that a California group plans to combine Walden Two living, predicated on and consecrated to the concept of the mindless person, with the use of consciousness-expanding drugs). It is a pity, therefore, to have to express the conviction that the bland bliss of Walden Two is probably unattainable. It is almost certainly unattainable by Skinner's means, since his principles of learning, while highly useful and correct for application to a narrow range of conditions, are inadequate and irrelevant for much of the important learning that goes on in life. Chomsky[36] has pointed out, for instance, that if one had to learn language according to Skinner's rules, a whole lifetime might go by before one acquired the simplest rudiments. Solomon's studies[37] on the effects of punishment yield results contrary to what Skinner would predict, and so on down the line. This is not to discourage people from seeking the Nirvana of Walden Two, but to apprise them that they may meet difficulties.

Skinner's system apart, by the late 1940's doctrinaire approaches to child-rearing were almost a thing of the past, and the needs-centered, down-to-earth, humane eclecticism of Benjamin Spock (a psychoanalytically trained but pragmatic pediatrician and psychiatrist) had swept the field. Spock's frequent injunction to "Enjoy your baby!" may smack of the fun morality we mentioned earlier, but it certainly makes a lot better sense than what has been dubbed "self-conscious parenthood," which smacks of drudgery and fear and indecision. For as various doctrines of development have threatened all sorts of dire consequences stemming from unfortunate infantile experiences, and as traditional ways have slipped out of the twentieth-century grasp, many parents have become unable to act without endless soul-searching and worrying about what later effects this or that way of acting will have. In general, parents who have a certain amount of confidence in themselves and in their babies operate every bit as well by intuition as the self-conscious parent who holds the baby with one hand, delaying a decision while the forefinger of the other hand runs through the index in Dr. Authoritative's *Manual of Expert Child Care.*

It comes as a surprise to many parents to realize that, if they know in general what to expect of a baby at different ages and what his needs and capabilities are, the baby pretty well instructs them what to do if they will only learn to read his "language of behavior." He will not automatically be "spoiled" by the attempt to understand him; automatic indulgence and unswerving habit-training are far greater dangers.

This language takes two forms. First, there is the expressive quality of the manifestations of the baby's distress. From a very early age, the baby's cries of hunger, fatigue, anger, pain, and so forth, are fairly easy to tell apart. Sometimes there are postural cues. For instance, it is sometimes hard to tell whether the baby's cries signify hunger or colic, but the baby tends to stretch out and arch his back when hungry, and to double up in the throes of colic. The second form of the language of behavior is the feedback a parent receives from the baby when trying to meet its needs. If the parent tries to feed a colicky baby, the baby may indeed try briefly to nurse, but after a few swallows will spit out the nipple and resume crying, indicating that the adult has not yet singled out the right need and its remedy. Of course, it is not merely the turning off of crying that guides parental behavior, but also the baby's smiles and gurgles of satisfaction.

By late infancy, the baby can make dialogues with his parents more nearly explicit. By reaching out his arms and straining in the general direction of something he wants, usually to the accompaniment of shrieks or murmurs, he can convey that he wants something and where the adult should look for it. Characteristically, the adult offers the baby likely objects; wrong guesses are met by brief, angry shrieks; when the right object is offered, the baby accepts it with a grunt of satisfaction. We have already spoken of how the baby becomes able to initiate social games. At a still more advanced, but still prelinguistic, stage, the baby can communicate with tokens. If he tries to climb into his feeding table, it signifies that he is hungry; he may bring a phonograph record that he wants to hear played; he brings his coat or sweater as a way of saying that he wants to go out. Notice the analogy here with the dog who brings his dish to announce his hunger, or his leash to request a walk, or a stick to be thrown and retrieved. Even the mooing of the cows as they crowd around the pasture gate at dusk tells us that they are ready to return to the barn for milking.

When we stop to think about it, we take it for granted that we can read the language of behavior of, for instance, cats, dogs, and horses, and respond appropriately, so it should hardly be surprising that the behavior of young human beings can make sense to us—especially since they have not yet learned our many devices for covering up our true feelings. In general, in all our roles as adult human beings we respond not only to the words people speak but to the total array of information they transmit in everything they do. We read their motives, pretensions, doubts, and hidden feelings in their gestures, posture, tone of voice, dress—in short, in their language of behavior—and we can in the same way take cues from the baby.

Issues in Infant Care

While the main aim of this book is descriptive rather than prescriptive—that is, it seeks to tell the reader what children are like and how they develop, rather than how to live with them or manage them or mold them—talking about practical applications should help clarify our particular way of looking at children. It is our conviction that a concern with practical questions keeps science alive and reality-bound, and even though we cannot claim omniscience, we can at least point out where some common practices are founded on fallacy. In addition, the discussion of practical problems is the best framework in which to present some further substantive facts of behavior and development.

ATTENTION, SPOILING, AND DISCIPLINE

Perhaps as a carry-over from the "habits" era, many parents still fear that they may give the baby too much attention, thereby spoiling him and giving him the upper hand in parent-child relations. And when it comes to discipline, the ambivalence of parents is enough to shake them in two. On the one hand, lack of discipline is thought to produce tyrannical, egotistical monsters with a whim of iron and a bulldozer approach to human relations. On the other hand, in keeping with the teachings of Romantic Naturalism, discipline will mar and embitter the child and teach him to be a cringing, obsequious authoritarian—and cause him to hate his parents, who seem to fear being found out by the analyst thirty years later.

When babies cry, it is because they need something, not that they (or we) always know what. Among the things they need is human attention, initially in great abundance. "Attention," after all, is nothing but the loving closeness and stimulation that we have been talking about. It is out of attention that powerful bonds grow up between adult and child, and it is these bonds that make later communication possible—including the communication involved in discipline. It is possible that some adults are put off by so intimate a relationship, even with a baby, or are afraid of the unfamiliar potency of the emotions that go with it, and it is for such reasons that they are reluctant to give the baby a full measure of "attention."

Usually, with the one exception of evening bedtime (once the baby has given evidence that he is ready to sleep the night through), spoiling does not seem to be an issue in infancy. Later in childhood, over-indulgence—particularly of an undiscriminating, buying-favor sort, un-related to the child's needs—can certainly have some untoward effects, but babies thrive on genuine attention and the handling, talking, singing, and all the rest, that go to make it up. As the baby becomes more secure about the solidity and reliability of his personal relations, he himself will be able to turn away from preoccupation with his parents and move into an active exploration of his nonhuman surroundings, returning from time to time to enjoy his parents' company on an ever more mature basis. It is a hangover of the habit-training view that sees the baby never stopping demanding what he is given now. If anything, the greatest danger at this age is probably the failure to satisfy the baby's cravings for attention, leading to an increased need which, like the neurotic needs of adults, becomes at the extreme insatiable. In other words, premature attempts to cultivate the baby's "powers of self-reliance" may have exactly the opposite effect.

In general, amply loved babies are not interested in getting the better of anybody. As we shall discuss later, our society teaches us two versions of human nature, and the one that many people seem to learn best is that human beings are innately selfish, competitive, and out to do in others before they get done in themselves. By the magic of the self-fulfilling prophecy, that is a kind of person our society produces in great plenty. However, there is nothing inherent in the baby that causes him to seek dominance over others. Basic trust works both ways, and parents have to have some faith in the baby. The self-fulfilling prophecy works both ways, too, and, as a rule, babies are loving, sympathetic, and generous in direct proportion to their having been treated lovingly, sympathetically, and generously—and in terms of their real needs. Hence, both Watson and Rousseau find justification—and contradiction. For there is a well-meaning but oversolicitous kind of mother who hurries to do something about every expression of discomfort before either the baby or mother has a chance to find out what, if anything, is really called for. Often she seems to be seeking the child's explicit gratitude for her maternal ministrations. In this way, the wrong need may get gratified, leaving the baby with a vague, restless dissatisfaction that may later come out as "spoiled" behavior. A similar pattern may originate in parental insecurity: The mother feels so inadequate, or is so afraid of losing the baby's love, or feels so guilty about a lack of genuine affection for him, that she gratifies his needs blindly. Spoiling may also result from capricious teasing, or consistent meetings of needs, leaving the child fearful that he may never get what he wants, and dissatisfied when he gets it. Teasing is usually described disapprovingly as what some other cultures do to babies, but it is only necessary to watch American parents and American visitors to see how much we enjoy getting a rise out of children of all ages, even though we are "only kidding."

Even if it is true that unstinting affection and need-gratification in infancy does produce a trusting, affectionate, essentially cooperative individual, parents tend to wonder, won't such an individual be so badly disqualified for life in our savagely competitive society that we will have done him a disservice? In answer, there is reason to think that warm-hearted people who are ready to like and trust other people need not always end up as victims. It is not usually the person who has developed self-respect who turns into a doormat or a punching-bag for others. There remains, besides, a question of values, of whether parents want their child to grow up pretty much like everybody else, even if they don't think very much of what everybody else is, or whether they want him to approach some ideal of the human condition, even at the risk of some strain and conflict with his surroundings. Conformity begins in infancy.

The bonds of trust and affection that grow out of attention and need-gratification greatly simplify problems of discipline in infancy. During the first year, discipline is largely a matter of keeping the child apart from things that might injure him or which he is likely to destroy. Infants have no sense of property, their own or other people's. They may develop fetishistic attachments to dolls and blankets, but their main concern with objects is having access to them so that they can explore them. The baby who has lots of opportunity to poke into things does not feel more than momentarily aggrieved when some things are forbidden to him. Nor does he cease loving the parents who remove forbidden objects from his grasp or tell him "No!" as he reaches for something that cannot be kept out of his grasp. In general, parents who love their baby and have their baby's welfare at heart need not fear losing the baby's love or doing him an injury by acting like strong adults. There is no doubt that child-rearing demands some self-sacrifice on the part of parents, but self-sacrifice has to be balanced by a decent respect for their own needs as adults.

FEEDING AND SCHEDULING

In other cultures, in the more ignorant and less expert-ridden areas of our own society, and even in middle-class American society fifty years ago, before the habit-formers proclaimed their doctrines of regularity, the usual practice was to feed babies when they were hungry, subject to the reservation that the mother's breast milk might not be ready at the time the baby grew hungry. In the past half century, middle-class society has been through a revolution and a counterrevolution, plus a few incidental upheavals. The habits approach, basing its dicta on some rather flimsy statistics purporting to show the average time it takes babies' stomachs to empty (not even the time the average baby's stomach takes to empty), called for a strict schedule, from the time the baby came home from the hospital, of feeding every four hours on the dot (some physicians prescribed three-hour intervals for very small or immature babies), whether the baby had been screaming with hunger for an hour past or was so sound asleep that he had to be jiggled and prodded awake. Beyond the daily timetable to which a mother was to adhere religiously, the authorities plotted out well in advance a calendar schedule telling when all babies were to be weaned and when introduced to which new foodstuffs.

Partly because the mechanistic rigidities of the habits approach went against the parental grain (although many parents went doggedly ahead applying the methods of "science," no matter what their own feelings might be, and others who departed from the Right Way felt guilty about their lack of character), and partly in response to the naturalistic teachings of the anthropologists, *demand feeding,* based on the parent's perceptions of when the baby is actually hungry, began to supersede scheduled feeding, both in what parents did and in what pediatricians prescribed. One of the discoveries that emerged is that demand feeding, with a very little assistance from parents, moves toward a stable schedule according to which the baby consumes more food at more widely spaced intervals until he comes into equilibrium with the accepted patterns of his culture. That is, social patterns set the cycle of hunger and satiety that are one component in his biological clock.

One incidental issue that has now been fairly well resolved in principle is the dispute between the breast-feeders and the bottle-feeders. We suspect that the evangelistic zeal of the bottle-feeders during the behaviorist era expressed a complex of attitudes. There may have been a conviction that bottle-feeding was sanitary, whereas breast-feeding was not. Bottle-feeding may have been one more means of taking parenthood away from parents and bringing it under medical control, and in many hospitals there were—and are—covert and open pressures by doctors or nurses to formula-feeding. A contributing value may have been that our society went through a period of machine-worship during which people dreamed of living in a world of pure reason uncluttered by the demands of biology. Women were to be liberated from the constant demands of motherhood and from the reminder of their animal and primitive natures. The Watsonian ethic would decry breast-feeding because it fostered the sentimentality and the mother love that were so dangerous to human welfare. Women themselves felt that breast-feeding tied them down, and they took to bottle-feeding to escape the fatigue and discomforts that go with breast-feeding and because of a conviction that breast-feeding would rob them of their figures, youth, beauty, and allure.

The breast-feeders, who, in this almost entirely bottle-fed nation, are nowadays the apostolic reformers, could invoke the argument of naturalness, plus the more practical ones of the superior nutritive value of human milk by comparison with cow's milk and the convenience of breast-feeding—no formula to be mixed, bottled, and stored, and no sterilization needed. Mother's milk is also thought to carry antibodies which enhance the baby's resistance to infection.[38] The psychiatrically and psychoanalytically oriented pressed the argument that breast-feeding gave mother and baby a chance to be alone together in close contact, where the mother could croon and whisper to the baby, and he, in turn, could stare at and learn to know his mother's face and feel close and warm and supported. But it is possible—and advisable—to give a bottle with exactly these same provisions, if the baby is held, rather than left in the bassinet or crib with a bottle propped next to his mouth. (One objection to leaving the baby with a bottle is that, unless his head is held slightly raised, there is danger that milk will enter the eustachian tubes and cause infection.) Finally, the irrefutable contention was advanced that, whatever breast-feeding meant for the baby, some mothers found in it a deeply pleasurable experience, taking satisfaction in the wholeness of their feminine biology.

It seems to us (and we believe we express a current consensus) that, for women living in good hygienic conditions, personal feelings are the only sensible criterion for deciding between breast and bottle. Where sanitation is unsatisfactory, or milk expensive or difficult to come by, breast-feeding is the only safe way to nourish a young baby, and the new popularity of bottle-feeding among women in technically less advanced societies has sometimes been ruinous for the health of their babies.

Another aspect of feeding is *weaning*, which refers both to the transition from breast or bottle to cup and to the transition from milk (or whatever milk substitutes are currently in vogue) to solids. The literature suggests that weaning too was once—and still is in some societies—a matter of bitter battles between mother and child, to the point where many American mothers felt it necessary to have the baby witness a ceremonial smashing of his bottles. Many cultures have special procedures for weaning: spreading bitter substances on the mother's nipples or, as in a number of African tribes, sending the baby on a long visit to grandmother. (We should say again that in many primitive societies weaning does not take place until age two or three or even four, and may be delayed as a crude contraceptive technique.)

Nowadays, in United States society, weaning seems to take place without trauma to mother or child, probably because modern pediatric practice makes the transition—both the presentation of the new and the withdrawal of the old—gradual and at first tentative, but beginning early, so that the baby comes to take it for granted that nourishment comes in a variety of flavors, textures, consistencies, temperatures, and containers. Due account is taken of the baby's readiness for change: his general emotional security, the absence of physical upsets (especially digestive), and the increased drooling that suggests new digestive capacities. There are also situational factors to be considered: The baby is most amenable to feeding innovations when he is wide awake and after his first, voracious hunger has been appeased. When he is tired or very hungry, the urge to suck is strong, and he will have little patience for spoons and cups. Individual differences show up, some babies taking to new food-stuffs and feeding methods with great gusto, some matter-of-factly, some cautiously, some not at all; some babies are ready at an early age, others not until much later, and parents can respond appropriately. Here again, a certain amount of trial and error is called for, which is no strain for the self-confident parent who can watch the baby's reactions and adapt to the messages transmitted via the language of behavior.

In the early decades of the century, experts on nutrition discovered some important principles of what constitutes a sound human diet. Unfortunately, in their application of these principles to the feeding of babies and children, the nutritionists were often as rigid, dogmatic, and magicalistic as their intuition-guided forerunners had been.

Perhaps the revolutionary turning point in dietetics came in the late

1930's with the publication of Clara Davis' findings[39] on the self-selection of diets by recently weaned infants. These babies of their own accord ate the proper proportions of the right food components: proteins, carbohydrates, fats, vitamins, minerals. It is important to stress that Davis' subjects did not ration their intake of different substances meal by meal after the manner of a dietician's chart; it was only in the long run of weeks that their diets balanced out in the correct proportions. Along the way, babies sometimes went on "jags," sticking to one food, such as bananas, for days at a time. A second essential point is that the babies ate needed foodstuffs even when these were patently distasteful, as in the case of salt, which some children took straight, grimacing all the while. In general, the babies were oblivious to what the adult would consider palatable or unpalatable combinations of foods, or the sequence in which foods should be eaten at a given meal. Because of its fundamental implications, Davis' study needs to be repeated with a larger sample of babies of different ages and with more varied and elaborate foodstuffs— caviar and salami, for instance, not to mention sweets—than the commonplace, bland staples she used in her original investigation.

It would be impractical for parents to feed their babies cafeteria-style in an attempt to apply Davis' findings literally. However, parents can learn from Davis' study not to be upset by a baby's aversion—usually temporary if it is not made an issue of—to particular foods, or to be alarmed when he goes on food jags. They can also try offering a widely variegated diet—perhaps in the form of morsels from the adults' plates— to babies from a young age, letting the baby decide which things he finds appetizing and which he wants second helpings of. (We assume a family with adequate means to afford varied and adequate fare. In cases of poverty and malnutrition there is a tendency after weaning for the child to share with the adults a diet of excessive carbohydrates and inadequate protein; and, for reasons we shall see, to prefer the familiar foods and resist innovations.) Actually, a relaxed attitude—within broad limits—about the baby's diet seems to be the rule nowadays, which may be one reason that so-called feeding problems, once common, have become a rarity in this country's middle class.

Davis' findings illustrate the principle which Cannon[40] called the *wisdom of the body.* Briefly put, this principle says that the organism has some capacity to recognize—not consciously or logically or analytically, but at the appetitive level of what seems attractive—those foodstuffs which contain nutrients in which the body is deficient. Such selection was first observed in cases of physiological malfunction. For instance, people suffering from Addison's disease, which affects the adrenal glands and so interferes with salt metabolism, spontaneously increase salt consumption to compensate. In the same way, rats with their adrenal glands removed become highly sensitive to the presence of salt and can detect extremely minute quantities dissolved in water, as shown by their greater consumption of weak saline than of plain water.[41] Again, children who eat plaster (which is rich in calcium) from the walls are sometimes found to be suffering from calcium deficiency. People have hypothesized that pregnant women who develop "cravings" do so in response to actual dietary lacks, but the evidence is slight.

Since some people have interpreted the wisdom of the body to mean that the child can safely be left to govern his own intake, we must emphasize that it is far from perfect. Although the wisdom of the body may steer us toward nourishing food, it does not warn us away from poisons. Children do not hesitate to sample the contents of medicine bottles and soap packages and pesticide canisters or lead-laden paint, as the regional poison control centers that have been established in the United States can testify. The wisdom of the body does not signal to us which is the delectable mushroom and which the deadly toadstool. Foods low in nutritive value may be more attractive than nourishing ones and may even block consumption of needed nutrients by dulling the appetite. This clearly happens in the case of those children who seem to live on potato chips, soda pop, and candy. It seems to be the case that a liking for a narrow and perhaps prestigeful range of European foodstuffs, to the abandonment of the local diet of fish, coconut, fruits, and taro, accounts for the fact that many Tahitians lose their permanent teeth by late adolescence. Culturally defined food habits tend to corrupt the body's wisdom. In many societies with inadequate diets, vital nutritional supplements are there for the taking but are ignored in favor of what the culture defines as food. Many Americans would rather suffer malnutrition than eat "trash" fish such as squid, octopus, eels, or sea urchins, or the recently created fish flour, or "exotic" cuts of meat such as sweetbreads, testicles, brains, or kidneys, or the fat and marrow that are so essential in Eskimo diet. Tomatoes, a valuable source of vitamins and minerals, were long shunned as poisonous.

A curious, sometimes individual but often cultural phenomenon is *pica*, the regular eating of non-nutritive substances.[42] For instance, a number of people in the southern United States regularly eat clay, now moist as it comes from the ground, now sun-dried, now oven-baked. Some like it in wafers, others prefer it in chunks. Some have a special penchant for the gray kind, others like the yellow or the red. All of us have probably known mild pica in the form of chewing the erasers off pencils or consuming small wads of paper, and some children seem to have cravings for wood or even soap. All such eating seems unrelated to or even at odds with the wisdom of the body.

THUMB-SUCKING AND COMFORT DEVICES

Sucking is an essential part of the neonate's equipment for survival. During infancy it becomes, in addition, a need which demands gratification in its own right. When the sucking need does not get gratified in the course of nursing, the baby makes up for it by sucking on other things— his thumb, a corner of his blanket, rattles, and so forth. A follower of David Levy, Ena Roberts,[43] found that finger-sucking was related to too-brief feeding time in the early months, or to an abrupt change from long feeding times to short ones. Unfortunately, Roberts' findings are equivocal, since she had no way to measure food intake to be sure that both thumb-suckers and nonsuckers were getting the same amount to eat. Levy[44] himself, in a classic series of studies, has demonstrated compensatory mouthing in puppies and pecking in chicks. Puppies fed from a free-flowing nipple, which gratified their hunger without gratifying their need to suck, sucked avidly at themselves, each other, curtain fringes, and proffered human fingers. Similarly, chicks given only a limited opportunity to peck, although adequately fed, pecked at each other's bodies until the feathers came out. A difficulty with this observation is that what looks like compensatory pecking may instead be the pecking that goes into establishing a dominance hierarchy, a pecking order, so we need a comparison with normally reared chicks before we can safely interpret Levy's findings. Another possibly relevant factor in such studies is that of space—a number of authors have pointed out that rearing animals in crowded conditions produces disturbed behavior of various kinds.[45] On the other hand, chicks fed by hand and thus completely deprived of pecking experience starved to death when later left to eat in the ordinary way. It appears that pecking may have to be stimulated during a critical period early in life to become functional. In the same way, Sears and associates[46] have evidence to suggest that if the human baby is cup-fed from the very beginning, the sucking need is never established. However, we can detect no visible benefit to either baby or mother in bypassing the usual sucking activity of infancy.

If we understand that sucking, beyond its role in feeding, is an autonomous need, then thumb-sucking in infancy no longer appears a dirty, disgusting "habit" which the child threatens to carry with him into adulthood and which must be stopped immediately, if need be with the help of the splints and cuffs and mittens and bitter-tasting medicines once featured in infant care manuals and mail-order catalogues. During infancy, thumb-sucking is not really a problem, and it usually stops spontaneously by the end of the preschool years. The relationship, if any, between thumb-sucking and malocclusion of the teeth is by no means clear, but it is likely that only the most persistent thumb-sucking—which may express other psychological needs, as for extra love and attention—is a menace to the dental arch.

One possible alternative to the readily available thumb if the baby needs extra sucking is a pacifier, provided it is kept reasonably clean. (In practice, it is usually a good idea to have several pacifiers ready for action.) It must be said, however, that some mothers and some babies prefer thumbs to pacifiers. But children who use pacifiers seem more willing to give up than thumb-suckers their thumbs, and very few children seem to begin thumb-sucking after relinquishing their pacifiers. In infancy, the pacifier (or the thumb) may also serve, perhaps in an illusory way, to allay hunger temporarily and so help in spacing out the baby's feedings.

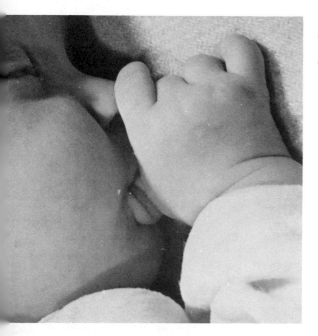

A major function of thumb-sucking seems to be that of closing off contact with the outside world at bedtime.
Wayne Miller

A major function of thumb-sucking seems to be that of closing off contact with the outside world at bedtime so that sleep can come. The parents can muffle the baby against noise, the baby can close his eyes against light, but the only way to desensitize those most vigilant receptors, the hand and the mouth, is to incorporate them into a closed circuit of internal activity. At bedtime, along with thumb-sucking, there often goes a great variety of other self-directed activities which are called comfort rituals. Some of the frequent ones are twisting a lock of hair, holding on to an ear, fingering a blanket, or cuddling a favorite—often tattered and disreputable—doll.

Fewer parents these days than formerly are likely to regard such behavior as symptoms of psychopathology, especially now that the Peanuts' blanket-trailing Linus has become a familiar figure around the world. Bedtime masturbation is quite common beginning late in the first year and can be seen as another way of shutting out the world to find sleep. Elaborate measures to curb infantile masturbation—even daytime masturbation—are probably inappropriate. The desirable course seems to be to give the baby a reasonable amount of freedom to find out about the body that he is, without unintentionally giving masturbation more importance than the parents really wish to. Too great a concern with controlling the baby's behavior can lead to such absurdities as keeping the baby's hands under the covers to prevent thumb-sucking and outside the covers to prevent masturbation.

TOILET TRAINING

As we suggested earlier, toilet training belongs in toddlerhood, but since one still hears that babies can be "trained" by age six months—or four months, or one month—it seems a good idea to say something about it here. Some babies, beginning at a very early age, have a very stable schedule of defecation. When this is the case, and if the baby defecates while awake (many have bowel movements predominantly in their sleep), parents can capitalize on the baby's schedule and, once he is old enough to sit up comfortably, put him on the pot when a bowel movement is due. Even when the baby has an irregular pattern of defecation, an alert mother can tell from his behavior and expression that a bowel movement is imminent and place him on the pot. But take note that it is the mother who is trained, not the baby. What this sort of procedure accomplishes is to save one or two soiled diapers and clean-ups a day and familiarize the baby with the toilet as a comfortable place to be. If the toilet becomes a prison, problems can arise. If the baby's spontaneous defecation schedule changes, as it is likely to do, or if the baby has no schedule to begin with, it is worse than useless to try to get him to eliminate on parental demand.

Ordinarily, bowel control comes after the child can walk, and bladder control somewhat later, with daytime bladder control preceding nighttime control. But while it is pointless and perhaps even injurious to begin toilet training before the child is able to learn, it is likewise not a good idea to postpone it too long. That is, there seems to be a critical period roughly between ages one and a half and two years or so in which toilet training happens quite easily (provided the baby's life is going well in general), and outside which it can be very strenuous. But as in feeding and weaning, the best results come from noting carefully the baby's response to tentative trials, and establishing toilet training with his interest and cooperation.

SLEEPING

The chief point about sleeping is that many healthy, lively babies past the age of a few months may never want to let go of the interesting world long enough to go to sleep, so it falls to the parents, supreme in their self-confidence, to create the occasion for naps and nighttime sleep. The baby provides abundant cues, by sagging, yawning, and irritability, when he needs to sleep. Once the baby has been put to bed and is asleep, how long he sleeps can usually be left up to him. But babies can be encouraged to conform to the patterns of early-rising or late-sleeping parents. Everyday observations indicate that most babies can learn to sleep in either noisy or quiet surroundings, but once they are used to one or the other, that is what they require. Many babies have a period of fussy crying before they fall asleep; this is easily distinguished from cries of genuine distress and does not call for any parental action. When babies are truly unhappy at bedtime, they have to be soothed and comforted in a way that does not provoke further wakefulness. In very young infants, this may take the form of rocking, crooning, stroking the head, or gently patting the back. Somewhat older infants may need to have a familiar adult stand by the crib for a few minutes, acting as a secure reference point before the baby can free himself from outside stimulation and let himself go into sleep. When the baby is taken visiting and put to bed in strange surroundings, extra measures will almost certainly have to be taken to permit him to get to sleep, and extra adult tolerance needed of the irritability and vulnerability that are likely to go with delayed or omitted naps.

EARLY CULTIVATION OF MOTOR SKILLS

As we have mentioned, there has recently been a vogue for teaching skills like swimming beginning at the age of a few months. We have often been asked our opinion about such practices, and we can only say that we see no harm in them—subject to some reservations. We have seen babies less than a year old minnowing happily through the water; we have watched babies younger than two on skis or getting the feel of a surfboard on a ripple of wave; we have seen three-year-olds pirouetting on tiptoe, and these youngsters seemed, to all outward appearances, psychologically unscarred.

One reservation that we have is that children may be cast prematurely in the role of performer, of the show-off and deliberate charmer who feeds on the audience's approval and applause. Another caution is that the child's skills may outrun his common sense. The baby who can swim may not know which water is safe to swim in and which water isn't. We recently witnessed a less-than-two-year-old happily pedaling his tricycle straight down the middle of a street, blithely riding through stop signs, to the verge of a major thoroughfare. A third warning is against forcing. Not only is there a threat to the baby's welfare in forcing him to persevere in an activity which he resists (at later ages, when the child can view events in better perspective, it may indeed be necessary at times to force him to do things like chores and homework), but forcing may boomerang and instill a lifelong loathing of what might have become an enjoyable activity if teaching it had been deferred to a later age. It may be worth emphasizing that babies given plenty of scope get abundant exercise on their own, and need no special encouragement to be active in the use of their bodies.

TOYS FOR BABIES

Normal cognitive development takes place in a series of interchanges between the baby and the world around him. He comes to a first basic organization of reality through watching, listening, tasting, smelling, touching, manipulating, and being acted on by the things he encounters. It is now well established, at least in the United States, that from an early age there are pronounced differences in cognitive competence between children of poor parents and children of the relatively well-to-do. It is likely that a comparable distinction would be evident in most societies, but we do not know. It is probable that the greater cognitive adequacy of middle-class children can be traced to the greater number, variety, and accessibility of the objects they encounter, though this is generally coupled with the greater availability of mothers or caretakers who make these available, respond to the child's use of them, encourage further experimentation, and talk to him about such objects. This becomes vital when we consider the problems of cognitive enrichment for poor or "culturally deprived" children. Such compensatory enrichment should probably begin in infancy rather than at age three or four, and people who want to enrich the cognitive experience of young babies should be aware of what kinds of materials are likely to work best.

Babies enjoy and benefit from the opportunity to handle (including mouthing and chewing on), to take apart, and eventually to put together all sorts of things. Many of the most educational materials and things occur as a matter of course in the environments of middle-class children. Among the important learning materials are very simple ones: paper to crumple and flatten and tear and suck and chew on; rags to use likewise; clothespins and teething rings to teethe on; plastic dishes to bang on table top or floor; mirrors in which to admire oneself; paper bags and empty boxes to put things in and things to put into them, including, in late infancy, grocery cartons the child can climb in and out of; and kitchen utensils and pots and pans to use in myriad ways. Parents can well consider household effects to be the baby's basic playthings, and access to them becomes more feasible as the family rises above the subsistence level. Freedom to dabble with his fingers in cooked cereal and other such foodstuffs is important in the baby's coming to know the world and its properties, even at the cost of some additional mess.

Besides what the regular household provides, toymakers have come up with some ingenious and useful devices (homemade equivalents are easy to make and just as good). Mobiles that hang above a bassinet or crib seem to fascinate very young babies, but very soon it is important to have things in reach. Babies who are reaching out to bat at and grasp dangling objects enjoy having an arrangement of curtain rings and horizontal bars to hit and tug at, especially if these are suspended on springs and even more especially if moving them actuates bells or rattles. Rattles and soft dolls suspended by lengths of elastic also give the baby something to set swaying, to grasp, to pull and release, and to mouth or chew on. Slightly older babies (past six months) can operate the kind of music box which is wound by means of a drawstring. There is no reason similar contrivances could not be built to yield all manner of sound effects. Other cultures may or may not deliberately provide playthings, depending on the established understandings of the meaning of infants' activities, the use of child nurses, and the like. In late infancy and early toddlerhood, blocks with holes and rods that fit through the holes get played with at successively more mature levels. By late infancy, when the child can creep, the spatial arrangements of house and furniture become playthings for the baby to explore with his whole body, weaving through chair rungs, squeezing into the space between stove and refrigerator, detouring around footstools, opening and emptying drawers, and clambering into low cupboards. So-called activity panels or gadget boards, equipped with knobs and cranks and gears, with doors that open to reveal mirrors or pictures or simply the world on the other side of the board, and miscellaneous locks and latches, are appealing to babies and young children, although most commercial versions are less imaginative than what an inspired father or mother could construct. A large transparent plastic bottle loosely filled with spools, blocks, clothespins, and such, makes an excellent plaything for babies a year and older.

We assume that no parent will ever think that playthings can take the place of human company and affection and the social games of infancy and early childhood, but as babies get older they increasingly like to explore the possibilities of raw materials and things and spatial and causal relations—particularly with the occasional involvement of the adult.

The Baby's Cultural Heritage

It is clear that the family a baby is born into has its own special characteristics. Any given family, though, is a part of a larger social unit whose members share characteristic ways of thinking, feeling, judging, and acting. Some of these ways are practical adaptations to the conditions of life: The Eskimo builds his house of snow, the dweller in the tropics one of thatch; the island or seacoast dweller evolves a lore of the sea, the inland dweller a lore of the mountains or forest; and so on. But interwoven with these ecologically practical arrangements are beliefs, assumptions, values, expectations, life styles, manners, and so on, that may have little to do with the immediate exigencies of food, shelter, health, safety, amusement, or procreation.

Collectively, the ways of a given society are called its *culture* (in large and complex societies, different groups are said to have their own subcultures). According to which culture he is born into, the child will learn a special, all-inclusive (but not necessarily, as we shall see in a moment, completely explicit or logically consistent) view of human nature and destiny, material reality, and—in most cultures—the workings of the supernatural. This view is communicated to the child explicitly in the teachings of his elders, but even more without any explicit justification or even statement, in the traditional ways of doing things, in ritual observances, in emotional reactions to events, in tones of voice, in fixed relationships to different people in the social structure, and in manner and style of movement.

We shall point out later in this chapter some of the things all cultures have in common, representing what we take to be some universals or imperatives of the human condition, but for the time being we want to stress that cultures differ, that the differences are many and deep, and are not something external to the individual person, or veneers overlying a common human nature. Rather, a particular culture is one special version of human nature, an orientation to life that is assimilated, so to speak, into the individual's very bones. It is because our culturally given outlook becomes so intimately ours that most people never discover that they share a culture. It is easy to grasp that other people have bizarre beliefs and outlandish practices and food and clothing, have delusions which we may label a culture, but for us our perceptions and beliefs and values are always obviously the factual and correct ones.

THE AMERICAN CULTURE

Until now, most anthropologists have been of European origin, and the logical thing for them to do was to travel afield and observe the behavior of "exotic," non-European people. For the purposes of this book, however, it may be more instructive to begin by pointing to some of the features of United States culture as various experts and amateurs, imported and domestic, have delineated it. Among the more astute observers of the American scene, past and present, have been Alexis de Tocqueville, Charles Dickens, Mrs. Trollope, Geoffrey Gorer, Cora Du Bois, David Riesman, Paul Goodman, and Russell Lynes.[47] Americans live in a highly technical, largely urban society, which already dictates some proportion of their behavior. They live in small nuclear families in sharply differentiated clumps and neighborhoods, whose design is largely accidental but follows economic lines. Their mechanized society depends on an intricate division of labor, which tends to demand highly specialized skills unlike the learning of an array of traditional crafts as in primitive societies. They travel and change abodes frequently, and are likely to prefer passive entertainment and the opinions transmitted by electronic mass media. Instead of exchanging news and gossip while they pound their washing on a rock or sit together plaiting mats and baskets, American women gather at the laundromat or the beauty parlor or supermarket. American men, because they work at specialized occupations, form friendships among members of the same guild. Only American school-age children are able to preserve some vestiges of tribal life, and even they, as Robert Paul Smith[48] has pointed out, are gradually being regimented not only into the ways of schools, but into the Little League, scouting, the use of prefabricated, highly complex play materials, summer camp, the round of after-school lessons, and regular visits to the orthodontist.

Americans value success, and assume that each generation will outstrip the one before it. There is very little sympathy for the failure, the ne'er-do-well, the underachiever, the dropout, the mendicant (be he priest or vagrant) unless he is a highly-paid professional fund-raiser, and the person who has stopped rising through the organization or system is discarded (or, more kindly, shunted into a dead-end sinecure which he and his fellows politely pretend is not the limbo of the might-have-beens). Americans believe in progress when it is measured by technical innovation. At the same time, they are conservative in their social views, which may account for some of their ambivalence about intellectuals, who are valued when they can solve practical problems but who are mistrusted because they are likely to harbor radical, hence disturbing, ideas. In the same way, they value education, but less because it enriches individual experience and liberates thinking than because it enhances earning power and gives access to the right circles. Americans tend to be optimistic, but their optimism sometimes overflows into feelings of omnipotence and then, when they find that a problem cannot be quickly solved, they may be plunged into total pessimistic impotence. Efficiency is highly esteemed, and with it an emphasis on hurry and working fast, which leaves little room for leisurely savoring of life, contemplation, and examination of goals.

A streak of violence runs through American culture, in the conduct of foreign policy, in the way police treat criminals, in the way southern—and northern—bigots treat Negroes and civil rights workers, in motion-picture and television dramas, on picket lines, and throughout the daily newspaper, though other cultures, to be sure, have been or are far more violent. American men and, even more, American women conceal their age, esteem youth, and look forward with reluctance and dread to maturity—let alone old age.

In former times, American society set great store by delay of gratification, on doing without immediate rewards for the sake of greater ones later on, but this value is being eroded both by the cult of youth, which says that one must snatch one's pleasures while they are still pleasurable, and by the credit-card and installment plan philosophy of enjoy-now-and-pay-later which helps keep the economy booming. For the economy not to expand steadily is considered disastrous, and other forms of stability are also often suspect.

Americans believe that marriage is good and that everybody should get married, preferably early, but this ethic is complicated by the fact that American men and women are strongly ambivalent about sexuality and about each other. It sometimes almost seems that American men would rather watch pornographic movies, which are purveyed in great profusion, than go to bed with an actual woman, and would rather go to bed with a casual pick-up or a prostitute (though prostitution is less institutionalized than in many other cultures) than with a woman with whom a genuine human relationship has to be formed. The much discussed, though probably not highly prevalent, vogue of mate-swapping and group sex seems to reflect the difficulty we have reconciling sex and marriage. Divorces are relatively frequent and an increasing number of children must cope with life in terms of a single parent or of shuttling between combinations of parents and stepparents.

If American culture is full of rifts and inconsistencies and incongruities, perhaps the most basic one is the two incompatible moral codes every American child learns—though such ambivalence also marks many other cultures. Whatever his religion, every American child is taught something akin to the Christian ethic, stressing such virtues as charity, forbearance, compassion, altruism, humility, and cooperation, and corresponding, as we have suggested, to an attitude of basic trust, perhaps with an ascetic overtone. But he also learns the American business ethic of dog eat dog, the survival of the fittest, which stresses and demands such traits as aggression, competitiveness, acquisitiveness, self-preservation, guile, and ruthlessness. It is interesting that those groups in American and European society who resisted Darwin's theory of evolution on religious grounds nonetheless embraced a social Darwinism that seemed to justify the law of the jungle as a governing principle in human affairs and further justified the established social hierarchy as naturally ordained. There were, of course, medieval antecedents for such views as well, as in the Divine Right of Kings. As it works out in practice, a majority of American women and a minority of American men come to espouse the Christian ethic; a larger number of American men live primarily by the business ethic, with some concessions to Christianity when dealing with their own kind of people and on Sundays, and sometimes with some grotesque rationalizations seeking to reconcile the Christian and business ethics ("How I Found Christ and Made a Million Dollars"). A great number of other American men, however, seem to live in perpetual and painful conflict, never quite sure how to act and never free of misgivings once they have acted. It may be that such moral conflicts find somatic expression, which would help account for the mass hypochondria of American society implied in gargantuan consumption of laxatives, stomach remedies, headache remedies, tonics, dietary supplements, health foods, and magical nostrums, without mention of recurring fads and cults.

A strange by-product of the rapid change in the material situation and in values has been the growth of a new sort of Protestant ethic. The original version, as set forth by Max Weber, saw the businessman as acting less for his own good than as God's agent, so that he preached and, in various degrees, practiced thrift, honesty, austerity, and chastity. Because he adhered to such virtues, he was justified in feeling that he was of the Lord's anointed and that he and a country dedicated to these principles could do no wrong. His contemporary descendant, while still preaching much the same fundamentalist theology, social conservatism, and blood-and-fire patriotism, has become a dedicated if sometimes frantic and frustrated hedonist, with life's great goods defined by sports cars, gadgets, swimming pools, Las Vegas, compulsive sex preoccupation, fine clothes, and luxury cruises.

Notice that this subculture, which characterizes many of our leading citizens, overlaps hardly at all with another which might be called radical, godless Christianity. The members of this group, who are mostly young but who have been inspired by such elders as Paul Goodman and Paul Jacobs, emphasize personal closeness, love, intensity of personal experience, sexual liberation, the use of drugs as a way of exploring the full range of feeling, internationalism, pacifism, and democratic socialism.

As we shall say again, not all American young people belong to this camp. A great many—probably most—have strongly identified with the new, inverted Protestant ethic; a few, particularly among the upwardly mobile lower classes and minority groups, still subscribe to the old Horatio Alger one; some, as in the surf-bum and ski-bum sets, follow a philosophy of psychopathic hedonism; others try to embrace an idealism uncluttered by economic and political considerations.

SOME UNIVERSALS OF CULTURE

Having taken a look at some aspects of a particular culture, let us go on to discuss some general implications. Any cultural orientation has its own logic, whereby certain conclusions follow "naturally" from a given set of premises. If one "knows" that babies are selfish, scheming creatures who with the slightest encouragement will become monsters of egotism, then it follows, as in fact it does for many people, that one must begin by "breaking the baby's spirit," on the analogy of breaking a wild horse. If one "knows" that heroin transforms human beings into wild beasts, then of course one must protect society by banishing heroin. If women exploit men, and men women, it is because each has a cultural version of maleness and femaleness that makes the opposite sex less than human and so something to be taken advantage of. Part of the task of education is to dissolve cultural stereotypes so that one can perceive and react to people as human beings, with a complete set of human characteristics, including frailties and vices, rather than as specimens defined by a single, conspicuous label (the social psychologist's stereotypes): Negro, Jew, Yankee, Beatnik, Rich Man, Astronaut, Movie Star, Undesirable, Welfare Recipient, Playboy, Sex Kitten, Dope Addict, School Dropout, Blind Person, Criminal, Primitive, Cripple, Star Athlete, or whatever.

Part of our problem in thinking about cultural differences is how to comprehend diversity within unity. For what we are saying is that all people (and peoples) are alike and that all people are different. All cultures, no matter how diverse, express a peculiarly human mode of existence of such universality that we cannot be sure whether it is learned or biologically determined. Certainly the human constitution is necessary to the distinctively human things we do. Speaking, as human beings practice it, seems to be intrinsically impossible for apes, as are pictorial representation (which excludes daubing at canvas, which apes can do), the making of fire, and, if not the use of tools, the use of tools to make tools, as George Gaylord Simpson[49] recently put it. On the other hand, we cannot predict from a person's having a human constitution precisely how he will behave, what his tastes and values and understandings and goals and competences will be. We know a great deal, for instance, about the structure of the human hand, its ability to grasp, knead, twist, and all the rest. But we cannot predict from our knowledge of the hand how the hand will be used: to build ham radio sets, to put a coin in a slot, to mold clay into works of art, to carve ivory, to make love, to clean wax out of an ear, or to shape a stone arrowhead. The potential functions are manifold, but the realized ones depend on the individual's history and the culture he is part of.

Nevertheless, all organisms sharing the human constitution also share certain forms of behavior. Some of these, of course, have analogs in infrahuman species, while some are exclusively human. All human beings, the occasional hermit apart, live in groups, and social contact and social learning are essential to the human condition. It takes a long time for the human infant to mature to the point of independence, and all societies accordingly have a highly developed *family life,* including quite intricate kinship systems, within which the child is given tutelage in the culture. The tutelage exists whether it is given in formal schooling or in the context of everyday activities. Babies and children everywhere have the same physical and psychological needs, and every society has selective priorities in its provisions for meeting these needs. How well is another question, since some societies—primitive and advanced—produce adults who can barely function well enough to keep the society going.

Central to human social life, inside and outside the family, is *language,* speaking and listening to speech. Other creatures, as we have noted, can make and modulate the necessary sounds, but only human beings have developed language beyond sheer emotional indicators and warnings. In some societies, of course, language is also written and read. To find universal features of different human languages is a task that has kept linguists busy and bewildered for many a long year,[50] but it is clear that all languages serve, by whatever linguistic means, the purposes of factual and mythic and affective communication within a given society. (Notice that two groups—say Americans and Britons—speaking the "same" language may attach quite different semantic and affective values to similar terms; in psychology, a behaviorist is one who espouses a particular doctrine, whereas in zoology, a behaviorist is a biologist who studies animal behavior; to the psychologist, ethology is the study of animal behavior by zoologists, whereas to the zoologist, ethology is a particular theoretical doctrine.) Not all languages contain the same "concepts" or lend themselves to the expression of the same ideas with equal ease. For instance, one would have to invent a whole new vocabulary of Choctaw to translate an English-language treatise on chemistry or sociology into that language. The Roman Catholic Church is kept busy coining new Latin words for atomic energy, solid-state electronics, gene drift, contraceptive devices, operant conditioning, and other things and ideas that played a minor role in the time of the Caesars.

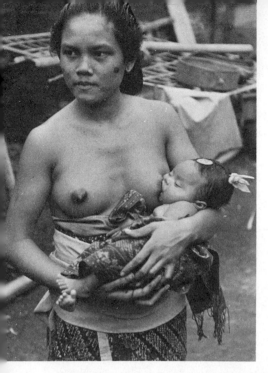

(*Left*) A Balinese mother suckles her baby.

Gregory Bateson and Margaret Mead, *Balinese Character*

(*Below*) Balinese babies are fed by having their mouths stuffed with pre-chewed food.

Gregory Bateson and Margaret Mead, *Balinese Character*

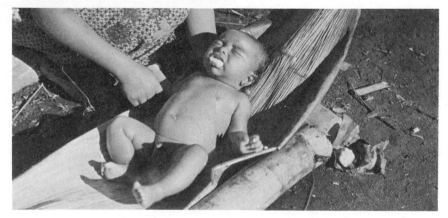

All people use *tools* of some complexity, whether hammers and chisels and plows and spear launchers or forceps or ultrasonic devices for cleaning the teeth. All human societies, as we have said, have systems for organizing *time* and *space*. Human beings everywhere share certain *emotions* such as anger, grief, dread, joy, and amusement, which seem to be human extensions of feeling states found in many vertebrate animals. Even though all people share a number of emotions, different cultures have different rules governing what occasions produce which emotions, how a given emotion is expressed, and toward whom which emotions may be directed. For instance, in the United States, it is considered unmanly to cry, and it is thought improper, outside certain detective stories, to use physical violence against a woman. By the same token, physical aggression is unwomanly (or at least not ladylike), as is the use of coarse language. We should further note that all societies have conventions for concealing emotions and for simulating emotions one may not necessarily feel, as when we enthusiastically congratulate someone for what we privately consider an unmerited triumph. It seems likely, too, that all societies practice *displacement*, the redirecting of feelings from a dangerous object to a safe one, as when we take out on our family the resentment we feel toward our boss. Since many people have fantasies of going to a place where people practice free, untrammeled love, it is as well to point out that all societies have regulations (some differing, some almost universal, as in the case of incest taboos) governing the *conduct of sex*—not that these are always obeyed. We do not want to discourage the romantic seeker after Eros entirely, and there certainly are people whose sexual practices are far more relaxed than our own, but here again the pilgrim should be reminded that these peoples too are people, not mere vehicles of erotic gratification.

Every society has been driven to examine its own existence and the environment in which that existence takes place, and to evolve a metaphysic, a general conception of reality, including nonhuman reality, human nature, tribal origins, and the supernatural, together with a supporting mythology which in turn implies codes of morals, ethics, good manners, and skills (both ritual and functional). The accumulated wisdom of the tribe is often summed up in maxims, aphorisms, and parables. The important thing to see is that even supposedly "simple" cultures are in fact quite elaborate and that a culture cannot be defined in terms of its quaint folkways, of the sort featured in travelogues, but only by its underlying assumptions about the nature of reality.

For our purposes, it is important to understand how culture is transmitted, how the child comes to think and feel and perceive and act like a Balinese, say, or a Maori or a Navaho or an American or a Greek. This, unfortunately, is a question about which very little is securely known. Whiting and Child[51] have pointed to some interesting statistical relationships between the economic level of societies and child-rearing practices, but such studies only hint at the processes of social learning involved.

Part of the difficulty is that so much of culture seems to be imparted implicitly, as we have said, without words, in manner and touch and tone of voice, and is learned incidentally, without any immediate behavioral echo, as a corollary of things learned explicitly. For example, if we could gather batches of American readers of this book into one room—as we sometimes do—and ask for a show of hands as to which was better, the natural or the artificial, we would get an overwhelming vote for all that is natural. This is an especially instructive example of the subtlety of implicit teaching and incidental learning since these lovers of the natural live lives founded on artifice—automobiles, television, air conditioning and central heating, the written word, logic and mathematics, the arts and decoration, and cosmetics and self-adornment. Here, as in many cases, the lessons of culture seem to be more potent than the evidence of the senses. By the same token, the value that youth is better than age is not something invented and propagated by young people, but has become a stable cultural tenet transmitted from generation to generation.

The implicit features of a culture are contained in the things its members take for granted, the "of courses." It is because so much of our culture is implicit that it is very hard for us to transcend our ethnocentrism and see our culture as from the outside. It is like coming to know our own bodies, which are simultaneously something to be known and the instrumentality by which we know them. In Heinz Werner's words, one cannot, from within, see one's own eyes. From the standpoint of our own culture, *of course* the mother wheels her baby about in a carriage instead of carrying him in a sling against her body or papoose-fashion on her back, of course new highways have to be built to relieve traffic congestion at the expense of trees and houses, of course cruelty to animals is wrong, of course one eats beef, of course one takes the baby to the doctor or clinic for a regular checkup. But from the perspective of other cultures, of course beetles are a great delicacy, of course pork is unclean, of course it is admirable and a sign of spiritual nobility to stand on one foot for twenty-four years, of course it is bad manners to watch a person eating, so of course one sits with one's back to the feast, of course it is your mother's brother whose authority you must obey.

The present era is unique in that, after centuries of stable continuity, cultures everywhere are changing rapidly, usually in the direction of Europeanization and Americanization. We can only assume, somewhat regretfully, that the rate of change will be accelerated until there is a relatively uniform culture—subject to limits imposed by climate and natural resources—the world around. Meanwhile, especially in societies like our own, and despite pressures to conformity, there are still recognizable subcultures.

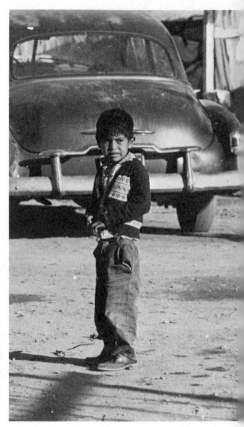

The culture of poverty.
(Below and right) Office of Economic Opportunity
(Far right and far right, below) Ken Heyman

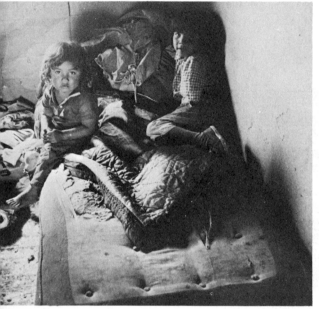

Most American subcultures were formed by the clustering together of people who separated themselves by preference or were segregated by external pressures from the larger society. Examples are the enclaves formed by groups of immigrants—Chinatown, Little Italy, Little Bohemia, and so on—and based on common language and customs differing from those of the rest of the United States. Some enclaves, of course, are ghettos into which are forced those whom the established society will not allow to live with its members. Harlem and the Negro districts of communities across the country are examples. We even have the phenomenon of the so-called Gilded Ghettos, opulent expanses of suburbia inhabited almost entirely by Jews who are unwelcome in Gentile-dominated suburbs. Back-country communities without modern roads and communications have likewise clung to and elaborated their familiar ways of doing things, with little regard to what was happening in the outside world.

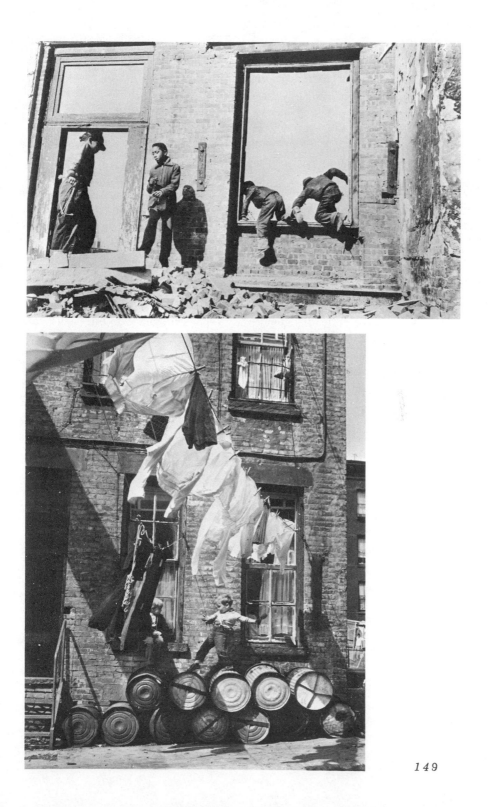

But now, as successive generations of the descendants of immigrants get assimilated into the economic and social life of the country (sometimes through the back door of crime and the rackets), as Negroes refuse to remain disenfranchised, oppressed, uneducated, and poor, as technologically sophisticated factory farming displaces family farming, as suburbs spread into and devour the country, as the rural poor are drawn to the cities, as electricity and bathtubs become more commonplace, as manufactured commodities displace homemade ones, and as radio, television, and magazines spread a common stock of knowledge, ideas, entertainment, and folk heroes, subcultural differences are remorselessly obliterated. Social class differences remain, but around a shared set of values and assumptions.

Insofar as the spread of uniform culture means the end of ignorance, superstition, xenophobia, moralism, and rigid ideologies, it is probably good. However, it usually also means the weakening or disappearance of local customs, special delicacies, and the skills and competences that get lost when mass-produced commodities replace homemade ones. We can still detect the differences between southern ways and northern, among east and plains and mountain and west coast, between the rural outlook and the urban, between slums and suburbs, and among ethnic and religious groups, but the rate of change is dizzying.

SOCIAL ROLES

Within any social group or subgroup, individuals play different *roles*, that is, they learn to perform in certain expected ways consonant with their position in life. Within the family, we have the roles of father, mother, wife, husband, son, daughter, brother, sister, and others depending on how the family is organized. At work, we have the roles played by certain specialists—doctor, lawyer, plumber, mechanic—as well as the roles that go with being owner, executive, subordinate, power behind the throne, union representative, and so forth. In the schools, we have the roles of principal, teacher, and pupil. There are roles that go with political office and participation in community affairs. Storekeeper and customer have roles to play. In social situations, people cast themselves, sometimes fleetingly, sometimes consistently, in the roles of virile sportsman, seductive siren, staunch friend, dispenser of sage counsel, and so forth. Indeed, some sociologists would go so far as to say that personal identity consists entirely of the roles a person plays. While most of us are not explicitly aware of role playing, we almost all recognize the special pleasure of those situations which allow us to "be ourselves," to "let our hair down," in sum, to leave off role playing. Every child, at every stage of his development, is being groomed more or less consciously for a particular set of social roles. Within a given society and subculture, each family has its own history, tradition, and values, and provides its own indoctrination, in terms of how it meets or fails to meet needs, the prevailing emotional climate, the games it plays, what experiences it exposes the child to and what it shields him from, what it doesn't know about, and the feelings it attaches to those things to which it exposes the child. What the child learns, we hope it is clear, is not a culture plus a subculture plus a social role, but a way of experiencing the world and himself in relation to it, generalizable or particularizable in these terms. Then, too, the family's general orientation is modified in action both by the child's qualities as an individual, whether boy or girl, whether he arrived at an opportune or inopportune time, whether he is firstborn or ninth-born, and also by the meaning that children have for this particular family.

People have children for a variety of reasons. Chief among these, we would like to believe, is the solid pleasure of parenthood, of having a child to share the family's triumphs and tribulations, to be partly a person of the parents' own creation whom they can love and cherish, and whom they can watch grow into a life which he will eventually create for himself. Even when the desire to have a child is extrinsic, or even when pregnancy is unplanned or unwanted, a real live baby, once born, can demolish all his parents' preconceptions and, once they master the mechanics of parenthood, arouse in them a fund of tenderness and protec-

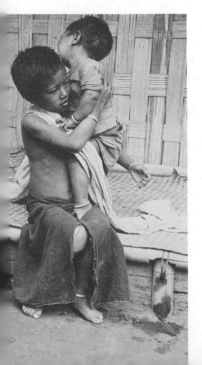

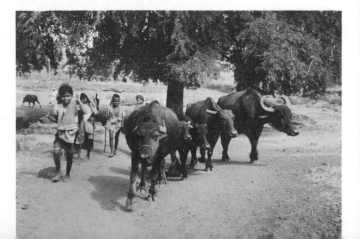

In some societies, older children are given genuine responsibility for the care of younger ones.
Gregory Bateson and Margaret Mead, *Balinese Character*

In India, as in many other societies, there is early assumption of adult responsibilities.
The Ford Foundation

tiveness and delight beyond anything they had ever dreamed of knowing. For some number of parents, the motivation to parenthood is the simple assumption that all normal people get married and then have children. Sad to state, as we know, some people find out after the fact that they did not really want to get married, or at least not now or to this particular person, and some find out—although they are not as likely to admit it since it is less readily undone—that parenthood was not for them. We may be approaching a time, of course, when contraception is so much the norm that having children will necessarily become a matter of deliberate planning.

Some people want children as a way of perpetuating the family name and fortune—in such cases, of course, role-grooming may be very explicit and sharply defined. In some societies, such as Japan, perpetuation of the family name is so important that if all the children are girls, one girl's husband is adopted into the family and given its name. For some people, having a child can be a way of projecting into the future the realization of their own frustrated dreams and ambitions, as though having a child gives the parent a second, vicarious chance at life. Sometimes a child is wanted to fill what feels like a vacancy in the parents' lives but may actually be only an emptiness in themselves. Children may be valued as potential contributors to the family economy or because they will look after their parents in their declining years.

For a number of people, parenthood is a necessary proof of their biological adequacy, and a man may need a son as testimony to his virility. Some parents may count so heavily on having a child of one sex rather than the other, sometimes without realizing it, that they only have one name ready. Or they may betray their bias by falling into the habit of referring to the unborn baby exclusively as "he" or as "she." If a child of the wrong sex arrives, they may have trouble adjusting to reality, and in a few extreme cases may treat the child in ways grossly inappropriate to its future sex role. Some children, of course, are valued hardly at all, and are just another mouth to feed, body to clothe, and bottom to wipe. It should go without saying that each of these attitudes has profound effects on the acts and feelings of parents, and hence on their young.

It makes a difference to a baby—and to the roles he comes to embody—whether he comes first in his family or follows other children. The first child typically "breaks trail"—that is, the parents learn about children the hard way, by practicing on their firstborn, who is on the receiving end not only of their fumblings, uncertainties, and downright mistakes, but may also bear the brunt of the excessive anxiety and overprotectiveness often expended on a first child. In spite of the seeming trials and vicissitudes of being first in the family, however, a good deal of recent research seems to indicate that firstborn children fare somewhat better than later-born ones.[52] (In-between children do least well, and the youngest fare second best; if the youngest is born after a long delay, he is likely to equal the achievement level of a firstborn.) This finding may reflect the need for as much adult attention as possible, as recently suggested by Rosenzweig.[53] Whatever the later outcomes, subsequent children are handled less anxiously and more casually, with greater reliance on the child's ability to manage some things for himself. This may mean, of course, that parents are less sensitive to cues from later-born babies so that less communication takes place. Often enough, parents expect a second baby to be just like the first, and are surprised— and sometimes resentful—to find him being his own individual self.

Depending on family variations, some children have to learn their manners early, some are valued for their personalities and others for their symbolic meaning or for their usefulness to the parents, some are initiated from the outset into the forms of religious observance, some are pressed to command and others to compete, or to cooperate or obey or fatalistically accept. Out of their early experience, including the traits of temperament and responsiveness that they bring to the situation, children may come to see the world as looming and ominous, or agitated and bewildering, or lively and exciting, or serene, or deadly dull. The baby's awareness of the world will not take final form for a number of years, but the emotional groundwork is laid down during infancy, so subtly and yet so pervasively that it appears to have been there all along, as though his special way of viewing the world were the only possible one.

It is interesting to note that cultural differences among biologically similar individuals are not restricted to human beings. The studies of animal development which we have mentioned show that members of infrahuman species cannot be thought of as having fixed white rat—or monkey or chicken or ant—natures, but that these natures take different shapes in different developmental contexts. Thus, Eleftheriou, studying the physiology of deermice, found himself hampered by the deermouse's savage tendency to bite. By the simple expedient of letting deermice be raised by white laboratory-mouse foster mothers, he was able to secure nonbiting deermice.[54] Naturalistic observations have indicated that complex behaviors such as hunting are taught to the young of some predatory species such as foxes; we have experimental evidence that mating behavior in white rats or rhesus monkeys cannot be taken for granted as innately given; and that many species of birds sing their characteristic song properly only by virtue of having been exposed to the singing of normal adult birds.

Thus, whatever generalizations we make about animal or human behavior, we are obliged to make them with reference to the particular social climate in which development takes place. We must also mention that as the child gets older, he learns a great many things on his own, without social mediation, on the basis of his encounters with objects, by solving the problems life puts in his way, and by puzzling out the things that perplex him. But his ways of benefiting from firsthand encounters, and the sorts of solutions he comes up with, are all conditioned upon his cultural experience and the things it has made him able to perceive, feel, learn, and reason about.

AN EXAMPLE OF CULTURAL SHAPING: SEX DIFFERENCES

We cannot in this short space hope to do full justice to the transmission and learning of culture—for one thing, not nearly enough is known about it, although its consequences are everywhere to be seen—so we shall dwell in some detail on one aspect of the totality, both as a general example and because of its significance in its own right. This is the way children are made aware of sex roles and sex differences, particularly in our own society.

Several things need to be said by way of preamble. Anatomical and physiological differences between the sexes are poorly correlated with sex roles, both vis-à-vis the opposite sex and in the culture at large. There is great human variation in sexual mating, in courtship patterns, sexual play, positions during intercourse, and alternate paths to orgasm. Needless to say, a culture which did not include in its definition of the sex act the ejaculation of sperm into the vagina would last only one generation. We cannot take it for granted that sexual motivation arises spontaneously, through simple physical maturation, since animal studies indicate that both drive level and mating patterns depend on early experience for normal development.[55] Nor can it be taken for granted that sexual experience is always defined as pleasant.[56] A culture's view of sexuality can weaken the intensity of sexual feelings, it can disguise them from the individual himself, it can intensify them to the point of making them frightening, it can attach bugaboos and strictures that make sex simultaneously pleasant and disagreeable, and it can define which acts, objects, partners, and settings produce agreeable sexual feelings, and which disagreeable ones. The culture defines which are permissible partners, which partner initiates sexual activity, the acceptability of homosexual behavior, and how private sexual activity should be. It also defines whether one should be made jealous by infidelity, and how jealousy is to be manifested.

Outside the sex act, there can be yet wider variations in the roles assigned to males and females with respect to such tasks as child-rearing (though to paraphrase Clyde Kluckhohn, we know of no society in which the father is expected to bear the children), housekeeping, discipline of children, tending the fields or the herds, marketing produce, managing the budget, handicrafts, hunting, fishing, participation in government and decision-making, and participation in recreational activities. Still further, there can be great variations among cultures in the traits ascribed to the two sexes: such things as bravery, loyalty, passionateness, deviousness, honesty, perseverance, generosity, cruelty, fortitude, sympathy, emotionality—the reader is invited to supply others. Somewhere on the boundary between roles (prescribed duties and competences) and traits are interests, tastes, and preferences that are assumed to go with being male or female. Thus, we assign playthings, foodstuffs, activities, occupations, and useful objects to the two sexes, with some overlap. Nobody has yet fully explored and catalogued all the cultural differences in definitions of masculinity and femininity, but a very small knowledge of anthropology is enough to show that they are considerable. Among the Yamana of South America, for instance, swimming is an exclusively female skill.[57] There seem to be some common threads, indicating that biological differences have some determining role, but much of what we take for granted as biologically founded turns out to be what our society is accustomed to think the biological differences mean.

We have already, many times over, changed our conceptions of sex roles, just as we have changed our thinking about human nature,[58] and we will almost certainly have to change them again. In our own relatively recent history, as we can see in eighteenth-century drawings and paintings, men had long, braided hair (or wigs in the same style) and wore ribbons and bows and long silk stockings. Now, when many young men are wearing their hair long and shaggy, their elders are likely to feel a sense of moral outrage at a departure from masculine propriety. Similarly, beards are nowadays seen as the mark of the dangerous radical (with connotations of free love and the use of drugs), whereas not so long ago beards were taken for granted as part of adult masculinity—as they still are for certain privileged groups such as explorers or sub-mariners. Females are taken to task for wearing male attire, for exposing their bodies, and for the use of zany maquillage.

One of the themes of this book is that children have only recently been discovered as human beings, with characteristics and needs and feelings and rights of their own. But it is only recently that women have begun to be (the process is by no means complete) accorded full human status—competent to vote, to hold office, to own property, to enter into legally binding contracts, to run businesses, to be able to learn mathematics and sciences, to think logically, and to have sexual needs and feelings analogous to men's. Many men in our society, but presumably not in the U.S.S.R., still feel uneasy about consulting a woman physician —as do many women. For it must be said that a great many women have been just as conservative as men about accepting a change in the status of women, while others seem to see the liberation of womankind as a chance to revenge themselves for all the slights accumulated during the centuries of bondage and can resist no opportunity to belittle or degrade the male. The war between the sexes has not yet been settled, and both men and women are by no means sure what life style, what role or combination of roles, is appropriate to the female of the species. But by the same token, a change in the female role calls for corresponding changes in the male role, and it still has not been settled how the male role is to be defined. A further ramification is that parents are increasingly uncertain what sex-related values they should be conveying to their children, boys and girls.

In any case, all parents recognize the importance of sex differences. Note that the first question parents ask, if the obstetrician hasn't already made haste to tell them, is "Is it a boy or a girl?" When they know the answer, and not before, there is language available to talk about the baby—up to now, whatever their hopes, the baby has been an ambiguity, an *it*. Once they know the sex of the child, the appropriate set of attitudes comes to the fore—and the baby's role begins to take shape. Indecision aside, how are these conceptions of masculinity and femininity transmitted to an infant who doesn't yet know that he exists, let alone that he has a body which places him forever in the category of male or female? (We shall take up in Chapter 13 the matters of transvestism and homosexuality, which involve identification with the opposite biological sex.) These conceptions are transmitted not as intellectual knowledge but as dispositions, attitudes, feelings. Parents treat boys and girls differently because they, the parents, have acquired from their own upbringings a set of expectations, of inclinations to respond to and stimulate boys and girls differentially.[59] Kagan and his co-workers report that upper-middle-class American mothers, at least, treat infant boys and girls differently, particularly in responding with more vocalizing to baby girls' vocalizations.[60] Thus, usually without thinking, they express their expectations through manner, through the things they do, through the sorts of objects with which they surround the baby and toward which they direct his attention and feelings. In short, they enclose the baby within a material, social, and emotional environment which tells him what his capacities for action and feeling are.

More concretely, American boys get blue things, girls get pink. Friends and relatives give the boy tiny trousers to grow into, and the girl frilly frocks. Boys get the playthings labeled masculine, girls feminine ones. This difference is not so marked in early infancy, when both boys and girls are given, for instance, stuffed animals to cuddle, but it exists, and it becomes even more pronounced when babies become able to manipulate objects. From toddlerhood onward, many parents forbid little boys to play with "girl's things," as though implying that masculinity is a fragile state of being, easily undermined by any deviation from the ideal. Boy babies can be handled boisterously; with girls one tends to be gentle. One takes pleasure in the delicate contour of a daughter's mouth; in a son one takes delight in how vigorous and husky he is. Some mothers have even reported that they find it less disagreeable to change a baby girl's dirty diapers than a little boy's.

It should not be necessary to labor further the point that boys and girls grow up in different, culturally determined emotional atmospheres from the beginning. As they become able to act for themselves and to move around, their initiatives meet with quite different responses, whether indifference, amusement, tolerance, anger, sympathy, punishment, or alarm. It requires no great powers of observation to conclude that it may make a difference whether, as a little boy, it is the female parent who shows great indulgence, or, as a little girl, the male parent. (In the next chapter, we shall have something to say about possible sexual components in the relations of parents and children of opposite sexes.) All the far-reaching implications for feeling and behavior that go with being male or female require years of elaboration, but it is as a baby that one receives one's first lessons in being a boy or a girl. Perhaps the strength of parental attitudes toward the sex of their child can be seen in these lines from Ogden Nash's "Song to Be Sung by the Father of Infant Female Children":

My heart leaps up when I behold
A rainbow in the sky;
Contrariwise, my blood runs cold
When little boys go by.
For little boys as little boys,
No special hate I carry,
But now and then they grow to men,
And when they do, they marry.
No matter how they tarry,
Eventually they marry.
And, swine among the pearls,
They marry little girls.*[61]

IMPLICATIONS OF CULTURAL SHAPING

It is an uncomfortable notion for many people that they would have been quite different individuals had they grown up in a different family or subcultural or cultural context, yet the conclusion seems inescapable. In the first place, there is no escaping the process of cultural learning. A child can develop normally only in contact with adults during a long apprenticeship, and there are no culture-free adults. As long as a mother is reacting to a child, whom she inevitably perceives in ways at least partially dictated by her cultural outlook, they are linked in a circuit of interpersonal exchange in which the mother is imparting and getting information about herself, the child, and the world in general.

All cultures work, at least until they disintegrate. But not all work equally well in producing members who are fully human and humane. It is perfectly clear that some cultures shape people in ways that produce endless social frictions, that set individuals at odds with each other, and that set up internal conflicts and dissatisfaction. Most cultures rely on tradition and precedent for solving problems, instead of encouraging inventiveness, innovation, and fresh approaches. Culture may warp or stultify or stunt our humanity. But the answer does not seem to be to do away with culture, even if we could. We have the dire example of what happens to "primitive" peoples when Europeans, sometimes with the best of intentions (or ingenious rationalizations), destroy established cultural forms without providing time, opportunity, and tutelage for the development and assimilation of new forms. In our own country, we have the plight of Negroes uprooted from Africa, held in slavery, where family ties were systematically destroyed, and then emancipated into prolonged lack

---

* Copyright, 1933, by Ogden Nash.

of identity with either the old or new way of life; of the American Indians; the Americans of Latin-American origin; the Eskimos; and the Polynesians of Hawaii and Samoa, all of whom, at least at the economically depressed levels, have been condemned to personal and social rot. Rather, we are in this generation in a unique position because we are coming to understand, as previous cultures could not, how culture operates, how we might remake culture, designing a new version of human nature and rearing our children in approximation of an ideal. Those most entrenched in our present cultural orientation, in other words the most ethnocentric among us, secure in a conviction that what we have is both right and inevitable—the product of human nature rather than its shaper—and that all else is destructive subversion, resist this view as unrealistic Utopianism. It seems to us, on the other hand, that the evidence suggests a great deal of plasticity in the human organism, and that we have a beginning understanding of what to do—and what not to do—if we are to raise our children to be humane, decent citizens of the world. This is not to say that it would be easy, but only that it is possible. And, we would add, highly desirable if we are to eliminate the worst miseries of being human.

Unfortunately, we know more about how to change human nature than about how to change the framework of social institutions within which human beings have to operate. And the more human human beings become, the greater the contrast between their humanity and the inhuman and dehumanizing institutions to which in most modern societies they are expected to adapt. Perhaps the best we can do at this stage of social evolution is to concentrate, in the family and in the schools, on producing trustful, autonomous, intelligent, compassionate, cooperative young people with a sense of humanity, and hope that they will in time reshape the society which they inherit. The anthropologists have taught us about ourselves, and we have the opportunity and the responsibility to make wise use of their teachings.[62]

REFERENCES / Chapter 3

[1] Bowlby, J. *Child Care and the Growth of Love.* London: Pelican, 1965; Goldfarb, W. Psychological privation in infancy and subsequent adjustment. *American Journal of Orthopsychiatry,* 1945, 15, 247–255; Ribble, M. A. *The Rights of Infants.* New York: Columbia University, 1943, revised edition, 1965; Spitz, R. A. The psychogenic diseases in infancy: An attempt at their etiologic classification. *Psychoanalytic Study of the Child,* 1951, 6, 255–275.

For more general discussions see: Ainsworth, M. D. The effects of maternal deprivation. *Public Health Papers,* no. 14. Geneva: World Health Organization, 1962; Stone, L. J. A critique of studies of infant isolation. *Child Development,* 1954, 25, 9–20; Spitz, R. A. *The First Year of Life.* New York: International Universities, 1965.

2 Provence, S., and Lipton, R. *Children in Institutions.* New York: International Universities, 1962.

3 White, B. L. The development of perception during the first six months of life. Paper read at meetings of the American Association for the Advancement of Science, 1963.

4 Dennis, W., and Najarian, P. Infant development under environmental handicap. *Psychological Monographs,* 1957, 71, no. 7.

5 Ross, J. B., and McLaughlin, M. M. (eds.) *A Portable Medieval Reader.* New York: Viking, 1949.

6 Harlow, H. F. The nature of love. *American Psychologist,* 1958, 13, 673–685; Harlow, H. F. The heterosexual affectional system in monkeys. *American Psychologist,* 1962, 17, 1–9. Research findings from Harlow's laboratory have been summarized by Sackett, G. P. Effect of rearing conditions upon the behavior of rhesus monkeys. *Child Development,* 1965, 36, 855–868.

7 Igel, G. J., and Calvin, A. D. The development of affectional responses in infant dogs. *Journal of Comparative and Physiological Psychology,* 1960, 53, 302–305.

8 Denenberg, V. H., Hudgens, G. A., and Zarrow, M. X. Mice reared with rats: Modification of behavior by early experience with another species. *Science,* 1963, 143, 380–381.

9 Forgays, D. G., and Forgays, J. W. The nature of the effect of free environmental experience in the rat. *Journal of Comparative and Physiological Psychology,* 1952, 45, 322–328.

10 Smith, C. J. Mass action and early environment in the rat. *Journal of Comparative and Physiological Psychology,* 1959, 52, 154–156.

11 Bennett, E. L., Diamond, M. C., Krech, D., and Rosenzweig, M. R. Chemical and anatomical plasticity of brain. *Science,* 1964, 146, 610–619.

12 Thompson, W. R., and Schaefer, T. Early environmental stimulation. In Fiske, D. W., and Maddi, S. R. (eds.) *Functions of Varied Experience.* Homewood, Ill.: Dorsey, 1961.

13 Levine, S. Psychophysiological effects of infantile stimulation. In Bliss, E. D. (ed.) *Roots of Behavior.* New York: Harper, 1962.

14 Rosenblatt, J. S., Turkevitz, G., and Schneirla, T. C. Early socialization in the domestic cat as based on feeding and other relationships between female and young. In Foss, B. M. (ed.) *Determinants of Infant Behavior.* New York: Wiley, 1961.

15 Scott, J. P. Critical periods in behavioral development. *Science,* 1962, 138, 949–958; Scott, J. P., and Fuller, J. L. *Genetics and the Social Behavior of the Dog.* Chicago: University of Chicago, 1965, Part II.

16 Ader, R. F. Social factors affecting emotionality and resistance to disease in animals: III. Early weaning and susceptibility to gastric ulcers in the

rat. A control for nutritional factors. *Journal of Comparative and Physiological Psychology,* 1962, 55, 600–602.

[17] Denenberg, V. H., and Whimbey, A. E. Infantile stimulation and animal husbandry: A methodological study. *Journal of Comparative and Physiological Psychology,* 1963, 56, 877–878.

[18] Hatch, A., Balazs, T., Wiberg, G. S., and Grice, H. C. Long-term isolation stress in rats. *Science,* 1963, 142, 507.

[19] Evans, B. *The Natural History of Nonsense.* New York: Vintage, 1958 (originally published in 1946); Ogburn, W. F., and Bose, N. K. On the trail of the wolf-children. *Genetic Psychology Monographs,* 1959, 60, 117–193.

[20] Montagu, M. F. A. *The Direction of Human Development.* New York: Harper, 1955, Chapter 11.

[21] Caldwell, B. M. The effects of infant care. In Hoffman, M. L., and Hoffman, L. W. (eds.) *Review of Child Development Research.* New York: Russell Sage, vol. I, 1964.

[22] Klatskin, E. H., Jackson, E. B., and Wilkin, L. C. The influence of degree of flexibility in maternal child care practices on early child behavior. *American Journal of Orthopsychiatry,* 1956, 26, 79–93.

[23] Haggard, E. A., Brekstad, A., and Skard, A. G. On the reliability of the anamnestic interview. *Journal of Abnormal and Social Psychology,* 1960, 61, 311–318; Pyles, M. K., Stolz, H. R., and Macfarlane, J. S. The accuracy of mothers' reports on birth and developmental data. *Child Development,* 1935, 6, 165–176.

[24] Schaefer, E. S. A circumplex model for maternal behavior. *Journal of Abnormal and Social Psychology,* 1959, 59, 226–235.

[25] Yarrow, L. J. Separation from parents during early childhood. In Hoffman, M. L., and Hoffman, L. W. *op. cit.*

[26] U. S. Department of Health, Education, and Welfare, Social Security Administration, Children's Bureau. *Bibliography on the Battered Child.* Washington: U. S. Government Printing Office, 1961 (mimeographed).

[27] Levy, D. M. Advice and reassurance. *American Journal of Public Health,* 1954, 44, 1113–1118.

[28] Clock, R. O. *Our Baby.* New York and London: Appleton, 1912. For a still earlier, and still more disaster-fraught account, see Ashby, H. *Health in the Nursery.* London: Longmans, Green, 1898.

[29] U. S. Dept. of Health, Education, and Welfare, Children's Bureau. *Infant Care.* Washington: U. S. Government Printing Office (periodically revised).

[30] Wolfenstein, M. The emergence of fun morality. *Journal of Social Issues,* 1951, 7, 15–25.

[31] Watson, J. B. *Psychological Care of Infant and Child.* New York: Norton, 1928.

[32] U. S. Dept. of H. E. W. *Infant Care,* 1938 edition, p. 3.

[33] Watson, *op. cit.,* p. 87.

[34] *Ibid.,* p. 186.

[35] Skinner, B. F. *Walden Two.* New York: Macmillan, 1948.

36 Chomsky, N. Review of *Verbal Behavior*, by B. F. Skinner. *Language*, 1959, 35, 26–58.

37 Solomon, R. L. Punishment. *American Psychologist*, 1963, 18, 239–253.

38 Gyorgy, P., Dhanamitta, S., and Steers, E. Protective effects of human milk in experimental staphylococcus infection. *Science*, 1962, 137, 338–340.

39 Davis, C. M. Results of the self-selection of diets by young children. *Canadian Medical Association Journal*, 1939, 41, 257–261.

40 Cannon, W. B. *Wisdom of the Body*. New York: Norton, 1939.

41 Richter, C. P. Total self-regulatory functions in animals and human beings. *Harvey Lectures*, 1942–43, 38, 63–103.

42 Kessler, J. W. *Psychopathology of Childhood*. Englewood Cliffs: Prentice-Hall, 1966, pp. 106–108.

43 Roberts, E. Thumb and finger sucking in relation to feeding in early infancy. *American Journal of Diseases of Children*, 1944, 68, 7–8.

44 Levy, D. M. Experiments on the sucking reflex and social behavior in dogs. *American Journal of Orthopsychiatry*, 1934, 4, 203–224; Levy, D. M. On the instinct-satiation: An experiment on the pecking behavior of chickens. *Journal of Genetic Psychology*, 1938, 18, 327–348.

45 Calhoun, J. G. Population density and social pathology. *Scientific American*, February, 1962, pp. 139–148; Thiessen, D. D., and Rodgers, D. A. Population density and endocrine function. *Psychological Bulletin*, 1961, 58, 441–451.

46 Davis, H. V., Sears, R. R., Miller, H. C., and Brodbeck, A. J. Effects of cup, bottle, and breast feeding on oral activities of newborn infants. *Pediatrics*, 1948, 2, 549–558.

47 Commager, H. S. (ed.) *America in Perspective*. New York: New American Library, 1947; DuBois, C. The dominant value profile of American culture. *American Anthropologist*, 1955, 57, 1232–1239; Goodman, P. *Growing Up Absurd*. New York: Random House, 1960; Lynes, R. *A Surfeit of Honey*. New York: Harper, 1957; Riesman, D., in collaboration with Reuel Denny and Nathan Glazer. *The Lonely Crowd*. New Haven: Yale, 1950.

48 Smith, R. P. *"Where Did You Go?" "Out." "What Did You Do?" "Nothing."* New York: Norton, 1957. (Also available in paperback.)

49 Simpson, G. G. The biological nature of man. *Science*, 1966, 152, 472–478.

50 Weinreich, U. On the semantic structure of language. In Greenberg, J. H. (ed.) *Universals of Language*. Cambridge: M.I.T., 1963.

51 Whiting, J. S. M., and Child, I. L. *Child Training and Personality*. New Haven: Yale, 1953.

52 Altus, W. D. Birth order and its sequelae. *Science*, 1966, 151, 44–49; Altus, W. D. First born and last born children in a child development clinic. *Journal of Individual Psychology*, 1964, 20, 179–182; Ring, K., Lipinski, C. E., and Braginsky, D. The relationship of birth order to self-evaluation, anxiety reduction, and susceptibility to emotional contagion. *Psychological Monographs*, 1965, 79, no. 10; Sampson, E. E. The study of ordinal position: Antecedents and outcomes (1964, mimeographed); Stotland, E., and Dunn, R. E. Identification, "oppositeness," authoritarianism, self-esteem, and birth

order. *Psychological Monographs,* 1962, 76, no. 9. These titles are only a sample of the recent voluminous research on this subject.

[53] Rosenzweig, M. R. Environmental complexity, cerebral change, and behavior. *American Psychologist,* 1966, 21, 321–332.

[54] Eleftheriou, B. E. Unpublished doctoral dissertation, Purdue University, 1961.

[55] Altmann, S. A. (ed.) *Social Communication among Primates.* Chicago: University of Chicago, 1966.

[56] Church, J., and Insko, C. A. Ethnic and sex differences in sexual values. *Psychologia,* 1965, 8, 153–157.

[57] Lowie, R. H. Review of Gusinde, M. *Die Feuerlander Indianer.* Mödling bei Wein: Anthropos, 1937. *American Anthropologist,* 1938, 40, 495–503.

[58] Van den Berg, J. H. *The Changing Nature of Man.* New York: Dell, 1964; Platt, J. R. The step to man. *Science,* 1965, 149, 607–613.

[59] Rothbart, M. K., and Maccoby, E. E. Parents' differential reactions to sons and daughters. *Journal of Personality and Social Psychology,* 1966, 4, 237–243.

[60] Levine, J., Fishman, C., and Kagan, J. Social class and sex as determinants of maternal behavior. Paper read at meetings of the American Orthopsychiatric Association, 1967. An unpublished study in 1967, by Henrietta T. Smith, of institutional infants at "Metera," in Athens, shows that nurses tend to reward girls' positive social overtures but to respond to boys' negative behavior.

[61] From *Many Long Years Ago,* by Ogden Nash, by permission of Little, Brown & Co.

[62] L. K. Frank gives an interesting overview of infancy, including the anthropological approach, in *On the Importance of Infancy.* New York: Random House, 1966. PP 32; see also Ainsworth, M. D. S. *Infancy in Uganda.* Baltimore: Johns Hopkins University, 1967.

4 *Developmental Principles and Approaches*

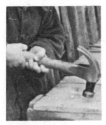The study of human behavior and development is not merely a search for facts. It also involves finding a pattern in the facts, general principles that will enable us both to understand how we as adults got to be the way we are and to know how to guide the development of children sensibly. In the first three chapters, we set forth a great many facts and suggested some key principles. It is now time to try to pull together what we know, so as to make sense of what has gone before and to prepare for what is still to come.

Some Representative Theoretical Orientations

PSYCHOANALYTIC THEORIES

Let us begin by taking a somewhat closer look at a few of the more salient views of human nature, starting with the views of Sigmund Freud, who was a major modern contributor to the discovery of human childhood as an area of serious investigation. The reader should remember that Freud had very little direct contact with children and constructed his account of development from self-observations, some observations of his own children, and the reconstructions and recollections of his adult patients—his one famous child patient, Little Hans, was treated indirectly, through Hans' father. Freud's was primarily a dynamic, that is, motivational, theory of behavior, although, as we shall see, it always had cognitive and intellectual components. These were later elaborated on by some of Freud's followers, such as Ernst Kris, Heinz Hartmann, David Rapaport, Erik Erikson, and Freud's own daughter, Anna, all of whom became known as psychoanalytic ego psychologists. Freud acknowledged a wide variety of human motives, or drives, but in the end he concerned himself mainly with two: libido, or sexual energy, and the death wish, or a drive to destruction of self or others (these two motivational forces have been dubbed Eros and Thanatos, from the Greek words for [carnal] love and death).

Freud proposed a three-way conceptual partition of the person into *id*, the blind strivings of Eros and Thanatos and the source of all the person's motives and energies; *ego*, the rational, reality-oriented part of the person (whence ego psychology); and *superego*, corresponding approximately to the conscience, the moral and ethical part of the person's make-up. Developmentally, the baby at birth is considered to be pure id, a seething mass of passions governed exclusively by what Freud called the *pleasure principle*, unbridled seeking for immediate gratification. Needless to say, the baby's greedy id-strivings collide almost at once with an only partially yielding reality, and out of this collision of forces and frustrations there develops a layer of ego, constituting the practical strategies and the capacity for delay and detour by which the developing person can take account of reality in the quest for id gratification. The ego, that is, is governed by the *reality principle* taking account of what is already possible or of the means of making gratification possible. The kinds of thinking that accompany the id-based, pleasure principle in its search for immediate gratification, whether in the young baby, in adult dreams, in daydreams or fantasies, or in psychosis, are called *primary-process* thought, whereas the reality-oriented thinking associated with the ego is called *secondary process*. Finally, not in infancy but in early childhood, and in ways that we shall discuss shortly, a portion of the ego becomes further differentiated as superego, imparting an ethical-moral, socially responsible dimension, in addition to the purely pragmatic reality principle, to the search for gratification of the id-impulses.

The differentiation of some of the id into ego and of ego into superego can be seen as a process of cognitive development. Side by side with it goes a series of motivational changes in what Freud called the *psychosexual stages* of development. Note that the motivations remain the same throughout life; it is the manner of their expression that changes. Psychosexual development refers to shifts in the channels or zones of the body through which id gratification is sought and obtained, and in the objects which serve as gratifiers.

4 Psychosexual Stages *#1* The first of the psychosexual stages is called the *oral phase,* during infancy, when the main channel of gratification is the mouth and upper digestive tract, and the gratifying objects are the nipple and the mother who provides it—plus, to a lesser extent, the thumb, pacifier, or whatever else the baby puts in his mouth. In the Freudian view, the infant's eating is not merely a matter of appeasing hunger and assuring organic survival, but also a source of proto-erotic satisfaction. Furthermore, since the baby destroys what he has consumed, he is simultaneously satisfying his death wish. Early infancy, before the baby's teeth have sprouted, is called the *oral-passive* period. Later, when he has acquired enough teeth to begin to bite, he enters the *oral-sadistic* period in which the aggressive (Thanatos) component becomes even more conspicuous.

#2 In the period we call toddlerhood, according to Freud, the main channel of gratification, subject to some restrictions we shall touch on later, ceases to be the mouth and becomes the lower digestive tract and anus, and the baby enters the *anal stage* of psychosexual development. This period, in which the baby gains control over the anal sphincter and the process of holding on to and expelling bowel movements, is supposedly marked by preoccupation with anal functions, to the point where having his bottom spanked may be pleasurable to the baby. The anal period was thought of by Freud as a time of inevitable conflict between parents and child over who shall regulate the time and place of defecation, and the baby gets ample exercise of his destructive tendencies in withholding bowel movements when his parents want him to let go, by expelling feces when his parents want him to hold on, and by smearing his feces in an act of defiance.

#3 If all goes normally during the anal period, the source of gratification shifts to the genitals, and the preschool years are described as the *phallic stage*—a designation betraying Freud's male-centered view of behavior. The phallic stage, in which gratification is sought without concern for the feelings of other people, is distinguished from the *genital stage* of adolescence and adulthood, characterized not only by mature sexuality in the usual sense but also by love and a concern for others' feelings.

The phallic stage evolves into and culminates in the *Oedipus complex,* named for the tragic hero of Greek legend, King Oedipus, who unwittingly but in fulfillment of a prophecy made at his birth slew his father and married his mother. According to Freud, the boy (we shall talk in a moment about the girl's Oedipus—or, as it is sometimes called, Electra—complex) directs his phallic strivings toward the mother, putting himself in direct rivalry with the father, whom he ambivalently both hates and loves. The father is seen as retaliating with an open or implied threat to injure or cut off the boy's penis—a threat of castration. This threat is usually viewed as being expressed in the context of punishing the boy's masturbation: In actuality such threats are made by some parents, and were doubtless more prevalent in Freud's day.

The child, by now about age five, moved both by fear of castration and by love for his father, capitulates, renouncing his claim on the mother's favors and at the same time *repressing* (forcing out of consciousness) all sexual cravings. This renunciation of sexuality brings the child into the stage of psychosexual *latency*, corresponding to the middle years of childhood, which ends only when the physiological developments of adolescence bring a new upsurge of more mature sexual feelings, destroying the quiescence of latency. Furthermore, in capitulating to the father, the son is said to *identify* with him, to take on his styles of action, and to *internalize*, to make a part of himself, his father's moral values, which form the basis of the superego. That is, the parental prescriptions and proscriptions that formerly came to him as "thou shalt" and "thou shalt not" now speak to him in his own voice, saying, "*I* must" and "*I* must not," and arouse feelings of *guilt* when violated. To keep sexuality (and excessive aggression) at bay, the ego brings into play several of the *mechanisms of defense*, one of which is repression, already mentioned, and other stratagems by which one reinforces the repression of dangerous cravings and impulses.

The superego is initially a rigid, tyrannical sort of conscience, which only later becomes more flexible and tolerant (corresponding accurately to empirical findings that children shift from literal to relative concepts of morality), and the ego is hard put to mediate among the insistent clamor of the id, the harsh moralism of the superego, and the realities of the outside world. For Freud, a psychiatrist oriented to disturbed—particularly neurotic—forms of behavior, the defense mechanisms were always defenses against oneself, not the world outside. For instance, the child engages in *reaction formation*, a going to the opposite extreme, as when he rejects not only sexuality but the opposite sex in general—middle-years boys notoriously will have nothing to do with girls or "sissy stuff." By the mechanism of *sublimation*, the id-energies are transformed into socially acceptable drives, as, for example, the school-age child's new concern with intellectual, objective learning—Freudians would say that it is the resolution of the Oedipus complex that makes children ready for school, and that some of those children who do badly in school are suffering from an unresolved Oedipus complex.

The *obsessive-compulsive* mechanisms found in adult neurotics (extremes of meticulousness, repetitive hand-washing, and so on) have their counterparts in the *repetition* and *ritual* of the normal child as seen in such activities as counting all the cars of a freight train, having to touch every lamppost, holding one's breath until one reaches the corner, or avoiding the cracks in the sidewalk to the tune of "Step on a crack, break your mother's back"—which Freudians would interpret as a disguised expression of ambivalent hostility (and associated guilt and fear) against the now unattainable mother. Other well-known defense mechanisms are *projection,* whereby one ascribes one's own unconscious motivations to other people, and *rationalization,* whereby one justifies evilly motivated behavior in terms of some virtuous or neutral purpose.

Freud never formulated to his own satisfaction the course of the Oedipus complex in girls, but offered the following sketch. Initially, the girl's Oedipus complex is identical with the boy's: The girl, considered to assume that she has a penis, addresses her attentions to the mother in competition with the father. For the girl, however, the crisis comes not with the threat of castration at the hands of the father but with the dreadful discovery that she has been castrated (and amputated)—presumably her interpretation of the female genitalia. At this juncture, the girl can react in either of two ways. Ordinarily she is seen as now identifying with the mother, and competing for the father—seeking a baby from him in fantasy as a substitute counterpart of the lost penis. In the face of reality she then will shift from actual striving for the father's favors to substitute father-figures, repressing her impulses as she reaches latency. The girl's (less common) alternative reaction to castration is called the *masculine protest,* a persistent if symbolic denial of the loss of the penis and the pursuit of an essentially masculine style of life (whether or not involving the practice of Lesbianism), with a more or less permanent inability to play a feminine role in love or marriage. Such women are called by Freudians "castrating females," possessed by *penis envy,* as though seeking to take away from men what rightfully belongs to women.

Both boys and girls, reaching maturity, are seen as seeking mates with whom (in part) to reenact their earlier Oedipal attachments—"I want a girl just like the girl who married dear old Dad." Indeed, all close attachments, including that formed to the psychoanalyst in therapy (*transference*), are viewed as partial reenactments of the ambivalent relations to the parents formed in infancy and early childhood.

It is worth mentioning parenthetically that Freudians invoke the repression that climaxes the Oedipal drama to explain *infantile amnesia,* the fact that we find it hard or impossible to remember anything more than disconnected fragments of events happening before age five or six. It is as though the repressed sexual feelings took with them all the associated events, to be recaptured only in the special condition of hypnosis or the *abreaction*—the reliving process—of psychoanalytic psychotherapy.

We should note that normal psychosexual development requires the enactment by child and parents alike of strictly fixed roles in the psychosexual drama. These roles are thought of as instinctive, and so are considered *biological imperatives.* Any departure from the biological imperatives is considered to lead to more or less serious disturbances of functioning.

Before discussing some of the more common departures from the normal course, we must introduce another Freudian concept, that of *cathexis.* At each psychosexual stage, one's supply of libidinal energy is said to be invested, or *cathected,* in the relevant channel and the important gratifying objects associated with that stage. Thus, in the oral stage of infancy, the child's mouth is said to be libidinized (that is, it has acquired erotic meaning), and the bottle or breast—and, by extension, the mother—cathected (has erotic meaning attached to it). When the needs associated with a given stage are gratified, the child is said to withdraw his cathexes and reinvest his energy in the new zones and objects of the next stage. If, however, inadequate gratification is given, all or part of the child's cathexes may remain *fixated* at that stage, that is, the child may still go on seeking the gratifications appropriate to a stage which he is supposed to have outgrown. Paradoxically, fixation can be produced both by insufficient gratification, which leaves him ever hungering, or by overgratification, which leaves the child so well satisfied with his present mode of existence that he is, so to speak, reluctant to move on. But assuming that a child has found satisfaction at one level and moved on, if he then encounters excessive frustration at a later stage, he may *regress*—that is, go back—to the last earlier stage at which he found satisfaction, so that the baby who finds the demands of toilet training in toddlerhood, say, too taxing, may revert to the clinging helplessness and orality of infancy.

Now it is clear that total fixation at or permanent regression to childhood patterns of behavior would be a rare and profoundly pathological style of life. However, the Freudians have a system of adult character types said to express partial fixations at early levels of psychosexual development. Thus, the adult "oral character" is marked by infantile, dependent, demanding behavior, and by a preoccupation with oral gratifications: eating, gum-chewing, smoking, nail-biting, drinking, pencil-chewing, garrulous talking, and whatever. Oral sadism, deriving from the second oral stage, would be shown not only in a literal tendency to bite but in the symbolic biting expressed in harsh words. Fixation at the anal stage might be expressed in either the "anal-retentive character," who seems to have learned too well the lessons of control, orderliness, and regularity associated with bowel training, and whose behavior is marked by stinginess, accumulating and collecting of money or other valuables, rigid adherence to forms and routines, suspicion, legalistic ways of thinking, and what has been described as "emotional constipa- tion"; or the "anal-aggressive character," who seems still to be fighting the battle of bowel control and who expresses his rebellion against authority by extreme messiness in personal habits and grooming, by indifference to routines and schedules, and even by the tendency to "dirty" language, which can be seen as a symbolic befouling or "soiling" of the environment or those around him. The "phallic character" would be one who selfishly exploits others sexually, without regard to their needs, concerns, or feelings—in males, the Don Juan or the sexual psychopath or the rapist, in females the self-centered nymphomaniac.

A few other features of the Freudian system should be mentioned. For Freud, significant motivations and their alterations by defense mechanisms were primarily unconscious, and the true mainsprings of behavior lay deep in organic nature. In the course of ego development, some features of experience enter consciousness, including a certain limited knowledge of oneself and one's motives. The knowledge that is not conscious at the moment but is available to consciousness is said to reside in the *preconscious,* as in the case of all those things we can easily remember. The *unconscious* is thought to contain both those strivings that have never been conscious and those that have started forth and then been repressed, for instance, the Oedipal impulses. The pres- ence of unconscious strivings is inferred from evidence of the operation of defense mechanisms, from self-betrayals in such forms as selective forgetting, making meaningful mistakes and slips of the tongue, and from the content of dreams, which are supposed to be symbolic, more or less disguised representations of all the unfulfilled cravings that come out of hiding during sleep, when the person's defenses are down. In short, people constantly do things for reasons that they do not recognize and may even deny.

Having sketched the formal elements of the Freudian system, let us say that Freud made a monumental contribution to our understanding of human behavior. Certainly we can see something like oral preoccupations in infancy—people sometimes describe the baby as being "all mouth." Certainly we can see Oedipus-like or Electra-like behavior in the preschool years, as when the child lavishes affection on the opposite-sex parent, even inviting that parent to share the child's bed, meanwhile telling the same-sex parent to go away, or turning that parent's picture to the wall. (In adults, we can see persistent Oedipal tendencies in people who marry mother-surrogates or father-surrogates.) Certainly we can see people living at odds with their own motives, practicing self-deception (which may deceive no one else) on a staggering scale, and in general struggling to get loose from leftover problems of childhood, including overinvolvement with parents. Certainly we can see ambivalence, strong hostility as well as strong affection to parents and to others who are very close—and certainly the hostility is sometimes veiled and indirect though indubitably there. We can see Freudian symbolism not only in our dreams (one six-year-old girl dreamed that a raging bull trampled down a fence and gored her in the bottom, but, strangely enough, it was "sort of pleasant"), but in myths and fairy tales. Consider the symbolism of the ogre in "Jack and the Beanstalk," of the oven in which the ogre's wife hides Jack, of Jack's cutting down the beanstalk, and of his using the gold stolen from the slain ogre to live alone with his mother. Irrationality and absurdity are everywhere around us, and Freud has taught us to look beyond face values.

Nevertheless, we feel that Freud's brilliant contribution has serious shortcomings, some of them acknowledged by his less orthodox followers. It accounts much better for pathological behavior than for normality, and almost not at all for what we consider superior styles of life. It is possible that babies born in nineteenth- and early twentieth-century Vienna were turbulent bundles of id—or were made so by parental practices—but the babies we know are not only intent on immediate gratifications and sometimes perverse but also cheerful, curious, playful, often affectionate without detectable undertones of salacious desire, and given to joyously pursuing and practicing mastery of skills and objects.

In general, like most drive theories, Freud's deals with unsatisfied (and even insatiable) instincts, but, as Robert W. White[1] has pointed out, a complete psychology has to deal also with the behavior of organisms which are awake and in reasonable equilibrium, free from the goading of deficiency drives. Indeed, one may say that human beings are at their most human when their basic biological needs are least involved.

The behavior of a human being in the throes of asphyxiating, choking, starving, or parching is not much different from that of any other animal. And when biological needs are satisfied, they cannot be invoked to account for love, curiosity, the higher learning, imagination, humor, foresight, symbolic activity, and all else that is distinctively human. Just as the old economics of scarcity, in which there is not enough to go around, must yield, in an age of mechanized production and population control, to an economics of abundance, so in the behavioral sciences must deficiency theories yield to accounts of the behavior of organisms whose basic needs have been satisfied. For the replete organism, as White says, does not invariably drift off into the blissful Nirvana of semicoma, but looks around to see what there is to do next. (This Nirvana concept of motivation is the psychological extension of the physiological concept of homeostasis—seeking the resting-state.) In White's view, boredom becomes as great a spur to action as lust or hunger.

In terms of development, Freud laid more stress on the determining power of biology (in his own version), and less on the influence of experience with people and things (except for the preordained acting out of the biological imperatives), than present evidence on the effects of early experience makes tenable. But whatever the flaws in Freud's formulations, we can see them only because Freud himself opened our eyes (in Erich Fromm's phrase, people stand on Freud's shoulders and, because they can see so much farther than he, consider him a pigmy; this is a variant of the usual figure of speech, which has the modern pigmy standing on the shoulders of giants.[2]), and he showed us phenomena that any adequate theory of behavior is going to have to include. While it may be that Freud's theory was too intricate and complex to lend itself easily to empirical verification or disproof, he at least tried to deal with the full richness of human behavior as it is known to the dramatist, to the novelist, and to the painter.

Freud was the father of psychoanalysis, but his was not the only analytic school. There are several varieties, most of them founded by former colleagues of Freud's as schismatic movements which Freud himself considered heretical. Carl Jung, of Switzerland, presided over a religiously oriented school which lays much stress on the *racial* or *collective unconscious* (an idea found in Freud, too), the basic patterns or structures which guide ideation. These supposedly universal patterns are called *archetypes,* and, as Jung has shown, are found in many cultures. In this view, life is more a search for understanding (as of the way archetypes shape behavior) than for direct or indirect carnal gratifications.

Otto Rank originally built his system around the *trauma of birth,* a lifelong attempt to return to the warm, safe nothingness of intrauterine existence, from which the newborn babe is cast into a cold, hostile, and unmanageable world. As Rank's thinking evolved, he became more concerned with *will therapy,* designed to help people know what they really wanted, instead of living with the agony of formless dissatisfactions, and to feel free to want it. Rank's influence is still visible in several current versions, including the *non-directive therapy* of Carl Rogers, which places responsibility for his own psychological welfare on the client rather than the therapist, and, more explicitly, in the teachings of many schools of social work.

Alfred Adler, a Viennese socialist, was far more concerned than Freud with social influences on development, in keeping with his Marxian orientation. To Adler we owe such notions as *sibling rivalry,* the warfare among brothers and sisters for the affection of the parents, with much emphasis on the dethronement of the firstborn child from his place of unique eminence by the arrival of younger children. Adler also gave us the concept of masculine protest, already mentioned, and of *organ inferiority,* the sense of weakness or inadequacy (beginning with every child's smallness and helplessness) that keeps people striving and drives them to extremes of *compensation* to make up for their real or imagined insufficiencies in stature or competence. Organ inferiority was the basis of Adler's concept of "inferiority complex." Basically, Adler's is a more optimistic, problem-solving view of man than is Freud's.

In the United States, as we have said, a school of anthropologically and sociologically oriented psychoanalysis has developed alongside the orthodox one. The roster of this group includes such names as Harry Stack Sullivan, Karen Horney, and Erich Fromm. Horney and Fromm have been extremely critical of modern civilization and the social and personal ills it begets. Where Freud saw civilization as a painfully and partially attained modification of the violence of the id, in their view, modern society is itself inhuman and dehumanizing, and those who try to live lives of love and virtue, representing man's basic strivings, will inevitably find themselves in torment. We have already mentioned the work of Erik Erikson, who perhaps comes closest to bridging the Freudian and post-Freudian approaches. Erikson evolved a scheme of considerable use in the study of development, describing the eight stages of man, which are a more generalized statement of the Freudian psychosexual stages. Thus, as we have seen, the oral stage of infancy becomes for Erikson the period for the formation of basic trust or mistrust, which are seen as closely implicated with the oral experience of hunger and feeding but which are also related to the dependability with which other basic needs are met. As we shall see in the next chapter, Freud's anal period of toddlerhood is elaborated by Erikson as the time for the development of either autonomy or attitudes of shame and doubt.

LEARNING THEORIES OF DEVELOPMENT

The learning-theory tradition, which lays heavy emphasis on the role of the environment in shaping modes of behavior, has two main antecedents. The first of these is British associationism, characterized by John Locke's doctrine of the newborn as a *tabula rasa,* a clean slate (literally, a wax tablet shaved clean) on which the world writes or impresses its message. The message the world writes on the individual consists of associations, a set of connections between events that occur together in time and space. Associationism found its scientific expression in the second major forebear of learning theories, Ivan Pavlov's conditioned reflex theory.

The basic tenet of learning theories is that the elaboration of behavior observable in the course of development can be explained, apart from a few concessions to physical growth and maturation, as the continuous formation of connections among stimuli and responses. Pavlov, as is widely known, demonstrated that one can link arbitrary, experimentally manipulated stimuli (called *conditioned* or *conditional* stimuli) to already existing "natural," *unconditioned* stimuli that reliably elicit a fixed, *unconditioned* response. This is accomplished by introducing the conditioned stimulus just prior to the natural, unconditioned one. Thus, if food is an unconditioned stimulus for salivation, sounding a bell immediately before giving a dog food causes the bell alone to become the stimulus, after a few pairings, for salivation, even when no food is given. One can, in the laboratory, establish a great many conditioned associations, limited only by the number of unconditioned stimulus-response sequences one can identify. One can make some arbitrary event cause the pupil to contract as though a bright light were about to flash, or the eye to blink as though it were about to be subjected to a puff of air.

Pavlov and his contemporary, Bekhterev, for the most part, studied the conditioning of simple reflexes, the way the organism reacts to having something done to it—secretory responses, muscle twitch or limb flexion to vibration or electric shock, and so forth—many of them describable as vegetative responses mediated through the autonomic nervous system. In contrast to reflex reactions, there are also instrumental acts, the things the organism does in response to its own inner states, such as the hungry rat's looking for food in a maze. American behaviorists such as Watson extended Pavlov's *classical conditioning* model to include instrumental, goal-directed behavior. As we shall see shortly, another branch of American behaviorism provides separate accounts for classical and instrumental conditioning. The classical conditioning technique has proved very useful in the study of perceptual discrimination and generalization. For instance, one can sound one particular tone as a signal for food, and introduce a different tone unrelated to feeding, and the animal learns to react to the relevant tone and to disregard the irrelevant one. As the difference between the tones is reduced, the animal's responses allow us to infer the limits of discrimination. On the other hand, if only a single tone is used in a conditioning experiment, the animal will "generalize" his response to a great variety of tones introduced later on.

The fundamental form of classical conditioning is between a stimulus and a response, but repeated associations of stimuli can lead to stimulus-stimulus conditioning, as when Tristram Shandy's mother formed a connection between the periodic conjunction of her husband's winding the clock and then having intercourse with her, causing her to cry out at a delicate moment, "Pray, my Dear, have you not forgot to wind up the clock?" One can also form response-response connections, as in the habitual sequence of actions by which one gets dressed—here we have the phenomenon of "equivalent acts" which may be substituted in a response-response sequence, so that if the child asks his father to tie his shoes just as the father is about to tie his own shoes, the father may go forth with his shoelaces dangling. Response-response conditioning can be invoked to account for behavior when no external stimulus can be found to explain it. Thus, in the language of associationism, states of the organism such as hunger, thirst, sexual arousal, attitudes, or expectations can be described as responses which in turn stimulate yet other responses.

Associationism has been a potent force in American psychology. In the Pavlovian tradition, Clark Hull and his students, notably Kenneth Spence, have greatly elaborated on the classical conditioning model to take account of more subtle learning such as the formation of concepts and latent learning.

In this view, *concept formation* is seen as establishing an equivalence among a group of stimuli on the basis of the number of "identical elements" the stimuli have in common. Thus, the concept "man" includes all those beings who share such identical elements as deep voices, facial hair, masculine styles of dress and haircuts, and so forth. (Later in this book [see page 312], we shall propose a similar view which relies not so much on specific identical elements as on equivalence, first, of global physiognomies and, at a more advanced stage, of logical relatedness: a signal flare and a telephone have little perceptual similarity, but we can recognize that they both are equivalent to the extent of being "means of communication.")

Latent (incidental) *learning* takes place in the absence of any demonstrable motivation or reinforcement (reward), as when the hungry white rat, exploring the maze for food, also learns incidentally where water is to be found in the maze, so that he goes directly to the water when he is placed in the maze thirsty instead of hungry. A great deal of our learning, such as our learning about space and time, about values, and, indeed, the cultural learning we have already described, seems to be of this latent, incidental sort. The fact of latent learning was long used to counter association theory, and for a time associationists denied its very existence. Now, the Hull-Spence position seems to be that latent learning follows the same course as overt stimulus-response learning, except that the motivation, response, and reinforcement are fractional rather than full-blown, so that the somewhat thirsty animal, even if he does not actually drink the water, is nevertheless partially reinforced by the mere sight of it. Hull evolved a whole set of axioms to describe the learning process, including a set of propositions about the strength of drives and inhibitions, habit-family hierarchies (the likelihood that any one of a group of competing responses would be released in given circumstances), and secondary or substitute reinforcers (the tokens that can appease the animal without actually satisfying his physical needs, as a pacifier lessens hunger pangs). The Hull-Spence model (the axioms and the predictions derived from them) gives a fairly good account of some cases of learning, but its predictions have been disappointed in numerous other cases, even after much tinkering with the basic axioms and the adding of new assumptions (such as those used to account for latent learning). The reader who wishes a detailed discussion is referred to Hilgard.[3] In general, the system has become more cumbersome than the facts it sets out to explain, and so has little utility. Shortly before his death, however, Spence published papers assigning much greater weight to cognitive factors than a strict behaviorism would allow, which may signal a decided change in the learning-theory camp.[4]

A number of Hull's collaborators, including John Dollard, Neal Miller (whose more recent work has been in brain biochemistry), and Robert Sears, have sought to fuse Hullian learning theory and Freudian psychodynamics with a particular view to showing the learned (as opposed to instinctive) basis of motives. Their best-known contribution has been the hypothesis that aggression is always produced by frustration, and, conversely, that frustration always leads to aggression. The hypothesis was fruitful in inspiring research, and many of the predictions derived from it were verified. However, while it can be shown that in certain circumstances, frustration and aggression do go together, the generality of the hypothesis has been mooted by numerous observations. A famous study by Barker, Dembo, and Lewin,[5] for instance, showed that one possible outcome of frustration is regression, behavior at a less mature level than before frustration was introduced. Rosenzweig[6] has shown the variety of reactions frustration may produce. Common-sense observation suggests that one can sometimes react to frustration constructively, as by seeking new solutions to a problem.

Another way of looking at instrumental acts, in addition to the stimuli with which they are associated, is in terms of their outcomes, the practical consequences they produce. In classical instrumental conditioning, the experimenter provides rewards if the animal behaves properly, for example, there is food waiting if the animal goes to the correct arm of the maze. A second kind of instrumental conditioning, made prominent initially by E. L. Thorndike, arranges things so that the animal itself makes things happen and is rewarded as an intrinsic result of doing the right thing. Thus, if the animal can learn to work the latch on the cage door, he is rewarded by being liberated from the cage. Thorndike phrased this relationship between the animal's own activity and the rewarding results it produces as the *law of effect*, which says simply that those behaviors that lead to satisfying consequences tend to be repeated under like circumstances. Initially, the law of effect went parallel with another that said that annoyance (equivalent to punishment) as a consequence of behavior tended to weaken and, eventually, to *extinguish* the behavior, but later observations led Thorndike to drop this part of his formulation. Instead, the extinction of behavior is said to occur simply because of the lack of satisfying consequences, the lack of reinforcement.

As we have said, Solomon[7] has collected evidence suggesting that Thorndike and his followers may have been too hasty in abandoning the

177

principle of annoyance, since it seems to be the timing of punishment that determines whether it inhibits behavior. Thus, punishment given at the very inception of an act thoroughly inhibits its repetition, while punishment given immediately on completion of an act is a somewhat less effective deterrent. The longer punishment is delayed after completion of the act, the less effective it becomes. This formulation might serve to explain why punishment rarely deters criminals. In fact, the criminal act itself, such as committing a burglary, may be successful and thus get reinforced, whereas it is behavior later in the total sequence, such as trying to dispose of the stolen goods or confiding to a girl friend, that gets punished. Strictly by theory, the criminal would be encouraged by the reinforcement of the act of burglary to try again, whereas the punishment would teach him to modify his post-burglary behavior. In Thorndike's view, behavior was essentially shapeless and random, being produced by a diffuse state of disequilibrium, such as that engendered by hunger or fear. Those components of random behavior that happened to produce satisfying effects were retained, whereas those that did not were not. In this way, amorphous behavior could be given shape and made to appear as though it were directed from within, whereas in fact it was the pattern of effects that was responsible. Reinforcement can be thought of as effective either because it is rewarding (that is, because it satisfies some need and reduces tension) or because it supplies information, akin to feedback, that guides the organism in intelligent action. Estes and his collaborators[8] have devised techniques to assess separately the relative contributions of reward and information to the learning process, and it appears, as in Spence's findings mentioned earlier, that information is at least as important as need reduction.

Work on the law of effect has been carried forward by B. F. Skinner, whose prescriptions for child-rearing we have already outlined, and his collaborators. Skinner prefers to speak of *operant* learning or conditioning instead of instrumental, an operant being a whole class of instrumental acts which may differ in the way they are performed but still produce the same effect. Thus, the somewhat different instrumental acts of saying at the dinner table, "Please pass the salt," "Give me the salt, please," and "May I please have the salt?" all produce the same result and so belong to the operant class of asking-for-the-salt. Skinner's radical behaviorism goes beyond Thorndike also in its doctrine of the empty organism (the ultimate *tabula rasa*), according to which the newborn baby can be described entirely in terms of the capacities for action built into his physical constitution, the reflexes that enter into classical conditioning, and the motivational states that will set the baby in random motion. From there on, the law of effect takes over to give shape to the baby's behavior and can be exploited by the parent or educator to make of the child what he will—likewise the trainer of animals.

Among the specific contributions of Skinner and his co-workers is the analysis of *schedules of reinforcement*. Instead of reinforcing the animal (usually a pigeon in Skinner's laboratory) every time he gives the correct response, one can reinforce some fixed percentage of occurrences of a particular response, or space reinforcements according to some average time interval. Some interesting findings emerge from this sort of analysis. For instance, if reinforcement is given consistently and then discontinued, the reinforced response extinguishes very rapidly; but if reinforcement has been given only intermittently, extinction is greatly attenuated. However, this principle does not seem to hold, as we have seen, when it comes to extinguishing bedtime crying in young infants. Skinner has also demonstrated a phenomenon he calls "superstition"—a completely irrelevant act occurring just prior to a reinforced relevant one may also be reinforced and thus be incorporated into the total response, so that the pigeon invariably stretches its neck or pirouettes before pecking the key that brings it food. Skinner has also demonstrated the possibility of teaching an animal behavioral *chains*, elaborate sequences of actions which bring the animal reinforcement.

Skinner shares with S. L. Pressey the paternity of the teaching-machine and programed-instruction movement in the United States. In programed instruction (whether or not presented via a machine) an area of knowledge is broken down into small steps or units which are presented one at a time in logical order, each presentation being followed by one or more opportunities for the learner to apply his learning, as by answering a question, with immediate knowledge of results (usually, knowing that one is right is sufficient reinforcement). Programed instruction has proved fairly useful with some subject matters, such as arithmetic, and with some subjects, particularly children who find it hard to pay attention and to learn in regular classroom settings. A learning program can be attacked in solitude, at one's own pace, away from distractions, and the manipulation of the materials, especially on a machine, provides an additional incentive.

As a technique for total education, however, programed instruction has disappointed the original high hopes of its proponents, at least partly because some of its assumptions about how people learn seem to be in error. Some forward-looking technicians, let it be said, anticipate the day when a whole field of learning, including original documents, pictures, tables, charts, diagrams, and movie footage, can be put on a reel of videotape, or, more flexibly, entered in the memory of a computer, together with a highly flexible program that permits the learner to move about through the material according to his own interests, to be used on the individual's private viewing machine.[9]

The principles of operant conditioning have also had some application in psychotherapy for a few conditions and in the treatment of minor problems such as shyness or timidity.[10] The technique here is to discover what will serve as a reinforcer for the individual whose behavior is to be modified—such things as expressions of approval, or pieces of candy, or money—and then to use these to reinforce successively closer approximations to the desired behavior. Zeaman and House[11] have used operant techniques to good effect in experiments with the mentally retarded, suggesting applications to their education.

In spite of its contributions, the learning-theory tradition, in all its variations and expressions, fails in our view as a general account of human behavior. This is not because of its environmentalism—if there is any hope of improving humankind, it lies in the manipulation of the environment, and learning theory is pushing hard to test the limits of environmental manipulation. Learning theory is weak because it ignores so many areas of learning. It is concerned hardly at all, or at most programmatically, with knowledge, with the broad interconnected system of facts and ideas and meanings and values that school learning is supposed to deal with. It has very little patience with the learning of concepts and relations and principles, with thinking, reasoning, and insight, or with the consequences of learning—for instance, how learning contributes to the development of intelligence or honesty or sympathy or friendliness, or how it can serve to make a person less egocentric or ethnocentric. Learning theorists sometimes go to extravagant lengths to avoid coming to grips with phenomena that do not fit their conceptions. One device is expressed in *Maier's Law:*[12] if you can't explain it, call it something else. The child's acquisition of his native tongue does not happen in ways that fit the usual conceptions of learning, so it has come to be called what we have called it—"acquisition."

Another area in which learning theory is unsatisfactory is that of unlearning, which is something different from simple forgetting. The child must unlearn, in due time, such beliefs as fairies or Santa Claus, or that babies come by stork, not to mention the many superstitions he invents or accumulates. Indeed, one of the chief problems of higher education is to discover what misinformation or misconceptions the student brings to college so that they can be untaught. Learning theory remains silent on how, in the first place, one can learn things that are not so, such as a belief in Santa Claus, and all the other phantom entities and forces with which people populate the natural order. Nor does learning theory tell us any more about learning through language, by having things described to us, than it does about learning language itself. In general, learning theorists concentrate on the externals of learning, on the easily measurable atomistic indices, such as changes in skin conductivity, salivation, muscle twitches, bar-pressing, or moving from place to place. When they look beneath the surface, it is usually for mediating processes in the central nervous system, bypassing the subjective realm of knowing, wanting, and feeling, as in the accounts of thinking by Osgood[13] and by Miller, Galanter, and Pribram,[14] or in the work of Pavlov and his followers. This criticism is not to say that learning is independent of the nervous system, but that the facts of learning transcend our knowledge of nervous system functioning, and even where correspondences can be found, learning still exists on its own level and can be studied in its own right, regardless of what the neural processes may be.

Let us point out that there are other learning theorists who work outside the Pavlovian and Thorndikean mainstreams, and in some cases even contrary to them. Howard and Tracy Kendler[15] study the role of cognitive or verbal mediation, rather than neural mediation, in learning. Their favored technique is to compare the learning of *reversal shifts* and *nonreversal shifts*, by which the animal is taught a discrimination and then has to learn a new discrimination. A reversal shift is learning that the same dimension of discrimination continues to be the relevant one, but it is now the previously unrewarded stimulus that gets reinforced; thus if color is the relevant dimension, the animal is first rewarded for responding, say, to the blue stimulus and not the red, and then has to learn to respond to the red and not the blue. A nonreversal shift involves changing the basis of reinforcement to a completely different, previously irrelevant dimension. Thus, if the animal first learns to respond on the basis of color, he then must learn to respond on the basis of size or shape or whatever. Interestingly enough, white rats, young children, and young monkeys, but not older monkeys and people, find reversal shifts much more difficult than nonreversal.[16] That is, it is harder to unlearn to respond to one end of a dimension than to unlearn the whole dimension and shift to another. The Kendlers interpret such findings to mean that linguistic mediation is the key to reversal shifts. While it seems likely that

181

verbal analysis facilitates reversal shifts, perhaps by making possible the framing of hypotheses about what the rules of the game have now become, it is not the whole story, since nonlinguistic organisms like rats and monkeys do, with however much difficulty, eventually learn to make reversal shifts.

Another student of learning who escapes the objections we have entered against learning theorists in general is Harry Harlow,[17] who studies *learning set* (also called learning to learn), the fact that the animal generalizes principles to new learning situations, instead of learning a specific response to a specific stimulus. For instance, in so-called oddity learning, the child or animal has to learn to respond to the stimulus that is different from the rest of the set. Having done so, he can then transfer the general principle of oddity to a new oddities problem, as when he first learns to pick the block that is a different color from the rest, and then has to learn to select the block that is different in shape from the others.

Harlow has also stressed that curiosity (without other reward) is a sufficient motivation for learning, and that solving problems is intrinsically satisfying, and not merely a means to satisfying some physical need. We have already mentioned Harlow's research with surrogate mothers, which had as its original aim to disprove the learning-theory hypothesis that the mother comes to be valued as a conditioned stimulus for the satisfaction of physical needs: The monkeys, it will be recalled, preferred the terrycloth mother, who did not feed them, to the bare wire mother who did.

It is an assumption of learning theory that the basic processes of learning are the same in all animal species, but M. E. Bitterman and associates[18] have shown that there are qualitative differences among animals of different species in their performance on standard learning tasks such as reversal shifts and probability learning, lending support to the discontinuity hypothesis (to be discussed later in this chapter) as it applies to evolutionary differences, if not directly to individual development.

A number of students of learning have addressed themselves to the question of learning by imitation, with findings that go counter to the usual learning-theoretical formulation that imitation itself is learned as an operant out of an accidental coincidence of doing something just after somebody else has done it and then being rewarded for it. One incidental finding, by Darby and Riopelle,[19] is that monkeys who learn by watching the behavior of other monkeys learn better from another monkey's errors than from his correct responses, indicating that nonimitation is an important part of observational learning.

MATURATIONAL THEORIES

The usual textbook formulation of developmental change is that psychological development is a product of learning and *maturation*. Maturation includes but is not the same as growth, which refers primarily to changes in size. Maturation is the continuation of the prenatal developmental processes which produce qualitative changes in tissues or in anatomical and physiological organization. Thus, cartilage ossifies into true bone, myelin sheaths come to cover the peripheral nerves, new enzymes arise in the digestive tract, the body changes in proportions, the endocrine glands change in relative size and activity, yielding new organizations. The thymus gland, for instance, atrophies during childhood, and the decrease in thymus activity, long a riddle, is now seen as important to the development of somatic individuality, the idiosyncratic tissue composition that makes tissue grafts between individuals impossible (although progress has been made in circumventing the body's immune response to permit organ transplants, and even in utilizing the immune response to combat cancer). The pituitary gland has periods of greater and lesser activity during development, and the gonads do not mature until adolescence.

There is no doubt that maturation of the somatic equipment takes place and that it affects our capacities for acting and reacting. A whole group of theorists has seen in maturation the chief explanation for behavioral changes in the course of development. While such theorists grant that learning takes place, learning is thought of primarily as the activation of structures that have already taken shape in the given organism. It is as though the nervous system becomes a coded or pictorial replica of the outside world, so that perceiving is a matching of neural structure with object, and thinking a running off in miniature of events in the real world. Since it is the organization of the nervous system that structures thought, language is not a mechanism of thinking but only its accompaniment.

Some of the chief proponents of this viewpoint have been Gesell, Montagu, Carmichael, the great Swiss psychologist Jean Piaget, whose thinking has become influential in this country only in the last decade but who began his researches forty-odd years ago, Kurt Goldstein, Martin Scheerer, and Heinz Werner. Characteristically, these writers have been more concerned with cognitive processes than with emotion or motivation, and have postulated sets of polar opposites defining the differences between immature and mature behavior. The progression from immature to mature is usually described in terms of stages, epochs in the child's life characterized by particular themes or modes of operation, as in Freud's psychosexual stages, although the exact age periods differ from authority to authority. We shall give only a sampling of the principles and polarities set forth by these theorists

Gesell proposed a principle of *reciprocal interweaving* which seems to mean a shuttlelike pattern of movement into the future, as though the child takes two steps forward to gain new experience, and then one step back while he consolidates his gains and integrates them with the past. For Gesell, the child's overt behavior is an expression of reciprocal interweaving in nervous system maturation. Gesell's principle of *epigenesis* was simply his statement of the principle of discontinuity, the idea that the individual undergoes qualitative reorganizations as he develops.

Goldstein is best known for the polarity of *concrete* and *abstract* behavior, which he proposed first in connection with his studies of the effects of brain injury. Concreteness means being bound to the present situation and its sometimes irrelevant dynamics, as when the patient sorts a collection of blocks according to color and then is unable to make a new sorting on some other basis such as shape, or when he cannot gratuitously go through the motions of knocking on an imaginary door, or is unable to name a comb until he actually uses it to comb his hair. Abstract behavior requires detachment from the immediacies, consideration of alternative modes of action, and thinking and acting in terms of general principles and future outcomes. Goldstein's formulation is also relevant to normal human development which can be viewed as a progression from concrete to abstract modes of functioning.

Piaget has contributed such notions as egocentrism, already discussed, and its polar opposite, *relativism*, the ability to shift perspectives and see how a situation appears to someone else. He has given the name *primary adualism*—that is, lack of two-ness, or nondifferentiatedness—to the baby's initial inability to distinguish clearly between events happening inside himself and those originating in the outside environment, so that he experiences dreams as happening in the outside world and acts as though he could control external events by wishing, by sympathetic magic. Two major notions in Piaget's system are *assimilation* and *accommodation*. Assimilation refers to the way the child reshapes his experience to fit his own level of functioning. Accommodation, by contrast, refers to the way the child's experience reshapes his style of operation.

Piaget has given us a sequence of ways in which the child is supposed to perceive causal relations. The first of these is *animism,* whereby material objects, living or not, are regarded as having an animal spirit that makes them behave as they do. Animism may be implicit, as when the child simply acts as though something were alive, as when he shows sympathy to a broken plaything, or explicit, as when the child says that the broken plaything hurts. The next is *artificialism,* according to which all events are regulated by some humanlike entity, as when the child asks, "Why do they have thunder?" At a more advanced level comes *naturalism,* the acceptance of impersonal natural forces as the governing agent in many events, including some portion of human behavior, as in scientific accounts. We have already mentioned Piaget's notions of the nonconservation and conservation of objects. Piaget has also defined a number of stages in the development of logical thinking, such as the sensori-motor stage of babyhood, when all behavior is assumed to be stimulated reflex-fashion from without, and the impulsive *pre-operational* stage of early childhood, which yields to the more systematic, analytical approach of the *operational* stage. Piaget has embellished his stages with descriptive terms drawn from symbolic logic and esoteric branches of mathematics. In addition, he has supplied a model of brain organization to account for the operations of thought and how they change with age.

Piaget's thinking, even after many decades of study, is still evolving and changing, notably in the direction of giving more weight to learning and of making the learning and use of language and symbolic forms a major component in the development of thinking.[20] His astute observations and ingenious task-setting have worked a revolution in the study of psychological development and made this a significant segment of general psychology. The authors, over the years, have assimilated and accommodated to much of Piaget's thinking, and his ideas are implicit in many parts of this book.

Heinz Werner was dedicated to making the principles of individual psychological development the key to a general philosophy embracing animal evolution, historical change, cultural differences, and psychopathology. Werner incorporated Goldstein's abstract-concrete and Piaget's egocentric-relativistic polarities into his view in addition to several developmental polarities of his own. One such dimension is development from syncretic (global), undifferentiated functioning, in which perception and thought resemble what William James called a "blooming, buzzing confusion," to differentiated and articulated functioning. Whenever the child or adult meets a new situation he may have to recapitulate this sequence. Many of us can remember the first time we ever saw the engine of a car. At first encounter, it appears as a syncretic, poorly differentiated, burbling, throbbing, ticking, whirring, faintly ominous metal mass enmeshed in a tangle of wires and pipes and hoses and protuberances—although this description is already too well articulated to convey our first global impression. With experience, we become able to sort out—to differentiate—the visible components: the engine block, the manifolds, the carburetor and air cleaner, the fuel pump, the distributor, the generator, the water pump, the radiator and connections, and so forth. And as we are instructed in the engine's functioning, including the movement of parts hidden from view—the rotor, the pistons and rods, the crankshaft, the camshaft, the valves, the timing gear, and so on—we become able to see the engine as an intelligible, orderly, stable, integrally functioning unit: but this now differentiated and articulated whole is quite different from the global, undifferentiated whole with which we began. In the chapters that follow we will point out a number of phenomena that seem to follow the pattern of differentiation and higher-order, emergent integration expressed in the *syncretic-articulated* polarity.

Two other polarities of development are closely linked in Werner's system. These are development from *rigidity* to *flexibility* of thought and action, and from living in a *labile* world to inhabiting a *stable* one. In the unstable world of the young child, where feelings mingle with objects and the spirit world coexists with the material, where meanings and identities change without warning, and where there are no limits on what is possible, stability can be achieved only by adhering to rigid, habit-bound, and ritualistic patterns of behavior. We find similar behavior in adults who, faced with the flux and complexities and perplexities of life, take refuge in tradition and simplistic slogans and dogmas and formulas. As and if the world becomes more stable, reliable, orderly, and predictable, more possibilities for effective action become apparent and behavior can be increasingly flexible and varied.

Werner also had a special interest in language, in both its factual, descriptive, propositional functions and its evocative, affective, expressive ones, as in poetry and metaphor. Some of his ideas in this area are expressed in the account of language learning in the next chapter.

It might be supposed that psychoanalytic theories, which are concerned primarily with motivation and emotion, and maturational theories, which focus on cognition, could simply be combined to give a reasonably complete picture of the individual and his development. The thought has occurred to quite a few people, for the most part originally of a psycho-analytical persuasion, including Silvano Arieti, E. J. Anthony, René Spitz, Peter Wolff, Ernest Schachtel, and David Rapaport, all of whom have sought to integrate the two approaches, largely in terms of parallels between Freud's primary-process thinking and the primitive (egocentric, concrete, rigid, syncretic) thinking described by maturational theorists. It seems to us that these attempts have been abortive, perhaps because psychoanalysts find it hard to cope with the emergentism of maturational theories, and because neither psychoanalysis nor maturational theory makes sufficient provision for learning and the role of context on be-havior. Werner, for instance, talked a great deal about cultural differ-ences, but had almost nothing to say about how one comes to assimilate a particular cultural outlook.

KURT LEWIN'S FIELD THEORY

Maturational theories came out of one branch of *Gestalt psychology*. Whereas other psychologies tried to analyze psychological functions in terms of their elements, Gestalt psychology was concerned with the qualities of organized things-as-a-whole. The Gestalt psychologist would point out that a square constructed of either dots or lines is perceived in terms of its squareness, which is designated a *whole-quality,* rather than in terms of the particular elements that go to make it up.

It is hard to summarize the Gestalt position because it contains a number of contradictions. On the one hand, the Gestaltists insisted upon the distinctive human qualities of human beings, complaining that asso-ciationism dealt with "mere facts" to the neglect of values. On the other hand, Wolfgang Köhler (who, along with Max Wertheimer and Kurt Koffka, was one of the fathers of the Berlin school of Gestalt, the one best known in the United States) vigorously denies the possibility of qualita-tive transformations in the course of either normal evolution or individual human development. At the same time, he emphasizes the role of *insight* (understanding, often rapid, as expressed in "Eureka!" or the "Aha experience") in learning and the discontinuous learning curves that are produced when the organism arrives at insightful understanding of the task. Köhler is a reductionist (for a definition of reductionism see page 190), and seeks to explain behavior and perception in terms of maplike representations of situations in the brain. Although much of his work was concerned with perception and the effects of different organizations of stimuli on perception, Köhler staunchly maintains that the real world is in principle unknowable, holding that what we take to be reality is only something that we infer or reconstruct out of discharges in the nervous system.

Although both Wertheimer and Koffka were interested in work with children, the Berlin school was nondevelopmental in its orientation, but it produced one psychologist, Kurt Lewin, who was at least partly developmental in his outlook and who did considerable research with children. Lewin's point of view is called *topological field theory*, and is based on his concept of *life space*. The life space consists of those aspects of the environment which stand out for the individual as psychologically relevant. Lewin represented the life space diagrammatically as a potato-shaped region of space marked off with routes and barriers representing types of activity allowed and available, or prohibited and blocked. The routes in this life space lead to goal objects with positive and negative valences which indicate whether the objects are attractive or repulsive. The person in the field (which may itself be something thought about as well as the person's perceived world) is moved or immobilized by the action of these valences along the pathways that are open to him, representing courses of action. In this way one can represent a number of classical situations. Frustration, for instance, can be shown as an attractive goal across an insurmountable barrier. Various states of conflict can be represented, as when the person is torn between two competing but incompatible attractions, or when a negatively valenced object lies across the path to an attractive one, or the condition of ambivalence, when a goal has both positive and negative valences. Lewin was avowedly "ahistorical" in his approach; that is, he was less interested in how a life space comes to be constituted as it is than in its structure at the moment of action. He did say, however, that the life space becomes progressively more differentiated in the course of development, and, as suggested earlier, he conceived of regression as a de-differentiation of the life space. And it does not seem incompatible with his views to assume that the life space also undergoes qualitative reorganizations and reintegrations as development proceeds.

Lewin represented the person in the life space's field of forces as an empty circle, reminiscent of Skinner's empty organism, so that people are no longer described in terms of their own capacities but in terms of their environments. Thus, instead of talking about stupid and intelligent people, we can talk about stupid or intelligent life spaces. Or, if we want to drop Lewin's terminology, we can talk about more or less intelligent environments. Thus, intelligence is not a property of nervous systems but of how the world appears to people, its qualities and flavors and meanings and possibilities for action. If we adopt this view of intellectual differences, then the goal of education becomes that of making people more intelligent by teaching them what the environment consists of and how it operates (and how they can interact with it), including the action of forces and agents lying beyond perception, whether x-rays or infrared or molecular structure or ultrasound or viruses or RNA or human physiology or the law of supply and demand. For the life space changes as we come to understand the principles by which we and the world work, including the fact that different cultures shape the life space of people in very different ways, including the moral, esthetic, and emotional valences it assigns to things. We shall return to the topic of intelligence and how it develops at the end of Chapter 7.

Characteristics of Theories of Development

It is our aim in this section to look at some of the broader assumptions about human nature that underlie the psychological theories we have just described. That they are all deficient in various important ways does not make them useless—even an erroneous theory can lead the investigator to new and otherwise unsuspected facts and relations.

REDUCTIONISM AND MECHANISM

It used to be that theories were meant to explain phenomena in the sense of saying how they were possible. Nowadays, most theorists have concluded that explanation in this sense is out of the question. As soon as we try to understand how living organisms are different from inert matter, how they metabolize, reproduce, maintain physiological equilibrium (*homeostasis*), move about (in the case of those organisms that move under their own power), adapt to stimulation, and so forth, we are at a loss. And when we move to the psychological level and examine such phenomena as consciousness, attention, love, sympathy, thought, perception, self-knowledge, self-control, and the like, our powers of conceptualization break down.

What most theorists now profess is to have abandoned explanation in favor of description, systematic statements of cause and effect, correlations, and analyses. However, we still find many remnants of explanatory thinking and even of the metaphysics that prevailed before science came into its own. For instance, there are those who still insist upon the existence of instincts, which, since no one is prepared to say what an instinct is, is no more helpful than invoking phlogiston or animal magnetism.

A common substitute for explanation is found in *reductionism:* Instead of explaining the phenomena themselves, one seeks to account for them by events at a "lower"—meaning simpler or more physically tangible—and hence more manageable level. In the case of psychological phenomena, this means "explanation" at the level of physiology, anatomy, or biochemistry. Or, alternatively, one can construct a "model," in the form of an analogy or metaphor, a mathematical equation of broad generality, or a mechanical equivalent such as a computer. The hidden motive in such explanations often seems to be to explain away rather than explain, to get rid of the intangible phenomena and with them the uncomfortable notion that in actuality they perhaps cannot be explained. In their desire to emulate the more precise and rigorous physical sciences, many biologists and psychologists seem to fear that admitting the facts of human behavior opens the door to vitalism or even mysticism. Most scientists of behavior seek a naturalistic conception of the facts, without recourse to such entities or substances as "spirit," "mind," "élan vital" (which translates roughly as "life force"), or anything else added on to the material organism which lives and acts.

Here we have the recurring conflict between *dualism,* which says that mind and body are distinct, and *monism,* which says that mind and body are merely aspects of the same organism. The authors are sympathetic to a naturalistic monism which recognizes that the organism has *different levels of functioning,* including the psychological. Our brand of monism sees the psychological level in the organism's congress with objects and their meanings and qualities, including the self as object and the symbolic objects that people construct with words, numbers, and the like.

Reductionism has gone hand in hand with *mechanism,* a more or less explicit assumption that the ideal model for organic and psychological functioning is the machine. The mechanistic tradition received its greatest impetus from the French mathematician-philosopher Descartes, who conjured an image of a machine-man operated by levers and pulleys and valves and conduits through which pneumatic fluids or vapors could travel. Note that this conception is not wholly absurd; our bones and joints and muscles do operate this way, and who is to deny the mechanical pumplike action of the heart and circulatory system? Modern theories of nerve action have simply substituted electrochemical transmission of impulses for Descartes' humoral flow. The absurdity comes when we try to extend this model (which Descartes seems to have meant not as an analogy but as the literal truth, although he had to tread softly lest he offend the religious authorities) to other functions, as in the TV-commercial version of the digestive tract as a series of vats, beakers, retorts, and connecting tubes, with stopcocks to control the flow of gastric juices. Or we have the standard model of perception according to which nerves act like wires bringing information into the brain; once the codified information is in the brain, it has to be decoded, interpreted and made sense out of, to which end the model-makers provide something like a cathode-ray screen containing the decoded image and a homunculus (sometimes acknowledged, more often not) to read off the picture and activate the nerves which carry information to the glands and muscles. This miniature person in the brain is the modern-day descendant of the soul, and seems to be the mechanist's device for handling consciousness or mind. In this case, it would seem reductionism breeds dualism, or even multiplism. For, as Skinner[21] has pointed out, the homunculus too needs his own perceptual apparatus to read off the cathode-ray tube display, which logically implies that he must have a homunculus in his brain, and that homunculus another homunculus, and so on without end.

The mechanistic approach has found its most sophisticated modern expression in *information theory,* which seeks to describe human functioning in the language of digital computers.[22] The information-theory model is sometimes helpful and has given us such concepts as *feedback* and *signal-to-noise ratio* and *reverberating circuit.* In the strict computer sense, feedback consists of a yes or no response to a single operation or part operation. In terms of behavior, it means that any action by the organism has effects which feed back to the organism and serve to regulate the next act, and so on. We have already given the example of how the ground feeds back information to our feet in walking. Similarly, the play of facial expression on someone to whom we are talking can serve as feedback that modifies what we say next—in experimental situations, the experimenter can steer and shape what the subject is saying by reacting in a predetermined, arbitrary way that the subject may have no inkling of.[23] The signal-to-noise ratio seeks to specify how clearly important information—the "message"—stands out from the background or is camouflaged by irrelevant, distracting "noise"—the concept of noise can be applied in any sense modality (it is analogous to visual clutter), and not only to hearing. The reverberating circuit is one way to account for memory or learning or "information storage" by imagining that events set up continuing circuits of neural activity which can be called upon and combined for purposes of thinking and acting.

There seem to be at least three things wrong, however, with information theory as a general account of behavior. First of all, the evidence that mammalian (or even vertebrate) nervous systems operate according to the same principles as a digital computer is very slim indeed.[24] Second, the computer model requires that complex acts which occur simultaneously in the living organism be strung out in time, even though it be micro-time. For instance, one can teach a two-year-old to recognize the letters of the alphabet at a glance. To enable the computer to distinguish letters of the alphabet requires a whole system of explicit analyses in which all the ways letters are composed and differ from each other have to be spelled out and programed into the machine. Generation after generation of two-year-olds continue to recognize letters, geometric forms, people, animals, facial expressions, words, sentences, voices, odors, and melodies, while computer engineers are still struggling to teach their machines the simplest sorts of pattern discriminations. Computers are extremely inefficient, but their inefficiency is compensated for by the phenomenal speed with which successive single operations are performed. Third, the computer model leaves no room for perversity or inventiveness or meaningful errors, for values or moods or motivational states which any psychologist has to weight in making descriptions and predictions.

FIELD THEORIES AND EMERGENCE

The nonvitalistic alternative to mechanism has traditionally been holistic theories (in recent years more commonly called *field theories*), which take their analogies and metaphors from those areas of physics dealing with field effects—hydraulics, electricity, magnetism, gravity— from chemistry with its qualitative transformations (as in John Stuart Mill's "mental chemistry"[25]), and from biology with its notions of growth, homeostasis, metamorphosis, and systems. But note that this approach, while perhaps more intuitively congenial to common-sense understanding of human nature, is still a form of reductionism—it makes no provision for consciousness, self-knowledge, self-control, originality, fantasy, symbolic activity, in short, what are regarded as the "higher mental processes."

The philosophical alternative to reductionism is the doctrine of *emergence*: It seeks to define different levels of analysis or "orders of reality" or complexity, each with its own set of governing principles that transcend the principles regulating the simpler levels. As applied to human beings, the doctrine of emergence would distinguish such successively more complex levels as the behavior of the atomic particles of which we are composed; the chemical and biochemical level, including gene action and functions like metabolism and nerve-fiber action; the macrophysical, including the mechanics of movement and the hydrodynamics of circulation; the physiological, including processes like homeostasis, digestion, sickness and recovery from sickness; the psychological realm of subjective feeling, including thought, emotions, and awareness of body states; the person, with attitudes and goals and values and attachments; and, at still higher levels, man as an element in a team, a group, or a society; or a society as one element in the stream of history; on the cosmic scale of the astronomer, of course, man disappears from view.

Emergence does not deny that events at one level may be coordinated with events at another. Obviously, we can have a psychological existence only by virtue of our material bodies. It does, however, say that each class of events can be described in its own right, without reference to other levels, and that corresponding events on two levels may each need its own set of principles. For instance, we know that perceived color depends on the wave length of light, but whereas wave length varies continuously, hue varies discontinuously, as in a rainbow. Now it is customary to speak of the biological basis of behavior, which is accurate in the sense that without an organism there would be no behavior, and that the way an organism is constituted sets bounds on its behavior. But we can with equal truth speak of the psychological foundations of biology, in that our physiological functioning is responsive both to internal thought and to perceptual stimulation from without, and in that our personal and social experience can, in time, alter even our anatomy, as seen in studies of the effects of enrichment and deprivation and stress on animal development.

Continuity and Discontinuity. When we talk about psychological development, the contrasting doctrines of reductionism and emergence go by the names of *continuity theory* and *discontinuity theory.* Continuity theory, which is reductionistic, holds that development is simply an accumulation of skills, habits, discriminations, without anything new appearing in the make-up of the individual. By contrast, the discontinuity view, based on the doctrine of emergence, holds that in the course of development the organism undergoes genuine transformations—that is, reaches successively higher, emergent levels of organization—on the model of biological metamorphosis. Thus, in human development, walking is seen as discontinuous with (but emergent from) creeping; talking as discontinuous with babbling; drawing pictures as discontinuous with scribbling; and so on through a hierarchy of emergent functions. Lewin, and from a quite different theoretical standpoint, Zing-Yang Kuo, have stressed the transformation of the organism as it takes each developmental step.[26]

These differences are not the mere quibblings of theologians. One's whole view of child-rearing and education depends on whether one takes a continuity or discontinuity position, with very real consequences for what kind of people one perceives or produces. The continuity theorist stresses training, the cultivation of skills and stimulus-response relations, whereas the discontinuity theorist stresses the cultivation of insight, understanding, self-knowledge, imagination, and a broad perspective out of which new organizations of behavior and meaning can emerge.

Determinism and Voluntarism. Tied in here, as suggested earlier, is a further split between doctrines of *determinism,* associated with reductionism and continuity theory, and *voluntarism* (or the exercise of will), associated with emergence and discontinuity theory. The determinist holds that the individual is helpless to control his own behavior and destiny, that he cannot behave in the present with a view to future outcomes, and that if he has an intimation of self-regulation this is nothing but delusion since he is in fact a prisoner of the accidents of his past history.

Few emergence theorists nowadays would dare to counter this view with a doctrine of free will, because we know too much about how far our characters and motives and abilities and tastes and outlooks are shaped by events that happen during early periods of our lives when we are essentially helpless. We also know too much about social and natural forces and how these can act without regard to individual plans and wishes. Nonetheless, discontinuity theorists would say that, given favorable rearing conditions, human beings acquire a perspective on the world and on themselves that permits them to some extent to anticipate the future, to think for themselves, to inhibit some forms of activity and to force themselves to engage in others, and above all to reason out their situation so as to frame their own set of ethical and moral principles for the conduct of life, instead of blindly obeying all the rules ordained by their culture. The discontinuity theorist would also have to concede that a great many people, by virtue of less favorable histories, show a low degree of self-determination and seem to lead lives governed by the push and pull of circumstance, or at best grumble against fate or strike out in rage against a world in whose workings they have no say.

To understand this issue fully we need to be aware of the concept of *teleology*—which we are not advocating—which says that natural events move toward a goal or purpose, as though in fulfillment of some master plan. The master plan can be thought of as imposed from above, as by a deity, or somehow coded into life so as to predetermine the direction of evolution, development, and behavior. Now it is one thing to say that natural evolution has a direction, which is not hard to define and describe, but quite another to say that it has a prior purpose or meaning. Unfortunately, though, many of those who denounce this teleology extend their denunciation to deny the possibility of individual human purposes and goals, which is quite a different matter. For there can be no denying, it seems to us, that individuals do formulate designs for living, and work hard to fulfill those designs, or that groups of individuals define and execute social policies, some of which, as in agricultural or conservation measures, can influence natural evolution. As Bruner[27] points out, man, as far as we know, is the only species in which individuals anticipate their own death. The purposive view acknowledges that people in planning their lives may be deceived about their own motivations, or may think, often, that they are acting autonomously when in fact the whole pattern was subtly laid down for them in infancy, or may come up with some wholly bizarre designs, or that circumstances may change in ways that make the original plan obsolete. It only says that, for better or for worse, people can have an orientation toward the future and are able to adapt present action to anticipated outcomes, and that they can act ethically, taking account of other people's purposes and values as well as of their own.

NATURE AND NURTURE, OPTIMISM AND PESSIMISM

Two more sets of contrasts remain to be mentioned as relevant to the specific theories that have been put forward to make sense of the facts of human development and behavior. The first of these is the ever-recurring *nature-nurture* controversy, the question of whether human behavior can best be accounted for in terms of biologically given structures, motives, abilities, propensities, or instincts, or in terms of those qualities acquired through experience in a particular material, personal, and cultural setting. (Those who uphold the nature side in the controversy are called *nativists* or *instinct theorists* or *genetic determinists.* Those who plump for nurture are called *environmentalists.*)

On this dichotomy and the one that follows, we shall not take sides, preferring to seek a synthesis of nature and nurture. Anastasi[28] has pointed out that the meaningful question is not whether nature or nurture gets the credit or the blame, or even how much each contributes to development, but how they interact in the formation of an individual with thus-and-such characteristics. The two areas in which the nature-nurture controversy has raged most fiercely are those of morality and intelligence. Psychologists have pretty much abandoned hope of finding any biological correlates of virtue or wickedness (though echoes are found in current descriptions of schizophrenia, alcohol and drug addiction, and criminality), but the origin of intelligence is still an embattled topic. It is a vital one, since our whole approach to education (which supposedly provides an environment conducive to the development of intelligence) can hinge on whether we think ways and means can be found to make everybody bright or whether we are resigned to letting children sort themselves out in keeping with their native (and hence presumably fixed or only slightly alterable) endowments.

The other remaining major contrast we shall point to is between *optimism* and *pessimism,* between those who have seen human nature as intrinsically virtuous, so that the child comes into the world trailing clouds of glory, and needs above all else to be protected against corruption by a wicked world, and those who have seen the newborn babe as steeped in original sin and pervasive evil, so that the task of child-rearing becomes that of beating the devil out of the child to make room for a socially given morality. To this polarity of good and evil must be counterposed the more modern view of *neutralism,* that the child is neither virtuous nor wicked by nature but can become either—or in various proportions both—according to his experience.

Now if we combine these two dimensions of optimism-neutralism-pessimism and biologism-environmentalism, we can construct a table with six cells, each representing the conjunction of two positions, one from each of the two dimensions, as shown in Table 1.

It turns out that most major theorists can fairly readily be assigned to one of these six cells. (We could, of course, complicate our scheme by adding the dimensions of reductionism-emergence and determinism-voluntarism, but such a complication seems unnecessary. All these theorists have a more or less reductionistic and deterministic outlook, at least as regards the early years.) The cell at the intersection of optimism and

TABLE 1 / **A Taxonomy of Theories**

	Biologistic	Environmentalistic
Optimistic	Jean-Jacques Rousseau	John Locke
	Arnold Gesell	Karl Marx
	M.F.A. Montagu	Ivan Pavlov
Neutralistic	Jean Piaget	E. L. Thorndike
	Leonard Carmichael	J. B. Watson
	Heinz Werner	B. F. Skinner
		Clark Hull
Pessimistic	Sigmund Freud	Thomas Hobbes

biologism contains such names as that of Jean-Jacques Rousseau, with his doctrine of romantic naturalism, and those of his modern successors such as Arnold Gesell and Ashley Montagu, the latter of whom finds love and cooperation as basic ingredients of the natural order. The neutralist-biologist cell contains the names—again, among others—of Jean Piaget, Leonard Carmichael, and Heinz Werner. Piaget has studied moral development as one aspect of cognitive development, which he sees as dictated by biological maturation, but contemplates morality only with the detached eye of the scientist. Carmichael is an evolutionary theorist who sees a decided progression toward intellectual mastery over the environment but remains largely uncommitted on the subject of good and evil. The outstanding pessimistic biologist of our era was Sigmund Freud, who saw human nature as essentially vile, with some faint hope in the corrective forces of socialization and education, especially as their effects became part of human heredity (Freud subscribed more or less explicitly to Lamarck's—and, at first, Darwin's—belief in the inheritance of acquired characteristics). Moving to the environmentalist column, the optimistic empiricists include the seventeenth-century British philosopher John Locke, with his doctrines of the *tabula rasa,* the neonate as a clean slate on which experience writes or impresses its lessons, and of the *association of ideas,* according to which those events which repeatedly occur together become linked in thought. Karl Marx, the author of economic determinism and dialectical materialism, was likewise an optimistic environmentalist, as was the renowned Russian physiologist Ivan Pavlov, who gave us the conditioned reflex, a more rigorous statement of the association of ideas. Note that Pavlov's system included an emergent something called the *second signal system,* by which human beings are

197

enabled to learn language and transcend their animal nature. The American associationists, such as Edward Thorndike, J. B. Watson, Clark Hull, and B. F. Skinner, have tended to be neutralist-environmentalists and, in their reductionistic way, have had rather less faith than Marx and Pavlov in human beings' capacity for virtue. One might even doubt that virtue seemed to them a relevant topic for psychological consideration. Finally, if only for the sake of logical completeness, in the pessimistic-environmentalist cell we may place the name of the British philosopher Thomas Hobbes, for whom the environment had to redeem a primitive condition of life which he characterized in a famous quotation as "solitary, poor, nasty, brutish, and short."

Developmental Principles

All the theories we have discussed suffer, perhaps inevitably, from the flaw of egocentrism. In each case, that is, the theorist and his fellows have adopted a single perspective on the human condition and assumed that they were seeing it in its entirety, in the round. Now it is perfectly clear that these various perspectives yield information so diverse that it seems hard to believe that all the theorists are talking about the same creature, who is now angelic and now depraved, now a black-box robot shaped by reinforcers, and now a shaper of his own destiny, now devious and involved in a life of self-deception and now straightforward, now lust-driven and now serene, now hardheadedly oriented to solid reality, now adrift in a miasma of ignorance and superstition tricked out as philosophy. And yet we know that man is all of these and that any final theory is going to have to reconcile all these incompatibles, that it will have to account for man at his most heavenly and his most bestial, man the passive automaton and man the striver and doer, man at his most deluded and most penetrating.

The authors do not claim to be ready to accomplish this ultimate synthesis, but we do feel that the study of development will reveal man's plasticity, the way experience can bring forth a variety of human natures, and that a few fortunate individuals can be given the psychological means for reconciling and mastering their own conflicting tendencies and finding a meaning in life. Meanwhile, the best we can hope for is to indicate what seem to be some durable and useful principles of human development and to suggest where researchers might look for further enlightenment. *Eclecticism* is usually taken to mean a more or less uncritical piecing together of theories or fragments of theories, and in this sense becomes a term of opprobrium. But we are seeking, along with Gardner Murphy, Gordon Allport,[29] and others, a synthetic eclecticism whereby all the seemingly paradoxical aspects of human functioning can be subordinated in an emergent conception of man. We refuse to be committed to any orthodoxy, our only commitment being to the humanity of human beings: We have already clearly emphasized that we are more hospitable to some theories and assumptions and more hostile to others. For perhaps the most important single principle of human development is what Ralph Linton calls the *self-fulfilling prophecy,* which says simply that our children become what we expect them to become, whether our expectations be phrased as hopes or fears, left implicit or made explicit. Especially with our fears, we are likely to adopt a defensive, preventive, punitive approach to child-rearing, and the harder we work to stave off this or that dire possibility, the more likely it is that the possibility will become a reality.

GROWTH GRADIENTS

The first pair of principles to be discussed has to do with the directional flow of physical development. In those organisms which have a head and a tail, growth invariably proceeds in two related directions. The *cephalo-caudal growth gradient* refers to the fact that the head end of the organism develops first, in prenatal growth, with the lower portions taking shape at later periods. This same principle seems to apply to postnatal behavioral development, in that the baby's head becomes functional before his hands, that is, he uses mouth, eyes, and ears before he grasps; and his hands before his feet, that is, the baby is a skilled manipulator with his hands before his feet come into focus as playthings, prehensile instruments, or, later, things to walk with. Similarly, like the legendary ostrich, the baby at first seems to consider himself invisible as long as his head is covered, as in a game of peek-a-boo.

The *proximo-distal* growth gradient says that growth proceeds outward, from the central axis of the body toward the periphery. The proximo-distal gradient is most conspicuous prenatally in the development of the limb buds from the trunk and, in turn, of the still more remote hands and fingers and feet and toes from the limb buds. Postnatally, the child uses his whole hand as a unit before he can control his several fingers. In general, somatic and functional development seems to grow like an inverted tree, downward from the head and outward from the trunk, organized around the internal branchings of the nervous and circulatory systems and digestive tract.

DIFFERENTIATION AND FUNCTIONAL SUBORDINATION

The principle of *differentiation* says that development proceeds from the simple to the complex, from the homogeneous to the heterogeneous, from general to specific. From a single-celled zygote there develop by differentiation an immense number of cells of highly varied structure and function. The first cells formed by division of the zygote are all of the same kind, differing only in their position with respect to each other. As differentiation proceeds, the cells change in character, forming different kinds of tissues with *specialized* functions: nerves, skin, bone, blood, muscle, and so on. In turn, differentiated structures and functions become integrated into new, more inclusive, emergent patterns, yielding a simplicity with many components. Because the differentiated components are submerged in the new organization, losing their separate identities, we have called this process *functional subordination*—that is, the part-functions are subordinated to the emergent whole-function. (Other writers, notably Werner, refer to the same process as *hierarchization* or *hierarchic integration*.)

We can see the themes of differentiation and functional subordination running through all of behavioral as well as physiological development. At first, the baby cries with his whole body; later, his crying becomes more circumscribed. His distress reactions are initially all of a

An example of functional subordination: Hammering for its own sake becomes hammering in order to make something.
L. Joseph Stone

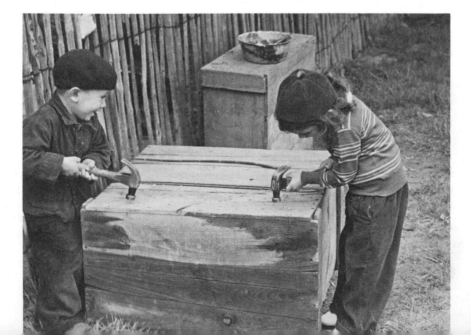

kind, whereas later they take on greater specificity, so that he has distinctive cries for hunger, pain, anger, and loneliness. When the baby begins to walk, the more differentiated gaits like striding, hopping, trotting, galloping, running, and skipping all lie ahead. Walking is at first a sufficient occupation in its own right, but later becomes subordinated to the end of getting from one place to another. Soon after he begins to walk, the baby or young toddler loves to carry things as he walks, but not until later with a view to conveying something to a particular location in order to use it. Speaking begins with single words (or word-clusters), but after a period of speaking in single differentiated word units, the child begins combining words into higher-order sentences. For a toddler, hammering as banging is enough; when, as a preschool child, he becomes able to use a hammer and nails, driving nails is a sufficient occupation; at a more advanced stage, hammering or nail-driving is functionally subordinated to making specific things.

ASYNCHRONOUS GROWTH AND DISCONTINUITY OF GROWTH RATE

The principle of *asynchronous growth* summarizes the way the focus of development shifts at successive periods in development. If one imagines a baby the size of an adult, the result is grotesque, for babies are not miniature adults. It immediately becomes obvious that the whole body does not grow at once, but that different regions and subsystems develop at different rates and different times. In looking at prenatal development, we saw how during the germinal period the baby's placental structures came first, while the embryo itself lay dormant in the germinal disk. Later, there was an interval devoted mainly to a preliminary formation of the cranial structures, while the other body parts marked time. Thereafter, now the heart, now the limbs, now the respiratory system took the lead. Asynchronous growth after birth accounts for shifts in the relative size of head, trunk, and extremities, and for the underlying changes in glandular patterns. Voices and faces are different in infancy, childhood, adolescence, and maturity. Consider alone the extent to which the nose is submerged or dominant at various ages. Even during adulthood and old age, body proportions keep changing, as clothing manufacturers know.

What we have just said refers to the growth of subsystems of the body. The subsystems, of course, grow in the context of the whole body, which itself changes in overall size and weight, but in spurts, not in a smooth curve of increase. The fact that the rate of growth changes at different periods is expressed in the principle of *discontinuity of growth rate*. Growth is very rapid in early infancy but levels off gradually through the preschool years and goes on at a relatively slow pace during the so-called middle years of childhood. The beginning of adolescence, is marked by a new spurt of growth which levels off in early adulthood.

We are not sure what the psychological equivalents of asynchronous growth and discontinuity of growth may be, but it is certain that children do have periods of greater receptivity to certain kinds of learning and thinking, and times of intense preoccupation with one kind of behavior or area of experience, which they then leave to go on to something else. We shall talk more about such patterns shortly in our discussion of competence motivation. There is also some reason to believe that new phases of psychological development may be signaled by periods of disruption and turbulence.

The developmental principles we have set forth so far are largely descriptive and generally accepted. The ones that follow are more inferential, and have more to do with the subjective experience of the developing person, and so are more open to controversy and debate. They strike us as useful principles for the understanding of behavior, and necessary if one is going to consider behavior in all its subtlety and variety.

DEVELOPMENT TOWARD SELF-KNOWLEDGE AND AUTONOMY

The principle of *development toward self-knowledge and autonomy* points to the progressive differentiation of self from environment, and of various aspects of self from the totality, and to the integration of self-awareness into an emergent self-image or self-schema. It also points to the child's increasing ability to regulate his own behavior and to think and act on his own. We have already sketched in some highlights of the development of self-awareness (see page 101). Here we want to make explicit that such development is a general trend (complicated by our tendencies to self-deception), accompanied by increasing autonomy, ability to think, decide, and act for oneself, to consider one's own actions in perspective, and to find original modes of acting. Now it is obvious that some of what we experience as self-determination or "will" had its actual beginnings outside ourselves, in the knowledge and understanding and values that other people taught us. But it is possible also to make other people's teachings truly one's own, so that they cease to be external to oneself and instead are part of one's own equipment for behavior.

The development of self-awareness involves several sorts of differentiation. There is differentiation of self from environment, there is differentiation of self as knower from self as thing known—consider the statement "I am thinking about myself"—and there comes to be a differentiation of private self and public self. Here we have a sub-principle of *duplicity*, of being able to think one thing and say another, to have an inner life, and eventually to dissemble and to lie. It sometimes seems that middle-years children go through a period of deliberate lying, not so much to deceive as to test their powers of deception. Perhaps the first manifestation of duplicity appears in late infancy or early toddlerhood with the child's playful simulation of an emotion, as when he pretends to be hurt so as to be cuddled and soothed, or with his playful adoption of an identity not his own, as when he pretends to be a dog. As we shall see in the next chapter, autonomy—establishing an independent self—is a dominant theme in toddlerhood.

COMPETENCE MOTIVATION

As we said earlier, psychologists and psychiatrists have too long tended to think in terms of deficiency motivations, whereby some lack or imbalance must be invoked to account for behavior. However, as thinkers (who are also skilled observers) like Barbara Biber and Gardner and Lois Murphy have pointed out, such a formulation does not account for the fact that children brought up in a warm, supporting, and stimulating environment show from an early age a pleasure in exploration, manipulation, and mastery of the new things they encounter.

Robert White[30] has suggested the name of *competence motivation* for the child's curiosity about things and what they are like and his drive to acquire and exercise skills in dealing with the world, whether at the level of stacking rings on a peg, learning and using new words, or learning to ride a tricycle, perhaps in the same way that adults do puzzles. Human behavior is not all describable in terms of biological imbalances, or even in terms of need for affiliation with other creatures, but includes in addition something like cognitive needs or strivings— needs to know, to find out, to be interested.

Whether, along with White and conventional psychological thinking, we want to locate this motive force inside the organism, or whether, like D. O. Hebb and Mary Henle and some others, we want to give more attention to the motivating and mobilizing power of objects and their demand qualities, we must take account of behavior which does not seem to be activated by physical or interpersonal disequilibrium but by the enjoyment of doing what is near the edge of ability—the ability to be tantalized. Indeed, as we have said, disequilibrium interferes with such behavior. Competence motivation becomes an important developmental principle because the behavior it produces leads to learning, and learning to change. Competence motivation has obvious links to Harlow's curiosity drive and to his notion of learning sets, learning to learn (see page 182). Since much of development is built on the accumulation and integration of knowledge and understanding, learning sets must be considered an important factor in development. Learning sets may also help us understand how children become able to perform perfectly novel, emergent acts unprecedented in their own experience—for instance, every normal child says things that he has never heard said (see page 232).

AMBIVALENCE, GROWTH AMBIVALENCE, AND DUAL AMBIVALENCE

We have already mentioned the fact of *ambivalence*, of how one can be of two minds about someone or something, finding it simultaneously or in alternation both attractive and repellent. Often we try to conceal one of these minds from ourselves and admit only to the attitude we consider acceptable. Ambivalence describes our feelings about many of the people and situations we meet in life, and sometimes our feelings about ourselves. It also seems to characterize how children feel about growing up, as though there were considerable conflict between a progressive urge, which tells the child to venture forth, to explore, to try new things, and a conservative one, which tells the child to preserve the status quo, to play it safe, to avoid ventures into the dangerous unknown, or even a reactionary one that lures the child back to still earlier stages of immaturity. This conflict is called *growth ambivalence*.

There is little evidence of growth ambivalence in infancy, but it becomes prominent in toddlerhood, where the child at one moment is all autonomy, competence, and bluster, and the next moment is asking to be babied, to be rocked, petted, and fed. Obviously, the weight is usually on the side of progress, since most people do grow up, but not wholly, which may be why so many of us, even as adults, quail and wobble whenever there is a major decision to be made, even when change is obviously in the direction of improvement.

Now, it is bad enough that the child is plagued by growth ambivalence, but to make matters worse, so are his parents. That is, they applaud every step of his development—his first smile, his first participation in family games, his first walking, his first word—but each such step brings an increasing and disagreeable appreciation that the parents are losing their baby, that the child is moving toward self-sufficiency and defiance, away from innocence and into the harsh reality of the outside world. The combined ambivalences of child and parents about growth we have called *dual ambivalence*. Dual ambivalence reaches an acute climax, as we shall see, at adolescence, when the youngster is making his final move away from the family and into mature independence, but it crops up at every stage and transition. The child's first day at school is a moment of excitement but trepidation for the child, and of pride but regret for the parent.

MATURATION, EXPERIENCE, AND LEARNING

Physical maturation is a fact. The child does go through somatic transformations and metamorphoses which have profound effects on his psychological functioning. It is important to understand how maturational changes arise and what their implications are for behavior. It is obvious, first of all, that all of maturation is instigated (and realized with reasonable environmental support) by the genetic material contained in the cell nuclei, and its capacities for processing environmental information so as to manufacture an organism. We have seen how, at the plastic, embryonic stage of development, the introduction of abnormal information in the form of viruses, x-rays, chemicals, temperature changes, and so forth, evokes teratogenic expressions of a bizarre kind. Once certain alternatives are chosen however, they are generally irreversible, so that the organism becomes less and less plastic, in the sense of having fewer and fewer alternative potentialities. We know about some obvious influences on postnatal physical development—diet, fresh air and sunshine, illness, exercise—but the psychological relevance of these is obscure. There is good reason to think that autonomic nervous system and endocrine functioning can be shaped by emotional experience, and through them both the vegetative functions that they regulate—digestion, circulation, respiration, sweating, sex, and so on—and associated patterns of temperament and motivation. At least since Freud, we have come to take for granted the notion of psychosomatic illness, the physical malfunctions and lesions produced by chronic emotional stress. It is possible that normal maturation is in part a psychosomatic effect, governed both by stressful emotions and pleasant ones, and hence by the environmental circumstances that produce them. It is tempting to think that cognitive-intellectual experience, and the demonstrable residue of learning that it leaves behind, also has psychosomatic consequences. In fact, as we have seen, enriched cognitive experience does alter brain biochemistry in the rat, and C. J. Smith[31] has shown that the brains of rats raised in "rich" environments develop areas of specialized function, whereas the brains of rats raised in ordinary laboratory conditions do not, acting instead according to the "law of mass action." The findings from animal research are reviving interest in a once-discarded concept, what Wheeler called *stimulation-induced maturation.* We know, because as educators we do it all the time, that we can teach people to make new perceptual discriminations, to perceive new patterns of figure-ground organization, and to perceive previously hidden spatial and functional relations, but we do not know whether we have thereby altered the structure of the sense receptors. We do know, though, that sense receptors deprived of stimulation early in life atrophy and may become nonfunctional.

The chief effect of maturational changes seems to be to make new kinds of behavior possible. That is, *maturation* and *experience* seem to stand in a circular relationship, each feeding into the other. Thus, it is only at a given stage of maturation that the baby becomes able to roll over, to walk, to control his sphincters. Another way of saying the same thing is that a maturational change brings with it a *readiness* for the appearance of a given kind of behavior. The new behavior may appear almost spontaneously—in Wayne Dennis's term, *autogenously,* that is, self-generated—with a minimum of specific preparation, practice, stimulation, or support. Or it may require special environmental stimulation of some sort, as in the case of learning to talk. Now in general, the mere fact of maturation having taken place does not guarantee that the associated behavior will take place. If, for instance, a seemingly autogenous behavior like walking is delayed artificially beyond its normal time of appearance, as by prolonged illness or an injury that keeps a baby bedridden, walking comes with greater difficulty than under normal conditions. On the other hand, deprivation of proto-walking activities up to that time seems to have little effect. We have already mentioned, too, that no one has yet studied the contribution of spatial orientation, particularly to the vertical, to the development of walking, although we know that blind babies walk later than seeing ones. In the same way, the maturational changes of puberty do not automatically bring with them sexual lusts and strivings—experimental evidence indicates that white rats and monkeys who have had socially-deprived prepubertal histories are sexually inadequate, and anecdotal evidence indicates that many physically normal adult human beings have a low level of sexual drive. Many sorts of readiness, moreover, such as readiness to learn to read or to use numbers, seem to depend at least as much on prior experience as on any particular maturational states. Obviously, maturation and amount of experience are both highly correlated with how long a child has lived, and it is logically very difficult to disentangle the relative contribution of each to a state of readiness.

While maturation, whether proceeding naturally in the course of growth or produced by psychologically meaningful stimulation, defines the beginning of a period of readiness, such periods may also have an end. That is, maturation may bring *critical* or *sensitive periods,* analogous to those of prenatal development, during which a given function is most responsive to cultivation, trauma, or neglect. We do not know enough about what brings a critical period to an end, whether some maturational change or a conflicting bit of learning, or just what the consequences are of delaying learning beyond the end of a critical period. We do know or suspect a few things. Such evidence as we have suggests that delaying the formation of close social attachments much beyond the age of six months may impair the baby's ability to form such attachments. There is good experimental evidence that puppies kept from human contact during their first nine to fourteen weeks of life are permanently unable to become attached to humans.[32] The evidence is less good, but there is some reason to believe that some chronic bedwetters had their toilet training delayed too long, say past age three. We have already mentioned that interfering with walking during and beyond the normal period of beginning to walk may have adverse effects. On the other hand, we know that some skills ordinarily acquired fairly early in life, such as reading, can still be learned late in life, although perhaps not so easily. Much work remains to be done to clarify the nature of critical periods and their generality for all of postnatal development. Meanwhile a good rule for parents and teachers seems to be that when a child seems refractory to being taught something, they should consider whether it is because he is not yet ready to learn it. They should also bear in mind that premature pressure may arouse antipathy and so yield results opposite to those they are seeking.

The fact that accumulated experience—*learning*—and maturation blend so inextricably and circularly into each other poses problems for the usual conception of associative learning. There are yet other difficulties, since conventional learning theories are concerned only with the acquisition of single responses, and take little account of how learning affects the individual's total cognitive-affective-motivational organization. It takes no account of learning by absorption, the taking in of broad patterns of knowledge about one's surroundings by simple exposure, from learning to recognize the members of one's family to learning about spatial relations, to taking on the styles of movement and intonations and values of the people around about. Most learning theories take no account of the way empathy and participation enter into learning about things and learning how to do things, or how learning broadens the range of the things we can empathize with or participate in. Little attention is given to emotional learning, learning to love and hate things, to develop a complex emotional repertory, to care, which we take to be at the heart of psychological development. Learning theories seem not to be concerned with the contribution of learning to thinking, reasoning, problem solving, the integration of experience and the construction of new versions of the world, whether playful or serious. They say little about mislearning, or, as we have noted, about unlearning. In short, they say little about the implications of learning for the development of intelligence, conceived not as coldly rational information-processing but as a capacity—in addition—for warm, feeling-laden, sensitive, relativistic, imaginative thinking. In the same vein, learning theory takes no account of how mislearning may impair the development of intelligence.

THE SCHEMATIZATION OF EXPERIENCE

A component of development is the acquisition of knowledge, a set of more or less patterned, integrated *schemata* (singular, *schema*). A schema is a conception of what something or a group of things is like. Ordinarily, schemata are implicit, although they can often be verbalized, and are experienced mostly as vague feelings. It is when our schemata clash with reality that they become most easily perceptible. Such clashes surprise us and can produce laughter, bewilderment, or terror, or various combinations of feelings, depending on the nature of the discrepancy. When the burly male speaks in a piping falsetto, or the wispy female in a booming voice, when the naked savage discourses knowingly on Proust and Ionesco and constructivism, when the magician pulls endless yards of fabric out of a thimble, when the nice young honor student down the block turns out to be a sex murderer, previously implicit schemata are brought into jarring contrast with new ones. Sometimes our schemata are so strong that they interfere with our perceptions; we call such schemata preconceptions, prejudices, stereotypes, or superstitions.

The schematization of the body can produce vivid schematic experience when a limb is amputated, leaving behind a "phantom limb" which, until it gradually shrinks away, feels as though it is really there.[33] One can even suffer pain or discomfort in a missing extremity. Apparently the parts of our own body are not automatically given to us by virtue of some sort of built-in representation in the nervous system, since phantom limbs do go away, and since people born with an extremity missing, but with intact brains, seem never to experience phantoms.[34] Instead, the composition and reach and other knowledge of our own bodies seem to be built up through early experience and feedback to our activities consolidated as a schema which tells us what our bodies are doing and where they are, both the whole body in space and the various parts relative to each other and to the total schema. Most of the time we know automatically and semiconsciously what our bodies are up to—we do not have to stop and wonder where a hand is before we can use it—but the major surface regions of the body can be brought into awareness at will.

The phantom limb has its schematic counterpart in what the authors choose to call "phantom environments," that is, animals and people sometimes go on acting in terms of the way things used to be, apparently unaware that circumstances have changed. In an experiment by Carr and Watson,[35] a maze alley that had previously led to food was blocked off, but rats which had learned to turn into the alley thereafter persistently and interminably continued trying to enter the now nonexistent pathway. Skinner[36] says that if one encloses a flock of sheep with electrified wire, after a while one can remove the wire and substitute string, and the sheep will continue to avoid the string as though it were wire. People, too, in their thinking about social issues such as sex, birth control, economics, conservation, pollution, transportation, international relations, the reapportionment of state legislatures, racial integration, education, or whatever, often act as though they were living in the phantom environments of bygone centuries. Nostalgia, of course, expresses a yearning for a phantom environment, one which may in fact never have existed.

Our better-defined and better reality-related schemata are sometimes called "concepts," especially when we can name them and talk about them. Our general schema of reality can be said to include more restricted, specialized schemata such as a spatial schema, a schema of time, and schemata of social roles, causation, life, death, sickness and health, procreation, body functions, esthetics, morality, social organization, human nature, shape, color, numbers and numerical relations, history, and so on through all the domains of knowledge.

CANALIZATION

One other variety of learning that we have touched on and which does not fit exactly either the classical or the operant conditioning model is called *canalization*, a term that Gardner Murphy[37] took over from the French psychologist Pierre Janet. When the organism is in a state of need, there are for many need states a variety of possible satisfiers. Thus, hunger, or even a special appetite or craving as for sweets, in principle can be satisfied by any number of different foodstuffs. Usually, though, a given culture decrees that only a few of the many potential satisfiers are acceptable, and after a while the individual develops a taste for and comes to think of the accustomed satisfiers as the only possible ones, rejecting the others as unfit. That is, he canalizes on what his culture defines as the proper satisfiers of needs. The Eskimo child learns to relish whale blubber, the southern child hominy grits, the Rhode Island child johnnycakes, the Philadelphia child scrapple, the Hawaiian child smoked fish and poi, the Oriental child rice, and so on around the world. And the child simultaneously learns not to like various other, equally nourishing foods. Most Americans quail at eating raw fish (although they will eat raw oysters), horse meat, or pickled bees. In a recent study by Burghardt and Hess,[38] young turtles fed consistently for their first few days on particular foods, all of them part of most adult turtle diets, thereafter consistently chose the specific food each had started with. Our many canalizations amount to a schematization of the familiar as "natural" and "good" and "human," with an accompanying distrust of anything that does not match such schemata as alien and hence "inferior." It is our feeling that parents would do well to give their children early in life experience with highly variegated need satisfiers, including people, to forestall the formation of narrow and rigid canalizations which may prevent openness to new experiences. This is not to speak of occasional distinctly deviant canalizations—in the realm of sexuality, for instance, we have homosexuality, in which the satisfier of sexual needs is a person of the same sex, and fetishism, in which objects like shoes or underwear or stuffed seagulls become invested with sexual meaning.

It will be seen that there is a kinship between canalization and both imprinting and cathexis. In Murphy's view, canalization is the more general, inclusive mechanism, with imprinting and cathexis as special instances. Burghardt and Hess, however, in the study mentioned above, have completely reversed this relationship, and describe food canalization as food-imprinting, and the difference may be merely one of choice of words for the same concepts. Since the authors early imprinted or canalized on the thinking of Murphy, we shall continue from his viewpoint. Imprinting, then, would be canalization of response to the mother (or surrogate) as the gratifier of something like a "need-for-affiliation." A difficulty with this position, of course, is that imprinting takes place before there is any opportunity to learn about the need-gratifying potentialities of the mother figure.

Cathexis likewise is seen as canalization on particular objects out of a potentially large array that gratify erotic needs, and in this respect is closer to standard notions of learning. However, cathexis includes not only the gratifying objects but also the zones and channels—mouth, anus, genitals—of satisfaction and, in addition, the activities—sucking, biting, chewing, expelling, rubbing, thrusting, handling—that bring the person into contact with satisfiers. Thus, to make cathexis a special case of canalization requires broadening of the original concept. To make canalization a general principle of character-formation, we should be prepared to include in it such things as hammock-sleeping, as contrasted with ground-sleeping or mat-sleeping or bed-sleeping, as a means for satisfying a need for rest. Whether such a broadening weakens the power of the concept by making it synonymous with *taste* or *preference* is something the reader is free to decide.

In any event, canalization shares with learning theory and psychoanalysis its dependence on needs as a basis for learning, whereas in our view cultural learning is in large part motivation-free. Let us make clear that we are not rejecting the usual principles of learning, such as those having to do with the pairings of events, reward and punishment, primacy and recency, massed and spaced practice, retroactive and proactive inhibition, schedules of reinforcement, and so on, as these apply to a particular item of learning. Rather, we want to emphasize that there are other mechanisms for learning as well, and that the point of understanding learning is for its effect on development, the way experience gives us a progressively better-articulated knowledge of the world and of ourselves, and the conceptual and symbolic tools with which to think about the world and thus to transform our perceiving, feeling, thinking, and acting.

ROLE PLAYING

Yet another way that learning influences development is through the child's imitation of the people, real and imagined, whom he observes and hears about. Such *role playing*, sometimes in a spirit of travesty, sometimes as outright make-believe, and sometimes in an earnest attempt to find and convey an identity, includes the infant's imitation of simple actions and of adult gestures, expressions, and styles of movement, the toddler's taking on of domestic activities, the preschool child's dramatic play, the middle-years child's playing at pirates or spacemen (but in many cultures taking on serious roles as assistants to men and women), the adolescent's performance as whatever the current version of sophistication may be, and so on to the adult's being Pillar of the Community, or Learned Professor, or Captain of Industry, or Prominent Clubwoman, or pleasure-loving Femme Fatale. One of the more interesting things about role playing is the way middle-years and adolescent youngsters play the role of being their age. One eight-year-old boy, for instance, avidly collected baseball cards and kept track of games and team standings in the sports pages in accordance with the mores of his neighborhood, even though he had never seen a baseball game or expressed the slightest interest in attending one.

However trivial or specious role playing may seem, it gives the individual a chance to try on styles of life and the values they contain, and thereby to discover those modes of being that he or she finds most congenial and meaningful. It is worth mentioning that advertisers often play on the wish to try on attractive roles, implying that the buyers of their products will gain access to new realms of being. Opinion-leaders and trend-setters seem to be effective because they offer a role model with which people can identify. In general, as we shall say again, role playing is one of the ways one takes on a cultural identity. Obviously, role playing implies that one perceives the role. Mary Ellen Goodman[39] reports that Japanese urban middle-class five-year-olds were able to describe some sixty social role categories, defined by age, sex, kinship, and occupation, together with typical behavior or traits.

The Scientific Method

There seem to be three main approaches to the teaching of psychology. One is to teach it as subject matter, as an accumulation of facts and principles. Another is to teach it as method, the established techniques by which psychologists obtain information, with the subject matter of psychology defined as the problems susceptible to study by the available methods. Third is the teaching of psychology as quest, as an attempt to define the central issues and enigmas of human development and behavior and then to devise methods by which to study these problems.

While the older sciences tend to be taught by the first approach, the methods approach looms large in United States psychology, which, self-conscious about its scientific status, has striven to become an experimental science on the analogy of physics and to stress the description of the scientific process laid down by philosophers of science. So it is that most respectable textbooks of psychology have a chapter or more on the scientific method, how one deduces hypotheses from theories, tests hypotheses by an experiment, including the control and manipulation of relevant or potentially relevant independent variables, how one measures operationally defined dependent variables, applies statistical tests of the reliability of observed differences between experimental and control conditions, and revises theory in the light of the distilled experimental findings. The more rigorous of the experimentalists would banish into outer darkness information gathered outside the framework of the scientific method. Thus, "attention" and "consciousness" were outlaw concepts in psychology until biologists brought them back into favor. Much of our recent knowledge about animal development is only an experimental verification of what animal breeders and caretakers have long known and biologically-oriented ethologists have forced psychology to examine.

For a number of reasons, this book will be an exception to the general rule. One reason is that many of its readers will already have had an adequate introduction to scientific method, as in a beginning psychology course. Another is that actual scientific research, as a number of leading investigators have pointed out,[40] seldom conforms to the ideal set forth in textbooks, and is actually a somewhat disorderly procedure involving curiosity (independent of any particular theory), hunches, intuitions, trial and error, false starts, spoiled trials, lost subjects, concern with practical problems as well as abstract theories, and a large dose of serendipity—the happy accident. (Harlow's discovery of the sexual inadequacy of his surrogate-reared monkeys came about only when he tried to breed them for the purpose of procuring more laboratory monkeys.) Fine as it is for the study of many problems, the experimental method is simply not suited to many important issues in human development, if only because of the ethical implications of manipulating the fate of children.

There is the further problem that human development is a slow process, and our experimental manipulations and evaluation of effects may take years, whereas the experimentalist is oriented to the short-term study which yields rapid results. It is considerations of ethics and time which have helped make the study of animal development recently so popular, since we can place infrahuman infants in controlled environments in a way unthinkable for human babies (although, to be sure, some people have expressed misgivings about inflicting physically or psychologically traumatic treatments on the higher vertebrates, most especially monkeys and apes) and get information relatively quickly. We should note that students of animal development often use a technique to control for genetic effects, called *cross-fostering*. That is, the young are exchanged between mothers right after birth, so that their later behavior can be related to the characteristics both of the biological mother and of the foster mother who reared them. This control is preferable to the so-called *split litter* method, because there is great genetic diversity within litters, even in inbred stocks. Techniques have even been developed for trading babies between mothers right after conception. This technique is called *cross-implantation.*

One can experimentally study the short-range effects of nontraumatic treatments, as in learning experiments, on matched groups of human subjects. One sort of quasi-experimental study using variations not created by the experimenter but seized on by him is the comparison of institutionalized and noninstitutionalized children. More directly under experimental control, and an approach that is becoming increasingly widespread, is the enrichment of experience of institutionalized or otherwise severely deprived children. The scientific purist might be offended by such studies, in which "enrichment" consists of numerous, diverse, and more or less simultaneous treatments (human contact, linguistic stimulation, teaching sensory discriminations, music and art, access to a variety of play materials, and so forth), making it extremely difficult to assess the impact of any one. On the other hand, we consider that rigorous adherence to experimental control of variables can produce a caricature of enrichment, as in one recent study in which the experimenter recited to babies, "in an impersonal fashion," the numbers one to five, ten minutes twice a day, five days a week for ten weeks.[41] However, when one chooses and compares conditions over which the experimenter has no control, such as age, sex, social class, cultural and subcultural differences, child care practices, or illness or physical impairment, one is obliged to use the method of the *natural experiment,* the chief method of disciplines like astronomy where intervention is out of the question. But notice that natural experiments can follow the laboratory paradigm, except that it is the real world rather than the experimenter that manipulates the independent variable. The natural experiment is usually concerned with outcomes; with functions and abilities such as perception or intelligence or thinking or attitudes, as they are found in subjects from the different comparison groups. The experimenter provides the stimulus and records the response, but he is mainly interested in the way the antecedent variable mediates the response. Thus, for instance, if a researcher wanted to compare human figure drawings by lower-class and middle-class children, he would supply the paper and pencil and instructions, which would be a constant factor for all subjects, while the variation would come from social-class differences over which he has no control, but representatives of which he would have carefully selected for comparison.

A once-fashionable method in child psychology was the *normative study,* the recording by age of those changes in functioning that occur in the course of development. Nowadays, our awareness of the impact of different approaches to child-rearing makes us question the universality of almost any age-normative findings. That is, the age at which a new competence first emerges, and with what intensity or in what quantity, or even whether it occurs at all, seems to vary with the developmental context. This does not mean that normative studies are useless, but only that one has to specify the conditions in which the norms can be expected to apply. Normative techniques can be very useful in comparing the effects of sex differences, cultural and social class differences, and home versus institutional rearing on development.

While the canons of scientific method stress measurement, the fundamental technique of the developmental psychologist is *observation,* watching children in action to see what they do and how they go about it in homes, supermarkets, playgrounds, nursery schools, and other settings. It is through observation, often combined with some variant of Piaget's *"clinical"* method, by which one discusses with a child his thoughts and activities, that one comes to a first intuitive comprehension of what children are like. An astute observer can learn a great deal simply by watching and listening to and talking with children, after the manner of the naturalist observing the behavior of antelopes or ants or baboons. The power of naturalistic observation is attested by a review comparing two compendia of the behavior of primates, one based on laboratory studies and the other on field studies, which points out that the contents of the two volumes contain virtually no overlapping information.[42] Observations can be made in free situations or in carefully arranged ones, and can be oriented toward recording behavior in general or only some selected aspect of behavior. We can observe with a view to learning about children in general (the *nomothetic* approach) or to capturing the idiosyncratic uniqueness of a particular child (the *idiographic* approach).[43] The *case study* approach, particularly as it applies to normal individuals, has fallen into neglect in recent years, but there is still much to be learned from the intensive study of individual lives.[44] Investigations which study the same individuals repeatedly at different stages of their lives are called *longitudinal* studies; the longitudinal method is usually contrasted with the *cross-sectional* method, which compares the characteristics of different ages by studying different groups of children representing the various ages but presumably similar with respect to such other important variables as sex, socioeconomic status, and so forth.

Among the special environments in which we observe subjects, whether for idiographic or nomothetic purposes, are those provided by *tests*, which permit comparison of the child's performance with some reference group. There are two main sorts of tests, the *psychometric*, which yield a numerical score, or a collection of scores, called a *profile*, and the *projective*, which are scored qualitatively, in terms of the personality traits revealed.

The psychometric instruments include *intelligence tests* (of which more later), *aptitude tests* of special abilities such as arithmetic, mechanical relations, dexterity, clerical skills, and so on, *achievement tests* which tell how much the child has learned following exposure to a

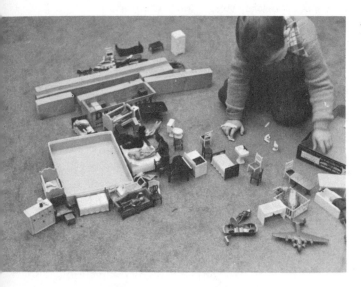

Projective play techniques.
L. Joseph Stone

course of instruction, and *personality tests* which measure the "amount" a child possesses of various traits such as hostility, anxiety, defensiveness, or whatever. Psychometric instruments can be either of the *paper-and-pencil* variety (once the child is literate), which can be given to a large number of subjects at the same time, or *individual* tests, which may be given orally, but which may also involve the subject's writing or drawing something, or assembling puzzles in a way that the examiner has to record.

Like psychometric tests, projective tests provide stimuli for the subject to respond to, but the stimuli permit a much wider range of appropriate responses, which are not "right" and "wrong" but rather are taken as samples of characteristic behavior or style of thinking and response. The stimuli may have a low degree of structure, as in the case of finger paints or the famous Rorschach ink blots, which invite the subject to supply his own structure; or they may be highly structured, like the dolls and house furnishings of Lois Murphy's Miniature Life Toys, which the subject is free to organize in ways that seem meaningful to him. Presumably the use the child makes of projective materials reveals something about his inner workings, but the interpretation of his performance has a large component of subjectivity, and attempts to objectify scoring have not been altogether satisfactory. Projective methods should not be thought of as tests in the strict sense, but as semistandardized settings in which to make observations of the kinds considered below.

Allied to tests are *questionnaires,* inviting the subject to supply information about himself, first used by G. Stanley Hall, one of the fathers of child psychology. We can also get information through *interviews,* a more or less formal or fixed series of factual or attitudinal questions asked orally. The interview gives the subject more scope to elaborate on his answers than does the questionnaire, and also permits the interviewer to explore what look like promising byways. Notice that interviews can be used not only with the child himself but also with parents, teachers, or other people who know the child.

Tests and interview questions give the subject's behavior a focus, but there are also devices that let the subject run free but that sharpen the process of observation. First of all, there are *anecdotal reports* of behavior, which may take such forms as a continuous, narrative *running record* or a more global, summary *impression record.* We can prepare tally sheets telling the observer exactly what items or aspects of behavior to be on the lookout for. When we want to compare the incidence of certain behavior, such as nose-picking, teasing, or sandbox play, from child to child or group to group, we can arrange schedules of observation (*time samples*) such that all subjects will be observed for comparable periods. We can construct *rating scales* by which an observer assigns numerical weights to behavior in terms either of general characteristics such as kind-cruel or of more circumscribed specific behaviors like crying or asking for help. Notice that ratings of this sort always imply a frame of reference, and it must be made explicit whether a child is being rated relative to "children the rater has known," "children of this age," "boys in general," "girls in general," "the child's brothers and sisters," or other children, say, in this child's preschool class. Parents and older children can make ratings of themselves, of other children or parents, of their own children or parents, of schools and teachers, of TV programs, and so forth indefinitely. Rating scales can also be used in the evaluation of things children do or make, such as maturity of play, masculinity of style, imaginativeness of language, or quality of paintings.

For the study of group organization we have such techniques as *sociometry,* by which each member of the group is asked which members of the group he would most or least like to have share in some specific activity. The compiling of such choices gives us a good picture of the group's status hierarchy, who the often-chosen stars are, who the choosing but unchosen hangers-on, who the nonselected outcasts. The patterning of reciprocal choices gives us a picture of group solidarity and reveals the clusterings that are cliques. A way of studying the personality characteristics that go with status in the group is the *guess-who* technique, which gives the child a trait description—for example, "this child is always showing off"—and asks the child to guess which member of the group it is.

We can extend our own powers of observation, by the use of one-way screens which remove the observer from the child's ken, along with his possible interference in the very events he wants to study, with cameras, binoculars, parabolic microphones, tape recorders, and endless gadgetry. The use of recording devices also permits us to observe the same bit of behavior repeatedly for detailed analysis. But the ingenuity of the psychologist's observing techniques, whether using the naked eye or telephoto lens, along with his real need to study unselfconscious behavior, raises grave questions about invasion of privacy and just what it is about an individual's (and his family's) life that a psychologist has a right to know—especially if the individual does not realize how much he is revealing or to what use the information is to be put. It is because these are such grave problems, and because we feel that the welfare of the individual has to come first, that beginning students in our laboratories are repeatedly cautioned to keep strictly confidential what they have learned about particular individuals, and not to convert their privileged knowledge into idle gossip. Children may inadvertently expose not only themselves but also all kinds of family secrets, and the student, researcher, or teacher who is made privy to such secrets has a solemn obligation to see that they stay secret. Publications, it need hardly be added, must always conceal the identity of individual subjects. Research on sensitive questions such as personal relations and attitudes may be stressful, and the experimenter must do everything possible to minimize stress and to assure that any temporary dislocations are set right. This is particularly important where for serious experimental purposes the experimenter in some way misleads or misinforms his subjects.

In closing this section, let us remind the reader that he or she will find abundant examples of research applications throughout this book. Let us also say that many problems are waiting to be studied, and in order to study some of them, we will almost certainly have to find new techniques.

While we have been talking about theory and techniques, our infant has pulled himself to his feet and toddled into a new stage of development, where we must make haste to follow him—at this age, he is moving very fast.

REFERENCES / Chapter 4

[1] White, R. W. Motivation reconsidered: The concept of competence. *Psychological Review*, 1959, 66, 297–333 and Ego and reality in psychoanalytic theory. *Psychological Issues*, 1963, Monograph No. 11; Smith, M. B. Socialization for competence. *Social Science Research Council Items*, 1965, 19, 17–23; see also Chodoff, P. A critique of Freud's theory of infantile sexuality. *American Journal of Psychiatry*, 1966, 123, 507–518.

[2] Merton, R. K. *On The Shoulders of Giants*. New York: Free Press, 1965.

[3] Hilgard, E. R., and Bower, G. H. *Theories of Learning*. New York: Appleton-Century-Crofts, third edition, 1966.

[4] Spence, K. W. Cognitive factors in the extinction of the conditioned eyelid response in humans. *Science*, 1963, 140, 1224–1225.

[5] Barker, R. G., Dembo, T., and Lewin, K. Frustration and regression: An experiment with children. *University of Iowa Studies in Child Welfare*, 1941, 18, no. 1.

[6] Rosenzweig, S., and Kogan, K. L. *Psychodiagnostics*. New York: Grune & Stratton, 1949.

[7] Solomon, R. L. Punishment. *American Psychologist,* 1963, 18, 239–253.

[8] Keller, L., Cole, M., Burke, C. J., and Estes, W. K. Reward and information values of trial outcomes in paired-associate learning. *Psychological Monographs,* 1965, 79, no. 12.

[9] Nelson, T. H. The Hypertext. International Federation for Documentation: *Abstracts, 1965 Congress,* p. 80.

[10] Allen, K. E., Hart, B., Buell, J. S., Harris, F. R., and Wolf, M. M. Effects of social reinforcement on isolate behavior of a nursery school child. *Child Development,* 1964, 35, 511–518.

[11] House, B. J., and Zeaman, D. Reward and nonreward in the discrimination learning of imbeciles. *Journal of Comparative and Physiological Psychology,* 1958, 51, 614–618.

[12] Maier, N. R. F. Maier's Law. *American Psychologist,* 1960, 15, 208–212.

[13] Osgood, C. E. On understanding and creating sentences. *American Psychologist,* 1963, 18, 735–751.

[14] Miller, G. A., Galanter, E., and Pribram, K. H. *Plans and the Structure of Behavior.* New York: Holt, 1960.

[15] Kendler, T. S., and Kendler, H. H. Reversal and nonreversal shifts in kindergarten children. *Journal of Experimental Psychology,* 1959, 58, 56–60.

[16] Tighe, T. J. Reversal and nonreversal shifts in monkeys. *Journal of Comparative and Physiological Psychology,* 1964, 58, 324–326.

[17] Harlow, H. F., and Kuenne, M. Learning to think. *Scientific American,* 1949, 181, 36–39.

[18] Bitterman, M. E., Wodinsky, J., and Candland, D. K. Some comparative psychology. *American Journal of Psychology,* 1958, 71, 94–110.

[19] Darby, C. L., and Riopelle, A. J. Observational learning in the rhesus monkey. *Journal of Comparative and Physiological Psychology,* 1959, 52, 94–98; Riopelle, A. J. Observational learning of a position habit by monkeys. *Journal of Comparative and Physiological Psychology,* 1960, 53, 426–428.

[20] Inhelder, B., and Piaget, J. *The Early Growth of Logic in the Child.* New York: Harper & Row, 1964.

[21] Skinner, B. F. Behaviorism at fifty. *Science,* 1963, 140, 951–958.

[22] Miller, Galanter, and Pribram, *op. cit.*

[23] Krasner, L. Studies of the conditioning of verbal behavior. *Psychological Bulletin,* 1958, 55, 148–170.

[24] Sperry, R. W. Summation. In Kimble, D. P. (ed.) *The Anatomy of Memory.* Palo Alto: Science and Behavior Books, 1965, pp. 140–177.

[25] Boring, E. G. *A History of Experimental Psychology.* New York: Appleton-Century-Crofts, second edition, 1950, pp. 229–231.

[26] Lewin, K. *A Dynamic Theory of Personality.* New York: McGraw-Hill, 1935; Kuo, Z.-Y. *The Dynamics of Behavior Development: An Epigenetic View.* New York: Random House, 1967. PP 34.

[27] Bruner, J. S. *On Knowing.* Cambridge: Harvard-Belknap, 1962.

[28] Anastasi, A. Heredity, environment, and the question "How?" *Psychological Review,* 1958, 65, 197–208.

[29] Allport, G. W. The fruits of eclecticism—bitter or sweet? *Psychologia,* 1964, 7, 1–14.

[30] White, *op. cit.*

[31] Smith, C. J. Mass action and early environment in the rat. *Journal of Comparative and Physiological Psychology*, 1959, 52, 154–156.

[32] Freedman, D. G., King, J. A., and Elliot, O. Critical period in the social development of dogs. *Science*, 1961, 133, 1016.

[33] Haber, W. B. Reactions to loss of limb: Physiological and psychological aspects. *Annals of the New York Academy of Sciences*, 1958, 74, 14–24.

[34] Simmel, M. L. The absence of phantoms for congenitally missing limbs. *American Journal of Psychology*, 1961, 74, 467–470; Wilson, J. J., Wilson, B. C., and Swinyard, C. A. Two-point discrimination in congenital amputees. *Journal of Comparative and Physiological Psychology*, 1962, 55, 482–485.

[35] Carr, H. A., and Watson, J. B. Orientation in the white rat. *Journal of Comparative Neurology*, 1908, 18, 27–44.

[36] Skinner, B. F. *Walden Two*. New York: Macmillan, 1948.

[37] Murphy, G. *Human Potentialities*. New York: *Basic Books*, 1958, Chapter 5.

[38] Burghardt, G. M., and Hess, E. H. Food imprinting in the snapping turtle, Chelydra serpentina. *Science*, 1966, 151, 108–109.

[39] Goodman, M. E. Child's-eye views of the world of people. *Wheelock Alumnae Quarterly*, Winter 1965, pp. 7–10.

[40] American Psychological Association. Education for research in psychology. *American Psychologist*, 1960, 15, 158–159.

[41] Casler, L. The effects of supplementary verbal stimulation on a group of institutionalized infants. *American Psychologist*, 1965, 20, 476 (abstract).

[42] Altmann, S. A. Primate behavior in review. *Science*, 1965, 150, 1440–1442. (Reviews of Schrier, Harlow, and Stollnitz's *Behavior of Non-human Primates* and DeVore's *Primate Behavior*.)

[43] Allport, G. W. *The Use of Personal Documents in Psychological Science*. New York: Social Science Research Council, 1942.

[44] See Allport, *supra;* Church, J. (ed). *Three Babies*. New York: Random House, 1966; Dukes, W. F. N = 1. *Psychological Bulletin*, 1965, 64, 74–79; Garraty, J. A. The interrelations of psychology and biography. *Psychological Bulletin*, 1954, 51, 569–582; Langness, L. L. *The Life History in Anthropological Science*. New York: Holt, Rinehart, & Winston, 1965; White, R. W. *Lives in Progress*. New York: Holt, Rinehart, & Winston, second edition, 1966.

5 *The Toddler*

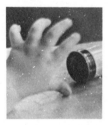

Between the ages of about fifteen months and two and a half years, the child lives a style of life that is called by some toddlerhood. Not all authorities recognize toddlerhood as a distinct period in development, preferring to assign the months before age two to infancy, and the months thereafter to the so-called preschool years. This seems to us a debatable course on several grounds. First, it seems inappropriate to call a child who can talk, often very proficiently, an *infant,* or unspeaking one. Second, even though he has become a walking and speaking baby, he is still a baby, very different in manner and appearance and competence from what he will become around age two and a half. Most important of all, toddlerhood is marked by its own very special emergents: completing the transition from quadruped to biped, the development of psychological autonomy, beginning to speak, and sphincter control. We, along with a lot of other people, object to the cuteness of "toddler," but we have not found a better name. Some writers, particularly the British, speak of the "run-about baby," but this is more cumbersome and does not lend itself easily to a designation of the period—that is, "run-about babyhood"—as well as of the child himself.

Behavioral Development in Toddlerhood

Even before he came to be a toddler, the baby may have been walking for some time, but he had probably done so uncertainly, with arms held high for balance—he was so involved with maintaining vertical equilibrium that his hands could not be used for any other purpose, such as carrying things or scratching an itch, while he was walking. When in a real hurry to get someplace, he was likely to revert to the speed and security of travel on all fours. But now he is truly up and away— exuberantly, doggedly, or timidly, according to his temperament—his legs spread apart but pumping steadily. Many toddlers fall down a great deal, tripping or stumbling or simply losing their balance, but they rarely hurt themselves seriously; this is because they have not yet learned the maladaptive reaction, found in older children and adults, of going stiff when they fall. Instead, they tumble limp and relaxed and resilient. In any case, they haven't far to fall. A toddler's legs are still short, by adult standards, in proportion to his trunk and head, giving him a bottom-heavy look which is further enhanced by the bulky diapers that will soon, in keeping with his new estate, give way to training pants. In appearance, as we have said, the toddler is still a baby, and one can follow his growth in Western homes as his head begins to rise above the top of the dining table until he can see what is on its surface, and as he reaches toward and eventually becomes able to grasp doorknobs. (Readers from cultural settings in which these are inappropriate measuring instruments are invited to devise their own yardsticks.) The toddler's babyish charm is indicated by the fact that he, more than the infant, was the model for the cherubim and cupids of Renaissance paintings. His small size means, of course, that he views much of the adult-scale world in terms of the undersides of things—the bathroom sink, for instance, with its water pipes and drain and the rust and scale and cobwebs that are masked from adult vision.

In much of his behavior, too, the toddler is still a baby. Every new object is seized, inspected, waved about as though to sample its heft and whatever sounds it produces, and as often as not stuffed as far as it will go into his mouth. He may be content to sit on the floor for long periods —for him—banging and tinkering with pots and pans and utensils while his mother goes about her work. He is still a baby, at least in early toddlerhood, in being more motor than verbal in his dealings with people. As in late infancy, the toddler probably takes two naps a day, switching to a single nap before age two. With time out for naps, the toddler's waking day now stretches from perhaps five in the morning to as late as eight in the evening. Nevertheless, he manifests new and unbabylike competences.

We shall describe shortly some of the major developments of

toddlerhood, but here we might mention some minor acquisitions found in children in United States culture. It is during toddlerhood that the child becomes able to chew gum without swallowing it, to drink through a straw, to eat with a spoon (we have not been able to find out at what age Chinese and Japanese children master chopsticks, but Indian toddlers have learned to use only the right hand for eating), to blow his nose into a handkerchief or tissue held by an adult (he may try to blow his own nose, too, with rather messy results), and to eat an ice-cream cone—a skill best acquired in warm weather outdoors, where the problems of mopping up are reduced. By age two, he may become able to work a simple record player, switching it on, selecting a particular record (which he seems to distinguish by the physiognomy of the label or even part of the label) and placing it on the turntable, moving the tone arm into position, and adjusting the volume—he generally keeps it turned low, suggesting that his hearing may be extremely acute. He may learn to ride a tricycle or a pedal-less kiddy-car, although on a tricycle he may at first try to push with both feet at once and have some trouble getting the knack of alternate thrusts. Also, his skill may outrun his judgment, and he has to be restrained from riding his tricycle into the street. He will probably not learn to put on and fasten his own clothes until the preschool years, but he early becomes adept at removing them, and an adult busy taking goods from the supermarket shelves may be startled to look down and discover a nude baby. The toddler imitates the superficial actions of grooming, chewing on toothbrush bristles or going through the motions of brushing and combing his hair—we even have a record of a seventeen-month-old trying to trim her nails with a pair of pruning shears.[1] Japanese babies by age two have learned to bow properly to an adult.

The toddler is moving rapidly away from babyhood and toward childhood in many other ways. Most generally, as Erikson says, the toddler is striving for *autonomy*, becoming aware of himself as a person among other people and wanting to do things for himself, with the developmental alternative of *shame and doubt* if conditions favorable to the development of autonomy are missing. The toddler demonstrates his beginning autonomy—and his desire for more of it—in every field: in the mastery of his own body (in walking, trotting, climbing up and climbing down, hopping and jumping, manipulating things, and in controlling his sphincters); in his mastery of objects (the toddler typically wants to push his stroller instead of riding in it, he wants to carry outsized things from place to place and back again, he becomes able not only to dismantle but also to reassemble various playthings, he becomes sensitive to attributes of objects such as their color or shape); in social relations (he learns language, he plays elaborate games, he begins to refuse parental commands and requests and offers of help, manifesting what is called *negativism*).

The toddler's push toward autonomy is by no means absolute and continuous, however. It seems to be greatest in Western societies and least in those cultures where the toddler still is regularly carried by the mother or baby-tender. Growth ambivalence shows up in the child's vacillating between dependence and independence, a conflict that will persist in various guises into adulthood. Out on a walk, the toddler may plunge off in pursuit of a pigeon, or go scuttling into a particularly alluring hallway, only to stop short and come hurtling back into his mother's arms. He may strike out on his own to explore the wonders of a store, and then burst into tears when he realizes the hand he is reaching for belongs to a stranger. When trying some new feat such as jumping from a step, he makes a great show of boldness but still clings tightly to an adult hand. In sum, he is still in the early stages of trying himself out, and it will be a long time before he achieves anything like true autonomy of thought and action. Also, in keeping with the principle of dual ambivalence, his parents, while taking pride and pleasure in each new step forward, both lament the movement away from infancy ("my baby!") and are unsure how much to trust the toddler's seeming competence, when to keep hands off and when to hover or intervene.

POSTURE, MOTOR BEHAVIOR, AND ORIENTATION IN SPACE

One of the key transitions of toddlerhood is from creeping to a pedestrian way of life, from quadrupedal to bipedal locomotion. It is true that the child begins walking while still an infant, but toddlerhood is marked by a qualitative change, shown by walking's being the normal mode of travel (although the toddler may still creep in a spirit of play), by the toddler's greater stability, and by his no longer needing his arms for balance, so that he can now carry things with him—as we said earlier, carrying things is a species of compulsion for the toddler. In spite of his new proficiency, the toddler up to about age two may still have to set himself in motion by rocking back and forth from foot to foot (such preludes to action are called *intention movements*, and are seen in a variety of situations, from the dog's circling before he lies down to the pitcher's winding up before he throws the ball).

Before long, the toddler not only walks but trots. In his bare feet, the toddler, like Tuesday's child, is full of grace. His toes are likely to be spread as he runs—and he is likely to run, and to run trippingly on his toes, far more than he is to walk or to use a sedate heel-and-toe movement. Once he has begun to run, he seldom moves in any other way, and one can see the beginning of later preschool styles of action, as in turning a corner—the toddler (and preschool child) typically turns a jog in a corridor by running straight ahead into the wall, bouncing off and changing direction, then resuming his run. He becomes able to hop on two feet, and perhaps to stand on one, although he certainly will not be able to hop on one foot much before age three. He learns to walk backward. He learns to pivot on one foot—at first he had to toddle laboriously around through a change of direction. He "dances" to music, at first by bobbing up and down in place, and then by moving his feet in a crude imitation of adult dancing—but note that children growing up in societies in which dancing is an intrinsic part of life become proficient dancers at an early age. Toddlers also enjoy being danced around in the arms of an adult to the tune of singing or humming or to music from phonograph or radio.

Here once again we must stress the great variety of individual styles, tempos, and temperaments that characterize the toddler's movements, in addition to variations of mood or transitory state (as a rule, "variety" refers to differences among individuals, "variation" to differences within an individual from time to time, or to ways in which an individual departs from the norm of his group). Some toddlers are bold, some are timid, some rough, others gentle, some are darting, some smoothly modulated, some graceful and others clumsy—but before describing a toddler as clumsy, we should make due allowance for the hampering effects of clothing, especially in those climes that demand heavy snowsuits and boots.

In new situations, most toddlers go through an initial phase of cautious quiescence, looking and listening and taking stock and staying in contact with the parent. Then, as they come to feel at home, they are likely to begin a hectic round of impulsive exploration, testing, and probing, pulled first this way and then that by the demand qualities of things and of spatial arrangements. In their familiar settings, by contrast, where the distracting effects of novelty are less potent, many toddlers can spend long periods of time engrossed in a single activity.

As we have said, toddlers love to carry, shove, haul, trundle, and otherwise set in motion things in the environment, the bigger the better.

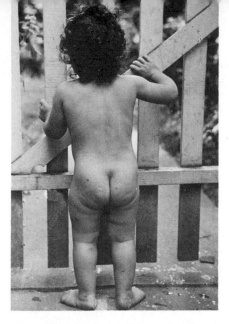

The toddler is the model for the cherubim and cupids of Renaissance painting.

Some toddlers devise elaborate ways of aiming themselves onto a seat.

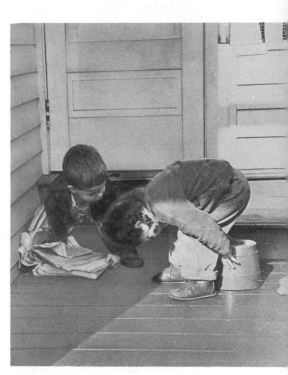

L. Joseph Stone

A toddler would rather carry something big, requiring two hands, than a small thing, and two small things, one for each hand, than a single small thing. This is the age at which the child trots about pulling or pushing the mechanical ducks or corn-poppers or other such toys that produce a pattern of sound and action. The toddler may try to give his dolls a ride in a coaster wagon and have trouble because the handle and pivoting front wheels are designed for pulling, not pushing, whereas the toddler wants to push so that he can see the dolls riding.

Almost from the time he first crept, the baby has been able to go up a flight of stairs on all fours (assuming that his world contains stairs). Going up, with the supporting stairs filling up his field of view, is fine; but when he turns around to go down, the stairs drop away beneath him, he faces the void, and the visual-cliff effect holds him fast and fear-stricken at the top of the stairs (although no amount of visual-cliff effect can guarantee against accidental tumbles). It is not usually until toddler-hood that the child learns how to get back down the stairs in one piece. One expedient is to go down in the same position that he went up, but in the reverse direction, feetfirst. This method entails a lot of hesitation, of

227

easing knees and hands warily from step to step, and of twisting and craning to see where he is and where he is going. Another technique is to sit on the steps and bump downward on his seat one step at a time. Somewhere around age two, the child may be able to walk downstairs clinging to an adult finger—but here, as at other times, he may be overwilling to surrender all his weight to the adult and simply dangle helplessly. Perhaps by age two and a half, he walks both up and down the stairs, one step at a time, holding on to a railing. Most children cannot climb a vertical ladder until about age three, at least partly because, apparently out of a fear of falling, they cannot release their grip to move their hands one by one in concert with their feet. (It would be interesting to know at what age children manage ladders in societies where, as in Manus, houses are set high on stilts.) By late infancy, the child can be taught to slide down feetfirst from a bed or couch or coffee table, and the toddler has no trouble descending in this manner from surfaces no more elevated than, say, his own head; even so, he still has to be watched when he is off the ground.

In early toddlerhood, the child has to climb up not only onto a full-sized chair but equally onto a toddler-sized one, by sprawling or kneeling on the seat and twisting himself around until, finally facing in the right direction, he gets his feet down and is triumphantly seated. This approach to small chairs, like his cautious feet-first descent of a staircase, indicates that space behind the toddler is less stable and differentiated than the visible space in front of him. The same ambiguity of rearward space is shown in the way he seats himself on a stool or low bench, which differ from a chair in not having a back to hold on to while climbing up and turning around. The toddler has to aim himself toward the seat edging backward and peering either over his shoulder or between his legs until he is in place, then letting himself down onto the seat. By late toddlerhood, the baby can, like an adult, plump confidently and casually down on a seat.

However, the toddler does not, by contrast, climb onto an adult lap, but offers himself to be drawn onto the adult's knees. Sometimes, of course, his frequent lap-sittings may mean that he wants to be snuggled and cuddled and petted and babied. As often as not, though, he is a very active lap-sitter: He seeks and delights in jiggling, bouncing, and dipping outward into space while lightly encircled by the adult's arm or firmly held by the hands. The adult has to do most of the work, but the activity originates in the toddler.

In all this activity and movement we see the toddler's increasing familiarization with and mastery of space and its possibilities. He knows by heart the layout of familiar regions, and may even cry out in protest when, on the way to Grandma's, his mother makes a left turn where she customarily makes a right. He knows where things are kept, including taboo things like medicines. It is important to try to understand in what sense the toddler knows a segment of space. He does not know it as one portion of a larger totality. He shows no surprise that one region of space adjoins or flows into another, but he seems to have no idea which regions are contiguous with which, or along which boundaries, or that other, unknown regions lie just out of view, awaiting discovery. Rather, he seems to know a great many specific locations, and a great many routes linking locations, without any notion of their overall organization. In this respect he is like many so-called "space-blind" adults, who learn to navigate from point to point but are incapable of inventing an alternate route or of drawing a coherent map. Nor does the toddler yet appreciate that one object cannot be in two places at the same time. For instance, the family of one two-year-old had a rather unusual automobile. One day, while out driving in it, they passed another car just like their own, provoking the father to remark jestingly, "Look, somebody stole our car." The two-year-old responded by bursting into tears, unmindful of the "obvious" fact that their car was still safely in the family's possession. The toddler's orientation to space can be summarized by saying that he lives in an *action space*, defined less by its formal relationships and coordinates than by its possibilities for movement, the dynamics that push and pull and steer and channel the toddler's active migrations. These dynamics are strictly equivalent to the demand qualities or the valences of objects, mentioned earlier.

His growing mastery over both the larger space in which he moves about and also of the spatial relations between objects or parts of objects is shown in his manipulation of playthings. Now, he not only takes things like cooking utensils apart but begins to put them back together as well. He becomes able to screw back on bottle caps of a size that he can manage. He can stack pierced blocks on a peg, but if they are graduated in size he cannot yet arrange them in the "right" order. Nor can he, much before age two, fit together a series of nesting boxes or "eggs." He perceives gross differences in size, but cannot yet reliably distinguish smaller ones, as seen in his stubborn attempts to put large things inside small ones. Also, when fitting together anything except circular forms, he has trouble aligning the forms correctly. He can, however, balance a stack of things, as related in this account:

229

[Debbie, seventeen months, two weeks] now stacks several objects (two to five of them), then stoops or squats, picks them up gently at the base of the pile, and proceeds to carry them elsewhere.

The note continues:

Refuses, however, to have anything to do with her small blocks, and either ignores them or flings them out of the box with fine vigor.[2]

Here we see the continuation from infancy of the toddler's preference for sizable playthings, such that one could postulate an inverse correlation between age of baby and size of playthings. Friends and relatives usually err in giving the baby presents of miniaturized bits of reality, which may well appeal to older children but whose charm is usually lost on the vigorous action-oriented younger one.

When, as sometimes happens, the toddler stays in one place, his posture is very different from that of younger and older children. As in the account above, when he wants to pick something up from the floor, he drops into an easy squat. He may sometimes stay squatting to play with toys on the floor, but more characteristically he sits with his legs straight out in front of him, with a book or plaything either on his lap or on the floor between his thighs. A typical toddler pose is to stand with legs straight and slightly spread, and to bend double at the hips and waist so that his head rests on the floor and the child can look out between his own legs at an upside-down world. One twenty-two-month-old girl of our acquaintance could edge herself forward from this position right into a somersault. Notice a difference, though: The toddler apparently finds it most enjoyable to be upside down in relation to the world, but he finds it disturbing when things—such as a photograph of his father—depart from their familiar up-down orientation in space.

When the toddler is keeping an adult company, he characteristically leans limply against the adult's knees or shoulder (depending on whether the adult is sitting in a chair or on the floor), so limply that he may slide into a heap on the floor. This draping of himself against adults may continue into the school years, although past toddlerhood the child maintains better muscle tone and keeps his balance better. When the toddler is not directly engaged with other people, he is likely to treat them less as people than as things: as obstacles to be shoved aside, as drums to be thumped or kicked, as climbing apparatuses, as resting places. In general, the toddler's posture and movements are marked by symmetry, a limited differentiation of the two sides of the body, so that when he beats time or kicks his heels against the side of a box on which he is sitting, both arms or legs move as one—indeed, if he gets a Band-Aid on one finger, he may demand another for the matching finger on the other hand.

THE BEGINNINGS OF LANGUAGE

While the child's new powers of bipedal locomotion may be the most striking manifestation of toddlerhood, probably more important psychologically is his beginning to speak in his mother tongue.[3] We must stress that use of language is not an isolated skill, like eating with a spoon or riding a tricycle, but brings with it an all-pervasive transformation of perceiving, feeling, thinking, and general intelligence. We might insist that it is only by becoming a linguistic organism, by understanding speech and by speaking, that the child gains access to full status as a human being. On the side of being able to understand language, the child becomes open to endless verbal instruction, he can learn vicariously, through the words of others, he can enter realms of knowledge, such as history, that he can never know at firsthand, he can dwell in the virtual realms created by writers of stories and poetry, and he can learn accessory means of expression and manipulation like drawing and arithmetic. On the side of coming to speak, the child can convey his thoughts and feelings and wishes to others, he can think and reason and make sense of and order his own experience, he can make original statements, and he can concoct fantasies, jokes, and works of imagination.

There are several general things to be said about learning language before we describe the actual stages of speaking that the child goes through. As the gifted amateur linguist Benjamin Lee Whorf[4] pointed out, the range of concepts or relations contained in the language we learn may impose a limit on what we are able to think about and on how effectively we think about those things we do think about. In other words, according to Whorf, a person's thought processes and perceptions can be no richer or more precise than the language he learns. Furthermore, most languages give us fallacious categories which hobble our thinking. We have, for instance, the whole array of explanatory entities that people once believed in and that science has had a hard time eradicating: the ether, phlogiston, animal magnetism, spontaneous generation, the miasma, poltergeists—some students of science suggest that the time may come when the gene and the atom will go the way of these older constructs. However, simply to recognize the problem of language-embedded thought implies that we have partly transcended it. That is, there are linguistic forms, such as oratorical slogans, catchwords, and scare-words, that impede clear thinking, and there are others that liberate us and make us capable of new insights and perceptions and ways of talking about them. It is obviously a task of education to impart language in its liberating forms, as in the language of science, rather than its constricting forms, as in the language of tradition and dogma. We can tell from the growth and change of a language like English that people keep breaking out of the old forms and finding new means of expression, especially in the sciences. The child himself gives evidence that he is not wholly bound by Whorf's hypothesis. While on the one hand the child lives safely within his linguistic means, in that he can always understand more than he can put into words, he also lives beyond his active-linguistic means, saying words that he cannot pronounce, as in baby talk, making up new words or stretching old ones to cover new situations, and finding ways to group words into sentences well before he knows the standard rules of composition.

STAGES IN LEARNING LANGUAGE

We know that babies vocalize a great deal from an early age, and it seems probable that preverbal vocalizing plays its part in readying the child to speak. The accompanying table, adapted from a doctoral dissertation by Sanger, traces the development of some key features of prelinguistic behavior. This table merits detailed study because it shows a regularity of preverbal behavior that most theorists of language learning do not recognize. Beginning at a very early age, the human voice, other people's and the baby's own, is a potent instrument. An interesting aspect of Sanger's observations is that a number of behaviors increase to a peak and then dwindle away—see, for instance, the entries for conversational babbles which are very prominent at eight to ten months, for vocalizing when alone, which has its peak at six to eight months, and for vocal accompaniment to nonsocial action, conspicuous between eight to twelve months. Note, however, that these infant vocalizations are not language in the usually accepted sense of the conventional symbols by which people in a society communicate with each other, including the special provisions for baby talk.

Before expanding on the stages in learning active language, let us present them in summary form. Toward the end of the first year or early in the second, the baby begins saying single words with which he

TABLE 2 / **Prelinguistic Behavior**

PERCENTAGE OF OBSERVATIONS AT SUCCESSIVE AGES
WHERE KINDS OF BEHAVIOR WERE NOTED

Behavior	Age (months)						
	0–2	2–4	4–6	6–8	8–10	10–12	12+
Stimulated nonvocal							
Turns to sound	0	16	18	21	7	11	0
Stops vocalizing to listen to adult	0	10	26	29	26	6	0
Responds to voice alone	20	16	18	21	26	17	7
Appropriate response to verbal cues	0	0	0	0	19	33	53
Stimulated vocal							
Smiles or vocalizes to adult imitation	0	23	26	8	19	22	7
Conversational babbles	0	3	4	4	44	22	13
Imitates a sound	0	0	0	4	26	22	13
Appropriate sound to verbal cues	0	0	0	0	14	33	22
Spontaneous vocal							
Vocalizes when alone	0	25	18	46	11	0	13
Vocal accompaniment to grasping	0	0	9	4	33	28	13
Vocal accompaniment to nonsocial action	0	0	4	29	67	61	33
Calls for adult attention	0	0	0	8	37	33	0
Stable nonverbal sounds	0	0	0	0	4	11	67

Source: Sanger, M. D. Language learning in infancy: A review of the autistic hypothesis and an observational study of infants. Unpublished Ed. D. Thesis, Harvard University, 1955.

communicates, largely in the form of commands and requests. He is word-hungry and seeks the names of things as though compiling a catalogue of his environment. The child's first attempts to go beyond single words into narration or description often take the form of what Gesell called "expressive jargon," a flow of gibberish obviously meant to convey meaning. Expressive jargon soon drops out, however, and the child begins to combine real words, at first two at a time and then in ever-longer strings. Initially, he omits all but the most essential words and makes sentences without regard to adult rules of grammar. Gradually, the missing parts of speech appear, the baby's sentence structure begins to resemble that of adults, and, by age two and a half or three, the foundations of language are firmly established.

The baby's learning of true language, the linguistic conventions with which people in a given setting communicate, begins underground. We know that it has happened from the fact that the baby responds appropriately to things that people say to him, even though he himself does not talk. The transition from *passive language* (understanding) to *active language* (talking) may take several forms. A few babies seem to wait until their passive listening has given them a good command of linguistic forms, whereupon they blossom forth with complex utterances—we are told that one bright ten-month-old girl's first speech occurred at the dinner table, when she said, "I want a taste." The far more usual pattern is to begin speaking in single words, which may, in fact, be fusions of two or more words, as in *awgone, yapu* (the French toddler's equivalent of *il n'y en a plus*), *whadda?, good-boy, not-in-the-mouth, what-a-pity, enough-is-enough* (pronounced "enuss-enuss").[5] Quite a few children, as we have noted, either before or after they have begun to use single words, speak in "expressive jargon," gibberish that imitates the sounds and cadences of adult speech, often with such fidelity that it seems, like the comedian's double-talk, tantalizingly on the verge of being comprehensible. In fact, from the context and from occasional real words embedded in the stream of jargon, one can get a pretty good idea of what the child is saying. However, expressive jargon is a shortcut of limited utility, and most children speak primarily in one-word sentences, or *holophrases* (singular, *holophrasis*). Although such utterances consist of a single word (or word-fusion), psychologically they function as complete statements: I want to go "Out!"; Lift me "Up!"; That is "Daddy"'s shoe; Time for a "Bath!" (We make no attempt to reproduce the toddler's pronunciation.) Concrete nouns loom large in the vocabulary of the toddler, but he also uses a fair number of interjections (*hi, bye-bye, ouch*), verbs (*go, carry, eat*), adverbs (*up, out, again, back*). Many children learn *hot* quite early, sometimes as a designation for all hot things and often as a general cry of warning. Missing at the one-word stage, at least as we know it in European languages, are most qualifying adjectives and adverbs, and all pronouns, articles, prepositions, and conjunctions. At first, there are no inflections designating plurals or verb tenses.

The toddler's holophrases serve a number of functions. Interjections are ordinarily used as greetings, but more than one toddler has been known to bring a visitor her purse and exclaim "Bye-bye" as a clear invitation to depart. In general, the toddler is liberal with imperatives, commands and demands, sometimes, in all likelihood, in imitation of the way he is addressed. Many times words pop out as automatic responses to things and actions. The child often seems to be rehearsing his repertory of labels, going from object to object and saying their names. The child may say the name of an object with an interrogatory ring, as though asking the adult to confirm that he has it right. The child's hunger for names is insatiable, suggesting the sense of power over reality that language gives the child.

Much thought and discussion have been given to the subject of the baby's first word, on the presumption that this would provide a clue to the understanding of language in general. The reader will recall Frederick II's ill-fated experiment, meant to discover the child's "natural" language, and the Greek historian Herodotus reports a similar venture. Many present-day theorists, from psychoanalysts to learning theorists, are committed to the view that the learning of language must be extrinsically motivated, as a way of reducing tissue needs. Such a view would predict that the child's first words would refer to need states and the things that gratify them. The facts remain ambiguous. Part of the difficulty is in knowing what to count as the first word. For one thing, the boundaries between *babbling*, the infant's preverbal vocalizations, and true speech are not always clear. For instance, *ma-ma* and *da-da* are standard babbles of late infancy—as far as we know, the world around. They are also the standard baby-talk words in many languages for mother and father. The problem is to know when the baby is merely babbling and when he is greeting or calling for his parents as need-gratifiers. A toddler may salute his bath or his bottle with a shout of "Bah!" but if his whole day is punctuated with *bahs*, it is hard to make a case for his speaking. Or a toddler may learn to reply "There!" (pronounced *dzare*) to questions of the form of "Where's the . . . ?" but again it is impossible to decide whether he is using a meaningful word or performing an empty ritual. A second kind of difficulty is to know whether to count as a word those sounds the child says in response to prompting ("Can you say *kitty?*").

The only safe course is to count only spontaneous naming accompanied by pointing to the object named (which automatically excludes interjections, verbs, and adverbs as first words), and we have so few reliable instances of such naming that we cannot support any theory. Our impression, however, is that spontaneous first words may have little to do with need states. It certainly seems to be the case that many babies call their parents *mama* and *dada* only at an advanced stage of speaking. In general, need states move the baby to tears or fussing or concrete action, and not to speech, and words referring to such states as hunger, thirst, fatigue, illness, and pain are very late in appearing. Obviously, both people and animals express their need states and emotions by postures, gestures, facial expressions, and vocal sounds, many of them highly specialized, but these must be considered symptomatic behavior rather than symbolic. From our own observations of children in the process of learning to speak, speaking seems to be intrinsically rewarding and hence self-motivating, and we see no need to invoke outside dynamics.

Once the toddler has a basic stock of words, he begins joining them into two-word sentences, simple statements or questions, usually a noun plus a predicate word, as in "Car, backing up" or "Baby, crying." In the first example, "backing up" seems to have been learned as a unit. In both examples, the comma indicates the laborious piecing together of statements which is characteristic of the toddler's early two-word sentences. As the baby becomes more proficient, his sentences grow in length, but initially still without benefit of articles, pronouns, connectives, and inflections, and in happy ignorance of the "correct" way to form sentences. Miller and Ervin[6] give the charming example of a two-year-old who, having seen her baby sister bite and break her own balloon, pointed to *her* own and said, "Baby other bite balloon no." In a sequence which no one has yet plotted out, the missing parts of speech begin to appear, words get inflected, and the order of words in sentences comes to approximate that of adult speech.

It is important to see that the child's learning of language takes place with a minimum of instruction. The baby learns language—including not only words but the grammatical and syntactical rules as well—by hearing it spoken in a concrete context of people, actions, gestures, and feelings. As D. T. Campbell[7] puts it, one cannot teach a child language over the telephone. Nor is it correct to say that the child learns language by simple imitation. Rather, it is as though he were abstracting the rules and applying and generalizing them to his own behavior. This comes out most clearly in the child's errors. Actually, children make remarkably few errors, but the ones they do make are illuminating because they reveal the processes of learning at work. For instance, many children at first learn the past tense of irregular verbs correctly, and then, when they have begun to abide by the rules, change to incorrect forms. The child may at first say *brought,* and then later switch to any one of various forms, or sometimes use several interchangeably: *bringed, brang, branged, broughted* (some of these forms persist into later childhood). A common misapplication of the rules is seen in displaced inflections, as in "He pick it ups" and "I walk homed." Several children, from different families, have come up with a system of construction derived from the adult form *each other:* "We're hugging our chothers," "Are you mad at your chother?" and "They're hitting their chothers." In addition to codified rules, children pick up the intonations that express banter, despair, sympathy, exasperation, puzzlement, disdain, disagreement, whatever. They also mimic their parents' affectations, as in the special telephone manner that most adults assume. It is often an embarrassing self-revelation to hear a child speaking in one's own voice and turns of speech.

The toddler learning to speak is amazingly accurate in his grasp of word meanings: what kinds of things, actions, properties, and relationships a given word refers to. For, proper names apart, a word (or phrase) can be thought of as a *concept* that designates a whole class or category of related things. One recent research finding is pertinent here. If adults are given a list of words to memorize and later asked to recall them, instead of repeating the words in the order they appeared in the list, subjects tend to regroup them into logically related categories. This tendency is called by Bousfield[8] *associative clustering.* Now, a study by Rossi and Rossi[9] indicates that associative clustering appears as early as age two, suggesting that language may exist for the child in an organized way almost from the beginning. In some sense, the child reacts to the words within a cluster as members of the same concept, even though he lacks a word with which to name the concept. For it is possible also, Whorf notwithstanding, to "have a concept" without words; the preverbal baby recognizes members of the class things to eat, or familiar people and unfamiliar people, or things that roll; the nonverbal infrahuman organism likewise recognizes foodstuffs, potential mates, sources of danger, and so forth, and even "generalizes" the stimuli to which he learns to respond in a conditioning experiment. In general, stimuli which elicit equivalent reactions, as when the chimpanzee reacts to a length of rope as though to a snake, can be considered as belonging to the same unverbalized concept. The toddler can learn makes of cars, for instance, with amazing accuracy. But sometimes he generalizes a word in ways that adults find surprising. For instance, many toddlers learn *heavy* in the sense of "hard to lift," but they seem to apply it to anything entailing strain or effort: Easing his way down a steep slope, a two-year-old observes, "This is a heavy hill"; vainly straining to reach something overhead, the two-year-old says, "That shelf is too heavy." Many toddlers use *strong* in exactly the same way, and *strong* and *heavy* interchangeably, as in "Is the ice heavy enough to walk on?" What seems to underlie such meanings is that the word refers simultaneously to the person acting, his action, and the thing being acted upon.

In much the same way, the toddler seems to learn attribute-dimensions as a whole before their extremes are clearly differentiated, as shown in the frequency with which he mixes up terms like *hot* and *cold, open* and *close, on* and *off*, and *up* and *down*. A toddler being handed some water in a glass shouts, "Too much! Too much!" and then, when the adult pours some off, screams in protest. In this case, it seems, *too much* is synonymous with *a lot*, which it is only partially in adult speech. An eighteen-month-old referred to all red motor vehicles as *engine*, which was his word for fire engine. It is interesting that redness was one of the two main organizing dimensions of this concept, even though the child at that time could not name colors or respond reliably to color names. We have encountered several children who referred to the adult's arm and leg hairs as *threads*, apparently not recognizing the kinship with head hair. A boy going on age three saw a covered wagon on television and called it a *mixer-truck*, apparently on the analogy of the cement-mixers that deliver ready-mixed concrete to construction projects.[10] This same boy, apparently lacking a word for bite or sting, told his parents through his tears, "Didja bump your toe on a fly?"[11] A mother gives this account of a toddler's generalization:

> Ruth pinched her finger in a door and I told her to come to Mommy and I would kiss it to make it feel better. She held out her finger to be kissed. The next time she hurt her finger she immediately ran to me and held out her finger to be kissed—I thought she remembered and understood. The next day she got a bump on the head and came running to me—with her *finger* held out for me to kiss. It was just a ritual.[12]

This same little girl also demonstrated on many occasions how the same object could be called by different names according to the function it was serving. For instance, a pillow on the bed was *pillow,* but balanced on top of her head it was *hat;* she scribbled with a *pencil,* but a pencil in her mouth was *cigar* or *pipe.*

Language as a Tool and a Toy. So far, we have spoken mostly of the processes by which the toddler acquires language and of how language exists for him. To fill in the picture we need to say something about how language is used, what functions it serves and what linguistic mechanisms are available to fulfill these functions. In a later section, we shall have something to say about some broader issues involved in linguistic behavior and its development.

It is commonplace to say that a primary function of language is communication, to exchange information about enduring or temporary states of affairs, about rules and procedures and expectations and values, and to share knowledge and experience. In general, presumably as part of a more general urge to social communion, most people have a strong urge to tell other people what they know, to surprise them, to act on their emotions, to make them laugh, and sometimes to tease them, but most basically for the satisfaction of social sharing. Part of the process of communication, of course, is asking questions: What is it?; What is it for?; How does it work?; For what reason?; and so forth. Obviously, too, a major form of communication is getting other people to do things, issuing orders of one sort or another, which the toddler frequently and imperiously does. By age two, the toddler does a great deal of verbal communicating, not only with adults but also with playthings and with himself. One special form of communication that should not be overlooked is deception, the giving of false or misleading information, whether playfully or in earnest. The toddler may begin to play simple jokes on his parents, announcing to his homecoming father that "Mommy go store," when in fact she is in the kitchen, or he may be able to lie to the extent of denying some accusation with a vigorous, head-shaking "No!" There is also, we should remember, the important issue of self-deception, which begins in the preschool years.

An often neglected form of communication is self-communication, talking to oneself. Self-communication has various guises: self-direction, as when the baby verbalizes the steps required in, say, playing a record; self-control, as when the child tells himself "No-no" or "Mustn't touch" as he approaches a forbidden object; and, at ever more sophisticated levels, making one's experience explicit for one's own benefit, as in analyzing, figuring things out, making generalizations, stating relationships, describing things to oneself, and in general giving order and coherence to one's knowledge. And we must mention again all the processes of rationalization and justification by which one makes one's own motives acceptable to other people and oneself. All these linguistic functions taken collectively add up to verbal thinking. We must also add reverie, daydreaming, imagining, and wishing to the array of self-communications. In the toddler, most forms of self-communication have to be mediated through an adult. That is, the child cannot think directly to himself, but thinks out loud to an adult, engaging in a dialogue which enables the child to formulate, catalogue, and systematize his experience. In much the same way, toddlers and children at the beginning of the preschool years find it next to impossible to talk directly to children their own age and communicate instead through an adult intermediary. Many adults, too, when wrestling with a problem, seek out a friend to act as sounding board on which to try out ideas that cannot be dealt with in solitude.

The language that a child learns contains a number of subvocabularies, referring to special, logically related "domains" of experience. For instance, there is the special vocabulary of number and quantitative relationships. Quite early in his speaking history, the baby learns to count one, two, *two* originally standing for any quantity greater than one. He then goes on to one, two, a lot; one, two, three, a lot. Many two-year-olds can count to five or ten or beyond, but this may be a mere recital of a learned sequence. For one thing, the child may count things correctly up to a point and then improvise: 1, 2, 3, 7, 5, 4. Furthermore, he does not adhere to a strict one-to-one correspondence between numbers and objects; thus, in counting, he may skip objects or count the same one repeatedly, so that his last number bears no relation to the size of the collection. Also, counting and summing seem to be psychologically different operations, with the ability to count coming before the realization that the last number counted is the sum; thus, the child may correctly count five things, but, when asked how many there are still reply, "Two." The use of standardized units of measurement, like inches and ounces, does not appear until the late preschool or early school years.

Another special vocabulary is that of metalanguage, language that describes language, as in such terms as *word, sentence, punctuation, verb tense,* and so forth. The toddler's metalinguistic vocabulary is ordinarily limited to *word,* a stage beyond which many of us never go until we reach school.

Yet another domain is that of time. It is clear that the baby's early orientation to time far outstrips his ability to talk about it. Even the infant develops a stable sense of the recurring events in his routines, and although he may not anticipate that night will fall, he is not surprised when it does. The toddler knows a number of time-related words, like *day, night, first,* and *now.* He shows signs of remembering past events, as when the mention of somebody's name evokes an association, such as "Baby sick. Poor baby." He can anticipate the near future, as when, having been told that he will visit his grandmother after his nap, he bounces awake shouting, "Now go Nana!" Late in toddlerhood, the baby may use such words as *yesterday, today,* and *tomorrow,* but he mixes them up, cannot tell in what sequence they come, and is likely to fasten on a single word, such as *tonight,* to designate any point in past or future time. He also parrots the adult's "Not now," "Soon," and "In a minute," to indicate delay. To the adult, the toddler is an exasperating dawdler, since he is blandly unmindful of time pressures, schedules, and the need to be in a particular place at a particular time, so that the grownup has to make generous allowances for luring him away from play and into his outdoor clothes. Even while being dressed, the toddler may resolutely persist in trying to build a block tower or look at a book. By the same token, of course, the adult, wrapped up in his or her obligations and preoccupations, may seem an equally exasperating dawdler to the toddler. The toddler shows some grasp of simultaneity, as when the adult tells him, "You go play while I write a letter," and can play synchronously with an adult, taking turns adding blocks to a pile or handing things to an adult engaged in a work project.

We have already mentioned the toddler's orientation in space, his mastery of familiar spaces such as his home, his knowing where things are kept or have been left, and his knowledge of often-traveled routes, such as the way to the park, to the doctor's, to the market, or to Grandma's house. We might stress, however, that his knowledge of extended routes is essentially passive; he watches them unroll with a sense of rightness, but he cannot himself lead the way. If, on a walk, he decides to go around a clump of bushes as though to rejoin the adult on the far side, he is likely to become disoriented and panicky as soon as he loses sight of the adult. His spatial vocabulary expands to include such words as *up* and *down, on, over,* and *under, in* and *out, forward* and *backward, beside, next to, far away,* and *against,* and *around.* He is very sensitive to the car's going *up the hill* and *down the hill.* On the other hand, he does not spontaneously perceive that a toy car will roll down a board propped at an incline, and he delights in having this spatial relation demonstrated to him. For reasons we do not understand, toddlers have difficulty learning the meaning of *corner,* whether of a block or a room.

The toddler begins learning the special vocabulary of shape, and can recognize and name such standard forms as cross, triangle, diamond, crescent (called *moon*), heart (called *Valentine* by many children), and star. But notice that his recognition is physiognomic in nature, that is, he does not know how these figures are composed. He does not know that a triangle has three sides or a star five points, he cannot draw these forms, and he cannot yet fit cut-out forms into a formboard. It is interesting that the toddler learns such seemingly obvious shapes as square and circle relatively late, probably because he sees them as concrete things, like ball or window, rather than as general designs corresponding to nothing special in the world of objects. Also, the toddler who grows up among written symbols learns very early to recognize letters and numerals as special classes of forms, as shown by his pointing and asking, "What's this *a*?" and "What's this *1*?", with *a* at first standing for all letters, and *1* for all numerals.

By age two, favored middle-class babies have learned the names for the standard colors, including black, white, and gray, and in many cases such special colors as pink, beige, and aquamarine. Color names are a domain in which there are striking cultural and subcultural differences. So-called culturally deprived children in our society may be greatly retarded in learning colors. Our chief system for coding colors is the solar spectrum (although surprisingly few people are aware of this organizing principle), but in other societies color names may be derived from the colors of the desert, from the plumage of birds, or whatever, and colors that to our eyes look wildly dissimilar may be given the same name. No one has yet found a satisfactory answer to whether distinct colors given the same name are perceived as being the same, or whether the person sees them as different even though he labels them identically. The most promising technique for finding out, it seems to us, is to condition an emotional reaction to one color and then see whether the reaction is generalized according to spectral relations or labels—or, conceivably, both.

One other major conceptual domain is that of causal relations, of how things work. The toddler, out of his experience, learns endless pragmatic sequences: He can turn lights on and off, he can work faucets, the radio, the TV set, and his phonograph, he knows that the cat scratches if you pull its tail, he knows how to tease his parents, but his vocabulary of cause and effect is minimal. He can say such things as "Make the car go," or "Make it work," or "Fix it," but he simply accepts the workings of things without surprise or curiosity, as though they were all to be taken for granted as the natural order of things. It is only later, in the preschool years, that he begins to wonder how the people get inside the television set, or where the musicians are hiding that he hears playing on the phonograph. We can think of only one exception to this general passivity. Two-year-old boys (but not girls in the sample we know), when they sit in a small rocking chair with a chime fastened under the seat, react by getting up and tipping over the chair to see where the sound is coming from. It is conceivable, of course, that we could elicit more such investigatory behavior by arranging situations in which the child's learned expectations were violated—if he were to work a light switch and produce the wailing of a siren, for instance, or turn on a faucet, releasing a flow of ink, or open a bureau drawer to liberate a flood of soapsuds. In general, however, although events may startle the toddler, as when the jack-in-the-box pops forth, they do not stir him to wonder. Later in toddlerhood, the child asks "Why?" but this query—when it is a genuine query and not just a device to maintain contact with the adult or to tease—seems addressed not so much to explanation of how things work as to motives and justifications: "for what reason?" or "on what grounds?" rather than "by what means?" or "in accordance with what principles?"

Among the numerous other domains of language and experience, some of which we shall discuss later, are: personal and group origins and history; birth; death; the workings of the body, including sickness; body sensations such as those of hunger, thirst, fatigue, pain, need to eliminate, and sensual pleasure; masculinity and femininity; morality, questions of right and wrong; emotions; manners, codes, and procedures; family relationships; authority and obedience; and the whole realm of hypothetical events, which the preschool child typically enters by playing the game of "What if?" ("What if Daddy died and we didn't have any money?" "What if you had wings and could fly?" The list is endless and heavily fraught with possible disasters.)

Notice that very little time is spent teaching the child language as such, getting him to say words or telling him correct phrasings. Rather, people talk and he listens, or half-listens, and on the basis of his listening he becomes able in turn to talk. But since he learns language in the practical context of people's linguistic dealings with the world, he simultaneously learns from what they say or imply a notion of how the world is, how things might be, how they ought to be, and what can and cannot be done about it. Likewise, what people say contains abundant implications about the child himself. Thus, the language he hears instructs him in how his culture views and values reality, and becomes an important instrument of cultural transmission.

Language, as we have said, consists not only of words and standard word-combinations, plus grammatical and syntactic rules for using words, but also a system (usually unformulated, but overlapping in part with grammatical rules) of logical operations by which we represent real or imagined states of affairs. The two sorts of operations the toddler first uses are imperatives and naming, or *denomination,* the simple act of labeling objects—"Baby." His two-word sentences are acts of *predication,* that is, of posing the existence of something and then designating one of its permanent or ephemeral attributes—"Baby crying." We know that the toddler becomes able to perform, at least in a rudimentary way, the operation of *counting.* We know, too, that the operation of *locating events in past or future time* becomes possible for the toddler, even though he may lack the standard tense forms. Here our knowledge about the order of emergence of operations ends. We know only that over the next several years the child becomes able to do such things as *summate* his counting, *evaluate* things, *compare* things along a number of dimensions such as size and color, *draw contrasts, contradict, brag, make rhymes, alliterate, tease, joke, lie, talk nonsense, make emphatic assertions* ("I am *so!*"), *make believe, make contingency statements* ("If it doesn't rain, we'll have a picnic"), and eventually statements of double and multiple contingency ("If it doesn't rain, and if Daddy doesn't have to work, and if we get home in time, then . . ."), *hypothesize, define words, draw inferen*ces ("She's a big girl, [therefore] she must go to school"), *find analogies, describe things,* and so forth. The various sorts of questions a child can ask also can be classified as embodying different sorts of operations—where, what, and which questions, for example. The things a child is asked to do on an intelligence test, such as to say in what way two things—for instance, an apple and a banana—are alike, are in many cases tests of his ability to perform well-defined operations.

In closing this first part of our discussion of language learning, we feel obliged to stress a few general principles which are often overlooked when dealing with this vital topic. First, it is obvious that all the words a baby uses, a few neologisms (invented terms) excepted, are in some sense imitations of words he has heard. But simple imitation is not enough to explain the acquisition of language. In the first place, we have no ready way to explain imitation itself, which as we have seen begins very early in life: the fact that an external stimulus gets translated into a series of internal motor events that produce a more or less accurate copy of the stimulus. Second, imitation may be long delayed, so that when a child first uses a word we may have no idea when he heard it originally. Furthermore, imitation is selective and relevant—the child imitates the right word for a given context and, for the most part, uses it aptly. Then again, it is hard to say what it is that the child is imitating when he applies an unspoken grammatical rule. In many cases, his learning requires a transposition of what he hears: The adult, speaking to the child, uses *I* to refer to himself and *you* to refer to the child, whereas the child must learn that he in turn uses *I* and addresses the adult as *you*. In general, learning the rules and learning to transpose imply an intelligent learning that is anything but a simple parroting. As we mentioned, even the child's errors tend to be intelligent errors—as in creating past tenses. We must note also the way the child drills himself in the use of language; Ruth Weir[13] has given us a charming account of the bedtime soliloquies of a two-year-old, many of which seem to be a quite conscious ringing of changes on standard linguistic forms. Finally, let us repeat that there seems to be no need to invoke extrinsic motivations for the learning of language—not only is speaking intrinsically rewarding, but a great deal of language learning seems to take place by unconscious absorption of words from the surroundings. It is conceivable and even probable, as Mowrer[14] has said, that the language some children hear is so heavily freighted with disagreeable content—taboos, scoldings, threats—that the whole idea of speaking becomes repellent, but this negative motivation tells us very little about the usual process of coming to speak.

It is because words have such power over reality that it is so much fun to play with language. Language play of a sort begins, as we have seen, with the babbling of infancy. In toddlerhood, some of the child's expressive jargon is a form of word play. The child spouts nonsense, partly for the sheer pleasure of hearing the sound patterns come out but partly also in a spirit of deliberate silliness, as though recognizing the absurdity of what he says: "Lig a loggie, dig a poggie, a la boggie poggie boggie."[15] Toddlers are not so likely to appreciate adults' verbal humor; if the adult, for instance, changes the wording or the sense of a favorite story with some idea of entertaining the toddler, he will probably encounter fierce indignation. It is not until the child has attained the relative sophistication of the preschool years that he can feel sufficiently master of his language to move on to the next stage, where sense and nonsense are consciously intermingled.

The toddler's language often accompanies and punctuates his other play, as mood music, as narration, as commands to himself and his playthings. As his play becomes more social and less solitary, true conversation plays in increasing role in it. His jokes are usually amused commentaries on events and incongruities—"Johnny pants off"—and do not yet include the banter, verbal teasing, and deliberate surprises and manufactured incongruities of which the preschooler is capable. When he does happen upon something that is funny, such as getting his overshoes on the wrong feet, he will repeat the joke, including appropriate expressions of mock dismay, until something new intervenes to break the spell. As we can see, the toddler's growing language skills are assimilated to everything he does; in addition, though, they open new realms of activity to him, in learning and thinking and in the social interchange that will come to occupy an ever-growing part of his still narrow existence. Meanwhile—and to some extent regrettably—he moves from the verbal music of infancy toward the still egocentric poetry of the preschool years and the communicative but often barren prose of adult discourse.

Play and Activities in Toddlerhood

A goodly proportion of the toddler's day is taken up by the mechanics of life—eating, napping, being bathed and cleansed and changed, dressing and undressing—but even so, he still has several hours a day free for other sorts of activities which we generally call play. The distinction here is that the sustenance-producing or otherwise useful activities of the adult are considered serious work, whereas the activities of the child are viewed as frivolous play. In part, such thinking is a residue from the days when hard manual labor, or drudgery, was the price one paid for sheer survival. In part it is a remnant of the Puritan ethic that man redeemed his essential sinfulness through work, and that to play was to flirt with the devil. Such a conception disregards the fact that in many societies, and increasingly in our own, no sharp line is drawn between work and play, so that one can perform life's chores in a spirit of good cheer and mix one's daily labors with other, intrinsically enjoyable activities. Furthermore, mechanization and automation have taken much of the drudgery out of life and have given us large amounts of leisure, and education has given us more scope both in choosing the kind of work we do and in using our leisure to good advantage. On the side of the baby, furthermore, his play is not exclusively frivolous. He works hard at mastering and perfecting new competences, and even those forms of play that seem aimless to the adult feed into his growing awareness of self and world. Notice that the baby is not oriented to achievement. He has no sense of any future benefits to be gained from his play here and now. Such benefits are incidental by-products. Nor does he, in his working toward mastery, feel any need to have final products as monuments to what he has done. The toddler (and older child) can abandon a project midway—he may abruptly abandon the doll he was putting to bed, or drop the crayon with which he was scribbling, or let the tune he was humming trail off—in a way that adults can find frustrating. But for the toddler the activity itself is what counts, not the completion of a total task.

It has been said earlier that the toddler prefers large-muscle activity to small-muscle, that he would rather deal with large things than small ones, that he would rather send his whole body hurtling through the channels and over the obstacles of action-space than engage in the sensitive manipulation of complex playthings, and in general this is true. In the park or on the nursery school playground, he loves the spring of a jumping-board under his feet (but he wants to hold an adult's fingers), the swooping movement of a swing (but not too high), the tug and jounce of riding in a wagon, the unwieldy weight of big objects to lift and haul and shove. He likes to hammer and pounds tirelessly at his pegboard. He trots about pushing or pulling a roll-toy. He revels in splashing in water, he explores tunnels and tries out—very tentatively when coming down—ramps and catwalks, he learns to ride a tricycle and to pull himself up a rung or two on a jungle gym. He digs in a sandbox, drifts about aimlessly, stares wide-eyed at other children at play, often moving empathically in rhythm with them, sets off in pursuit of a rolling ball, closes doors that he finds open or ajar and, when he is tall enough to reach the knob, opens closed doors. He squeezes into narrow crevices, steps up and down on large hollow blocks, and clusters with his fellows around every new activity.

But this is only part of the story. The toddler has his quiet moments, when he squats down to follow the progress of a beetle or an ant, or savors the feel and taste of snow, or listens to music (although he usually will bounce as he listens), or scribbles (it is a good idea to give the toddler drawing instruments only when there is an adult free to watch him; otherwise his experiments are likely to overflow to floor, walls, and furnishings), looks at picture books, spends long minutes in the examination and exploration of a new object, or relishes his food. By the time he is two, the American toddler may sit quietly hypnotized for a while in front of the television set, or trot in from the next room for a favorite commercial. There can be no doubt that the toddler finds certain sounds and images fascinating—he memorizes jingles from an early age—but there is reason to question how much sense television programs make to him. We even know of one two-year-old for whom watching television was a comfort device, and who, when he wanted to be quiet, sat on the

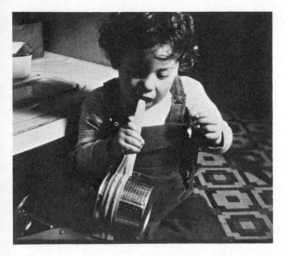

Pots and pans and utensils are standard playthings in late infancy and toddlerhood.

ABBY'S FIRST TWO YEARS/Vassar Film

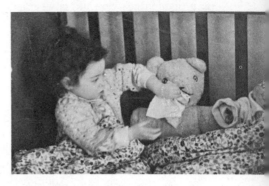

Early dramatic play.

L. Joseph Stone

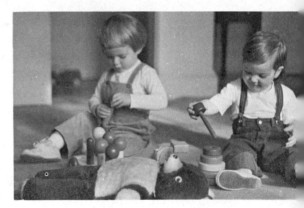

Parallel play.

Alexandria Church

couch, put his thumb in his mouth, and stared at the blank and silent television set.

The toddler, as the saying goes, is "into everything," and some part of his day is likely to be spent emptying toy-boxes, closets, and cupboards, sometimes with a view to playing with the contents—as when he drapes himself in oddments of clothing and parades around the house or admires himself in the mirror—but as often as not just for the inherent pleasure he finds in each step of the process, each novelty, each familiarity. From the time the child is a year old until almost school age, reasonably permissive parents must be resigned to a daily cleaning up chore in which the whole world seems to have disintegrated into minute fragments which must be collected, retrieved, sorted, reassembled, cleaned, and put away. The child may help, but his contribution is likely to be capricious and ineffective, and, if the adult is not vigilant, the child may take things out and apart faster than the adult can put them away. The toddler plays with his dolls, trundling them in their carriage, feeding them, petting them, admonishing them, wiping their noses, putting them to bed, and so forth. Let us stress that playing with dolls and stuffed animals, and taking one or more such to bed at night, is a part of the normal play of both boy and girl toddlers. Many parents—and aunts, uncles, grandparents, and neighbors—are aghast to see a little boy playing with his dolls, as though his very masculinity were in peril. As far as we know, there is no such danger; quite the contrary, it seems most important to give boys access to the social themes of dramatic play with dolls (of which more in a moment), and to encourage the development of feelings of tenderness, care, and protectiveness that dolls call forth.

In the toddler's play with dolls, we see one of the beginnings of *dramatic play,* the imitation or acting out of scenes and events of everyday life, in which the child tries out roles and identities drawn from the models he is exposed to. The first dramatic play of the toddler is likely to be episodic, confined to simple, unelaborated themes from domestic life: telephoning, answering the door, rocking the baby to sleep, shaving (little girls as well as little boys go through a pantomime of removing whiskers, and little boys as well as little girls may be observed "shaving" their legs and armpits), driving the car, drinking tea, smoking (more than one eighteen-month-old has been found with a cigarette or pipe or cigar shoved deep into his mouth and trying valiantly to strike a match), or fixing the car. In addition, he may trail his mother about the house, either playing on his own or imitating her activities, or even pitching in as best he can to help her with her chores. In some societies, of course, the child is expected actually to participate in family duties, and not simply to play at them.

Over the next few years, the child will weave such simple themes into more complex, sustained dramas. His reenactments tell us much about the things that stand out for him in his world, and about the affective significance things have for him. Common domestic matters, which are recurrent, simple, and easily grasped (at least in their externals), and which give him his first inkling of adult ways, are prominent, with the mother's activities taking precedence over the father's. The child's later dramatic play reaches ever further afield for its subject matter, into the realm of the filling station, the market, the construction project, the railway station and airport, the seashore, the circus, and, at still later stages, into the doings of cowboys and Indians, cops and robbers, spacemen, and, eventually, fairy tales and specially composed plays.

What we have said so far about play patterns in infancy and toddlerhood leads to a twofold developmental classification of play. The first classification is in terms of the *content of play*, what the child does. A classification in terms of content includes: *social-affective play, sense-pleasure play, dramatic play*, and *ritual* and *competitive games*. The second classification is in terms of the *social character of play*, who it is that the child plays with and the nature of their relationship. This classification of the development of plays gives us these categories: *play with adults, solitary play, parallel play, associative play*, and *cooperative play*. Now let us examine these two classifications in more detail.

THE CONTENT OF PLAY

As far as we can tell, play begins with *social-affective play*, taking pleasure in the manipulation of social relations and feelings. Such play begins with the adult, when he talks or croons to the baby, tickles him, works his hands and feet, nuzzles his belly, and generally acts in a way designed to elicit a positive emotional response from the baby. (Let us, however, signal a cultural difference. Caudill[16] reports that such stimulation is the norm in American families, whereas Japanese parents typically soothe the baby and avoid stimulating him.) The baby in turn learns to arouse parental emotion in a spirit of play, by simply smiling at the adult, by calling for attention, by initiating a particular game, by showing off his skills, by pretending not to hear when called, by feigning distress so as to be petted and reassured (adults do this, too, pretending that the baby has wounded them grievously, so that he will give them solace), and by teasing. American parents tease their children, but the teasing they practice is much milder than that found in numerous other societies, where teasing verges on the destructively malicious. Social-affective play implies the universal satisfaction found simply in being in communion with other people, but it also implies that there is a less benevolent pleasure just in getting a rise out of somebody. And, since we can observe teasing in primates, dogs, and other vertebrates, such behavior may be something of a biological imperative among social animals.

Quite early in life, the baby begins to enjoy nonsocial stimulation which produces something akin to early esthetic experience. We have called this kind of enjoyment *sense-pleasure play*. As with social-affective play, sense-pleasure play originates outside the baby, in the patterns of light and color and movement and sounds and rhythms and tastes and odors and textures and consistencies which attract his attention and give him pleasure. Later, in his explorations of object qualities and of his own body, the baby himself can govern his own sensual and esthetic experience. His play with raw materials—water, sand, mud, foodstuffs, whatever—can be viewed as sense-pleasure play, as can masturbation, swinging, bouncing, rocking, scribbling, humming, listening to music, and smelling flowers and other aromatic things. We can assume that the pleasure the toddler gets watching television comes largely under the heading of sense pleasure, more on the analogy of watching clothes tumble about in a washing machine than of watching a plot unfold. All the forms of play we are talking about can be combined—the toddler's lap-sitting, described earlier, seems to be a fusion of social-affective and of sense-pleasure play.

Once the baby has begun to reach out, to grasp and manipulate, we see the beginnings of *skill play,* consisting of the persistent exercise of newfound abilities, from making a doll dance by hitting it, to removing and reinserting the nipple, to dropping things from his feeding table, to walking, to carrying things, to piling blocks, and so on through his differentiating repertory. Obviously, there is often an element of sense pleasure in skill play, but there are abundant instances where the only point of an activity seems to be the practicing of a new ability—sometimes, in fact, with grim determination, as when a seven-year-old comes home at the end of the day a mass of scrapes, bruises, contusions, and tear-streaked dirt, but triumphantly at last master of his two-wheeler. We are not saying that the child has any notion that his mastery of a skill will be beneficial to him or even that he is motivated to become competent; he seems to be moved by the intrinsic fascination of the just-barely-able-to, which acts on people at all ages.

We have already described *dramatic play* as one of the emergents of toddlerhood, and need only add that it seems to be a vital ingredient in the child's process of identification, of learning to be a member of his family and society. After toddlerhood, in terms of the content of play, the child learns *formal games,* initially of a ritualistic, self-contained sort, like ring-around-a-rosy and London Bridge, in which there is no score, and eventually competitive ones, from parlor games to baseball. Here again there are cultural differences. In western Europe, winning at soccer may be a matter of life or death, but in the home, a friendly game of poker or Monopoly goes on indefinitely, since no one is allowed to lose.

It should not be necessary to point out that all these kinds of play extend into adulthood. Social-affective play is found in banter, teasing, practical jokes, flirtation, and the game of love. Sense-pleasure play has its counterparts in adult esthetic experience, in the enjoyment of art or music, in dancing, in the appreciation of spectacles, in the contemplation of natural beauty such as a sunset or a vista or waves breaking on a shore, or in watching the flames in a fireplace. The adult version of skill play can be seen in physical exercise, in practicing golf strokes or fly-casting, in maneuvering one's car adroitly through traffic, in whatever is done to gain or maintain proficiency. Dramatic play is most conspicuous in amateur and professional theatricals, but it also appears more subtly in the role playing of much of domestic, business, social, and community activities. Games, of course, have had an important place in adult life in every society we know of, although it is our impression that women have often been excluded from participation in formal games.

THE SOCIAL DIMENSION OF PLAY

The second major line of development in play is the social dimension. Most of the baby's early play is in interaction with an adult, and adult playmates continue to be important for some years. The toddler often wants the adult to be with him simply for company, and not necessarily for the sake of any interchange. Increasingly, the baby becomes able to play alone, or to play in a self-contained fashion as long as someone is near. When the toddler plays in a room by himself, he keeps the door open, and he periodically trots in to where the adult is, as often as not giving the adult's knees a fervent hug before returning to his solitary play.

At first, there is no play with *peers,* other children of the same age. Babies are curious about other babies, and will examine them carefully, with much poking, pinching, stroking, and pulling, while the other baby tries to do much the same, but with no observable recognition of kinship. Young toddlers circle each other warily, sometimes reaching out an investigative hand, but do not really make social contact. Late in toddlerhood, the child may suddenly show a wholesale affection for all other young children, hugging and kissing strange children on the street or in the store, as though in final recognition of a bond. At about this time (two or two and a half), the child makes a transition from solitary play to what is called *parallel play,* two or more children playing side by side, obviously taking pleasure in each other's companionship, but without any real exchange, unless it be a grim, silent tug-of-war for some coveted plaything.

The next step after parallel play, in which the activity of one child is unrelated to that of the other, is *associative play,* in which all the children are doing the same thing, such as telephoning or cooking or playing in the sandbox or swarming around the slide, but separately, still without any interchange. In a young nursery school group, one can watch an activity spread like an epidemic, as when one child decides to dress up and in no time at all the entire group is parading around in various get-ups.

In the preschool years, usually after age three, children move on to *cooperative play,* in which they can discuss and assign roles necessary to a joint venture, as when two children take turns pushing each other on a swing, or a group playing house decides who is to be the mommy, who the baby, and so forth. As we mentioned earlier, toddlers and young preschool children find it difficult to talk directly to each other, and prefer to have an adult act as middleman. When children do begin to converse, it is in the form of what Piaget calls *dual* or *collective monologue:* The children speak in turn, each apparently listening to what the other has to say, but each talking on a different topic, with little or no relevance to what the other is talking about (see page 282). Again, if one listens carefully to adult conversations, they, too, often seem to be collective monologues.

Autonomy and Self-Awareness

AUTONOMY

In Erikson's scheme of developmental alternatives, as we have said, the crisis in toddlerhood is between *autonomy,* the wish and, in a limited sense, the ability to be independent, and *shame and doubt,* feelings of worthlessness and incompetence. Out of his experience with people and things, the toddler is developing an ever more refined awareness of himself as a separate person, with his own budding wants and sensitivities and capacities. As he becomes aware of his new abilities, he wants to exercise them for himself, without help or hindrance or coercion from other people. Objectively, we know, the toddler has certain competences and certain limitations. The toddler himself, however, is an extremist: He seems to cherish a conviction of omnipotence, which may crumble totally when he comes up against overwhelming situations—or sometimes for no discernible reason—and give way to feelings of despair and impotence. Just as the toddler is most vigorously asserting his autonomy, he may suddenly want to be helped or carried, to be babied and cuddled and protected.

Perhaps the most dramatic manifestation of the toddler's growing autonomy is his intermittent *negativism,* variously expressed by "No!" (most toddlers learn to say *no* long before they say *yes*); by going rigid all over; by going limp all over; running away, kicking, biting, and scratching; and by temper tantrums. It seems to be a rule that strong parental upset in reaction to negativism acts as a reinforcer, increasing the likelihood that more negativism will be forthcoming. Most of the time, the toddler cooperates cheerfully with adults, automatically and casually, but negativistic behavior can erupt in the midst of conformity. Sometimes, as when the adult tries to do something for the child that the child would prefer to try on his own (signaled by a cry of "Me!"), negativism is real and intense but short-lived. Once the child has either acted for himself or satisfied himself that what he wants to do is indeed beyond his powers, normal relations can be resumed. Sometimes, of course, a real battle of wills emerges, in which case the adult has to be prepared to carry through with full authority, as when the child persists in trying to do something dangerous or destructive. In the aftermath, though, the adult has to be careful that the child does not suffer a damaging loss of face—which is possible at a very early age—and should ease the sting of authority with extra affection, a period of play, and the offering of a substitute activity. But many times the child's protests are little more than play-acting designed to find out how it feels to say no, and a parent who continues unperturbed to dress the child or tuck him into bed may well find the child still cooperating through a refrain of verbal resistance. If a parent fails to detect the playful quality of the child's negativism or disobedience, an actual crisis of authority may be generated where none existed before. Negativism is a normal and even essential part of development and, unless it is inflated into a major issue between parent and child, is soon assimilated to be the more constructive aspects of autonomy. In general, if the toddler has ample opportunity to explore and to practice things on his own, balanced by the support he sometimes needs and by a few necessary regulations, he will emerge from toddlerhood with a sound sense of his own abilities and a readiness to tackle the new problems of later ages.

Erikson's scheme of developmental alternatives is derived, as we have said, from the psychosexual stages of Freudian psychoanalysis. Thus, the crisis of autonomy versus shame and doubt corresponds to the anal stage; in which the battle between child and parents for control over elimination was the key issue. Freud, as we know, grew up in the Victorian era, when, in keeping with a widespread emphasis on public order and morality, such biological functions as elimination were thought of as "dirty"—disgusting, anxiety-producing, and perhaps even tinged with immorality. From which it flowed logically that toilet training was to be instituted early and accomplished quickly, with no questions asked and with whatever coercive or punitive measures seemed called for. It is small wonder, considering what we now know about the timing of developmental innovations, in keeping with the idea of critical periods, and about the child's own stake in finding autonomy, that toilet training so often became a battleground of wills, with the repercussions of unresolved conflicts reaching into adulthood, perhaps in the form of anal character traits (see page 170). There are still residues of Victorian moralism in thinking about toilet training, but in general nowadays people are more inclined to take a pragmatic, less emotional approach, minimizing stress and conflict and making learning easier. With the tension removed, even the subject of toilet training can become a theme of social-affective play, as seen in the following account by a mother of the behavior of her daughter, age fourteen months, three weeks:

> My mother must have told Ruth to say "Ach" when she was having a bowel movement. For a few days when Ruth had a bowel movement in her diaper, she'd say "Ach." One day she said "Ach" but she was clean so I put her on the toidy. She had a bowel movement there, pointed to it, and said "Ach." Since then she tells me "Ach," I put her on, and nothing happens. It has become a game, and Ruth knows how to get my attention.[17]

When we consider, too, that during toddlerhood several important functions are developing at once—notably language and bipedal locomotion in addition to bowel control—and that all these developing functions collectively feed into the child's feelings of self-worth at this stage, then it is easy to imagine that a disturbance in any of these areas would lead to an impairment of these feelings, or shame (as regards his value) and doubt (as regards his competence).

SELF-AWARENESS

Now it is time to look in somewhat more detail at the ingredients of the self-awareness that is so central to the toddler's autonomy. Let us begin with some of the ways the toddler, when focused on things outside himself, can egocentrically forget his own existence and his own role in situations. He seems, for instance, to have little awareness of his own weight, as when he flings himself about in the arms of an adult or tries to walk up a piece of cardboard propped up against a wall. He seems to have no notion of himself as obstacle, and does not move aside to let others pass. He even seems to have no idea of himself as obstacle to himself, since he will toil heroically to pick something up without realizing that he himself is standing on it. He often seems not to recognize that something is wrong with him, or if he does, to know what it is. Even when he clearly feels pain, as in the case of an insect bite, he cannot localize it accurately. Early in toddlerhood, the child may not be aware, even while it is happening, that he is wetting or soiling himself— or, afterward, that he has wet or soiled himself. It is interesting that he begins to localize seeing in the vicinity of his eyes, but when he is invited to peer through a cardboard tube, he plants it squarely between his eyes, as though in the center of a single Cyclopean orb. When we stop to think about it, even adults ordinarily experience the visual field as a unitary whole, and the toddler's attempt to look through the tube probably reflects the same unity of visual experience. What is interesting also is that this "Cyclops effect" persists after the child can say that he has two eyes, indicating that knowledge at the verbal level is not always perfectly coordinated with knowledge at the level of concrete experience.[18]

It often seems as though the toddler's bodily integrity were easily threatened, since he may react quite violently to breaking things or finding them broken, and may refuse ever again to play with a broken doll, even after it has been repaired. Here we see evidence of a close

Knowledge of body parts: This toddler can name all the major facial features.
ABBY'S FIRST TWO YEARS/Vassar Film

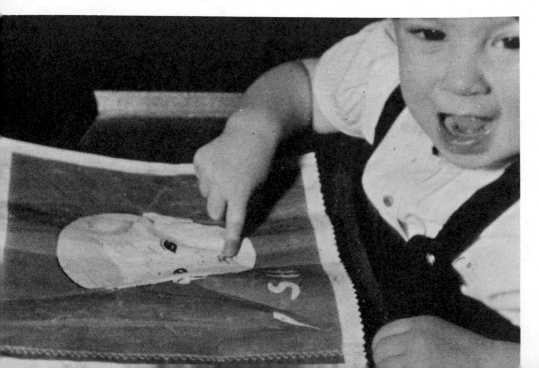

empathic identification with the things he deals with. Toddlers often manifest what looks like an almost compulsive neatness and cleanliness. Although he may enjoy dabbling in cereal or mud, the toddler afterward wants his fingers wiped clean. The Freudian theorist would say that the child's smearing of mud or milk is disguised play with his own feces, and that his desire for cleanliness expresses guilt. It seems simpler to assume that dirty or sticky fingers interrupt smooth communication with his playthings, and that the child wants the impediment removed.

In spite of gaps, the toddler has progressed far beyond infancy in self-awareness. His growing mastery first of defecation and then of urination, entailing recognition of the need to eliminate, the ability to restrain elimination by an act of will, and then to let go or actively expel, implies an expansion of bodily awareness. The toddler can name his major facial features and body parts (with only some confusions, as in the case of a two-year-old girl who, asked if she could point to her body, spread her legs and pointed to her genital region—some confusions, of course, are induced by adult euphemisms or ignorings), and becomes able to follow such instructions as "Let's see you open your mouth" or "Let's see you close your eyes." A few toddlers may be able to answer such questions as "What do you smell with?" and "What are your eyes for?" although verbal knowledge of sensory functions is more likely to appear in the preschool years. Furthermore, the child can begin to direct and instruct himself, to keep up a running commentary on his activities, and to regulate his own behavior verbally in terms of parental commandments and taboos, indicating a dawning conscience (even though the toddler—or older child—doesn't always obey himself).

Toddlers show a variety of reactions to being caught in some forbidden activity. They may, with fair individual consistency, burst out crying in either woe or anger, run and hide, feign sweet innocence, tense up and tremble, try to hide what they were doing, proffer the forbidden object to the adult, make a great display of affection as though to divert the adult, or even hurry to finish the activity before the adult can intervene. Many toddlers are vividly aware of ownership, may spend a large amount of time labeling objects with the names of their owner, and fiercely resist use of any object by someone who is not its owner. Such possessiveness may apply to other people's belongings before the toddler begins to defend his own against encroachment. Many parents with an altruistic bent try to bring up their children in a spirit of openhanded sharing, and are disappointed when a toddler seems to be selfish about his own possessions. It seems to be the case that almost all toddlers and young preschool children go through a period of possessiveness, which may be an important step in the definition of an identity and the articulation of relationships in the outside world, and which cannot be rushed.

Notice that two processes are at work in the formation of the toddler's self-awareness. First, there is the awareness that grows out of action, out of doing things and the feelings that go with particular activities. When he meets and masters a problem, he feels strong and competent and good. Second, there is the self-awareness that comes with other people's reactions to what he does. We have an example in the behavior of our articulate friend Ruth, just before her second birthday:

> I was telling Ruth how proud of her I was for going on the potty. She said, "Sometimes I wet my diaper and sometimes you are not proud of me. Now you are proud of me." She thought for a minute and added, "And I am proud of myself, too."[19]

Thus, an atmosphere of affection and applause (and when parents literally clap their hands in praise of the toddler's accomplishments, he joins in, too) fortify a sense of self as worthwhile and deserving of love. By contrast, an atmosphere of unrelenting reproach, disapproval, and exasperation keeps the toddler off balance, cripples his exploration, and reflects back to him an image of himself as unclean, inept, and beyond loving.

Let us emphasize that we do not advocate abandoning adult authority. The child who is loved and respected and valued can tolerate restraints and reproofs, and can even benefit from them in defining an identity. Once again Ruth, just under age two, gives us an illustration: "[She] got a scolding and started to cry. In the midst of her crying, she asked, 'Pick me up, please. I want to cry in the mirror.' "[20] For the child on the road to sound autonomy, the deformations of his self-image are temporary. Even as adults, we have moments of shame and embarrassment when we feel swollen and lumpy—or when, in dreams, we find ourselves walking agonizedly naked in a sumptuously attired crowd—but such feelings pass, leaving us at home with a body which, for all its shortcomings, is not such an unpleasant vessel to inhabit. In the same way, the toddler triumphant in his growing array of skills, causing his parents to laugh affectionately at his cute sayings, discovering in the world around him the new and fascinating wonders that are the external counterparts of his burgeoning sensitivities, soon forgets his setbacks in a larger sense of competence and self-esteem. And just as the toddler's self-respect depends on the world's respect for him, his esteem for others is contingent on his own self-esteem. Hostility, viciousness, and evil seem to originate in one's own sense of worthlessness, and whether one is caught in a vicious circle of hatred or a benign circle of love, we cannot escape the circularity of development.

The Regulation of Behavior in Toddlerhood

In talking about the major behavioral manifestations of toddlerhood, we have inevitably touched upon problems of authority and control. For the now-active toddler, in his pursuit of autonomy, by definition collides with the people and things around him. Collectively, the behaviors that parents try consciously to teach their children are known as the process of *socialization*—such things as good manners, eating in the proper way, speaking with respect to elders, chewing with one's mouth closed, modesty, and skills such as managing clothes. The explicit teachings of socialization are contrasted with the often unconscious transmission of culture. Before we discuss some of the specific major areas in which parents have to make decisions, a few general principles are worth mentioning.

First of all, many libertarian parents find the very idea of authority

Toddlers are traditionally "into everything."
L. Joseph Stone

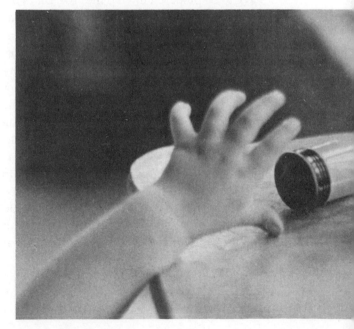

repugnant, as though to regulate a child will cripple his emotional freedom, deaden his creativity, and make him forevermore an abject puppet. The toddler represents in microcosm the perpetual problem of the individual versus society, of the way one person's striving after gratification or fulfillment can conflict with another's, and the need to find a *modus vivendi* with one's fellows that does not unduly stifle anybody's individuality. Among adults, we look for a certain degree of self-control and self-sacrifice, ability to postpone gratification, accommodation, give and take, cooperation, and a search for shared gratifications and fulfill- ments. The toddler, of course, is not an adult. Until he can exercise judgment, his parents have to exercise it for him. Furthermore, in keeping with the principle of growth ambivalence, the toddler dreads freedom almost as much as he resents restraints, and parents have to find a balance between, on the one hand, imposing limits that give the toddler a sense of stability and security and, on the other hand, encouraging exploration and venturesomeness. And parents who regret the necessity for control can console themselves that the most original, creative people have invariably been highly disciplined, not in the sense of being beaten into line, but in the sense of disciplined to take account of how things are. But just as there is danger in no control at all, so is there danger in overcontrol. At all stages, parents have to trust their children, and they have to be prepared to take the risks that go with freedom.

A second important consideration, implied by the first, is that of developmental *timing*. It is futile, and hence frustrating for parent and child alike, to expect of a child behavior of which he is not yet capable. Sometimes the child's readiness or unreadiness is a matter of motor con- trol or proficiency, sometimes a matter of how much and how well he can understand. Although developmental readiness is a necessary condition for learning certain things, two points should be emphasized. Sometimes the only way we can find out whether a child is ready is to try to teach him, being prepared to desist if it becomes evident that the child is not ready. A corollary of this point is that our attempts at teaching, if carried out in a relaxed way, may be what induces the readiness necessary to learning. The second point is that, from toddlerhood on, we must beware of the contrary tendency, holding the child back and denying him the ex- periences necessary to his development, overprotecting and "babying" him—the psychiatric term is *to infantilize*.

Another general principle is contained in the doctrine of *gradualism*. Babies tend to be conservative, to resist innovations, and in introducing something new, the transitions should not be unnecessarily abrupt, nor should we expect quick results. This does not mean that parents should be hesitant, which would be at odds with the principle that follows, but that they should watch the baby for feedback and adapt their tempos to his reactions. It is all right and probably even beneficial to push a little, as long as one knows when one is pushing too hard. In child-rearing, one makes haste slowly, in the sense that too hurried an approach to anything may defeat itself by the extreme resistances it provokes. Even the most cooperative of children need time to get used to new ways of doing things.

A further general principle is that of *parental self-confidence*. Parents must be able to act decisively, secure in their own maturity and wisdom and love for their child, and without undue concern for what The Neighbors will think. There will be times, too, when parents have to disregard to some extent what the child himself thinks. As we have suggested, there is a distinction between *needs*, which have to be met in the interests of sound development, and *wants*, which can sometimes be indulged but which sometimes have to yield to other considerations, of health, safety, parental convenience, or whatever. Parents who try to satisfy all a child's wants may soon find themselves at the mercy of a small tyrant who is no happier about his power than they are. There is still another aspect of parental self-confidence that should be mentioned: Parents should not be so afraid of losing a child's love that they hesitate to do anything that might antagonize him. The toddler cannot help getting angry when we thwart him, and parents have to accept the consequences of their decisions, without becoming dejected at the thought that the baby may cease to love them, and also without becoming indignant because he dares to react. An incidental feature of parental self-confidence is that it helps parents be relaxed, and not always on the alert for everything that might go wrong. For it is an important matter that parents should not create problems by seeing dread portents in everything the child does and reacting to the supposed portents as though the problem had already arisen. For instance, the mother who is afraid of having a "feeding problem," like the mother who feels it is her duty to fatten her child, puts so much emotion into every meal, and reacts with so much dismay to any balking on the child's part, that she spoils his appetite and manufactures a feeding problem. Here is one more instance of the self-fulfilling prophecy in development.

A final general principle in the care and rearing of toddlers is *avoidance of moralism*. This is not to suggest that parents should be indifferent to morality. But morality, like the rest of the child's psychological equipment, is something that develops, and there are appropriate and inappropriate moralities for different ages. The central core of any true morality, awareness of and concern for the feelings of others, has its beginnings early in life in the parents' love and respect for the child and for other creatures in the environment. The parents' attitudes are conveyed to the older infant and toddler both in their manner and in such words as "Gently" or "Easy" applied to the manipulation of vulnerable objects, whether pets or phonograph records. Toddler morality cannot extend far beyond this first stage, and it will be some time before such moral issues as generosity and selfishness, truthfulness, modesty, and so forth, can be meaningful to the child. With these general principles in mind, let us go on to examine some of the specific practical issues faced by parents of a toddler.

PHYSICAL SAFETY

Although both Freud's and Erikson's views of toddlerhood have their origins in the conception of the anal period, with its attendant matters of control, we prefer to begin our discussion of particular issues with questions of physical safety. For no matter how vital the proper resolution of successive crises, the child's first job is to survive in one piece. The toddler is a relentless explorer and tryer-out of things, and his enthusiasm and curiosity far outstrip his prudence. This is partly because his perceptual capacities and knowledge are still limited, and partly because he may egocentrically forget about himself as an object of harm. He may be so absorbed in watching the car backing out of the driveway that he fails to realize that he himself is in its path. In general, the toddler simply does not see the menace in speeding cars and their capacity for mangling flesh and bone, he loves water and has no idea that pond and ocean can engulf him and fill his lungs with unbreathable liquid, he does not sense the jolt of electricity lurking in a wall outlet or empty socket, or the incisive potentialities of a knife, or the toxicity of medicines or household chemicals. Adults, who adjust automatically to the changing field of forces inside a moving car, do not realize that the passive toddler may be flung across the car when it turns a corner, or sent hurtling against the windshield by a sudden application of the brakes.

Dangerous things and substances must be kept where they will not tempt the toddler to experiment. Their storage places—the medicine cabinet, the kitchen cabinet where the cleansing compounds are kept, the shelf for paints and solvents—have to be strictly taboo. Taboos are best conveyed by a bark of "No!" fortified, where necessary, by a slap on the outstretched hand; usually, though, the parent's tone of voice is enough. But since the toddler's still immature conscience is easily lulled, and since forbidden fruits are always the most alluring, a number of repetitions may be necessary. Also, the toddler is learning to tease, and he may continue to reach for proscribed objects, watching out of the corner of his eye for a reaction from the adult. When this happens, it may be well to remove the child from the site of temptation and get him started on something more constructive. As the toddler's vocabulary and under-standing increase, other, more precise words can be substituted for the original *no*, words like *hot, ouch,* and *cut.* Let us add that, the stronger the bonds of affection between parent and child, the easier it is to make taboos stick. Two additional points need to be made. Once the major hazards have been removed from the child's environment, parents should try to relax and not hover protectively over the child. In the first place, they do not want to make the child fragile-feeling and fearful. In the second place, he needs some scope to make mistakes and to learn from them, to tolerate a certain number of minor bumps and bruises and scrapes.

TOILET TRAINING

It is obvious that children in our predominantly urban-suburban society must learn, sooner or later, to use toilets. In some village or rural settings, when the weather is favorable, one can go off behind a con-venient bush, and even in the city it is not unusual for slum children to relieve themselves in an alley or between two parked cars; but by and large it is mandatory that our children stop soiling and wetting them-selves and use the elegant plumbing put at their disposal. There is a component of maturational readiness for *toilet training,* but maturation alone will not do the job. The parents must teach the child. This need not imply, however, a grim struggle for supremacy. The negativistic toddler may be on and off in his cooperation, but once he gets used to the idea and knows what is expected of him, he is usually willing to try out the process, if only because he wants to be like his parents.

Bowel and bladder training differ in both their timing and their methods, and so have to be discussed separately. Bowel training usually comes first, and control can often be established early in the second year. Training can be complicated, however, by the fact that many babies have their only bowel movements when asleep. Apart from this difficulty— which seems to go away without anything being done about it—bowel training can be effective when movements come on an approximate schedule and when there are advance warnings of which the baby himself seems to be aware. Even in late infancy, parents can see—and sometimes smell—a bowel movement approaching and, tactfully, put the baby on the potty-chair in time. (A potty-chair is recommended, rather than a seat that fits over the toilet, since the toddler can get into it himself, without help, and since quite a few children are frightened by the altitude of a toilet seat or by the turbulence of a flushing toilet.) But it is in toddlerhood, when the child can recognize the significance of certain interior stirrings and can perform the actions of holding on, relaxing, and expelling, that voluntary control becomes possible. Once the toddler is willing to try, further progress is more a matter of parental attitudes than of techniques. A casual, cheerful manner throughout, a concern for the child's comfort—like his elders, he may want to have something to read while sitting on the pot—a reasonable amount of praise when he does well, all contribute to the success of what should be a cooperative enterprise. Anxiety, prolonged confinement, strain, disgust, haste, and punishment or moral outrage when the child falters merely prolong and complicate the process. We should say, though, that an occasional child masters bowel control and then, satisfied, cannot be bothered to use the pot until some later age when he recognizes the inappropriateness of defecating in his clothing. It may be a good idea to let the child use his pot without the chair occasionally. This is because children sometimes fasten on one particular set of familiar conditions as appropriate to elimination and cannot function when these conditions are changed. One well-trained little girl, for instance, on a camping trip with her parents, was quite unable to eliminate, in spite of an obvious need, when supported comfortably on her mother's forearm. Next time, her parents took along her toilet seat, which, although it had to be held by an adult, was sufficiently familiar to permit her to move her bowels. To forestall such rigidity, in the interests of being free to take trips, it is sound practice to vary toilet conditions.

Bladder control comes in two stages, waking control and sleeping control. Waking control usually comes first, somewhere around age two, while sleeping control may lag some months behind. Since urination occurs more frequently than defecation, the opportunities for learning are greater. On the other hand, the premonitory feelings seem to be less distinct, and the mechanisms of muscular control more elusive. However, the baby's readiness becomes evident in his staying dry for ever-longer periods, and when he has not urinated for a while, parents can invite him to try. In the West, at first, both boys and girls urinate sitting down. In the case of boys, this means that the penis must be held pointed downward, especially if, as is often the case just before urination, the boy has an erection. Both boys and girls, when they have a chance to observe their parents in the bathroom, may want to try to urinate standing up, the way Daddy does. Explanations to the boy about his short stature relative to the height of the toilet, and to girls about anatomical differences, will probably have little effect, and both boys and girls may have to learn from sad, wet experience before they are willing to sit down again.

We should note in passing that bladder control appears somewhat earlier in girls than in boys, in keeping with the advanced developmental pace (including physical growth and maturation) set by females up to adolescence. As we might expect, bladder control is seldom established all at once, but takes time to become stabilized. There are occasional children who abruptly train themselves. One child, remarking spontaneously à propos of a baby sister that babies certainly wet a lot, thereafter stayed virtually dry. A little girl on a motor trip was fascinated by filling-station rest rooms and, after insisting on frequent visits to them, became completely trained. These, however, are the exceptions. Ordinarily, bladder training has to follow its on-and-off course while parents give the child ample opportunity to use the toilet—the light clothing of summer weather helps—but without making it the principal feature of his existence, offering praise for success, and taking accidents in stride. Even after the child has good control over his urinary sphincters, he may suffer brief relapses when tired or engrossed in play—all children seem reluctant to take time out to go to the bathroom—or more prolonged ones if he is sick or otherwise upset.

Nighttime bladder control follows almost automatically—but with some lag—as a consequence of daytime control. It appears that the child's practice in controlling his urinary sphincter reverses the reflexive response to bladder tension, from relaxation and expulsion to contraction and retention. It seems to make no great difference in establishing bladder control whether the child imbibes reasonable quantities of fluids at bedtime. It may help the process to awaken the child before the parents go to bed and allow him to urinate—in the case of a boy, the pot can be brought to him in his crib—but it is probably better not to do this unless it seems that nighttime control is becoming excessively delayed. In general, as in other areas, the less fuss, the easier the learning. Parents must expect occasional lapses, even in children who have good control, especially in times of illness, special excitement, or unusual strain. Even older children subjected to severe stress may revert to bedwetting. During the evacuation of London during World War II, school-age children separated from their mothers were said to wet their beds in such numbers that, as one observer put it, "half of England was awash."

An occasional child, of course, is unable because of some physical irregularity to control urination, and in such cases medical intervention may be necessary. Sometimes persistent emotional disturbances interfere with normal control, and parents have to do what they can—sometimes with professional medical or psychological help—to remove the causes of such disturbances. An occasional child seems to wet the bed for no reason except that he sleeps so deeply that normal controls are lost. Commercial devices are available for the treatment of chronic bed-wetting, that which persists beyond age four or five. Such devices seek to establish a conditioned response between bladder tension and awakening. When the child begins to wet, the urine bridges an electric circuit, causing an alarm bell to ring or giving the child a mild electric shock, thus waking him up. After a few repetitions, the need to urinate is supposed to act as a signal to awaken and go to the bathroom. Eventually, as control improves, it is enough that the child wake up only enough to tighten his sphincter but otherwise sleep on. We have heard of some successful use of these devices, and also of some failures, so we can recommend them only tentatively, and then only in serious cases where other means have been tried and found wanting.

SIBLING RIVALRY

Another area in which problems may arise during toddlerhood is that of *sibling rivalry*. There is a traditional belief, dating back to the story of Cain and Abel, and made into a formal psychological concept by Alfred Adler, that there necessarily exists among siblings—children of the same family—a spirit of competition, jealousy, and hostility. For instance, an older child, and especially a firstborn one who for a while was an only child, may feel that a new baby has deposed him from his reigning position in his parents' affections. A younger sibling, on the other hand, may feel resentfully envious of an older sibling's size, strength, and privileges. Adler and others have plotted out what they believe to be the typical patterns of sibling rivalry that go with particular birth orders (or positions in the "family constellation"), modified according to the sex of the siblings, but for our discussion here we need be concerned only with the particular circumstance that a toddler may be upset by the arrival of a new brother or sister.

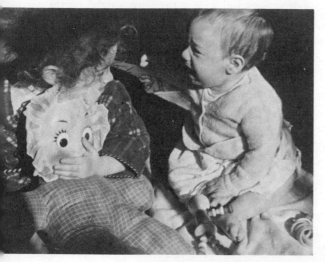

Sibling relations.
L. Joseph Stone

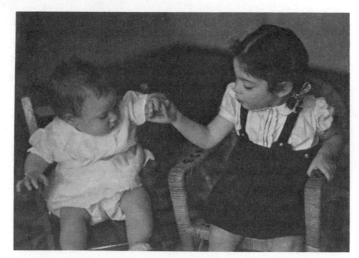

Experts have proposed various ways of forestalling or minimizing a toddler's jealousy toward a new baby. If the toddler is old enough—two and a half rather than one and a half—he should be told in advance so that the baby does not come as a total surprise, although not so far in advance that he forgets about it or that it becomes unreal with the slow passage of time. Within his restricted competence, the toddler can be given a share in the preparations for and cure of the newcomer, so that he can feel that the baby is in some sense his—or the family's—as well as his parents'. Most important, the parents should not become so engrossed in the care and appreciation of the new baby that they lose sight of the toddler's continuing need for affection and attention—the friends and relations who come to admire the new baby can help out in this respect, too. It is doubtful whether these and allied measures, no matter how assiduously and skillfully practiced, will altogether prevent the older child from becoming jealous of the new intruder. Nor is it certain that all jealousy should be prevented, if we want children to know a full range of emotions. We might also note in passing that the family dog or cat may exhibit a certain amount of jealousy toward a new baby as well.

A toddler may show jealousy of a new sibling in any of several ways. He may *regress*, turn back to more infantile ways of behaving. He may begin to whine or cry easily, he may cling to his parents, his speech may become more babyish or even disappear, he may lose control over his bladder. Such behavior often indicates that the toddler feels left out; it is as though he had concluded that the only way to get attention is to be a baby. If the toddler shows signs of regression, it may be necessary to give him an especially generous ration of love, together with whatever hints are possible that he can safely act his age. Another way in which the toddler may show his jealousy is by trying to injure or get rid of the newcomer. He may suggest to the parents that they somehow dispose of the baby (slightly older children have been known to propose flushing it down the toilet as a promising expedient), or that it is now quite time to return it to the hospital. Sometimes the toddler will try to take matters into his own hands with the sincere intention of doing away with the usurper. Here is one mother's account of the reaction of a seventeen-month-old boy to the arrival of a baby sister:

> When I came home with Jenny, Mark stared at me at first as though I were a complete stranger. He cried bitterly when his father carried Jenny from the car to the house. He was somewhat aloof for several hours. I was prepared to see some jealousy in Mark, but somehow I thought it would be subtle, or directed against me. Not so at all! The first chance he got, he went right for the baby, with the most agonized expression, and tried to sock her. He looked grimly determined to smash this little bundle of trouble, and yet he was obviously terribly upset by his own impulse and sobbed, "No, no," even as he went for her. . . . The ice finally broke one day perhaps a week after Jenny and I came home. I was diapering Jenny, and Mark was watching from his grandmother's arms. Jenny made some little noise. I imitated her and said to Mark, "Doesn't that baby make *silly* noises?" Suddenly Mark smiled broadly and said, "Silly!" It must have been a

revelation to him that I was on his side. Here we all were together, laughing at the baby. From then on, there was almost no more trouble. Gradually we let Mark loose in Jenny's presence, and it was practically no time before he was admiring her "tiny toes," kissing her, and patting her ("Gently, gently," he would remind himself).

Sometimes, of course, a peaceful solution such as this does not work, in which case the toddler must continue to be restrained from injuring the baby. But there need be no suggestion that the toddler is wicked or depraved. A formal, inflexible, categorical, and even angry prohibition can be imposed in full understanding of how justifiable the toddler's feelings are. Just as one can love a toddler—or any other person—and yet not approve of everything he does, so can one disapprove of something the toddler does, or wants to do, without ceasing to love him. As in all of discipline, the emphasis must be as much as possible on the act, and not on the toddler's worth as a total person. Especially in the matter of jealousy, an excessively moralistic approach can reinforce the toddler's conviction that he has been displaced. There are bound to be times when the new baby has to be given a disproportionate share of attention, as when he is sick, and when the toddler will inevitably feel that he has taken second place in his parents' affections. But such temporary strains, as long as they are the exception rather than the rule, will probably do as much to strengthen as to weaken the bonds between toddler and parents. It is when the toddler is consistently relegated to second place that he comes to think of love as something that has to be earned or stolen or fought for—or regressed for—rather than as something that is given as a matter of course in a free exchange. Sibling rivalry may be peculiar to small, nuclear families of the kind Europeans take for granted. In large, extended families, or in communal societies where the children belong to everybody, sibling rivalry may not develop or may take very different forms.

EATING

An area used to be of more concern than it is now is that of *eating*. On the practical side, parents, aware of the toddler's need for nourishment for growth and energy, sometimes are alarmed about whether the child is getting enough of the right foodstuffs. Their anxieties can be quite impervious to fact: They may consider that the child is wasting away, whereas he is clearly full of bounce and energy, and, as the pediatrician's records show, is growing normally and is no more subject to illness than the next child. But in addition to the practical aspects of eating, eating is closely bound up with cultural values as well. Some of us are heirs to the Puritan tradition that there must be no waste and that a clean plate is somehow a mark of virtue. In the same tradition, eating itself is not thought of as pleasurable, and dessert is frivolous and hence permissible only after the grim drudgery of meat and potatoes and spinach has been disposed of. In the Continental tradition, where food is to be enjoyed in its own right and good nutrition is incidental, the child who does not eat heartily is seen either as unhappy or as bearing a grudge against the provider of food. In some societies, from Germany to Italy to Greece to Polynesia, the bulk that comes with heavy eating is a sign of health, of prosperity and therefore of prestige, of happiness, and sometimes of beauty, and is moreover a tribute to the mother as loving and to the father as a good provider. As far as we know, parents everywhere tend to worry far less about overeating and possibly obesity—at least in the early years—than about lack of appetite, "fussy" eating, and the possibility that the child will become scrawny and debilitated.

Parental fears that the child will not eat enough of the right things are usually groundless and can be harmful. If the toddler has ample opportunity to choose from a varied and well-balanced diet, he is almost certain to get enough to eat, even if his intake appears to approach zero. We must remember that there are individual differences in metabolism, in need for particular nutrients, and in food preferences, and be prepared to make allowances for them. If, on the other hand, his mother becomes anxious and applies pressure, urging and cajoling and trying to force-feed, she can in her agitation make eating altogether disagreeable and create a true feeding problem where none existed. If it seems important that the toddler eat at mealtimes rather than at odd moments during the day, or if between-meals snacks throw his diet out of balance, he can do without snacks. If he then surprises his parents by turning ravenous at mealtimes, he can be fed a little early. Many toddlers and older children suffer a drop in blood sugar late in the day, giving rise to irritability and lack of concentration. This can be countered with a glass of juice, a bit of chocolate, or a lump of sugar, usually at no cost to the toddler's appetite.

SETTING LIMITS

Finally, we come to the problem of *setting limits,* which is closely related to the topic of safety with which we began this section, but with this difference: Here we are less concerned with the toddler's physical welfare than with the rights of others, with parental convenience and the preservation of property because of its economic, esthetic, or sentimental value. Inevitably, some household objects have to be forbidden to the toddler, because his competence is unequal to his curiosity and because he is blind to the values that adults see as obvious properties of objects. However, since a constant stream of "No!" and "Don't touch!" bewilders and paralyzes the child, and eventually loses all force, it is as well to reduce prohibitions to a necessary minimum. If fragile and precious objects are not needed for everyday use, they can be put safely out of the child's reach, and those that are needed can be grouped in a few locations, so that a few wholesale taboos can do the work of many specific ones. The knowing visitor can guess the age of the family's children by the "high-water mark" above which breakable possessions are kept. But there are two ways in which these prohibitions can be more flexible than those having to do with safety. First, the child can satisfy his curiosity about some objects by being allowed to handle them under supervision, holding them in his own or an adult lap to prevent breaking, and being given the caution of "Gently" or "Carefully." Second, some activities can be tolerated occasionally but not always. For instance, a tired mother can perfectly well decide that today is not the day for the toddler to empty out the bureau drawers, even though such behavior might be perfectly permissible another time. It should be clear that prohibitions work best in a context of freedom, so that the toddler has places he can go, things he can play with, times and places he can make a racket and run off steam. And if he is not allowed to tear up the first editions, there is no reason that he cannot have a collection of old magazines and telephone directories to do with as he will—he is perfectly capable of making and abiding by the discrimination. But the mother of a toddler learns to recognize long silences, which may at first seem blessedly peaceful but which become increasingly ominous and may end with a loud crash and a scream of distress.

When it is necessary to set limits, these should be firm and definite. The toddler has little comprehension of subtlety or tolerance of ambiguity, and finds comfort and security in clearcut guidelines. Tentative, hesitant admonitions invite the toddler to test the limits, to keep probing to see how far he can go and what he can get away with, behavior that is as trying for the toddler as it is for the adult. There is little place for "reasoning with" the toddler. Indeed, "reasoning" may be far less satisfying for the toddler than an abrupt command. The latent menace of much of the adult's reasoning is conveyed in a preschool child's tirade against a contemporary: "I'll hit you! I'll cut you up in little pieces! I'll— I'll—I'll *explain* it to you!"

Although parental definiteness can eliminate much resistance, testing of limits, and teasing, the child's striving for autonomy will not let him accept all authority passively. Sometimes the answer is in distracting the child, by changing the subject or introducing a new and attractive activity. Not every issue must be resolved, or every moral drawn, and we must remember the danger of the child's losing face. Sometimes a conflict of wills, or excessive pressure on the child, will result in tantrums. But even these are not always as serious as they may seem. Witness our friend Ruth at age fifteen months:

> Ruth has tried tantrums to get her way. She lies on the floor and cries. If I ignore her and leave the room she stops crying, comes to the room I am in, lies on the floor and screams. I go into another room and she follows. When she discovers she cannot get any attention this way, she comes over to me, puts her head in my lap and puts her arms around my legs and says, "Hug."[21]

In general, adult excitability tends to breed tantrums, which can make for a vicious circle where adult and child feed the flames of each other's passion, escalating to the breaking point. By contrast, tantrums that go unrewarded in terms of anger or dismay or surrender—or later moralizing—tend to subside more rapidly. If tantrumlike behavior persists in a given situation, the adult can only keep his head and carry on; if need be, a small and very angry child can be carried under one arm, his legs flailing behind the adult, without injury to either party. But as long as the bonds of basic trust are there, and if the adult respects the toddler's autonomy and makes allowance for differences of tempo, life with a toddler can be surprisingly serene. It is those adults who douse the toddler with cold water, or threaten him with loss of love or abandonment, who stoke the fires of tantrums.

REFERENCES / Chapter 5

[1] Church, J. (ed.) *Three Babies.* New York: Random House, 1966, p. 70.
[2] *Ibid.,* pp. 70–71.
[3] For a general discussion of the learning of language and of the role of language in development, see Church, J. *Language and the Discovery of Reality: A Developmental Psychology of Cognition.* New York: Random House, 1961.
[4] Whorf, B. L. *Language, Thought, and Reality.* Edited by J. B. Carroll. New York and Cambridge: Wiley and M.I.T., 1956.
[5] Church, *Three Babies,* p. 148.

6 Miller, W., and Ervin, S. The development of grammar in child language. In Bellugi, U., and Brown, R. (eds.) The acquisition of language. *Monographs of the Society for Research in Child Development*, 1964, 29, no. 1.

7 Campbell, D. T. Social attitudes and other acquired behavioral dispositions. In Koch, S. (ed.) *Psychology: A Study of a Science.* New York: McGraw-Hill, vol. 6, 1963.

8 Bousfield, W. A. The occurrence of clustering in the recall of randomly arranged associates. *Journal of General Psychology*, 1953, 49, 229–240.

9 Rossi, E. L., and Rossi, S. I. Concept utilization, serial order and recall in nursery-school children. *Child Development*, 1965, 36, 771–778.

10 Church, *Three Babies*, p. 161.

11 *Ibid.*, p. 160.

12 *Ibid.*, p. 229.

13 Weir, R. H. *Language in the Crib*. The Hague: Mouton, 1962.

14 Mowrer, O. H. *Learning Theory and the Symbolic Processes*. New York: Wiley, 1960.

15 Woodcock, L. P. *Life and Ways of the Two-Year-Old*. New York: Dutton, 1941, p. 94.

16 Caudill, W., and Weinstein, H. Maternal care and infant behavior in Japanese and American urban middle class families. In König, R., and Hill, R. (eds.) *Yearbook of the International Sociological Association*, 1966.

17 Church, *Three Babies*, p. 227.

18 Halpern, E. The effects of incompatibility between perception and logic in Piaget's stage of concrete operations. *Child Development*, 1965, 36, 491–497; Maccoby, E. E., and Bee, H. L. Some speculations concerning the lag between perceiving and performing. *Child Development*, 1965, 36, 368–377.

19 Church, *Three Babies*, p. 284.

20 *Ibid.*, p. 284.

21 *Ibid.*, p. 233.

6 *The Preschool Child: 1*

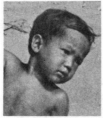

Between the ages of two and three, the child moves out of toddlerhood and becomes a preschool child. We can quarrel with this designation in two ways: Not all preschool children attend preschool; nor is there any reason to think, in the case of the child who does attend school, that either he or the school is "pre-" anything, any more than they are "post-" something else. It is true that every stage is marked by anticipations of things to come, just as it bears residues of what went before, but at the same time each period needs to be recognized in terms of its own identifying characteristics. However, the label "preschool" seems to be firmly fixed to the years from two and a half to five, and until a better one comes along we can only try to disregard its irrelevant connotations.

Until a very few years ago, the preschool years were the most intensively studied segment of childhood. As we have said, from the time the newborn baby leaves the hospital until he appears at nursery school, he is hidden away from the greedy clutches of the psychologist. Then, when he enters the first grade, he is once again barricaded behind the requirements of the school curriculum and the understandable reluctance of school administrators to have psychologists invade the classroom and disrupt routines—besides which, school-age children who have served as subjects for psychologists go home and tell their parents about the strange things they have been asked to do, and in less than no time the principal's phone is aclamor with demands for explanations. Thus, when the nursery-school movement got started in the United States in the

274

1920's, for the most part under college and university auspices, psychologists rushed to exploit the new pool of subjects thus made available. In recent years, the picture has come into better balance as psychologists have become more willing to leave their home base and study infants and toddlers in collaboration with pediatricians and public health nurses in pediatricians' offices and well-baby clinics, and even to go into the babies' homes. However, while a few communities and school systems have become more tolerant of psychological research in the schools, the study of school-age children and adolescents is still a difficult business, and psychologists on more than one occasion have met with embattled resistance from the community.

An Overview of the Preschool Years

The study of preschool children is rewarding not only from a scientific but also from a personal standpoint. For children of this age are, in the authors' biased view, delightful to work with and to know. The charm of this age may be evident even to harassed parents. The professional worker sees the preschool child as one who, not yet having learned the duplicity and guile, the masks and disguises and evasions of later ages, wears his personality on his sleeve: His thoughts and passions are instantly translated into words and deeds. His behavior is often colorful and sometimes violent, and, because of its transparency, easy to observe and record. His growing mastery of language and materials makes communication with him less demanding than with a toddler, but his very competence makes clearly evident his limitations, the gaps and misperceptions and miscomprehensions and erroneous assumptions that make his thought processes fascinating to follow, if sometimes baffling. But since his thinking is not restricted by adult considerations of logic, his utterances may have a quality of vivid imagination and even of refreshingly penetrating insight.

But let us add a caution: We are describing the child of educated parents who have time and energy and the inclination to talk with and listen to the child, who surround him with books and pictures and music and raw materials to be shaped as he sees fit, who can take him on excursions to the zoo and the farm and the seashore. The child of this age from a "deprived" background gives quite a different picture. He is likely to be fearful and inhibited, passive but explosive. He speaks grudgingly and with difficulty and, because he lacks words for many things, vaguely. His play consists mostly of formless rough and tumble. He eats greedily but without relish, and is loath to try unfamiliar foods. His diet is likely to be poor, his sleep patterns irregular, his skeletal development inadequate; he is likely to suffer serious decay even of his baby teeth, and to be highly vulnerable to infections of the eyes, skin, and respiratory and gastrointestinal tracts. It is important to bear these contrasts in mind as we talk about, for the most part, the happy, mischievous, energetic, bright, imaginative, voluble, knowledge-hungry American middle-class child.

During this time, the child's growth rate is leveling off from the first spurt of infancy. In his first two years, the "average child" added 14 or 15 inches (35 cm.) to his height; in the next three years he grows 9 or 10 inches or 25 cm. Nevertheless, around age three the baby reaches half his adult height. In his first year, the child gained some 15 pounds or 7 kg. (tripling his birth weight); thereafter, his rate of gain drops to about 5 pounds annually by age five. Indeed, growth in height may be nearly counterbalanced by the loss of baby fat (although his belly will stay rounded and his waist all but invisible throughout this period) so that he seems not to be gaining weight at all. His proportions are changing. His legs grow faster than the rest of him: at age two, they account for 34 per cent of his length; by age five, 44 per cent, which approaches the half-and-half proportions of the adult. (We are speaking here of North American children; we lack comparable data on Asian, African, and Latin-American children.) As his legs lengthen and head growth slows drastically, he loses the top-heavy look of infancy and toddlerhood. His full set of twenty baby teeth is usually completed by age two and a half—roughly the beginning of the preschool years. Similarly, the end of this period coincides approximately with the loss of the first of the baby teeth. As the cartilage and bones of his face develop and the fat pads in his cheek dwindle, his countenance loses its babyish cast and becomes better defined and more like his adult self. Sex differences in rate of growth are not very pronounced during the preschool years, although, as we shall see, boys and girls are following ever more widely divergent paths of psychological development.

Along with changes in size and proportion go changes in posture and locomotion and manipulation. Now, when he sits on the floor to play, his knees point forward but his forelegs are bent back along his thighs, and his buttocks rest on or between his heels. He loses his toddler ability to bend double at the waist, legs straight, and to rest his head on the ground, peering out at an inverted world between his legs. The high-stepping toddle of age two becomes a free-swinging stride. Over a period of several years, his one-stair-at-a-time approach to staircases yields to a continuous movement of ascending or descending, and he learns to scale ladders and jungle gyms and trees with low branches. When he wakes up from sleep, he may bounce to his feet, kick his feet out from under him and land seated at the edge of the bed, and, by straightening his body, allow himself to slide to the floor. (American middle-class children generally move from a crib to a bed around age three, although in some settings the child from early babyhood sleeps on a mat on the floor, in a hammock, or whatever.) The preschool child may still, as when he was a toddler, turn a corner by bouncing off a wall, or he may learn to hook his inside hand on a wall or piece of furniture and swing himself through the turn. He learns to spin about in one place to make himself enjoyably dizzy. When running along a smooth floor, he may stop to play with a toy by dropping abruptly to his knees and sliding to a standstill. In ordinary circumstances, he may move about with much swooping and twirling, flailing and flopping and tumbling until his parents wonder if he can possibly walk in a straight line. Actually, when the child does have a chance to clamber about on a rocky hillside, he may show surprisingly agile sure-footedness—which does not mean that he need not be watched and tended. The preschool child is still likely, just as when he was a toddler, to snuggle up to an adult knee or shoulder and gradually drape himself limply against the adult. Now, however, when he is carried, he takes some responsibility for holding on, wrapping an arm around the adult's neck or clamping his knees around the adult's waist, and plays some small part in keeping the child-adult totality in balance. From the people around him or from television, the child may pick up the idea of doing exercises, and performs a marvelous travesty of physical culture. He tries to do somersaults, sprawling sideways at the top of his turn. Similarly, he picks up styles of dancing, from ballet to ballroom to teen-age steps to tribal forms, and executes them in ways ranging from wild burlesque to smooth competence.

In the sphere of manipulation, the preschool child goes from clutching spoons and banging kitchenware to manipulating mechanical toys or hammers and saws. His use of materials is increasingly subordinated to making replicas of the world around him, and the making of replicas to their use in dramatic play. The blocks and boxes he likes to carry become building materials to be fitted into intricate and delicately balanced structures. With paint brush or crayon he progresses from scrawls and scribbles to lines and swirls and dots and cross-hatchings and color masses. Where first he used single colors arbitrarily selected, he goes on to single colors chosen with care, to combinations of colors kept well separated, to many colors freely intermingled, to colors used to identify specific areas. From the welter of his early experiments with line and form and color there emerge depictions of recognizable objects and activities. With a pencil or a ball-point pen, perhaps because they offer less opportunity for "abstract" explorations, the child is more likely to make an attempt at representation.

The preschool child's linguistic skills are expanding and elaborating. He acquires, at his own level, some of the skills of the contemplative philosopher. He brings language to bear on his busy taking in and digesting of the world—its color and flavors and textures and implications. He enters the realm of vicarious experience provided by written literature; he listens to and discusses stories and goes through the motions of reading, "saying" the text as he turns the pages. Indeed, quite a number of preschool children learn to recognize many printed words and may even in fact read. Some children are helped in learning to read by television, particularly the commercials with their many repeated conjunctions of printed and spoken brand names and slogans.

The preschool child has fewer internal limitations than when he was a toddler on his ability to formulate his experience, and knows fewer external, socially directed restraints than he will in the years ahead, which makes this a time of maximum spontaneity. In his openness, he often gives us striking insights into his own world and even ours—provided, of course, that we in our turn are prepared to be openly receptive to what the child has to tell us. All too often, we adults, instead of looking and listening and comprehending, laugh or admonish or shrug off or are seized with moral indignation.

As an infant and toddler, the child found an identity as a member of his family. Although the family continues to be his primary base and frame of reference for some years, now he begins the slow process of finding his place in humanity at large. He is exposed to more new things—real and imaginary—more new situations, more new people, more new roles, enlarging and complicating the possibilities for identification. He becomes aware of other children as people like himself and so becomes able to communicate with them directly, exchanging information and feelings and ideas. In his play with his peers, he moves from the parallel play of toddlerhood toward integrated and elaborate cooperative play projects. As his awareness of his body becomes more stable and better defined, so does his awareness of his own vulnerability, so that the preschool years witness the development of new fears about intactness.

Fears also increase as the child learns about the many menaces lying outside his ordinary experience, surgery and gangsters and war and kidnappers and ghosts and hobgoblins. During the preschool years, the child's personal style becomes more sharply articulated. Some styles can be defined fairly objectively in terms of traits or orientations such as leader, follower, participant, onlooker, outcast, or lone wolf. We can invoke such dimensions as energetic-sluggish, bold-timid, talkative-reticent, hostile-friendly, independent-demanding, imaginative-pedes-trian—the list goes on and on.

The preschool years do not lend themselves to a summary in a simple phrase of the kind we employed for infancy ("basic trust") or for toddlerhood ("autonomy"). For one thing, development goes on in too many directions at once. For another, the broad range of individual and group differences apparent at this age make generalizations shaky. Although Erikson has defined a set of developmental alternatives for this age (*initiative* versus *guilt*), just as he has for all the eight stages which he considers descriptive of the life cycle, he himself says that the preschool years are a time of rapid fluctuations, between overdependence and eager independence, between competence and ineptitude, between maturity and infantilism, between boyishness and girlishness, between winsome affection and sudden antisocial destructiveness. But just as the child is not all of a piece, neither are the preschool years themselves. Age five is a far cry from age two. Just as the toddler may retain many of the ways of an infant, so is the young preschool child in many respects still a toddler. Half-undressed for a nap, sucking his thumb or a pacifier, clutching a teddy bear or a frayed strip of blanket, he is revealed in all his tender immaturity. The young preschool child may still be incompletely toilet-trained. Observations by Roberts and Schoellkopf[1] indicate that at age two and a half, some 40 per cent of children have occasional daytime "accidents"; the child's sphincters are even more likely to betray him during sleep. By contrast, the five-year-old seems sophisticated, competent, and self-assured—and is twice as old.

Meeting People

In the young child's eyes, his parents are the repositories of all wisdom and strength and virtue, but during the preschool years his social horizons gradually broaden to include, on somewhat lower planes, people outside his immediate family. True, he has visited and been visited by numerous people during his early years, but, to judge by his behavior toward them and his later recollections, they have existed for him largely as curious, transitory apparitions without solid identities. Often, all the children he meets in a strange household are assumed to belong to the same family, and whatever adults he meets are assumed to be the parents of all the children. Now he begins to form genuine attachments to new adults such as a teacher, and then, through the teacher, to his contemporaries until, perhaps around age four, he can operate for fairly extended intervals in the company of his peers—although he still needs to have a familiar adult nearby to turn to in moments of perplexity or distress or crisis, or just because he wants some petting and cuddling. Some children, from babyhood on, have a variety of adult caretakers—grandmothers, neighbors, aunts, nursemaids, teen-age sitters—in which case it may be easy to accept new adults. Similarly, some children spend a good bit of time in the company of siblings close in age, cousins, and neighborhood children, and are likely to show a temporary advantage in social skills over children with less experience.

If the two- or three-year-old goes to nursery school, it is desirable that he be weaned over a period of some days from his mother to his teacher. As he becomes convinced that the teacher too is a human being, and that his mother will indeed return for him at the end of school, he can safely turn his attention first to the play materials and then to the other children. It is, of course, an individual decision whether a given child should go to nursery school and when he is emotionally ready to go, and if anxiety over being separated from his mother continues more than a week or so, the decision may have to be reconsidered. It is perhaps worth digressing to point out that there are special difficulties in establishing nursery schools for underprivileged children, as is now happening on a large scale under federal auspices. The poor child, whose early training is likely to include great stress on independence, may find it easier than the middle-class child to leave his mother. He may, however, find it very hard to accept his new teacher, who may have the handicaps —from his point of view—of the wrong color skin, unfamiliar accent and speech patterns, and a general behavioral style that he finds alien and unsettling. These difficulties can be overcome, but they require an extra ration of patience and understanding.

As we noted in the discussion of toddlerhood, young preschool children may at first treat each other like mere things. Before long, however, a reciprocal curiosity appears, manifested by a staring examination and a hesitant reaching out to touch each other's faces and bodies. Once the children have inspected and identified each other and learned each other's names, usually from the adults, they can exchange affection and play together. Their first play, of course, is likely to be of the parallel variety, in which there is little or no overt interchange—one child may hand the other a plaything, or take him by the hand to lead him to the swings or sandbox—but there is obvious satisfaction in the company of the other child. The children at first find it very hard to talk to each other except in imperatives, negatives ("No!" "Don't!"), and possessives ("Mine!"), and their first attempts at sustained conversations are likely to take the form of dual monologues. When explanations or the exchange of information are needed, the children are likely to call on an adult to act as their go-between.

Later on, the children begin to do things in bunches (*associative play*): A flock may congregate in the sandbox, or crowd into the rocking boat, or swarm over the climbing structures, shrilling together in an expression of shared feeling. Such behavior illustrates what the social psychologist calls *behavioral contagion,* the spread of an activity or a mood or an impulse through a group. Such contagion is a commonplace in the nursery school, where one can witness epidemics of telephoning, silliness, grotesque lurching about and collapsing to the floor, water play, tricycling—no sooner has one child begun something than everybody wants to do it. There is a growing willingness to look and admire—as when the teacher calls attention to somebody's new shoes or to the special plaything a child has brought from home—without, as yet, any need to compete for the center of the stage. Perhaps this is the place to say that there are qualities of children and their behavior that the printed word cannot fully convey, and that it is important for the student of human development to see and hear the activities of living children. If the student does not have access to a laboratory school, films (a list of recommended ones begins on page 565) and recordings may give some of the actuality that we can only suggest. Much can be learned, too, through discreet observation and eavesdropping in the playground or supermarket.

In their quieter moments together, young preschool children are likely to engage in "conversations" which seem to have as their aim less the exchange of information and ideas than the pleasure of affective communication. Such conversations, as we have said, are called *dual* or *collective monologues,* in that what one child says bears no relation, not even a tangential one, to what the other child says, the other's utterance serving simply as a springboard for a new line of thought. The following example of a dual monologue is between two four-year-olds, who are past the age at which such exchanges are common. Their teacher describes them as sitting cozily side by side, swinging their feet, waiting politely in conversational style for their turn to speak, and enjoying a feeling of "comfortable togetherness":

JENNY: They wiggle sideways when they kiss.

CHRIS: (*Vaguely*): What?

JENNY: My bunny slippers. They are brown and red and sort of yellow and white. And they have eyes and ears and these noses that wiggle sideways when they kiss.

CHRIS: I have a piece of sugar in a red piece of paper. I'm gonna eat it but maybe it's for a horse.

JENNY: We bought them. My mommy did. We couldn't find the old ones. These are like the old ones. They were not in the trunk.

CHRIS: Can't eat the piece of sugar, not unless you take the paper off.

JENNY: And we found Mother Lamb. Oh, she was in Poughkeepsie in the trunk in the house in the woods where Mrs. Tiddywinkle lives.

CHRIS: Do you like sugar? I do, and so do horses.

JENNY: I play with my bunnies. They are real. We play in the woods. They have eyes. We *all* go in the woods. My teddy bear and the bunnies and the duck, to visit Mrs. Tiddywinkle. We play and play.

CHRIS: I guess I'll eat my sugar at lunch time. I can get more for the horses. Besides, I don't have no horses now.*

Not all preschool conversations are of this kind. Many times the child is earnestly trying to get or give information, to communicate, and *non sequiturs* of the sort that occur in a collective monologue would be frustratingly infuriating. Even so, the preschool child's communication is far from perfect, although a sympathetic and patient adult can often divine what the child is driving at. One problem is that of egocentrism: The child simply does not recognize the need to provide the information necessary to know what he is trying to say. Another problem is that he may provide too much irrelevant information, so that his message is drowned in distracting "noise." Finally, he may not be able to maintain a single line of thought, so that he goes off on a succession of tangents. We recall a three-year-old boy who, having bowled over a little girl as he

---

* Most of the quotations from children were recorded at the Vassar College Nursery School. We are grateful for astute observations by Dorothy Call, Dr. Miriam F. Fiedler, Susan Fry, Cornelia Goldsmith, Agnes Griffiths, Dorothy Levens, Eveline B. Omwake, Lucretia Williams, and many others.

charged across the playroom, turned to her and said, "You should watch where you got what was coming to you!"

Needless to say, imperfect communication is not restricted to the early years of life, as the misunderstandings, cross-purposes, and confusions of much adult conversation demonstrate. It is worth emphasizing that many adults are guilty of egocentrism, and that many seeming conversations are in fact nothing more than collective monologues. But during the preschool years, children become better able to shape their thoughts to those of other people, to describe events comprehensibly, and use language to coordinate group activities in pursuit of some agreed-on goal, lapsing less often into blind self-assertion.

There are three other aspects of social relations with peers that emerge during the preschool years—sympathy, aggression, and leadership. As traits, though seemingly contradictory, these appear most clearly in the same individuals. Notice that the child is capable of sympathetic feeling toward members of his own family, at least from toddlerhood; the toddler may soothe an unhappy parent, or offer one of his toys to an ailing sibling. But the toddler's or young preschool child's first reaction to the distress of a child his own age is likely to be to burst out crying himself. Such crying is less a matter of sympathy, however, than an act of empathic participation, reflecting a lack of sharp boundaries between other people's feelings and his own—it is as though what hurts the other child hurts him, too, just as the adult can feel a jolt of pain when he sees someone fall down. Such reactions are another form of the behavioral contagion mentioned above. Sympathetic reactions to age-mates begin when the child pauses in his play to stare at another child who is suffering. Later in the preschool years we can see behavior akin to mature sympathy. One child will console another, or run to fetch the teacher to deal with an emergency, or rebuke a child who has been unkind. Of course, as Murphy[2] points out in her study of sympathy in young children, the child's motives may be less than pure, and his sympathy may be tainted with elements of patronizing superiority, guilt, anxiety, or disguised hostility. Observe, too, that the child who acts sympathetically in one situation may behave quite cruelly in another; this is particularly likely to be the case when the mob spirit takes over and children gang up to taunt and abuse a victim. Other times, a usually sympathetic child may simply not understand another's distress and so take pleasure in it as an amusing spectacle, as when he witnesses a tumble.

Authentic sympathy implies understanding of other people's feelings, both positive and negative, and it is perhaps for this reason that sympathy and leadership go hand in hand. At this age, group organization typically shifts from moment to moment, making sustained leadership difficult. Moreover, the child acting as leader often loses interest and slips out of his role. In spite of these impediments, a number of preschool children do show consistent leadership in one form or another. Some children impose their will by sheer force of muscle or character. Some become "bossy," identifying successfully with adult authority—it should be noted, though, that there is also the futile officiousness of the insecure child who is trying in vain to win the respect of his fellows. Some preschool children can play on the group like an organ. Some, remaining inconspicuous or aloof, can nevertheless exert a quiet but still potent authority as arbiter, adviser, or model.

The relationships between sympathy and leadership and between leadership and aggressiveness are fairly obvious. That between aggressiveness and sympathy is harder to fathom. It seems likely that they are found together in children who have strong feelings and are also responsive to the feelings of others, so that they know when to yield, to adapt, to be flexible. Successful leaders, child and adult, must know how to listen as well as command, or they soon find themselves leaders without a following. The correlation between sympathetic and aggressive styles is, of course, far from perfect. Some children who display little aggressiveness are capable of considerable sympathy—most of all, perhaps, in situations where they themselves feel imperiled. Other children are aggressive in ways that show no component of sympathy and in fact appear quite heartless; some aggression, of course, expresses serious psychological disturbance.

Regardless of their source, the preschool child's passions run high, even if, like summer squalls, they come and go quickly. For a young child, apparent acts of aggression may be more an exploration than an outburst of hostility. Yet in a flash of rage, if his strength were equal to his feelings, there is little doubt that he would kill without hesitation. But at this age, enmities are as unstable as friendships, so that, a moment later, the child may be showering endearments on the person he was just prepared to annihilate. Although as a rule friendships and enmities shift and change rapidly, in any one nursery-school group there are likely to be one or two children who are universally liked and admired, and another one or two who are just as pervasively disliked and shunned or picked on.

Like other forms of social behavior, children's quarrels and combats show developmental changes. To the best of our knowledge, there have been no recent studies of preschool children's fighting, but the findings from a classic study by Dawe[3] are probably still essentially correct. Although for most purposes we do not have to concern ourselves with sex differences during the preschool years, boys and girls show very different patterns of conflict after age three. Most notably, boys become increasingly combative between the ages of three and five, after which disputes fall off. Girls, on the other hand, quarrel less and less after age three. Boys engage in physical combat more than girls, who learn early to use their tongues as weapons, and both sexes try to settle property disputes by snatching and fleeing with the disputed article.

In general, combats develop from grim, wordless tugs of war over a contested plaything, typical of toddlers and young preschool children; to physical violence punctuated with angry cries and shouts; to violence displaced upon an enemy's property, as when a hat is trampled into the dirt, upon neutral objects, or upon weaker scapegoats. And physical clashes give way in turn to more "civilized" verbal ones. At younger ages, preschool children quarrel mainly over possessions. Then, unprovoked physical attacks, and retaliation, become common. Late in the preschool years, as at subsequent ages, social difficulties become the main source of conflict: who will play with whom, what they will play, who will take which roles, who will be included and who excluded, and who likes or dislikes whom. Note that four-year-olds are already adept at teasing and insults, and many a fight begins with a slur on a child's character or competence.

If we watch and listen carefully, however, we will discover that a lot of what looks and sounds like aggression is in reality nothing more than a part of the preschool child's constant role playing. We quote a lunch-table conversation which reveals a half-playful aggression reinforced by the four-year-old's love of language for its own sake and by a species of cooperative competition in which each child builds on the others' ideas in an effort to surpass them in outrageous fantasy:

JOHN: We'll cut off his arms.
ELLIE: We'll saw off his legs.
DON: Let's hang him up in a tree and tickle him.
JOHN: Let's poke him full of black and blue marks.
ELLIE: Let's cut off his hair and put it in the sandbox.
DON: Let's cut out his grunties.
JOHN: Let's smear him all over with grunties.
ELLIE: Let's make him eat lots of grunties.
JOHN: We'll wrap it up in some paper—not cellophane—some yellow paper, and then tie some string around it.

Two other preschool themes stand out in this passage. First, there is the large dose of scatology. Children very early learn the shock value of certain words, sometimes from having produced them accidentally in the course of making up nonsense words, and sometimes from hearing them used by older children in a tone of voice that conveyed their secret power. The child may have little or no idea what the words mean, but he knows very well that he can agitate his parents by saying them. Later in the preschool years, many children become temporarily addicted to "toilet talk," generously using words whose meaning they know quite well. Observe, though, that the preschool child's "bad language" deals only with superficial anatomy and with elimination; it is only in the middle years that the child begins to appreciate and exploit the special vocabulary of sexuality and its feelings and varieties, usually, of course, in its four-letter forms. Preschool children also pick up from the people around them such forms as *hell, damn, goddam,* and *son-of-a-bitch,* which they ordinarily use aptly, as expressions of displeasure, if ignorantly and, to the adult ear, jarringly. In general, adult outrage at the child's use of certain words only intensifies their value for the child, and they are best dealt with casually—their occurrence is more an esthetic abuse than a moral one. Some restrictions may be necessary, but these can be couched in terms of the times and places and audiences suited for such expressions.

The second theme is that of mutilation. As we have already noted about the toddler and as we shall see later, when we discuss self-awareness in the preschool child and the fears and conflicts he may have to deal with, body intactness is often of great concern to him. One way the child has of mastering his concerns about his body is to make sport of them in his play, just as the medical student affects an air of toughness or plays macabre jokes to help control his squeamishness about the sometimes sickening things he has to do.

The preschool child's social behavior, like much of his waking life, revolves around play. It is now time to examine in more detail what his play consists of, what it means to the child, what it tells us about him and his world, and what it tells us about *us*.

Play, Reality, and Fantasy

As we said in connection with toddlerhood, "play" is the term we use to describe whatever young children do that cannot be classified as the serious business of life—sleeping, eating, eliminating, getting dressed or undressed, getting washed, going to the doctor or the dentist, doing small chores. In the preschool years, though, play patterns change in at least four ways. First, play becomes more playful, to the point where the child makes a game of everything he does: He eats with the handle of his spoon or fork; he wants to wear his clothes turned front to back, or to wear his shirt as trousers; the boy, urinating, traces curlicues and arabesques in the toilet bowl (and sometimes, alas, outside it); he feigns hunger at bedtime and fatigue at the table; he "forgets" how to do things and makes "mistakes" so that he has to begin a project over again; he experiments with strange combinations of foodstuffs—one four-year-old boy invented a concoction he called (for reasons unknown) "Mexican soup," consisting of milk, chocolate ice cream, and mashed potatoes. Second, through the playfulness there seems to be a new earnestness in the preschool child's play, as though he is seriously trying on roles as a way of learning and experiencing the life styles they represent. Third, although the child can lose himself in his play to the extent that, for instance, he becomes angry with another child who will not play his part properly, or he actually tries to eat the mud pie he has fashioned, he nonetheless recognizes that playing—making believe or pretending—is a realm distinct from the real world in which genuine power is exercised and irreversible consequences follow from actions. He by no means understands how the real world works—he has no idea, for instance, of where money comes from and how it functions—but he knows that it falls very little under his influence. Fourth, the child's expanding emotional range and his ever-greater knowledge and skill in thinking give him new powers of imagination, both in the sense of playing with ideas and possibilities and of imagining entities and situations unlike any he has actually experienced. As we have said, his play becomes more and more social, collaborative, and, late in the preschool years, cooperative.

The preschool child continues unabated his earlier activities of sense-pleasure play, skill play, and social-affective play, and various combinations of these, but the dominant motif of the preschool years is dramatic play, the taking on of roles and the acting out of themes drawn first from domestic life and then increasingly from the world at large, including the world of fantasy. There is evidence from research by Singer[4] that a capacity for fantasy is one important way in which normal children differ from children who act out their every impulse, including impulses to violence and destruction. It is our further conviction that dramatic play is an important vehicle for learning, for identification, in the sense both of learning about other people and how to be like them and of coming to

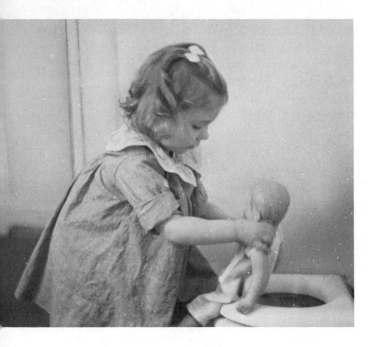

Dramatic play.
L. Joseph Stone

know oneself. But from the child's point of view, the satisfactions of dramatic play seem to lie in the magical sense of power and participation that are not yet his in the larger world. Let us remember, though, that we are talking about American middle-class children. We do not know how highly elaborated dramatic play becomes in other groups; certainly in many "primitive" societies, actual participation and apprenticeship in adult roles—as beggar, dancer, food-gatherer, cook, nursemaid, and so forth—begins at an early age.

In dramatic play, the child puts himself—sometimes literally—into other people's shoes. We see children dressing up in adult clothes, playing mother or baby or doctor, serving tea, acting the role of fireman or groceryman, pretending to be a rabbit or a tiger, and simultaneously being pilot and airplane, or steam shovel and operator. Roles which involve visible and clearly functional activities seem to appeal most to the child. The jobs of housewife, librarian, filling station attendant, carpenter, or bulldozer driver can be grasped instantly, at least in their externals, and emulated. Although it may chagrin the white-collar or professional father, it is not surprising that the child finds the role of office worker or attorney drab and unappealing. The child's literal adherence to the externals of a role, with little comprehension of its essence, shows up in the sometimes amusing mistakes he makes. For example, a child turns to his teacher and announces, "You know, I'm really desperate! Tell me how to play I'm desperate." Or a three-year-old girl, playing doctor with a doll as patient, says, "Now I have to test her kneeflexes." Or a boy, four, reports, "I'm afraid I have to tell you that I took out Jimmy's tonsils. It's all right, though—I put in some new ones." A five-year-old explains, "When my mummy hasn't any money my daddy runs and catches a check for her."[5]

In group dramatic play, young preschool children change roles rapidly, with no sense of strain, sometimes to meet the demands of the game and sometimes simply because they tire of a given role. The Baby may clamber out of his carriage and announce that he is going to be the Mommy; the erstwhile Mommy may then make herself comfortable in the carriage, or perhaps decide that she will be the Daddy, provided a third child will agree to be the Baby. Note that the children at first feel no need to adhere to roles of the same sex as their own. At age three, children are only beginning to be aware of physical differences between the sexes, and as yet have no stable notion of how biological differences are correlated with socially defined roles.

REFLECTIONS OF THE ADULT WORLD IN PLAY

Since so much of the child's dramatic play is modeled on the behavior of familiar adults, we can often gather from his reenactments the special qualities and meanings that the adult world has for him. It can be a revealing and chastening experience to have our gestures, postures, mannerisms, affectations, foibles, and turns of speech echoed back to us through the play of our children. Needless to say, we sometimes encounter reflections of parental tenderness, humor, good sense, and compassion. But the most striking insights come when we find ourselves projected as a scolding or whining voice, as a monument of pomposity, as a pettifogging tyrant, as a sleeping ogre who if disturbed snarls and gnashes his teeth. Much of the child's play is an unconscious caricature of adult ways, but a caricature that may be closer to the truth than we like to admit. Sometimes, of course, the parody becomes conscious, as in the following exchange between two four-year-olds perched atop a nursery school jungle gym and convulsed by their own cleverness:

JACK: It's *lovely* to see you!
DANNY: I'm so happy to see you!
JACK: How *are* you? How have you *been*?

DANNY: Sorry I have to go so quick.

JACK: I hope you have a good time falling down and bumping your head.

The caricature is less conscious, but no less telling, in a speech by Alice, age four and a half, as she tucks her doll into bed: "We like to have her, but I just want her to stop the nonsense. She wets the bed all the time. You *wicket* girl! You bad, *wicket* girl!" Another time, at age four years eight months, Alice, having been excused from naps, was alone with her teacher and decided to play school:

> "I'm going to be the teacher and I'll teach you how to write." *Takes pad and scribbles. Goes off across room to discipline a very noisy class (imaginary). Bawls out one child after another, ties them to their desks with long, long ropes so they can't get out, shuts the door firmly on them so she can't hear them crying. Throws arms around teacher's neck, kisses her, says,* "You're very, very good. Pretty soon you can go out and play with those recesses. That's really hard. It's really for older children."

Let it be noted that Alice was not necessarily mimicking the behavior of particular adults. In some cases, dramatic play is a fairly faithful copy of actual events, but in other cases it seems to reflect the child's perceptions of the adult world at large.

One thing that the child seems to be sensitive to in the adult world is the relative importance of different roles. It may be painful but illuminating to fathers to realize how often the mother, by virtue of her central role in household affairs, which of course are the area most visible to the child, assumes much greater prestige than the father, so that boys and girls alike may compete to take the part of mother in organized dramatic play. The behavior of a four-year-old girl with marked leadership qualities toward a boy whose standing in the group was low shows some of the status attached to particular roles in suburban society. The boy had been persistently trying to intrude on a game of house in which the little girl was Mommy. Finally, with subtle skill, she let him in and expelled him again in one smooth movement: "O.K. You be the Daddy. Finish your breakfast and I must drive you to the station. Here's your briefcase and you must get on the train. G'bye!"

Some revealing glimpses into the child's-eye view of the adult world come from the experimental or clinical use of toys which invite the child to construct scenes from family life. In his dramatizations, and in the very arrangement of the toys, the child may convey his conception of the relative significance of members of his family, the things which frighten children or disturb adults, or the weight of adult controls and impositions. He may depict himself hemmed in by threatening creatures or adrift in isolation, he may act out themes of sibling rivalry, or fantasy the revenge he would like to take against parental discipline.

REALITY AND FANTASY

Much of the play we have been describing can be viewed as a product of the child's fantasy life. Such a view, however, would be only partly correct. It assumes that reality and fantasy are two distinct realms, which is not altogether the case for the preschool child, for whom fact and fancy are likely to be interchangeable. The line between the two realms becomes more sharply defined during the preschool years—as when a four-year-old was heard to say to a playmate, "Let's pretend we're not playing pretend," or when another four-year-old asked his father about a cutout paper boat, "Would this *really* float on *pretend* water?"— but feelings, thoughts, and wishes continue to flow out into and influence the objective world, animating and coloring and shaping it in ways that adults may find surprising. Let it be said that in some respects the preschool child is in perfectly satisfactory contact with our "objective" world: He recognizes people and places and limits, he uses the tools and playthings available to him appropriately, he observes certain safety precautions, and so forth. But around and between and within objects all sorts of magical potentialities lurk.

To the preschool child, dreams are real events taking place in real space—a child may even balk at sleeping in his own room, on the grounds that it contains too many dreams. Stuart, a preschool child from whom we shall hear more, expressed puzzlement about dreams on highly realistic grounds: "How can I see the things in dreams unless my eyes are open?" Preschool children believe that the people they see on television are quite literally located inside the set, although it is not much before age four or five that it occurs to the child to wonder how they got there. And cartoon characters on TV are endowed with the same reality as the living people whose images he sees, and the activities and transformations seen on TV—like the metamorphosis of pumpkin into coach in "Cinderella"—are taken as possible and actual. Similarly, at some point the preschool child is likely to examine a radio or phonograph in search of the orchestra he hears playing.

The preschool child may nourish a firm conviction that he can magically influence events by an application of his will, just as he sees an adult "making" the car go. Observe that, as mentioned before, such a conviction is not too far removed from the "body English" that an adult exerts to steer or to propel a billiard ball or golf ball. This sort of conviction can also engender great guilt if, in a moment of anger, the child wishes somebody harm and that person subsequently suffers a mishap. Professional magicians are said to find preschool children an unresponsive audience. This seems to be because, in the child's own magical scheme of possibilities, there is nothing more remarkable in sawing a woman in half and then reuniting her than in the unanalyzed wonders of everyday life. For much the same reason, adults are far more likely to be entertained by *Alice in Wonderland* than are very young children.

Fantasy is related to, but different from, both humor and lying. The preschool child's humor is mostly a matter of burlesque, playing tricks on people, and talking nonsense, but it sometimes takes the form of pretending something that is not so, as when the child playfully denies his own identity and assumes another. Such a playful change of identity is quite different in character from the imaginary identities discussed below. It is worth noting in passing that adults' attempts to amuse the preschool child may be wasted or may backfire. For instance, one father thought it would be entertaining to tell his children that when he went to get a flu shot—which is briefly quite painful—he tried to run away, kicked and screamed in protest and had to be restrained by two nurses, and then fainted from the agony of the shot. This account was highly enjoyed by a school-age child, but the family four-year-old became seriously distressed, oblivious to the note of playful histrionics.

Lying does not appear in elaborated form until after the preschool years, but because the child's world is a mélange of the real and the fantastic, he may seem, to adults uninstructed in his ways, to be playing free and easy with the truth. In general, if the child's wishes conflict with reality, reality has to yield. For instance, a four-year-old looking for a particular television program brought the schedule to his father to find out when and where the program would be shown. Told that there was no mention of the program, he proclaimed, "They [i.e., the newspaper] ought to be punished for saying wrong things!" He tried again later in the day, and this time decided, "They must be crazy if they don't list it." Preschool—and older—children may become quite angry at a parent for not making the car go, even after it has been pointed out to them that the way is blocked by other cars.

At first, the lies a child tells seem to be an effort to remake reality so as to conform to a more desirable state of affairs. However, at least by age four, the child seems really to be trying to deceive his parents. He denies that he has performed certain misdeeds, such as using his mother's fountain pen to punch holes in cardboard, or claims that he has executed certain tasks, such as washing his hands for dinner, or he may displace responsibility to a sibling, the family cat, or persons unknown. By the end of the preschool years, he may be able to make up accounts of behavior designed to gain special merit for himself or to shed discredit on another, in at least a half-serious expectation of being believed.

When the child lies, though, or simply keeps his own counsel in hopes that he will not be discovered, or when he tries to keep a secret, he is at a double disadvantage. First, he is likely to feel that his thoughts, even the unspoken ones, are perceptible to adults—and perspicacious adults can in fact often guess what the young child is thinking—so that it is only a matter of time before some all-seeing adult will notice. Second, like other people, the preschool child feels a potent urge to share all his knowledge and ideas with someone—in the case of guilty knowledge, to confess and so to rid himself of a burden—and secrets are liable to come spilling out. ("You know what, Daddy? I have a secret. . . .") Even when the child does lie, it is probably good practice for parents to restrain their moral outrage and to treat the matter casually, indicating that they have some doubts, that they favor telling the truth, but that they have a general faith in the child's veracity. Certainly the preschool child's exaggerations and fantasies are not a moral issue, and parents have no reason to be concerned about them except in the rare, extreme case where they seem to threaten the child's grip on the real world. In the same way, it is only when the child's lying becomes so constant and pervasive that he seems to have lost trust either in his parents or in himself (as in mendacious bragging) that parents need become seriously concerned.

By the late preschool years or early school years, it becomes the child's turn to be morally outraged by adults' white lies, in ways that may be embarrassing when the child screams at full volume, "You're telling a lie, Mommy!" If truth-telling is represented as an absolute good, it is hard for a child to understand the distinction between lies told for personal advantage and those told to shield the sensibilities of other people. The child is as "realistic" in his morality as in his perceiving, and takes no account of motivation or extenuating circumstances. Piaget has devised several tests of moral realism for use with school-age children, in which the child is asked to judge which is the worse of two acts. These can also be used with four- and five-year-olds. If one asks the preschool child which is worse, the boy who, in trying to do a favor for his mother, smashes a stack of twelve plates, or the boy who, in stealing a cookie, breaks a single dish, he, like the young school-age child, is almost sure to censure the boy who broke the greater number of dishes. Such moral realism seems to be spontaneous although influenced by the absolutism or flexibility of parental attitudes.

Between the ages of two and five, the child increasingly demands realistic props for his fantasy play. For the young preschool child, a block can serve as a doll, a train, a building, or a cow. For the five-year-old, a block is strictly building material, and he wants some approximation of a real airplane to land at and take off from the airport he has constructed. The three-year-old can people a universe with sticks and stones and paper and rags—although he makes little effort to shape them into representational images. The four-year-old, to be a successful cowboy, wants some key accessory—a broad-brimmed hat, a cap pistol, or a neckerchief. For him, one element can stand for the whole configuration. The five-year-old is likely to feel dissatisfied in his role playing unless he can wear the full regalia of his part.

In older preschool children, there is also a striving after logical consistency in whatever roles they play, as though such consistency, like the use of props, is necessary to buttress their belief in their own fantasy. For example, the child playing the role of cowboy may not be able to go swimming until he has ascertained that cowboys sometimes shed their standard costume in favor of a bathing suit. A little girl playing a male role asks, "When I grow up to be a big man, will I have a penis like my Daddy's?" By age five, the child may be able to shape raw materials to make his own supporting props. He can lay out boxes and blocks to make a space ship, cut out pieces of wood and nail them together to make boats and airplanes, and improvise a costume out of oddments from the rag bag.

It is during the preschool years, especially at ages four and five, that *imaginary companions* most often appear. (We use the term generically to include not only imaginary playmates, animal or human, but also imaginary realms, identities, and playthings, as well as real playthings which seem to be treated as though they have an autonomous psychological existence.) One of the more careful studies, by Ames and Learned,[6] indicates that some 20 per cent of children may have imaginary companions of one sort or another. Our own inquiries, for the most part among female college students, suggest that the incidence may go as high as 50 per cent. Most imaginary companions seem to have vanished by age ten, although it is not unheard of for adults to have imaginary companions, and not only such fictional characters as the rabbit "Harvey." The authors know of an instance in which a military detachment at an air base during World War II shared an imaginary dog who, after the war, returned home with one of the men and became the pet both of his family and the neighborhood.

Imaginary companions are often experienced with all the vividness and solidity of real material objects, and children's families may find themselves making extravagant adjustments to the invisible (to them) visitor, taking care not to kick him or sit on him, and setting a place for him at table. Imaginary companions are sometimes born of a special need in a child's life, for a friend, a scapegoat, an extra conscience, a model, or an escape from either a stressful or a too dull reality. Frances Warfield's autobiographical account of her imaginary friend, Wrinkel, provides an excellent description both of the phenomenon itself and of one of the many functions an imaginary companion may serve. Wrinkel's behavior expressed the resentments and frustrations of a well-behaved hard-of-hearing girl who was afraid to acknowledge her handicap and therefore could not ask people to speak louder:

> Wrinkel came along at this time [*age six, according to her recollection, slightly beyond the preschool years*]. I wanted a close friend. Also, in my world of aunts and sisters, a boy was interesting.
>
> Wrinkel was invisible and inaudible, which left him free to do and say whatever he wanted. The first time he entered a room he found the exact center of the ceiling and drove in a large invisible staple. He tossed an invisible rope ladder through the staple, festooning it over the tops of pictures, curtain poles, and chandeliers, and climbed over people's heads, listening to their talk and making nonsense of it.
>
> Wrinkel was smarter than anybody—smarter than my sister Ann. For one thing, he was a boy. For another thing, though he could hear as perfectly as Ann could, he didn't care whether he heard perfectly or not. He chose to hear, and to act on what he heard, strictly as he had a mind to. . . .
>
> When people talked and talked and Wrinkel didn't make sense of what they said, that wasn't because he didn't hear it. It was because he liked to make nonsense by weaving his own name in and out of their sentences. . . .
>
> He killed people off for me all the time. He killed off all the ones I didn't like—the ones who cleared their throats pointedly or raised

their voices at me, as if they thought I might not hear them. He killed off deadpans, when they mumbled some question at me.[7]

Not all imaginary companions, it should be said, are as pleasant for the child to have around as was Wrinkel. Sometimes they are distinctly unwelcome, like the invading hallucinations of a schizophrenic, and seem to be the incarnation of some deep-rooted dread or guilt. For instance, while in some children a companion who acts as a conscience may be gently reproachful, in others such a companion can castigate the child into a frenzy of terror. On the other hand, imaginary companions need not serve any apparent motivation or embody a special problem. They simply appear on the scene, do what they do, and depart—sometimes fading away, sometimes dying a melodramatic death in a car crash or at the hands of pirates.

Other Activities of Preschool Children

It should not be supposed, for all this, that preschool children spend all their time in dramatic play or the exercise of fantasy, though they slide readily in and out of it. They spend time with their parents, in conversations, in trips to the park or the zoo, in playing rough-and-tumble games, in sledding or in sliding on the ice (some preschool children are able to skate or ski), splashing at the beach, building sand castles and digging tunnels in the sand, mock-wrestling, working around the house and yard, looking at books and being read to, listening to stories the parent makes up, studying leaves and stones and insects and birds' nests, working mechanical toys, and just observing and taking in. Some conversations with adults are serious and deal with such topics as tastes and preferences, feelings, age, geography, shared adventures, the existence and nature of God, elimination and other body functions, accidents and sickness and surgery and death, animals, Santa Claus (we are reminded of one four-year-old's account of all the things Santa Claus was going to bring him, after which his six-year-old brother shook his head in a mixture of pity and condescension, saying, "Oh, Richie, if you only knew what I know")—in sum, a huge array of things real and unreal. We must not forget that children love to confront their parents with hypothetical situations introduced by "What if": all the world were covered by water, people could fly, there were only men in the world, and so forth ad infinitum. Some conversations are built on frank absurdities—the nursery school director's spanking machine, for instance, or the child's deciding that he will play the role of adult.

Some four- and five-year-olds, once they have learned to count, can play simple board games such as Parcheesi with parents and older siblings. Notice, though, that the preschool child hates to lose and will cheat, fudge, stretch the rules, and demand endless exceptions and opportunities to change his mind when he has made a mistake. Sometimes one or more preschool children will play in a group with older children and be involved in such advanced games as cops-and-robbers (the small children are invariably cast in the role of victim, which often means being flung into jail or roped to a tree) or putting on a play or circus. (Staging a performance of this kind involves such interesting subsidiary—but still far from functionally subordinated—activities as making posters, selling tickets, and arranging scenery.) With peers or by himself, the child builds with blocks, draws and paints, cuts out and pastes, looks at pictures, saws and hammers, blows soap bubbles, listens to records, sails toy boats, and thinks about things.

THE MASTERY OF MATERIALS

In all his activities, the preschool child is interacting with things in the world, and we can see a steady progression in the direction of increasing appropriateness, ingenuity, imagination, and mastery in the way he uses the things and substances available to him. This is in keeping with a more general trend from impulsive activities under the control of the environment and its demand qualities toward planned, internally directed occupations. Of particular interest is the way the child uses raw materials to shape new products, from manipulating the materials for their own sake to the functional subordination of materials into emergent constructions. The child finds raw materials everywhere: Cleaning tissues are not merely something to blow one's nose with or to wipe up spilled liquids, they can be bunched together and secured with rubber bands to make a doll, they can be wrapped around a doll to make clothing, they can be spread over a doll as blankets. Paper clips, pipe cleaners, cotton wool, gummed reinforcements, cellophane tape, paper bags, metal foil, adhesive tape, rags, drinking straws, toothpicks, water, clay, and lumber are all grist to the preschool child's mill.

In shaping materials, the child uses such tools as scissors, saws, hammers, nails, drills, and staplers. He can make some limited use of screwdrivers and wrenches. With adult inspiration, he makes abstract collages of old wallpaper, leaves and twigs, and sculptured library paste. He makes constructions out of empty matchboxes, cereal boxes, cleaning-tissue boxes, and folded paper, decorated with sand, buttons, sea shells, junk jewelry, spangles, and so forth. Note that if one gives the child some version of Guilford's Unusual Uses Test[8]—designed as a test of creativity —which requires the subject to say all the ways he can think of to use, for instance, a common brick, at this age his responses will be few and uninspired. But when one actually gives him the materials to work with, he uses them in diverse and unexpected ways.

One of the more interesting lines of development is in the child's drawing and painting, which tells us less about his perceptual processes than about how his world is organized emotionally, in terms of significances. It makes a difference in how the child operates whether he is using paints, crayons, a pencil, or a ball-point pen. With a coarse medium, such as poster paint laid onto large sheets of manila paper with a wide brush, the child is likely to engage in experiments in pure form and color, in the spirit of sense-pleasure play, without any concern with depiction of objects. Indeed, at this age, it is only the most tactless of adults who would ask the silly question, "What is it?" On the other hand, one can perfectly well ask a child to "Tell me about your painting." Even when he does begin to paint pictorially, accidental effects may suggest new possibilities and divert him from his original purpose, so that what begins as a picture of a horse may midway become a picture of a house, which may then be transformed into a boat or may revert to an abstract exercise in design. Thus, what may look like an unrecognizable jumble of forms and colors may actually be a composite of many superimposed intentions. By age five, many children paint elaborate scenes containing complex events and activities set against detailed backgrounds of grass, trees, buildings, fences, animals, sky, clouds, and sun or moon or stars.

With a fine medium, by contrast, like a pencil or a ball-point pen, the child is likely to attempt pictorial representations, most typically first of people. The child's first drawings of people ordinarily consist of a roughly circular line enclosing marks standing for eyes, nose, and mouth—these may be in almost any position relative to each other. Even before he goes on to further elaboration, the child may draw an upturned or down-turned mouth to indicate happiness or sadness. The next step comes with the addition of ears and hair, the latter in the form of a scribble at the top of the head or a series of loops more or less encircling it. Next, stiff, sticklike arms sprout straight out from the sides of the head, ending in a club of a fist or a sunburst of fingers (if they happen to number five, it is probably accidental). Then legs grow downward, either directly from the head or from the arms near the head; the legs, too, are jointless and end in a ball of foot. The torso is likely to appear first as a disconnected whorl between the legs—to the oversensitive adult eye, this may look like an attempt to represent the genitalia, but in fact it seems to occur to very few preschool children to draw the sex organs. Then the torso takes shape as a crude oval or rectangle with the legs appended. For a while, even after the torso is represented, the arms may continue to grow out from the head; then they are attached to the torso, but only approximately in the shoulder region. Head and torso are likely to remain for some time juxtaposed, without an intervening neck. Implied action may be contained in the figure from an early age, but it usually has to be inferred, either from the inclusion of some additional form such as a shovel or car, or from the child's verbal description; to represent walking or running or sitting overtaxes the child's skills. Clothing and scenery may appear by age four. By age five, arms and legs, as well as the torso, may be represented by enclosed spaces.

Some children depict the complete human figure as an assemblage of discrete parts, like a piece of machinery, while others come to draw it as an ameboid whole. In general, heads loom disproportionately large, and people tower over trees and houses. Even though one figure overlaps another, both are usually shown in their entirety, as though the near figure were transparent. When the child first draws a house, he strives mightily to show all four walls, and usually ends up settling for three.

These are the stages that seem to characterize the figure drawings of middle-class American children given liberal access to paper and pencils and encouraged to scribble, trace, color, and draw. Our observations of twenty-eight lower-class four-year-old children indicate that their ability to represent people is, by comparison with a middle-class sample, significantly lower (although eight of the twenty-eight lower-class children made drawings as elaborate as those of the middle-class controls). Valid comparisons of drawings by children from different cultural backgrounds may be hard to make, since in some societies only a very few children may be given much opportunity to draw, and these few may be inducted early into a highly formalized system of representation and decoration.

Similar patterns of development can be observed in the use of other plastic materials, from modeling clay to building blocks. In his block play, the three-year-old is more concerned with problems of balance and shape and how big a structure he can erect than with combining blocks to make a particular *thing*. (Let the reader not be misled by our use of *he*—girls play with blocks, too.) The four-year-old functionally subordinates his use of blocks to make things, but his structures are usually sprawling, amorphous, loosely hung together, and easily toppled. By age five, the child can build highly integrated, tightly balanced block structures that may reach to phenomenal heights and are often baroque in their intricacy. His block constructions are in many cases functionally subordinated to dramatic play which may continue over a period of days.

The kind of block play we have been describing depends, of course, on the child's having lavish quantities of blocks at his disposal, in a variety of sizes and shapes; as in a well-equipped nursery school, to a degree impossible in many homes. The preschool child's carpentry develops in much the same way: The three-year-old takes pleasure in simply cutting and nailing pieces of wood, the four-year-old hastily slaps together crude and ramshackle airplanes and boats, while the five-year-old plans, measures, carefully joins together, and smooths and paints, returning to the same project, if necessary, again and again.

The competence in the use of materials found in middle-class American children dwindles into ineptitude by contrast with the skills found in many primitive societies. The old ways are changing, of course, with the ever-wider spread of Western practices and commodities, but one can probably still find relatively intact communities in which three-year-olds build functional traps to snare fish or birds or rodents, or in which five-year-olds can be trusted in their own canoes on the waters of the lagoon. Notice that the primitive child's situation is very different from that of the middle-class American child, whose life is culturally deprived by being tied into the market economy of the larger society. In the tribe, or in any small, self-contained setting, little girls participate early and actively in the woman's duties of child care, cooking, cleaning, weaving mats, and so forth, and little boys in hunting, fishing, making traps and weapons, gathering food, or whatever else may be the man's role, and it is hardly surprising that they develop a precocious competence in the skills of their society.

Awareness of Self

The description of self-awareness in infancy and toddlerhood was a relatively simple matter. We could speak of self-discovery, of abilities, of playfulness, of role playing, of basic trust and autonomy and negativism. By the preschool years, however, all the components of adult self-awareness (see page 101) are in operation, if only in a preliminary sort of way. Traditionally, adolescence is the time for shaping an identity, a sense of who one is and what one believes in, for defining values and

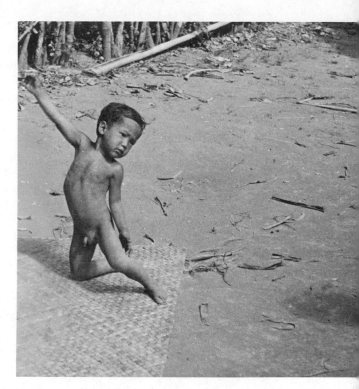

Balinese child trying to stand on his head: The child learns simultaneously about his own body and the space in which it orients itself.

Gregory Bateson and Margaret Mead, *Balinese Character*

goals and meanings. Many writers have spoken, with justice, of the preschool years as a first adolescence, a time for a first identity formation in preparation for moving away from the family into the world of school and peers and practical achievement. It should be remembered that the child's developing self-awareness is almost a special case of his developing awareness of things around him, particularly other people. His awareness both of himself and of the environment increases as he becomes psychologically more differentiated from his surroundings, as he comes to distinguish between external events and internal ones, and as he learns to suspend action in favor of contemplation, thought, and feeling.

Some musings by the child Stuart, whom we quoted earlier, at intervals during his fifth year help give the flavor of developing self-awareness in the preschool period.

> What is my back like, Miss Williams? (Nice, like other backs, etc.) *No!* Different. *Mine!* (Yes, but most backs are alike.) Like Mr. Stone's? Wide? (Like his and other people's.) Oh. (*He is thoughtful and slightly dashed.*)
>
> You can't see your own face, can you?

These observations remind us that in knowing one's own body one must coordinate two perspectives, one given from outside through sight and hearing and the other given through inner experience. The comments, occurring over a span of three days, of another boy, age four years and two months, give further insight:

> (*In the barber's chair*) Can you see your hair when you're not looking in the mirror?; (*next night in bed, calls father into room*) When I yawn [*opens mouth wide*] I can't sing. Why?; (*in bed the next night*) When I hold my nose and close my mouth [*demonstrates*]—see, I can't breathe. But when I hold my nose and open my mouth, then I can still breathe.

One would suspect that certain regions of the body are much more important for the child than others. For instance, when he washes his face, he washes only the frontal surface, and when he washes his hands, it is only the palms. We should also mention that older preschool children become very modest about exposing their bodies, even when their parents have set no particular example in this regard. One four-year-old girl, seeing a painting of a nude, asked, "Isn't she embarrassed?" It is in the school years, however, that modesty and privacy become a real issue. Now back to Stuart:

> (*Inspecting his abdomen as he dresses after nap.*) You know a thing? There is something funny about my skin. It fits all smooth mostly, but when I do this, there are extra skin in crumples. What is that for? (It's loose so you can move and stretch, etc.) No, it is not loose or it would show. It would hang down. It would be too big. (Like a rubber band.) Would it break if you pulled it too much? (Can stretch a lot.) I had this same skin when I was a baby. It fits very nice. It is me.

> Why have you a long head, and me a little round one?

> Sometimes I wonder about the blood in me. Inside me it is all wet and blood and moving and lots of insides, but outside is all dry and careful and you would never know about the inside part by looking at the outside part. Not unless you got a hole in you and some of the blood came out. All the people are like that. Their skins keep them in, but underneath their skins is such a lot. . . . Your insides never stops. . . . It is so funny to think of you being all wet inside and all dry outside. Everybody is like that. I am. Why, Miss Williams, *you* are (*laughs*). Did you ever think about it? (*Teacher offers to show him anatomical picture.*) A picture that would be for you would be for me, too? Then we are alike. You and me are alike.

Your insides is like if another person lived inside your skin.

Did you ever have a red pain in your throat? The pain it was there. I could not see it, but it was there. It is funny—I could not see it. . . . It is funny, it was *my* pain in my throat. Why could I not see it? I could feel it, it was mine, mine pain. . . .

Observe that Stuart's experience of pain is both synesthetic and intersensory. Pain produces a synesthetic effect of color, as it apparently did too in his description of the dentist's office (see below) and it seems to exist for him as something solid and potentially visible. This seems comparable to the infant's looking for the piano chord or the handclap, and is like another child's description of an electric shock to his hand: "It feels like a bone in your arm." We see the same tendency in Stuart's musings about speaking:

A voice is a fast thing, isn't it? Are other sounds voices of things? [*The reader is urged to dwell a moment on this insight.*] Is the day got a voice, a sound? Where is your voice? It comes out of your mouth? *Does* it, *is* it, *in* your mouth? (*Here Stuart begins to elaborate his idea half in play, half in earnest.*) Are all the words stored up some place in your mouth? How can you get food in if all those words are in your mouth? How much space does a word take? Words are thin little things. But some of them make a big noise. A sound—is it bigger than a word?

Stuart's growing awareness of common experience, including the recognition that adults not only have the same kind of bodies but that these towers of omnipotence and infallibility have feelings, doubts, and frailties akin to his own, is not limited to the human sphere and does not automatically lead to clarification in adult terms. Thus, on other occasions, Stuart wanted to know how it feels to be an earthworm and whether it hurts the ground to have holes gouged out of it.

Stuart's comments bring us back to another important strand of self-awareness, the problem of intactness of the emerging self. The more the child becomes aware of himself as an autonomous individual distinct from his surroundings, the more he is obliged to question his own identity and the more concerned he becomes about body integrity and intactness. This concern is not an altogether new development, but it becomes particularly acute late in the preschool years. Stuart, at age five, objected strenuously when his teacher appeared without her accustomed glasses and hence incomplete or damaged or deformed. These further quotations show how a visit to the dentist, blended with anticipations of a tonsillectomy, seems to have stirred up some of Stuart's feelings about staying intact:

> Once there was Stuart with a tooth and in it was a hole. So it was fixed. The man had many little streams there, very nice. There was a pain, a bright pain. It was bright when he pushed with a noise and a bar. But there was no blood. No blood. . . . Can I get a hole in my hand like the hole in my tooth? Will it have to be filled with a loud noise? . . . . The queen was in the garden hanging up her clothes, there came along a big thing to snap off her nose. . . . Her nose was not. It bled and bled and she died. Humpty Dumpty did die, too. He fell off and couldn't put together again. . . . When I have my tonsils out—what will happen when I have my tonsils out? Will it bleed? Will I be dead? [*Another four-year-old, not faced with a tonsillectomy but trying to make sense of things he heard, asked,* "You can't live without tonsils, can you?"] Being blood is being dead. Why do I have my tonsils out?
>
> *I do not like myself not to be myself, and that is what will happen if even my littlest tonsils is taken away from me.*
>
> . . . Sad it was to have a nose taken off. So it will be sad to have a tonsil out. Blood, blood, blood. When the nose—the tonsil is out.[9]

FEARS

The sense of vulnerability that accompanies growing self-awareness is often expressed in specific fears at ages four and five. A classic study by Macfarlane and associates[10] shows how patterns of fearfulness change with age and how widespread fears are in the late preschool years. Just as cognitive development depends on affective involvement with the world, so does fear develop out of knowledge of one's own vulnerability and an understanding of the potential dangers inherent in the environment. Note that fears need not be realistic: It is as easy to be afraid of ghosts or witches as of cars and undertow; kidnappers, though real, are rare, but this does not reduce the child's fear that he will be abducted. Moreover, the specific fears that a child may have may merely express a more general sense of menace. The swaying curtains in his room may take on monstrous aspects, and unnamed terrors may lurk under beds or in closets. It is for this reason that children may need to have a light left on when they go to bed. On the school playground, a child who snarlingly declares himself to be a tiger, or who pronounces his undulating arm a snake, may provoke genuine panic in his fellows. Their fright may be tinged with skepticism, but they would rather not take a chance on finding out. Freudian writers, of course, find in the fearfulness of the late preschool years an expression of Oedipal conflicts and castration anxiety.

Among other things, the child may develop a fear of death. This fear is not rooted in an abstract knowledge that all men are mortal, and that he himself will some day grow old and die, but simply in knowing that people do die and that something could happen to him—not eventually, but now. What dying means is likely to be uncertain and variable. At first, the child whose contact with death is likely to be a matter of dead insects or a mouse or frog found in the street may simply say that death means that "you put it in the garbage." In games death is reversible: "Bang! You're dead. O.K., now you must be alive again."

Children find it hard to grasp the blank finality of death—as do older people who, in self-pity, imagine themselves as able to witness the remorse of others when they themselves are dead. One child asked, "If you woke up one morning, and you were dead, would it hurt?" Stuart put it in these terms: "Being dead is like being blind, only *all* the time and the same feeling all over, everywhere, like blind in the eye." While the best analogy in life to death may be that of a continuing sleep, the child who is told this may become terrified of going to bed at night. Awareness of death as a threat to himself may come much later than a fear that one or both parents may die, and the child may violently resist any separation from a parent, lest it be final.

Middle-class American adults especially are inclined to shield young children from knowledge of death. This shielding is made easier by the separation of generations, so that many children never get to know their grandparents or other old people well, and so have little contact with dying. Not only do people put their elders in nursing homes or otherwise out of sight, but old people themselves collaborate by taking up residence in "retirement homes" or colonies for the aged. The general improvement in health has meant that relatively few children or young adults die any more—automobile accidents kill more people than any of the major diseases. Thus, parents may even deny the fact of death ("Grandpa's gone on a long trip"). They may try to disguise their own feelings (it is doubtful that even devout believers feel the supposed joy conveyed in "Grandpa is happy now in Heaven"). The child, however, with his acute emotional sensitivity, is not likely to be fooled. The unusual behavior of the adults, the air of mystery and exclusion, and the macabre atmosphere with which our society surrounds death will tell him that something is seriously wrong. And his piecing together of fragments of knowledge may produce fear and bewilderment far greater than he would feel in response to simple frankness about what has happened and how his parents feel about it.

The tendency to conceal death from the child rests on the same assumption of childish innocence that leads adults to try to insulate the child from other realities—sex, money, disagreements and animosities between adults, insanity, depravity, and the hard facts of power. In all of these areas, in the authors' view, children benefit from being given as much information as they can understand and manage, rather than inventions and evasions that needlessly confuse and complicate their feelings. Which does not deny to parents the right to say, "I'll tell you more about it when you're older." As we have said before, parents must be able to judge the timeliness of information.

AWARENESS OF GROWTH AND CONTINUITY

A further aspect of self-awareness is the child's growing recognition of himself as changing with the passage of time. Time is beginning to move—as we know, it slips away with ever greater velocity as we grow older—and the child begins to sense the transitory nature of his experience; as Stuart remarked, his birthday had come and gone and there was nothing left, but he was older. It sometimes appears that the child senses fleetingly that growing older brings with it not only competence and privileges and freedom but also responsibility and loneliness, which might explain otherwise seemingly unaccountable spells of babyishness, sulking, clinging, whining, and weepiness. The penalties of growth may be made especially prominent by the birth of a sibling, but even children without siblings show a certain amount of growth ambivalence, as when they play at being baby or ask the adult to "feed me" or "dress me." The child of preschool age delights in looking at the family photograph album, most of all at pictures of himself in earlier incarnations. Similarly, he likes to be told stories of his own now-dim past. This is not to say that preschool children do not remember anything. They can vividly recall isolated events or details of events that have escaped their parents, to the point where parents can use their children as memory storage machines, capable of recalling the name of the man who bought their car or what kind of dress Mrs. Jones wore when she came to tea. But their memories are spotty and lack continuity and organization. A three-year-old boy, passing a familiar landmark, comments, "Sally Smith cried and cried," recalling an event from six months before, but he cannot remember that the occasion was a trip to the beach. Or, a three-year-old girl, seeing a sample of wallpaper with a splatter design, observed, "Egg man"; the following week, when the egg man made his delivery, her parents for the first time noted that he wore a tweed coat remarkably similar in coloring to the wallpaper sample.

One way children cope with the problem of an ever-changing identity, as we have seen, is to assume a new one, to become somebody else. Our friend Stuart, for example, spent a number of months, when he was four, earnestly, doggedly, and skillfully being a particular nine-year-old boy whom he had heard of but never met. There is no evidence that he ever convinced anybody else that he was anyone but Stuart, but he nevertheless managed for a time to awe his peers with his patronizing manner and references to the school he attended, where they had real "lissons." Part of the temporal dimension of identity lies in the ability to do something now in anticipation of a future reward.[11] In experimental situations in which the subject can choose between an immediate small reward and a delayed larger reward, preschool children already show ability to delay gratification. Delay of gratification, however, is much more likely to be found in middle-class children than in lower-class ones.

Preschool children know the names for all the major external parts of the body, although there are striking social class differences in this respect. Poor children are at a special disadvantage when it comes to naming joints, such as wrist and ankle, and such adornments as eyebrows and eyelashes. The middle-class four-year-old can usually say, and the slum child usually cannot, that he smells with his nose, tastes with his tongue (or mouth), and touches with his fingers; that his eyes are to see with and his ears to hear with. The four-year-old has some vague idea of digestion but he seems not to take seriously the notion that food is transformed into feces. He is more willing to accept that the fluids he drinks are discharged as urine. As suggested earlier, he knows about air and breathing, and about the beating of his heart. As a study by Gellert[12] has shown, young children have little or no knowledge of their inner organs, how they are arranged, or how they function. The four-year-old may know that germs cause illness, but he doesn't know what a germ is.

It is interesting that, although the preschool child obviously is aware of himself and other people, he has a hard time keeping both kinds of awareness in mind at the same time. Asked how many people there are in his family, he may neglect, because he is counting from his own standpoint, to count himself. Asked if he has a brother, he will (assuming it is so) answer yes. Has his brother a brother? No. Is he his brother's brother? Yes. Has his brother a brother? No. The reader will not fail to notice the principle of egocentric thinking at work.

REFERENCES / Chapter 6

[1] Roberts, K. E., and Schoellkopf, J. A. Eating, sleeping, and elimination practices of a group of two-and-one-half-year-old children. *American Journal of Diseases of Children*, 1951, 92, 121–152.
[2] Murphy, L. B. *Social Behavior and Child Personality*. New York: Columbia University, 1937.
[3] Dawe, H. C. An analysis of two hundred quarrels of preschool children. *Child Development*, 1934, 5, 139–157.
[4] Singer, J. L. *Daydreaming*. New York: Random House, 1966, Chapter 6.
[5] Miller, L. Children and Money. *Redbook*, November, 1959, 39–41, 66, 68.
[6] Ames, L. B., and Learned, J. Imaginary companions and related phenomena. *Journal of Genetic Psychology*, 1946, 69, 147–167.
[7] Warfield, F. *Cotton in My Ears*. New York: Viking, 1948., pp. 8–9.
[8] Guilford, J. P. *The Nature of Human Intelligence*. New York: McGraw-Hill, 1967.
[9] A 52-page compilation of Stuart's comments has been mimeographed and may be obtained from L. J. Stone, Department of Psychology, Vassar College, Poughkeepsie, N.Y. 12601. ($2.)
[10] Macfarlane, J., Allen, L., and Honzik, M. P. *A Developmental Study of the Behavior Problems of Normal Children between Twenty-one Months and Fourteen Years*. Berkeley: University of California, 1954.
[11] Mischel, W., and Metzner, R. Preference for delayed reward as a function of age, intelligence and length of delay interval. *Journal of Abnormal and Social Psychology*, 1962, 64, 425–431.
[12] Gellert, E. Children's conceptions of the content and functions of the human body. *Genetic Psychology Monographs*, 1962, 65, 293–405.

7

The Preschool Child: 2

The Preschool Child's Thinking and Perceiving

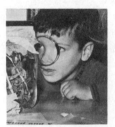 In this section, we shall try to deal systematically with how the world exists for the preschool child and how he thinks about it—in other words, with his *cognitive* functioning. In older, classical psychology, functioning was partitioned into the three areas of *cognition* (knowing, including perceiving and thinking), *affection* (feeling and emotion, including attitudes and values), and *conation* ("will," or as we would now express it, motivation). We now realize that these areas are far from distinct. The way a person cognizes the world necessarily includes his motivational states and his attitudes and feelings toward the things cognized. Feelings are closely implicated with drives and motives, and are always directed toward cognized objects of some sort. Perception, learning, and feelings are essentials in the development and arousal of motivations.

It follows, then, that the topics we have already discussed, such as play patterns, the mastery of materials, and self-awareness, can also be seen as aspects of cognitive functioning. In fact, our discussion in this chapter has an implied aim of showing how cognition may be the basis for integrating all of behavior and experience, that emotion and motivation can be seen as components in the way the individual cognizes objects and situations, including the self as object, and symbolic or imaginary situations. Notice that cognition, apart from the narrow aspects of it studied in psychophysics, as in the study of sensory thresholds, was for many years an outlaw subject in American behavioristic psychology (see the highly derogatory treatment by Verplanck[1]). Even the study of learning, which one would think has something to do with knowing, was in large part dedicated to showing that learning did not require cognition, that learning was a supremely noncognitive process. In recent years, thanks in part to the belated discovery of the work of Jean Piaget, Heinz Werner, and their collaborators, cognition is once more a respectable topic.

Let us note that our emphasis, in the discussion that follows, will be on shortcomings in the preschool child's cognition, not with the idea of holding him up to ridicule but to make graphic both how far he has come and how far he still has to go. Furthermore, those who have to deal practically with preschool children should appreciate how the child's still primitive grasp of reality may make communication difficult, and should be able better to take account of situations as the child sees them.

We must stress once again that we are describing the behavior of middle-class American children living in symbolically rich and complex environments. Lower-class children of this age show little of the inventiveness and playfulness and imagination found in the language of middle-class children. Bernstein[2] in the United Kingdom, Hess[3] in the United States, and Ortar[4] in Israel have attempted to relate social-class differences in children's linguistic patterns to the different ways their mothers speak to them. Bernstein draws a distinction between "elaborated codes," characteristic of middle-class mothers, in which status relations are minimized and full information is given, and "restricted codes," characteristic of lower-class mothers, in which status and authority are stressed and a minimum of information given. Hess has a similar distinction between, briefly, "instructive" (that is, informative and explanatory) and "directive" (with emphasis on telling the child what to do) styles of communication.

MASTERY OF LANGUAGE

Cognitive development, as we said earlier, is closely bound up with progress in the mastery of language and symbols, bearing in mind that language as it is handed down to the child may not only liberate his thinking but also constrict it by embalming experience in stale formulas and clichés, by providing false or nonexistent conceptual entities and explanations, by shunting certain interesting topics like sex and death off into the realm of euphemism or the unspeakable, and by deceiving him into thinking he has understood something just because he has labeled it and catalogued it. At its best, though, language can free the child's thinking by providing him with useful forms and operations.

The first steps in learning language have been accomplished by the early preschool years, and the three-year-old who comes from a normally stimulating background is a fluent talker. However, language learning is a lifelong process. We learn new words, we learn more about the scope and limits and the shadings and complexities of meaning of the words we already know. We learn to read, and to read at higher levels of sophistication as we learn about metaphor and imagery and allusion and reading between the lines. We learn to talk about painting and poetry and politics, and we learn the special vocabularies, syntaxes, and logics of such fields as mathematics, chemistry, and economics. Much of our school learning is by necessity vicarious, through words that tell us about long-gone events, distant places, the adventures of fictional people, and forces lying beyond direct perception. And even operations that seem wordless, as when we make pictures or look at them, or shape raw materials into a meaningful pattern, or react emotionally, are conditioned by language.

While the young preschool child has mastered many of the basic forms of language, the quotations we gave in the last chapter show that his mastery is incomplete. Some linguistic weaknesses persist well into the school years, not to mention the errors (and vulgarities) that school children teach each other. Phonetically, the speech of many preschool children shows residues of baby talk. Sounds and syllables are likely to get misplaced as in "aminal," "hangerburg," and "pisghetti." On the semantic side, the young English-speaking preschool child may still have trouble with pronouns and their shifting relativism. Even four-year-olds may mix up *he* and *she,* not because of any failure to distinguish the sexes but because they forget which pronoun goes with which sex. *We* may be learned as the first person plural but in addition function as a collective designation for the parents, who so often speak to the child in this form. Like the earlier difficulty with *you* and *I,* this one arises out of too-direct reflection of what the child hears. Thus, "Are we going out tonight?" is likely to mean "Are you and Daddy going out tonight?" Designations of time gradually become more precise, and by age four or five many middle-class American children know the days of the week and the seasons of the year, and some of the key holidays that fall in different seasons. Clock time ordinarily eludes the preschool child except for a few hours that mark turning points in the day's activities. Some especially verbal children may be able, by age five, to define words, particularly concrete nouns and usually in terms of action qualities: car—"You ride in it"; banana—"You eat it." Some five-year-olds can specify, at a primitive level, the defining attributes of a class of objects: An orange and a peach are alike "because they're both juicy"; a suit and a dress are alike "because they keep you warm." Even earlier, children can specify how two things are different, as in "Doggie bark, kitty meow." Needless to say, the child's ability to specify differences and similarities is far from absolute and depends on the nature of the contrast or resemblance—he may even have trouble with such a seemingly obvious difference as that between bread and cake.

Equivalences and Contrasts of Meaning. Some writers use terms like *abstraction, generalization,* and *concept* to describe the way people take note of similarities and differences among things. We prefer to reserve such terms for some precise technical applications and to speak instead, following Klüver,[5] of *equivalences;* it seems enough in speaking of the behavior of preschool children to say that they react to the members of certain classes of things as roughly equivalent, and are increasingly able to put into words the salient features of objects, actions, and relationships. Note that many equivalences appear without language, as when the male stickleback fish accepts a rounded block of wood as equivalent to a female; whereas others are wholly dependent on language, as when we say that coal and a muscle are both sources of energy. In fact, it appears from classical conditioning and other studies that human and infrahuman subjects "assume" equivalence until experience teaches them otherwise. The child's equivalences may surprise the adult. One toddler, having heard the label *windmill* given to a large, shingled, grain-grinding windmill, went on to apply it to a rambling, shingled house, a water-storage tank, a television antenna, and a small, skeletal, water-pumping windmill.

As we have said, children from an early age accurately differentiate the sexes, but on the basis of hairdo and clothing rather than anatomy. Even a five-year-old, looking at a photograph of a naked girl with a short haircut, may identify it as of a boy. By the same token, a boy seen in a television story set early in the century, when it was common for boys to wear their hair in a bob, may be misidentified as a girl, no matter how boyish his name or speech and manner and clothing—many children, unbeknownst to their parents, take it for granted that Christopher Robin is a girl. We have the account of a four-year-old girl reporting that a new family had moved in across the way, and that the newcomers had a baby.

Asked whether the baby was a boy or a girl, she replied, "I don't know. It's so hard to tell at that age, especially with their clothes off."

Sometimes the preschool child compensates for his linguistic deficiencies by stretching known terms to fit new situations—we have seen this at work in the use of *strong* and *heavy* (see page 238)—or by inventing new terms. A three-year-old girl hoped that the new baby would be "a boy-girl. You know, a girl with a penis." Children may invent antonyms to describe a contrast: "It has an upper part and a downer part"; "They're sure not slowpokes, they're fastpokes!"; "Sometimes nobody eats with me, and sometimes lots-of-bodies." Having spotted a berry and then being unable to find it again, a four-year-old remarks that he "must have undiscovered it." For some preschool children the very reasonable opposite of *O.K.* is *Nokay.* Observe that such drawing of contrasts comes well in advance of being able to learn to supply antonyms on demand, which typically appears at age seven but is found in bright children at age five or six.[6] A precocious boy, not quite four, observed a Jules Feiffer cartoon consisting of a series of profiles of the face only and accompanying text and asked, "What does this say?" Before his parents could reply he gave his own answer, "It says, 'If there aren't any heads, make them as good as you can,'" and then took a pencil and filled in the missing parts of the profiles. It appears that this obscure-sounding utterance was meant to say two things: "Those drawings look like the exercises in my older sister's school books," and "The task is to complete the drawings."

Preschool children come up with such inventions as the assertion of good behavior, "I am so being hāve" (we are reminded of a notice on a gate: "Be ware of dog"). In general, the verb *to be* has a dual existence for many preschool children, a duality formalized in some languages, including the Scandinavian. When describing an action, the child says, "He bēs quiet"; but to describe a state or attribute, he says, "He is sad." Some inventions are downright poetic: "Rounder is wider than longer"; "You don't look like you are"; one little girl liked to "secret around in the night"; held up in traffic, a boy complained to his mother, "Look at that old truck busying up the street so we can't get through." Sometimes the emotional meanings of a term dominate the strict semantic ones; for instance, one child climaxed a torrent of spluttering invective with ". . . you—you—you wrong number!" In spite of the metaphorical quality of these formulations, children of this age cannot grasp metaphors and other figures of speech, just as they miss irony and sarcasm (although they can certainly detect emotional tones of voice and expressions of feigned emotion). Analogies, however, may occur to the child, as when a four-year-old watching a cow being milked commented, "It's like a water pistol," or when a three-year-old girl, watching her mother hold some garment against Father's body to see if it was the right size, asked, "Is Daddy a paper doll?" Alice, age four and a half, produced this joyous combination of words and sounds, worthy of Lewis Carroll himself:

> "There's nothing true about that so don't be so glee." "I'm not full of glue, I'm just appearing to." Thumbly, thumbly, glantering damously. Clitter clatter, sing the clitter clatter and the violins some time over. . . . Sing the songs of meener, with the doors of the clitter and the marches too in the dark of the pleasantly opter.

Late in the preschool years, one finds the beginnings of philosophical wisdom, as when a four-and-a-half-year-old observes, "It doesn't matter, just the way it doesn't matter which sock your foot goes into."

Description, Narration, and Memorization. Preschool children's descriptions and narratives are rambling, loose-jointed, and circumstantial; they include endless detail, relevant or not—although they may omit key information—so that it takes a nicely attuned listener to disentangle the central theme and direction of what the child says. Beginning late in the preschool years and continuing well into the school years, we find accounts of movies or television dramas consisting of fragments linked by the all-purpose connective " 'n' then." The sequence of the narrative may correspond hardly at all with the actual sequence of events.

Young children memorize things in wholesale bunches and not in a systematic, organized way. Understanding is by no means necessary to memorization, as illustrated by the well-known hymn "Gladly the cross-eyed bear," the refrain of "Three chairs for the red, white, and blue," and the Pledge of Allegiance: ". . . to the Republic of Richard Stands . . . one naked individual. . . ." (For the benefit of readers outside the United States, the original reads "to the Republic for which it [the flag] stands" and "one nation indivisible.") Preschool children learn yard after yard of nursery rhymes, fairy tales, and advertising jingles, but they cannot paraphrase or summarize their undifferentiated knowledge. They can only recite it, and if they are interrupted in the middle of a recitation, they may find it impossible to resume where they left off, and so be obliged to go back and start all over again.

PERCEPTION

To move from language to perception, we get clues to the child's perceptual experience from his explicit verbalizations, from his concrete behavior with objects in the course of the day's occupations, and from his behavior in specially contrived test situations. The child gives voice to such discoveries as that distant objects look smaller than near ones, as shown by his ability to mask a person at a distance with his finger, or that his fears about being sucked down the bathtub drain are groundless because he is too big to fit. A five-year-old girl asks of a stained-glass window brightly lighted from behind by the setting sun, "Would it burn you if you touched it?"

We know further that some "obvious" properties of matter are by no means obvious to the preschool child. Both everyday observation and formal experiments make it clear that young children cannot reliably predict whether a cube of wood or iron will float or sink when placed in water. Once they have discovered empirically which will do which, the explanations they invoke may be wildly irrelevant, such as that things sink or float because they are dull or shiny. Nor does the child anticipate that to put an object in a full glass of water will cause an overflow. One of the best everyday indicators of the child's perceptual development is his progress in drawing, not only of people but of cars, houses, trees, and animals. His ability or inability to solve jigsaw puzzles and the way he uses blocks to build structures also give us information about how the child perceives.

Now let us look at some formal approaches to the study of perceptual development. Inhelder[7] has shown that if a young child is asked to draw a line representing the water surface in an outline drawing of a beaker, he draws it parallel to the bottom of the beaker, no matter whether the beaker is upright or tilted. Standard sensory illusions, such as the Müller-Lyer illusion, have been studied in children of various ages. The evidence from such studies with young children has been conflicting, partly, we suspect, because the magnitude judgments required are too fine or perhaps even meaningless to children of preschool age. However, Robinson[8] found that preschool children of high intelligence show the size-weight illusion (the size of an object influences our judgment of how heavy it is) and showed that two-year-olds could be taught to make weight discriminations which abolished the illusion. Stevenson and McBee[9] have found that preschool children make form discriminations more easily if the forms are solid cutouts than if they are simply printed on paper. It should be remembered that even though two-year-olds can learn the names of abstract geometric forms, it is not until age three or later that they can match cutout forms to the spaces in the form board. And even when they clearly match form to hole, they may have trouble orienting the form so that it will go into the space. Experiments by Ghent[10] and by Wohlwill and Wiener[11] have shown that four-year-olds are sensitive to the up-down orientation of abstract forms and show consistent preferences for one particular orientation of such forms. Furthermore, the preferred orientation for many forms is reversed between ages four and eight, with the change beginning around age six, perhaps, since some of the forms used resemble letters of the alphabet, in association with learning to read.

The authors have made some observations on perception in three-year-olds with a view to testing the relevance of the Gestalt laws of perceptual organization which describe the conditions under which objects and groups of objects cohere perceptually (the so-called autochthonous laws). The Gestalt psychologists assume, for example, that the chromatic kinship between adjacent hues on the solar spectrum, such as yellow and orange or orange and red, is innately given, so that the child would be expected to group colors spontaneously in the order of the spectrum (red-orange-yellow-green-blue-purple, or its reverse). Three-year-olds do not, and neither, surprisingly enough, do many educated adults. Another perceptual task is to trace a looping line. Most three-year-olds do not follow the line across its intersections with itself, but change direction and detour around the loop. Given the task of completing a geometric figure, such as a square or triangle, with a corner missing, children up to age five do not supply a corner but instead draw a single line joining the ends of the break. If one substitutes pictorial equivalents for the abstract forms, the results are the same.[12] Given the task of coloring a cross composed of one oblong overlapping another, some three-year-olds disregard the lines that separate the two oblongs and color the cross as a single mass. Those who do see the division apparently do not see the partially masked oblong as continuing out of sight behind the uninterrupted one, since they are as likely as not to color the two exposed ends different hues, as though they were unrelated shapes.

We still do not know as much as we should about the genesis of the child's perception of still pictures. Since pictures are a major medium of communication and education in our society, it is important as well as interesting to know what aspects of pictures the child responds to and how he makes sense out of them. We know that picture recognition begins in late infancy, and that toddlers recognize pictures of things and of particular people, and gross pictured emotions such as happiness and sadness. We have not been able to find out whether toddlers recognize real things, such as animals in the zoo, on the basis of having previously seen pictures of them. Toddlers can recognize pictures of familiar objects, like a horse or a particular make of car, taken from an unfamiliar angle, such as looking down from above. A study by Hunton[13] indicates that children may at first be indifferent to the inversion of pictures. Awareness of inversion may come in two stages: At first, the child may not see it as an upside-down picture of an upright object, but as an upright picture of an upside-down object.

We do not know very much about developing awareness of pictured actions, relationships among people and things, and overall themes and meanings. We do not know enough about perception of size and distance in pictures, although Wohlwill[14] has shown that children's awareness of size and distance in pictures can more easily be changed by varying the amount of information contained in the picture than can adults'. And still to be explored in the child's perception of pictures are the effects of color versus black and white, natural color versus arbitrary color, photographs versus drawings, line drawings versus chiaroscuro, naturalistic versus stylized, and so forth along all the possible dimensions of depiction.

SOCIAL AND SUBCULTURAL DIFFERENCES IN COGNITION

Responses on a number of cognitive tasks tell us both about pre-school children in general and about social class and subcultural differences. For instance, there are again significant differences in favor of middle-class children, as compared to "culturally deprived" children, on the task of completing a geometric figure with a piece missing, mentioned earlier. In addition, it appeared that some deprived children could not recognize the pictures.

Some other tasks on which middle-class four-year-olds perform significantly better than deprived children are: knowing color names, both in the passive sense of responding correctly to requests such as "Show me the *red* block" and in the active sense of being able to answer "What color is this block?" or "What color is the sky?"; copying geometric forms and block capital letters; drawing a picture of a person; "running" paper-and-pencil mazes; naming body parts; knowing sensory functions;

selecting the odd member from a set of three or five things, and verbalizing the nature of the oddity. Our investigations suggest that deprived and middle-class four-year-olds do about equally well when it comes to knowing the left and right sides of the body, dealing with such spatial relations as near and far, top and bottom, on and under, and knowing relative size terms.

Potentially useful techniques for studying age changes and cultural differences in cognition include jigsaw puzzles of appropriate levels of difficulty; describing pictured situations; and Guilford's Unusual Uses Test, mentioned earlier. Caldwell[15] and others are working to develop similar arrays of tasks, sometimes in the form of test batteries with normative data. Such efforts reflect dissatisfaction with the skimpy materials of established tests and their failure to take account of our growing knowledge of perceptual and cognitive development.

THE CONCRETE BASIS OF ABSTRACT THINKING

Most formal measures of cognitive functioning ask the child to detach himself from the personal, the emotional, and the pragmatically relevant, and to turn his attention to the abstract, logical, formal, analytical properties of things. Most of his life, however, is rooted and enacted in terms of personal relations, particularly family ones, and human behavior is the concrete prototype of all his understanding. Thus, when the child is given a formal classification test consisting of blocks that offer a number of abstract principles for grouping—color, shape, size—he may ignore all these and instead base his arrangement on the intimate, concrete scheme of his own existence and group the blocks into families, large ones being the "father" and "mother" and smaller ones the "babies." Here the child relies on the attribute of size, but size tied to emotionally important human relations. Nor should it be supposed that the child has any intellectual understanding of family organization. We have already said that he takes it for granted—equivalences, again—when he visits a strange household that all the people assembled under one roof constitute a family. A four-year-old who meets his teacher's husband is likely to ask, "Mr. Jones, are you Mrs. Jones' daddy?" and the next moment, with no sense of paradox, "Mrs. Jones, are you Mr. Jones' mommy?" A mere adult cannot really know, of course, whether the child is using *mommy* and *daddy* in the conventional sense or whether, lacking the words *husband* and *wife*, he is trying to ask something like "Are you the daddy in the family in which Mrs. Jones is the mommy?" Less ambiguous is the indignant retort of a five-year-old to the assertion that people in the same family cannot marry: "They can, too! My mommy married my daddy!"— though this involves the problem of time perspective and the virtually unimaginable time when mommy and daddy did not even know one another. (A further complication here, of course, is the possible Oedipal theme implied in many children's expressed intentions of growing up to marry the parent of the opposite sex.)

Children wrestle hard to understand the relationships implied in *grandfather, grandmother, uncle, aunt, cousin,* not to mention relatives-by-marriage, at least partly because they find it so difficult to realize that their own parents were once children. We must remember too that even the people the child knows well may not have a constant identity for him in changing circumstances. We have the case, all too poignantly familiar to nursery school teachers, of a child's failing, until prompted, to recognize his teacher one weekend when he met her on the street; the following Monday, after some deep and puzzled thought, he approached her and asked, "What's your name with your hat on?" This is only one instance of a general phenomenon known to adults: We may fail to recognize the corner storekeeper or policeman when we see him away from his familiar setting and wearing an unaccustomed costume.

Older preschool children are somewhat better able to detach their thinking from personal and affective considerations and to deal with the objective properties of things. In a classification test of the kind just mentioned, the five-year-old can sort blocks on the basis of such attributes as size, color, and shape—although he may not be able to make explicit what he is doing—but he cannot use these attributes consistently and systematically. Thus, he may produce groupings of the kind called a *cluster,* in which one key block serves as the point of reference, the other blocks being related to it in terms of some point of resemblance, but without any regard for how they may be related to each other. For example, if the key block, A, is a large red triangle, then block B may be attached to it on the basis of triangularity, C on the basis of redness, and D because it is big.

Another kind of grouping intermediate between the family and the formal is the *chain,* in which each successive block is related to the one that went before, but without regard to the overall organization. Thus, B goes with A because they are both squares, C with B because they are both blue, D with C because they are both small, and so forth. The available research findings are ambiguous about whether the child will prefer form or color or size as a basis on which to pair stimuli, and about age changes in such preferences. The ambiguity may be produced by group differences, individual differences, intraindividual differences, differences among test stimuli, and differences in instructions. Only research which controls all these sources of variance—and perhaps others—can answer this question. Our findings with respect to the ability to select the odd block from a set of three, tested with middle-class three- and four-year-olds and deprived four-year-olds, suggest that color is an easier basis of discrimination than size or shape, but this is by no means conclusive. Inhelder and Piaget[16] report that their subjects rarely attempted any sort of classification before age five, instead using the blocks to make designs ("graphic collections"); the first attempts at classification used shifting criteria, like the chain arrangements mentioned above.

CAUSATION

We have already touched briefly on some central areas of cognitive organization, such as time, space, and causation. It is now appropriate to look at each of these more closely. We have pointed out that young children do not inquire closely into causation, but seem to accept cause and effect as given—obviously, children may be angered or amused by departures from expectation. The child asks about motives—for what reason?—but not about processes—by what means did this come to pass? To turn on a television set and watch the screen light up into a segment of life complete with sound effects, to hold a piece of ice in one's hand and watch it melt, to trust a knife to the support of a magnetic holder, to follow the budding of a flower, these are not effects in the realm of physics or biochemistry but simply how things are.

According to Piaget, the child's first perception of causal relations is *animistic:* Things are seen to move, act, and react in terms of their own built-in thoughts, feelings, purposes, volition, moral judgment, and power of spontaneous movement and change. It seems clear, from the love and care that the child can shower on dolls or stuffed animals, the worry or compassion he can feel for a broken plaything, and the anger he can show toward some inanimate thing that will not do his bidding, that the child often perceives things animistically.

A number of anthropologists have questioned whether animism is a universal of childhood or whether it appears in Western societies as a result of adult tutelage. It seems clear that we do much to make animism explicit, whereas in other societies animism as such remains at the implicit level of the dynamism we spoke of earlier (page 101). Older children, and even college students,[17] often are willing to say that they think of things like fire or the moon as being alive. Every society we know of has a mystique of certain inanimate things like fire, the moon, the sea, the wind, and nature in general. Thus, it is less important to know whether animism as such is a universal than to understand the dynamism and magicalism resident in universal human experience. The child's animism—in our society—is unstable: He shifts back and forth between an affect-charged animistic orientation and a materialistic and pragmatic one, just as he does with respect to reality and fantasy. A doll may at one moment be an animate, sentient participant in his play, only to be indifferently tossed aside, lifeless and inert, a moment later. Stuart conveys something of the animistic outlook when he speaks of "discouraged songs" and "tired songs" and "happy houses," when he asks what it feels like to be a stick of wood, whether it hurts the ground to have holes dug in it, and when he tells how the hands of his clock move in response to changes in his activities.

According to Piaget, animism is succeeded in the child's perceiving and thinking by *artificialism,* the assumption that all events are to be explained by the action of some humanlike agent or entity or force which wills things to happen in fulfillment of some purpose of its own. Thus, the child's early causal questions—the animistic attitude does not lead to questions—are likely to ask about personal agents and motives or reasons: "Who did it?" "For what reason?" "Why that way?" For example, a child seeing the ground blanketed with pine needles asked, "Why did they put these here?" making quite clear the assumption of a conscious, purposive agency. In general, as we have said, children perceive purpose and meaning in everything and find it hard to view occurrences in terms of accident, coincidence, or the action of material, impersonal forces. But let us note that adult society does little to convey a naturalistic view of the world to the child. A few advanced nursery schools introduce the child to science, but most of what we explicitly or implicitly tell the child is couched in the language of dynamism, artificialism, and moralism.

If dynamism is the basic mode of perception, so that we naïvely experience space and the objects that occupy it as held together and activated by a nameless general energy, we can understand how perceptual development consists of the progressive differentiation of objects, attributes, and relationships, and their integrative schematization according to various principles which may or may not be articulated and which may or may not correspond to the realities. The role of language in perceptual development then becomes that of a device which focuses attention on this or that aspect of the world, differentiating it and integrating differentiated features. It is the dynamistic substructure of perception that allows the child to accept the world's marvels without surprise or wonder or any seeking for detailed, systematic explanations. It may be dynamism that makes us mistake contiguity for causation: A boy struck a utility pole with a stick at the exact moment of a power failure, and was thoroughly and guiltily convinced that he had blacked out the city. Many scientific principles are simply articulated and quantified dynamisms. We can sum up the action of gravity in a formula, we can state Newton's laws of motion, we can describe the release of nuclear energy, the replication of a DNA molecule, phosphorescence, and so forth, but the exact causes of these events elude us. This may be why, of course, people find mechanistic explanations appealing, since the pushes and pulls and frictions of mechanical systems are so easy to comprehend.

The Belgian psychologist Michotte[18] has constructed an apparatus for studying the perception of causality. Two squares of different colors are set in motion relative to each other (the "squares" are in fact the exposed portions of solid lines traced on a revolving disk), and by varying the temporal relations between the movement of the squares, one can produce the impression that one square is acting on the other in various ways. One can produce such effects as *launching*, where one square sets the other in motion the way a golf club does a ball; *triggering*, where one square seems to release a power of autonomous motion in the other, as though it had tripped a switch; and *carrying*, as though one square were pulling or pushing the other, so that one square seems to be moving actively and the other passively.

To the best of our knowledge, Michotte's techniques have never been used with preschool children, but Olum[19] has used them to study causal perception in seven-year-olds and finds two main effects never reported by adults. She describes these as *mutual approach*, where the stationary member of the pair is seen as moving to meet the other, and *passing*, where the moving square is seen as going behind or in front of the stationary one, even though such a passing never in fact takes place. It would be interesting to take such observations down to still earlier ages, although we can foresee some difficulties in getting younger children to make intelligible reports. In the same area, we might mention in passing Heider and Simmel's film[20] of "apparent behavior," which shows geometric shapes in motion in a way that conveys almost inescapably an impression of purposes, attitudes, and emotions. Again, as far as we know, no one has yet studied young children's reactions to this film.

It is apparent that the preschool child is in transition toward the more stable, orderly world of adulthood. It is obvious that a predominantly dynamistic outlook permits the creation of the phantoms and hobgoblins that befuddle serious, rational thinking about human affairs and social problems, and so must be outgrown. It is likewise obvious that adults never fully grow out of the magical world of childhood. The authors like to think that this is as it should be. Most of our verbal play requires that we be able to straddle the worlds of magic and reality, as the child is beginning to do when he deliberately toys with the idea of growing up in reverse, starting as an adult and becoming a baby, and even when he collaborates in the prefabricated fantasies of an animated cartoon. For the adult, music and art and literature and love, and even science and mathematics, have no meaning without magic. Without magic, we are cut off from our roots in universal human experience and wander forever homeless.

TIME

Time is a dimension in cause and effect, but more generally it provides one of the frameworks within which we orient and organize and coordinate our lives. We regulate our behavior according to clocks and calendars and schedules, we remember and anticipate and plan. But we also have a personal time which is only partially correlated with formal time schemes, as when time drags or flies, when we feel leisurely or under pressure, or when we feel that we are losing time, wasting time, saving time, or using time wisely. Personal time is closely related to our sense of our own mortality, and we have already mentioned how having a sense of a goal or direction is an intimate part of our self-awareness. In our experience of personal time, we dream of time machines, fountains of youth (and estrogen treatment during and after menopause may indeed offer women a fountain of youth), getting a fresh start, perpetual motion machines (again, solar batteries and radioactivity-powered machines give us a fair approximation), and eternal bliss or damnation in an afterlife. We try to capture time in such images as Old Father Time, the Grim Reaper, and relentlessly flowing rivers.

We must remember that our familiar ways of partitioning and ordering the passage of time, no matter how logically self-evident they seem to us, are not the only possible ones. The Balinese, for instance, have, or had a few years ago, ". . . a complex cyclical system of days, grouped into concurrent weeks. . . . And of these weeks they have a complete series from a two-day week to a ten-day week."[21] Unless a Balinese knows where he stands with respect to all these weeks at any given moment, he feels badly disoriented, just as we do when we suddenly discover that today is actually Thursday whereas we have been acting as though it were Friday. Unlike us, the Balinese have little regard for keeping track of elapsed time. They know precisely when, in terms of their several calendars, a child's birthday falls, but they are not likely to know, or care, exactly how old he is. (Needless to say, they know what general age period a child is in, that it is time he was weaned, or that it is no longer appropriate to carry him, or that he is old enough to run with the other children, or that he is about ready for the transition to adulthood, but these are not tied to particular chronological ages.)

There are pronounced cultural differences in the value assigned to time. In our highly scheduled society, punctuality and regularity are esteemed. In other societies, though, an appointment is kept only if the parties thereto are so inclined, work patterns are casual and impulsive, and the spirit of leave-it-to-the-morrow prevails. As E. T. Hall[22] has pointed out, attitudes to time may reflect status relationships, as in who is allowed to keep whom waiting, and for how long. Obviously, in such settings, children's time concepts and the role of these in their thinking will be different from those found in our society. Even when non-European peoples adopt the European time scheme, they are likely to modify it in unexpected ways. For instance, we have a calendar from India in which the horizontal rows consist not of weeks but of fortnights, and it requires a conceptual wrench to be able to use such an arrangement. We must also note that our system of seasons assumes the changes that take place in the earth's temperate zones, whereas in the tropics or the frigid regions people may get along very well with no seasons or only two. The tenacity of cultural time orientations is illustrated by the Australians, who celebrate Christmas in the full heat of the summer with a traditional heavy meal of goose or turkey. Even well-educated people may have a conception of historical time in which eras and events and personalities are hopelessly jumbled, in which Napoleon may trade remarks with Charlemagne on the eve of the Battle of Hastings.

The young child, who has no knowledge of history, whose clearly remembered past can be measured in hours, and whose future is a vague abstraction he has to accept on the word of adults, may understandably have some difficulty coming to terms with the formal time schemes of his society. Even when he has learned some key words, these may not yet have their conventional meanings. One four-year-old insisted, for instance, "It is not today! My mommy said it was Monday!" An understanding of the sequence yesterday-today-tomorrow may be delayed until the school years, although we know of one preschool child who announced to her dumbfounded parents, "Today is yesterday's tomorrow." Most four-year-olds, as we see in their play patterns, are very much creatures of the moment, whereas by age five, many children can engage in planned projects extending over many days.

As we said in connection with the child's self-awareness, many preschool children are entranced to learn of their own unremembered past and beg their parents to tell them about "when I was little." Let us point out that, in our view, past eras in one's own development are lost to memory not because they are repressed, but because they are assimilated and submerged in new organizations of knowledge of one's self and world, such that we become new people capable of recapturing former modes of being only in special circumstances—dreams, hypnosis, or in response to associative cues, whether the taste or odor of some bygone substance (witness Marcel Proust), an old photograph or letter, a visit to the haunts of our childhood, or the rediscovery of a once-cherished plaything (witness the powerful film "Citizen Kane"). Which is one reason people write and read books about child psychology.

Children, as we have said, have a hard time conceiving of their parents' ever having been little, and seem to entertain two quite paradoxical notions about their parents' past. On the one hand, the parental past seems to reach into prehistory, as implied in the often-heard request, "Tell me how it was in the olden days," as though the parents had known dragons and giants. On the other hand, children find it hard to accept that the world was ever essentially different from the way it is now, and listen incredulously when a parent says that he or she remembers the introduction of the jet airplane, commercial television, transistor radios, and the picture window, or, to go a little further back, zippers, cellophane, and commercial radio. A statement by one four-year-old suggests that he planned to grow up backward in time so as to join those who were already mature: "Pretty soon this will be the olden days and I'll be a man." Numerous children, as we have said, expect to catch up with their parents and marry them.

The preschool child is far more aware of his own growth than of changes in adults, if only because parents celebrate the child's alterations in size and competence, while trying their best to ignore or conceal their own changes. Just as his parents' lives stretch endlessly into the past, so do they promise to extend changelessly into the future, even though the child may know, but without much conviction, that his parents will someday be *very* old. It follows, then, that catching up is possible. Disillusionment on this score came to Stuart as early as age five, and we are fortunate to have a record of the very moment when he first realized that time is the same for everybody:

> It would be funny if I was big and you were little. I wouldn't pay any attention to you and I'd make you do things you didn't like to. [*Here Stuart is playing a favorite game of the preschool years, reversing the roles of child and adult, and, in the process, giving us yet one more glimpse of how grownups may appear to preschool children.*] But I guess I won't ever be able to do that to you 'cause I won't ever be able to catch up to you. I won't ever be able to be the same as you at the same time.

Closely tied in with the child's awareness of time in relation to growth and change is, of course, his awareness of his own and his parents' mortality, again perhaps tempered by a sense of immortality.

SPACE

Our civilization's ways of organizing space—at least on a terrestrial scale—are quite simple, even though some people have trouble with geometry or road maps. For large segments of territory, we use compass bearings and coordinates of latitude and longitude—bearing in mind that the impossibility of mapping a spherical surface on a flat plane, together with habits of thought left over from the days when surface travel was the norm, may leave us with outmoded forms of spatial thinking: It is difficult for many people to grasp that the shortest route east or west may in actuality be north or south, over the poles. For shorter distances, we are used to dealing in routes, the particular pathways, cues, and landmarks ("Bear left at the broken-down stone church"), and the behavior involved in getting from one place to another. In dealing with concretely perceived space (as contrasted with space that unreels a bit at a time as we navigate through it), we have a vocabulary of adjectives (high, low, outer, inner), adverbs (here, there, where), and prepositions (on, under, around, behind). Such indicators are tied to the pull of the earth, to the polarities of our bodies, and relations among things and locations. Some spatial relations, like up-down, are fixed (until we take off into interplanetary travel), while others, after the manner of first- and second-person pronouns, may be tied to the standpoint of the observer—if two people are facing each other, what is left for one person is right for the other, and what is in front of one person may be partly behind the other.

Simple and obvious though these notions seem, other societies may organize space quite differently and assign different values to spatial relations. The Balinese is as strictly oriented to space as to time, and cannot act without knowing how he is facing with respect to the cardinal directions and such key reference points as temple and graveyard and, within the home, kitchen and latrine. To sleep, one must align oneself just so. In Bali, as in most island cultures, a key organizing principle is the dimension of inland-seaward. Around the periphery of the island, directions refer to settlements or distinctive terrain features, so that the reference points change as one moves. The Eskimos of eastern Canada, who live in a world of ever-changing landmarks, navigate over long distances seemingly on the basis of a few stable terrain features and also on the basis of wind directions and temperatures, and perhaps even qualities of humidity and the smells characteristic of particular regions.[23] Needless to say, non-European cultures provide versions quite different from our own of what the earth as a whole is like.

We have already seen how, in infancy and toddlerhood, spatial relations are linked to the baby's own actions and migrations, with only a beginning notion of how things and places are related to each other. The preschool child develops a considerable vocabulary of concrete spatial relations, but he moves slowly away from an orientation in what we call *action-space* toward a more organized *map-space*. Maier[24] performed a classical experiment in which children learned all the particular routes within a swastika-shaped maze and then were tested for their grasp of the layout of the maze as a whole. It was not until the late preschool years or early school years that children formed an inclusive "map" of the maze. We can see the contrast between the child's practical command of space and his knowledge of spatial relations at about age five when he spontaneously or on request tries to draw maps of familiar areas such as his own house. Figure 3 is a map by a five-year-old, together with the actual floor plan, of a house in which he had lived just over a year.

Beyond map-space lies *abstract space* of the kind involved in geometries of two and more dimensions. Such notions are completely closed to the preschool child, and for the most part to the school-age child, but it is interesting that many adults are perfectly able to deal with abstruse geometries without ever having mastered the rudiments of map-space. All of us know people who are "space blind," who get lost whenever they depart from familiar pathways and who find it almost impossible to find their way to a new location alone, even with the help of elaborate and specific directions. We find it curious that such people need not be handicapped in their dealings with abstract space.

In general, then, preschool children are largely tied to action-space,

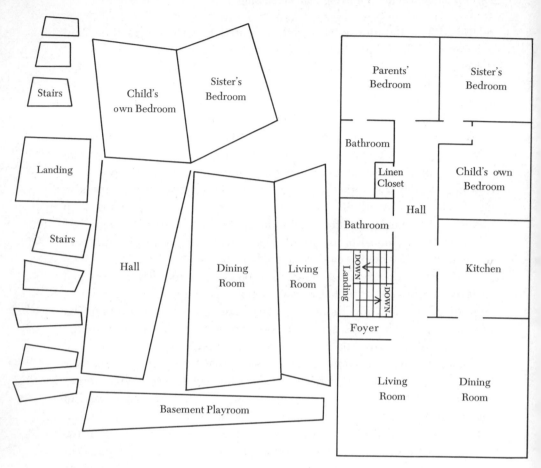

FIGURE 3. *A five-year-old's spontaneous map of the house in which he had lived a year and four months; on the right is the actual floor plan of the house. Both drawings are somewhat simplified; the child's original drawing includes the location of furniture.*

with a beginning awareness of map-space. Even so they may be able to grasp the notion of the world as round, as shown in this quotation from Stuart, at age four and a half, trying to disentangle a temporal idea which he has understood as spatial (note that the vocabularies of space and time overlap, as in *before, after,* and, in the present instance, *end*):

> Miss Williams, what is the end of the world? . . . I don't see how it is a *place,* because my mommy says the world is round, and so there could not be any end where the world stops, or where you could

fall off. It goes around, and then when you get to where you start, it goes round again.

As Stuart himself added, the problem again boils down partly to making sense of adult vocabularies: "I wish the grownups would say the same thing so I could know."

In this section, we have been talking about three-dimensional space, the space in which material beings exist and move and exert causal action. Earlier, in talking about perceptual organization, we touched upon problems in two-dimensional space, perceiving meanings and relations in designs traced on a flat surface. Note that the experimental psychology of perception has dealt almost exclusively with the perception of two-dimensional arrays, as though such perception were basic. In fact, however, it is three-dimensional perception which is fundamental, with the ability to comprehend two-dimensional patterns coming later, and sometimes not at all. A study by Hochberg and Brooks,[25] using a single subject who was not exposed to pictures for the first two years of life, sought to demonstrate that pictorial perception was as "natural" as the perception of voluminous space. Unfortunately—from a scientific standpoint, not the individual child's—there seems to have been no attempt to shield the child from all the other two-dimensional patterns that are commonly found in middle-class settings—wallpaper, fabrics, book covers, and so forth.

The behavior of culturally deprived children seems to suggest that they find little meaning in two-dimensional patterns, such as pictures. It is not that the children cannot see such patterns, but that they fail to perceive the message they contain. It is our belief, subject to further empirical study, that it requires practice to see the meanings and the spatial relations in two-dimensional representations and designs. This is not an abstract theoretical argument, but one that has serious implications for understanding the effects of cultural deprivation and what one has to do to counteract such effects.

Notice, too, that ideas of size and quantity can be viewed as special cases of spatial extent and organization, whereas ordinal numbers—first, second, last—can refer to temporal organization, spatial organization, or simultaneously both, as when children line up in the order in which they will have a turn at pinning the tail on the donkey, or when turns in a table game are dictated by the clockwise spatial disposition of the players. But measurement, expressing size and weight and duration and velocity in terms of conventional standards, is beyond the preschool child. The child says that something is very heavy or very light, or that something is going very fast, but pounds and miles per hour—and dollars and cents—are not part of his cognitive repertory.

A School for the Preschool Child

The idea of providing for the daytime care of children too old to be treated as babies but too young to be admitted to regular schools had diverse origins. Many of the first preschools and day care centers were inspired by considerations of social welfare, to take poor children out of the slums and off the streets, to shelter them, warm them, feed them, and keep them constructively occupied. Maria Montessori, who founded a whole movement in education, wanted to go further and salvage the intellectual abilities of poor children; ironically enough, in the United States, until the last few years it was primarily a few children of affluent parents who were taught by the Montessori method. American nursery schools, by and large, have developed in a different tradition, that of Harriet Johnson, Lucy Sprague Mitchell, Katherine Read, and others, and have grown independently of the more formally organized, less child-development-oriented public-school kindergarten movement. Nursery-school education was given a major thrust by the Head Start program, beginning in 1965, and seems well on its way to becoming an accepted part of public education. Since the spirit of the nursery-school tradition is quite different from that prevailing in public schools, the assimilation is not likely to be easy.

In their earlier, more specialized versions, nursery schools have taken on a variety of shapes. Some, more or less in the naturalistic tradition of Jean-Jacques Rousseau, have viewed preschool education as a vehicle of social reform, whereby children's natural virtue was to be let flower uncorrupted by the values of adult culture. In urban settings and in a context of small, nuclear families, many educators have seen in the preschool a chance to give the child access to space, time, and things offered in an earlier day in rural life and the extended family. Other nursery schools seem to have had as their chief goal to provide a pool of subjects for psychological research. Many nursery schools and day care centers have existed chiefly as baby-sitting services or parking lots so that mothers would be free to work or to spend their time otherwise than in child care. In general, facilities for preschool children have catered either to the poor or the well-to-do, but rarely both together. The parent-cooperative nursery school, however, is largely a middle-class phenomenon. Indeed, in the big cities and in prosperous suburbs, certain nursery schools are seen as training grounds for the better colleges, and competition to get one's child entered is as keen as for admission to the more prestigeful institutions of higher learning—and parents whose child has been turned away may feel that he is handicapped for life.

In recent years, for both rich and poor children, the preschool has often become a place for early coaching in intellectual skills in preparation for the formal schooling to follow. It is our opinion that much of the intellectual force-feeding and pressure to early reading that goes on in certain nursery schools today is irrelevant, poorly managed, and potentially a menace to sound intellectual development. At the same time, these new rigidities have their counterparts in traditional ways of thinking about preschool children. All too often nursery-school educators, in the interest of protecting children against forcing, may underestimate the intellectual capabilities of a young child and block him from learning things within his capacities but outside the accustomed province of the preschool. The resistance of some preschool educators is epitomized in the cry that one can never—or must never—teach a four-year-old to read, ignoring the ones who do read. Such teaching, it is sometimes seriously claimed, may wreck the child's nervous system, or turn him into a bookworm who neglects social participation and physical exercise, or, *horribile dictu,* destroy the traditional curriculum of the early school grades, as though these represent the organically right sort of education for all children. Such views are founded on the assumption of biologically fixed and universal timetables for the maturation of learning abilities, an assumption which is at best very fragile, and leads to the equally untenable view that everyone who has not learned to read by the age of seven is some sort of lost soul. Moreover, it seems to overlook the distinction between forcing formal learning and permitting and encouraging genuine curiosity and discovery.

We take the stand that nursery schools and kindergartens should foster all aspects of development, including intellectual development, without forcing and with full sensitivity to each child's interests and status. We further believe that, for most preschool children, formal learning should proceed from the child's concrete transactions with people, other living creatures, things, and materials, and should be taught as occasions offer rather than as organized group "lessons." At the same time, a good teacher can make sure that some occasions for learning come to pass, by sound planning, shrewd choice of materials and activities, and alertness to the child's reactions. Ordinarily, we think of preschools in terms of the way they serve the educational needs of children, but a good preschool also maintains close liaison with parents and can serve as a valuable source of parental education. It is often possible, too, for parents to participate directly in the classroom work of the school.

THE RAW MATERIALS OF A PRESCHOOL

We will not linger over the need for a preschool to have a sound, safe building with furnishings and equipment scaled to the children's size and proportions—adults visiting a nursery school for the first time may have the sensation of entering a Lilliputian universe where everything,

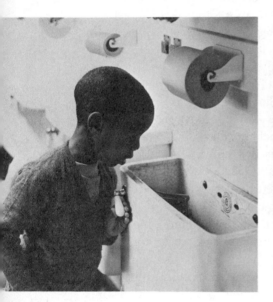

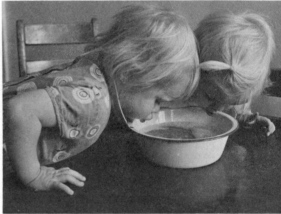

A Lilliputian universe where everything, including washbasins and toilets, is in miniature —with areas set aside for domestic play, for music, for water play, for painting, for table top activities, for block building, for carpentry, and so forth . . .

(Left) Dorothy Levens; (above) *Children in Community*; (below) Dorothy Levens; (above right) STARTING NURSERY SCHOOL/Vassar Film; (below right) Dorothy Levens; (below, far right) Irene Bayer/Monkmeyer

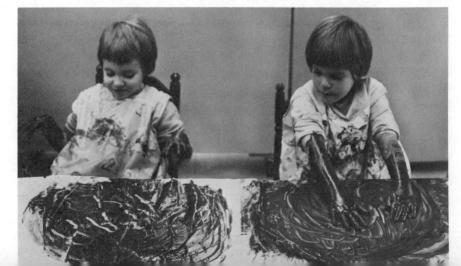

including washbasins and toilets, is in miniature—with areas set aside for domestic play, for music, for water play, for painting, for table top activities, for block building, for carpentry, and so forth; and to have protected play yards with a proper complement of swings, slides, jungle gyms and other climbing apparatus, pits to dig in, wagons, tricycles, large hollow blocks, boxes, and all the rest. Sometimes indoor space for climbing, jumping, and tumbling can also be provided. These are important, but their importance lies in their contribution to the school's more general educational functions of meeting needs and providing scope for

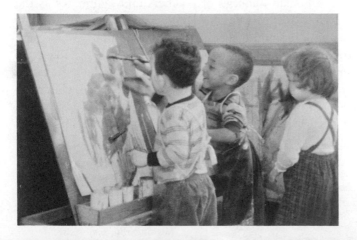

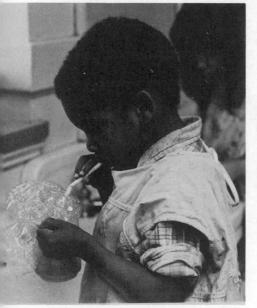

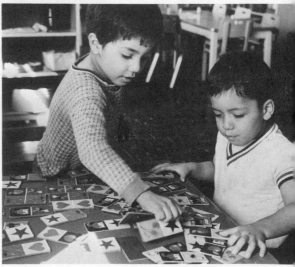

emotional, social, and cognitive development. (We should also point out that when children move out of the family and into the larger world of school, whether at age two or age seven, they encounter a whole array of unaccustomed bacteria and viruses, and the more vulnerable may have bouts of sickness, although, in the long run, they develop solid immunities.)

First on our list of basic ingredients come space and time, free space and free time to move about in freely, but also articulated space and time to provide a stable yet variable framework which gives the child a sense of order and organization.

Second come the human qualities of teachers and age mates as the child works his way into a broader pattern of social relations. It seems to us desirable to mix children and teachers of diverse cultural, ethnic, and economic backgrounds, so that they can learn from each other about the varieties of the human condition. It also seems desirable to include, as the opportunity presents itself, some proportion of handicapped children—those with motor or with sensory disabilities like impaired vision and hearing—for their own sake and for the sake of the physically normal children who may thus learn early to accept the handicapped as fellow

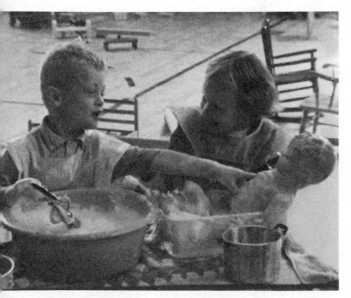

"She's blowing a bubble!" A basic form of learning comes from the exploration of qualities and raw materials.
Organizing Free Play/OEO Film

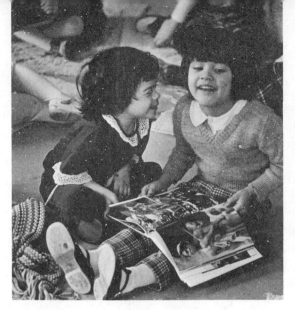

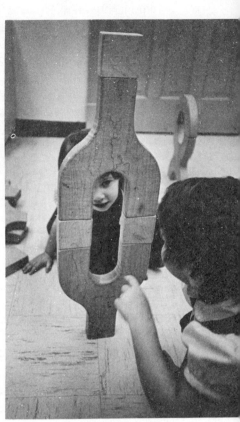

Learning materials: blocks, . . . props for dramatic play, a wide array of books, pictures, charts, and science materials.

(Top and right) Myron Papiz; (left below) Burke Uzzle; (below) Bettye Caldwell

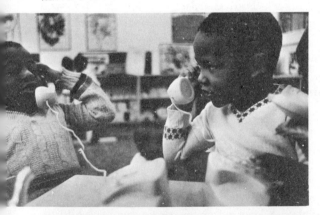

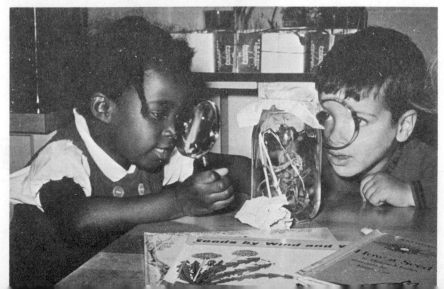

human beings. There is evidence, as from a recent study by Chesler,[26] that the handicapped constitute a minority group against which the majority is prejudiced. However, lack of prejudice is not an automatic consequence of early exposure; careful explanations are needed, and active intermixing of the children to help the normal child overcome any spontaneous distaste and also any vulnerabilities that get stirred up by the sight of abnormalities. Obviously, children with major impairments need extra care and attention, and a school should be staffed accordingly.

Third come learning materials: play equipment, blocks, plastic materials (paint, water, clay, dough, lumber, cooking ingredients, and so forth, and all the tools, utensils, and instruments that go with them); props and dolls and figurines for dramatic play, especially on domestic themes, and clothes and accessories for dressing up; a wide array of books and pictures and charts; Montessori-like "educational" playthings such as puzzles, picture lotto, mosaic design kits, and science materials like magnets and dry-cell batteries; musical equipment ranging from percussion blocks through melodic instruments like xylophones, autoharps, and pianos to record players and records; pet animals (birds and fowl, fish, frogs, guinea pigs, rabbits, turtles, and, in season, tadpoles); the foods and beverages served at lunch and snack time (too often, in our preoccupation with vision, hearing, touch, and kinesthetic experience, we neglect the cultivation of taste and smell); and the resources of the actual community—visits to farms, factories, stores, firehouses, railroad stations and airports, docks, woods, brooks, and lakes.

Fourth and finally, and involved in all that we have been saying, is language, the formulation and elaboration of experience in words and numbers which become a part of the child's working equipment for understanding and ordering events and in logical and imaginative thinking. In programs for deprived children, the emphasis on symbolic formulations has to loom proportionately larger than in programs for children from rich verbal environments. Two sharply contrasting approaches to linguistic enrichment can be found in the work of Minuchin and Biber, on the one hand, and Bereiter and Engelmann, on the other.[27]

These resources are not used singly or haphazardly, but are woven into a curriculum. But before we go on to discuss their organized patterning, let us look more closely at their individual importance. In its use of free time and space, the preschool gives children an all too rare scope to wander and explore, to follow their own thoughts through, whether in conversation or alone, to be aware and to be made aware of changing vistas and the changing lights of days and seasons, to watch events unfold and to follow them from origin to conclusion. Needless to say, freedom of space in a preschool is always freedom within limits: The yards are stoutly fenced, gates and doors and windows have child-proof latches, stairways are protected, there are things to climb but they are not sky-high—although they may well seem so to a 3-foot-child. Too free a space, apart from exposing children to physical dangers, leaves them disoriented and anxious. Outdoors, space is structured by fences and gates, by walkways and trees and grass and dirt, by the contours of the ground, by the fixed play equipment, and by equipment sheds and playhouses. Indoors, the spatial organization of shelves, partitions, equipment, and furniture sets up fascinating mazes whose mysteries the children can unravel and wonder at. Spatial arrangements define areas for particular kinds of activities. In buildings not excessively "modern," there are corners to which a child can retire and feel snugly alone. Systematic and stable arrangements of space invite children to discover for themselves the many polarizations of space into up and down, forward and sideways and backward, over and under and around, and so on. By structuring time into dependable but unhurried schedules and routines, the preschool gives a sense of recurrences and stability and predictability.

The preschool tries to treat space and time as a city does—or should—treat its parks, leaving some areas in their wild state, trimming and formalizing others, and clearing or paving still other areas for specified purposes such as bridle trails, athletic fields, and playgrounds. However, there is one fault with our analogy. When one paves a tennis court, it is lost to nature. But when a preschool sets up a schedule, it can do so provisionally and revocably. A flexible preschool can set its schedule aside to capitalize on a mood or an idea, to take advantage of a snowfall or a large patch of ice, to witness a special event; in short, a good program leaves room for surprises and improvisation and spontaneity.

The human resources of the preschool, as we have said, include both the teachers and the other children. A good preschool needs teachers in great plenty, for it is to them that the child must shift some of his attachment to his family before he can form relations with his peers. The teacher, however, is not a substitute parent—save for occasional crises—nor is he or she (we would like to see broken the stereotype of preschool teaching as an exclusively female function) simply a warder. Dealing with children so young, the teacher must be prepared to give affection freely, but without infantilizing the child or intruding on him. The good teacher is attuned to the preschool child's vacillation between assertive

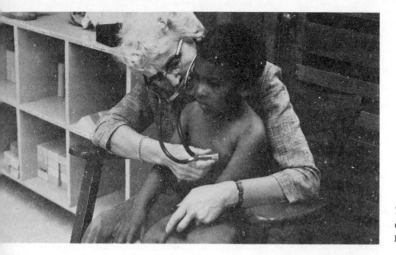

*The human resources
of the preschool.*
Dorothy Levens

*The preschool child vacillates
between assertive maturity and
clinging babyishness.*
Dorothy Levens

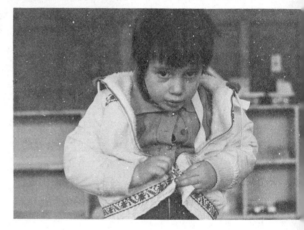

maturity and clinging babyishness, and can respond in ways that seem
suited to this child at this moment. The teacher has to perform such
maternal functions as helping the child with his clothes, with eating,
toileting (and toilet accidents), and naps. The teacher has to protect the
child from aggression by other children, from impersonal dangers, and,
sometimes, from his own impulses. The preschool child's passions, as we
said earlier, can become violent, so violent indeed as to frighten even
himself; when his passions threaten to run rampant, the teacher has to
intervene to comfort or soothe or restrain, to help the child understand
and control the forces that rage within him. And, perhaps above all, the
teacher is a source of ideas, knowledge, hypotheses, and comment, and a
model for curiosity and compassion.

The experience of cooperative nursery schools, college laboratory schools, and Head Start groups has shown that aides and students and volunteers, under the supervision of well-trained teachers, can extend and enrich a program. One reason for the success of Head Start, even when staff and facilities have been less ·than ideal, appears to be the assignment of a teacher, a paid aide, and a volunteer to each group of fifteen children. In our experience, the chief problem in the indoctrination of untrained assistants has been to help them overcome fear of the children and learn not to react moralistically and punitively to the children's childish ways.

The other children of his own age give the preschooler an introduction to social adaptation. Preschools in general have tended to group children in narrow age bands, a practice which has some virtues. It means that older children do not have to be stopped from picking on younger ones, or younger children protected from older ones. With children at his own level in size and strength, the child can safely fight out minor battles. He can try out his feelings and ideas on people who think the way he does. Among his peers, he can learn to cooperate and to share—not only material things but sympathies, antipathies, fears, interests, enthusiasms, and thoughts as well.

But, as we have said, a preschool with a mixed population teaches the child simultaneously that humankind is all one while being infinitely diverse. Thus, one can also make a case for more experimentation with grouping together children over the whole range of the preschool years, or beyond, family style, so that the older children can share their knowledge and know-how with the younger ones, and can themselves benefit by taking a protective and helping role with the little ones. (There is some reason to believe that children in certain institutions benefit from such groupings.) It is possible, of course, to combine groupings of both sorts, segregating the ages for some kinds of activities, such as outdoor play, where older and younger children need quite different equipment, and mixing them for others, such as (some) story-telling, singing, and meals.

The learning materials of the preschool can be infinitely varied. Books provide the children with vicarious emotional experience, with ideas, with experience in the possibilities of language, factual information, and opportunity to exercise creative imagination. Stories read aloud to a group provide a fine occasion for shared feelings, for getting to know each other as well as what is in the story. The skilled teacher reads so as to allow children to respond and question, to look at the pictures and chime in. With three-year-olds, reading groups should be small when possible, even two or three children; with four- and five-year-olds, larger groups are possible. Here we note an irony: The literature available to preschool children has been so superior in content, style, and quality of illustrations and design to what, until recently at least, they were likely to encounter in standard school textbooks, that for children who have been to a good nursery school entering the grades in schools which tend to limit the child's reading to those texts is an intellectual and esthetic step backward.

Listening to music, making music (however crudely), moving to music, and singing together are an essential part of preschool life. Plastic materials such as paints and clay and specially mixed and colored dough—and sticks and stones, and dirt, mud, sand, and snow—have a double importance. At first, the child likes to explore and manipulate them for their sensory qualities alone, without any thought of making anything with them. Later, he learns to shape and combine and decorate them to give solid external expression to his thoughts and feelings and perceptions.

The domestic play corner, with its dolls, toy furnishings and kitchen-ware, and a rack of men's and women's clothes for dressing up, provides the settings and materials for many of the ever-recurring themes of dramatic play. Domestic play can be given a realistic turn by letting the children take part, at their various levels of competence, in cooking

The skilled teacher reads so as to allow children to respond and question, to look at the pictures and chime in.
Organizing Free Play/OEO Film

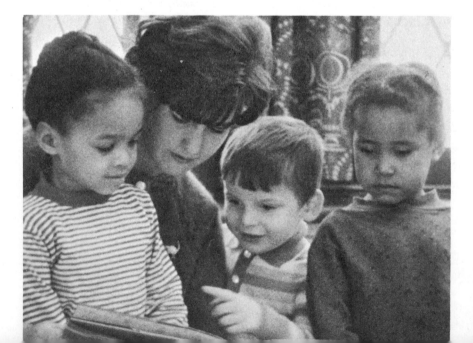

projects. The youngest children can shell peas and squeeze oranges with a fair amount of adult help and supervision. Slightly older children can make fruit gelatine and instant puddings. Still older children can try their hands at scrambled eggs, meat balls, fruit salads, cookies, and perhaps even birthday cupcakes. (We should make it clear that the nursery-school teacher has an obligation at least to go through the motions of sampling the results of the children's cooking; while it would be less than humane on some occasions to expect her to eat them, and she may resort to a promise to save them for home, usually such simple enterprises produce distinctly edible products.)

As themes drawn from the outside world begin to emerge in dra-

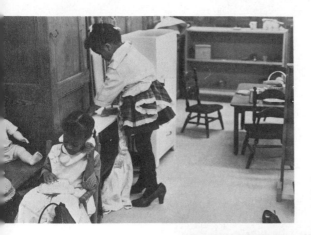

The domestic play corner provides the settings and materials for many of the ever-recurring themes of dramatic play.
Dorothy Levens

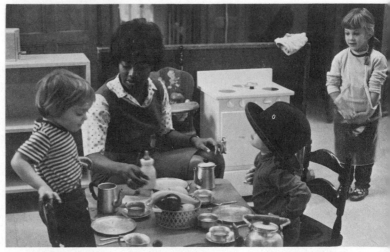

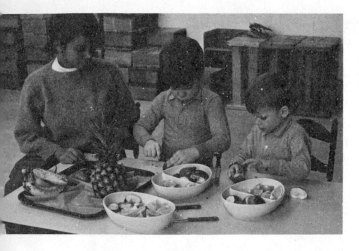

Domestic play can be given a realistic turn by letting the children take part, at their various levels of competence, in cooking projects.
Dorothy Levens

matic play, blocks and boxes and formal toys such as trucks and bulldozers, rubber animals and people, and real, functioning stethoscopes take on increasing importance as props. Animals kept in the school invite observation and curiosity; they may supply a lesson in procreation and animal maternity, if not paternity, as in the laying and hatching of eggs, or the litter of guinea pigs, and in growth and development, with chicks and tadpoles as subjects; and they can be used to teach gentleness and compassion. The use of animals seems especially important in enrichment programs for deprived children: Urban poor children seem to know animals only as vermin or as something to be feared, and to help them come to terms with a parakeet or white laboratory rat or hamster seems to give the children a whole new set of emotions. In this matter, of course the educators of nursery-school teachers may have to battle some deeply ingrained prejudices, since a great many people feel that any animal other than a dog, cat, horse, or cow is a loathsome object and find it unthinkable that anyone could pick up a horned toad or pet mouse, never mind a beetle, earthworm, or garter snake.

For a preschool in a rural or semirural setting the natural surroundings, manicured or left wild, provide spaces to traverse, things to climb and swing from, and places to run and hide and look. In addition, the leaves that fall from the trees in autumn, the squirrels busily gathering nuts and seeds, the rabbits and pheasants that leave tracks in the snow, the sap rising in the trees, and the woodchuck emerging from sleep in the spring, all are the stuff of a first venture into natural science. In spring, the children can plant their own flower and vegetable seeds and watch them grow. (Readers from very different climes will have to rework these passages.) Even in city schools, glimpses of nature are available in parks, and field trips to farms and open country can often be arranged. What city schools lack in raw nature can be compensated for by rich materials available for social sciences. If the country child can see food being grown and harvested, the city child can see it being marketed. Older preschoolers can also visit the gas station down the street, the museums of art and history and natural history, the garbage trucks, even the dynamos humming in the local power station. They can observe snow plows and pavement mending and seasonal changes of uniforms and store fronts.

Running through all the child's encounters with the living and inert materials of the preschool is the flow of words. The teacher, as interpreter, is telling the child about things, supplying names for events and objects, answering his questions and stimulating him to ask more, and the child is taking in and digesting information, asking questions, and

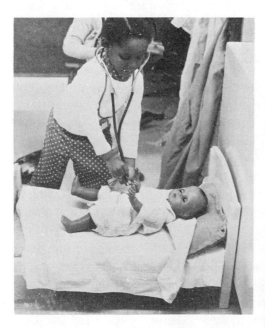

As themes drawn from the outside world begin to emerge in dramatic play, blocks and boxes and formal toys, and real, functioning stethoscopes take on increasing importance as props.
Dorothy Levins

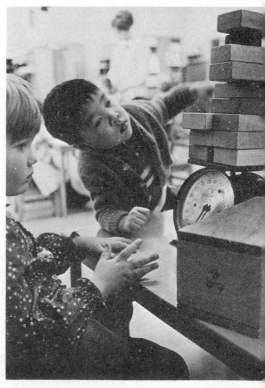

Learning formal relationships.
Myron Papiz

trying out his own formulations and hypotheses. This calls for a model of teacher behavior very different from the folded-arms bystander who merely oversees or referees. Out of the child's observations, his movements through space, his successes and failures in trying to make things happen, and out of the flow of human communication, factual, whimsical, speculative, imaginative, systematic, emotional, he begins to form ever more integrated conceptions of what reality as a whole is and how it works, and of ways of thinking about it and acting on it symbolically and concretely. The teacher's phrasing of reality is of considerable importance, both in terms of the information (and sometimes, alas, misinformation) she conveys and in terms of the attitudes and values she expresses, including prejudices and assumptions which she may not realize she holds.

CURRICULUM IN THE PRESCHOOL

The resources we have discussed are not merely made available to the child to use at odd moments, as the impulse takes him, and neither are they flung wholesale at the child with the expectation that he will pay full attention and take in and retain everything. The use of materials is planned and scheduled in keeping with the children's receptiveness and interest, in ways that provide variety both from day to day and within a given day, and in ways that promise to link separate experiences and make them part of a meaningful whole. We have to remember, in thinking about the organization of a preschool curriculum, that the child may be bursting with physical energy at one moment and with ideas the next, that he now feels sociable and now craves solitude. In general, a plan of activities tries to balance listening with talking, action with contemplation, application with relaxation, regulation with freedom, and boisterous with quiet play, and must be flexibly responsive to the situation and state of the children.

The preschool's curriculum is built around its routines, the stable sequences, known to the child and dependable, that punctuate the daily cycle: outdoor time, juice time, music time, bathroom time, story time, lunchtime, bathroom time, nap time, bathroom time, free play time (to paint, block-build, play with water, and so forth). Except for the times set aside for such biological necessities as eating, elimination, and rest, the pattern of activities can be varied from day to day.

Let us say, though, that we are of several minds about how long a preschool day can or should be. Through age four, if the child has a functioning home to go home to, we favor a morning program, dismissing children right after lunch. We see lunch as an integral part of a preschool curriculum, both for the sake of educating taste and smell and because it is often a time of easy sociability when ideas flow freely and experiences can be compared. For children on substandard diets at home, of course, lunch can be important nutritionally as well. However, the school day may have to be lengthened for the children of working mothers and for children from unfavorable home environments. The essential thing is that a long school day not be allowed to deteriorate into a daylong dreary custodial operation or one in which the children become surfeited with too many planned and organized activities, or—particularly in northern winters—a mere holding operation as the shades of night start closing in.

We also have to remember that good preschool teaching is grueling work, and too long a day will take its toll on teachers, who may have family responsibilities of their own and who certainly have to have time to attend to administrative chores. In a college or university setting, preschool teachers are often teachers of college students, too, and the preschool schedule has to allow time for teachers to meet with students. Preschool education seems to work best when parents can be involved, as welcome visitors or as participants, and time must be provided for parent conferences and for the writing of meaningful reports for parents and for the record. In general, then, the younger the child and the longer the school day, the more complicated life becomes, the more elaborate the provisions which have to be made to make such complications bearable, and the larger the available staff must be.

It is important for all education to be individualized: It seems particularly important in the preschool for teachers to be able to take account of individual needs or shifts of mood, to respond to individual queries or insights at the crucial moment, and for the child to know the benefits of sustained communication with an adult who takes him seriously. There are several ways in which a stable curriculum can be adapted to meet the individual needs of the children. Sometimes it is a good idea to divide the group among several activities. A teacher or student teacher or aide may take small groups on excursions: a walk, a visit to the school kitchen or boiler room, an outing to watch a construction project or to see the tree-trimmers at work. Seldom, of course, are all the children in a preschool class doing the same thing at the same time. Even when some whole-group activity, such as musical games, is in progress, some stalwart individualists may continue with a block-building

345

project, or ask a teacher to read a story, or blow soap bubbles in the washroom, or even sit on the sidelines, thumb in mouth.

Obviously, if nonparticipation seems to be too much the rule for a given child—because of pervasive homesickness, because he lacks interest in his fellows, or is afraid of them, or is an outcast—ways must be found to draw him into contact with the others. Operant conditioning methods, long used unlabeled by skillful teachers, have proved useful for this purpose, a favored adult "reinforcing," via expressions of affection and approval, any moves the child makes toward involvement with his peers. In most cases, once the child has begun making contact, peer relations prove to be intrinsically satisfying and adult reinforcement is no longer necessary. Sometimes it is a matter of deliberately forming small groups, including the solitary child, to read or to carry on a particular enterprise, on the grounds that it may be easier for him to form one-to-one attachments before venturing into the group as a whole, and that it may be easier for the other children to be friendly when the competition is reduced and in the context of a special and enjoyable project. This, too, is part of the curriculum.

Holidays, birthdays, or perhaps only an unusually festive spirit may call for a departure from routines. With the youngest preschool children, a minimum of planning and anticipation is possible. By age five, however, children can embark on long-range undertakings that may supersede the regular schedule. The Christmas party (now often combined with Hannukah celebrations, sometimes to the dismay of both Christian and Jewish purists), a puppet show, a play based ,on a favorite story are among the possible enterprises. Older children may initiate a sustained play project such as the building of a block city or, outdoors, a playhouse or network of canals. It is a good idea, when feasible, to let children pursue such inventions to a logical conclusion, even if it means encumbering a playroom floor area with semipermanent block structures or carving up a section of the playground with gaping trenches. A certain amount of mess and clutter is inevitable in a lively program. Field trips are also likely to interrupt routines. Such outings may be suggested by a story or by one child's experiences, or it may simply occur to the teacher that a particular trip would be especially relevant at this juncture. Field trips are valuable because they give substance to things the child may know about only verbally. Then, in discussions after the trip, the child is stimulated to further verbal elaborations. From such discussions may come ideas for still other field trips.

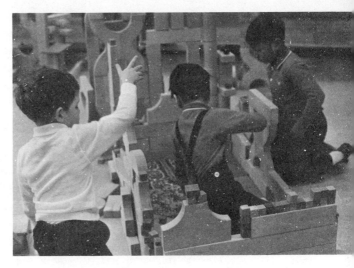

Older children may initiate a sustained play project such as the building of a block city.
Dorothy Levens

For all this flexibility, however, the basic framework of routines has to be there. It is both educational and reassuring to preschool children, who need stabilizing landmarks to which they can orient themselves. Amidst the round of activities and projects, children need relatively static periods of digestion, recapitulation, repose, and just plain enjoyment. The varied curriculum should be seen as an introductory survey of the universe, and not as a collection of lesson units that the child is supposed to retain. The value of the curriculum lies in the delight of knowing—if only for a fleeting while—that such things exist; it is in the raising of questions that the child can ask his teachers, his parents, and himself; it is in the orientation to learning and knowing and understanding as one of life's great satisfactions and as a lifelong spiritual adventure.

Premature demands that specific learning be retained may spoil the delight of learning. This does not mean that one never reminds a preschool child of something he has known and forgotten, or never encourages him to apply past learning to the solution of present problems, though with no implication or tone of voice of chiding. It does mean that one understands the value of preschool experience in the child's own terms, and in the perspective of all the long years it will take him to arrive at a mature grasp of the world he lives in. As Bruner[28] has pointed out, we can not only settle for half-learnings and half-comprehensions but value them, secure that the child will cover the same ground time after time, each time at a more sophisticated level of understanding and expertness.

347

A TEACHER FOR THE PRESCHOOL CHILD

What we have said so far implies that the preschool teacher—certainly the head teacher for each group—needs extraordinary personal and professional qualifications. It is our conviction that if we could put our very best teachers into the preschool and early grades, learning could be made functionally autonomous (that is, self-motivating and self-sustaining) so that later schooling could be organized around the library and the laboratories and the discussion table, instead of being the dreary, regimented, syllabus-bound thing it has so largely become, even at the college and increasingly at the graduate level. Pending Utopia, let us talk about what we can hope for in the teacher of preschool children. Since it is almost impossible to arrive at any objective weighting of virtues, the order in which we discuss them does not reflect an order of priority.

It is certainly important that a teacher—at whatever level—like children. As a human being, she (we yield, temporarily, to the facts of contemporary life) will not like all children equally, but she will not let the children become too aware of the fact. As in any occupation, one

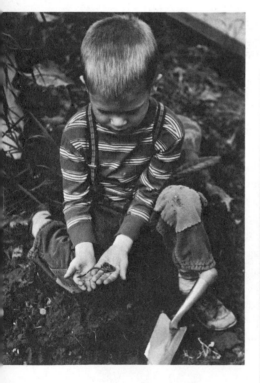

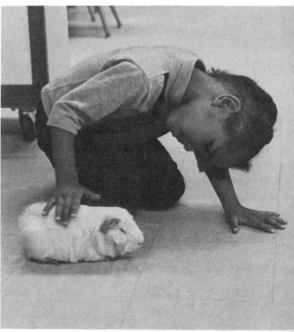

Children do not spontaneously share adult repugnance for the "lower" forms of animal life.
(Left) *Children in Community;* (below) Dorothy Levens

works best when one's job brings pleasure, and the surest way to enjoy teaching is to enjoy watching children in action. But enjoyment and effectiveness in teaching, as in parenthood, are vastly enhanced when liking for children is coupled with a thorough and differentiated understanding of how they operate. Again, though, as in parenthood, understanding does not mean that the adult relinquishes adulthood to become once more a child. It is important to be able to share the child's wonder and confusions and grief, but from a secure standpoint in adulthood where one can help the child straighten out and manage his feelings; to enjoy his growth and his discoveries and even some of his mistakes.

It marked a revolution in the education of teachers when it came to be accepted that teachers should understand the special ways of children, to facilitate communication between adult and child. But teachers also need a great fund of information about things in general. Furthermore, it should be information that they have made their own, and not merely facts and formulas parroted from textbooks. If the teacher is going to deal with the cosmic questions her pupils raise in a wide-open preschool curriculum—about God, Santa Claus, Jesus, death, and life—she must be prepared in advance. Apart from metaphysics, she will have to cope clearly and honestly with such issues as where Mommy has gone and when she will return, why people are different colors, what is a cocoon, what makes lightning, what is a fever, what happens when you flush the toilet, tell me about when I was a baby, can I look under your dress, and a host of others impossible to predict but vital to anticipate. The teacher not only conveys knowledge, but with it orientations to knowledge, that learning is exciting, or that grownups are stupid, or that the world is full of fascinating mysteries, or that curiosity is dangerous and the child had better learn to keep his ideas and questions to himself. The teacher needs to be an alert observer, but a participant observer who can interpret and clarify the child's intellectual and emotional experiences, and who capitalizes on the fortuitous occasions for learning which arise.

It is evident that the teacher needs more than intellectual qualifications. She needs physical stamina. Keeping pace with a pack of preschool children can be strenuous work, especially at those moments when they decide to scatter in all directions at top speed. Like athletes, many preschool teachers burn out early (or, as in other fields, find that the accretion of years does not bring a corresponding growth in income) and move on into administration, library work, or teaching the less mercurial children in the older grades. The teacher must be prepared, as we have said, to suppress her fears and revulsions when children hand her their beloved pet frogs, snakes, or other fauna, or pieces of them. She must be more or less shockproof, but this implies neither moral neutrality nor lack of emotion. She will have occasion to become angry, but in an adult fashion. She will inevitably be moved to delight and also to occasional laughter, but a sympathetic laughter that children can share, not a derisive or contemptuous laughter that humiliates. She will have her irritable days and her depressed days, but without imposing her moods on the children or expecting them to be especially sympathetic or considerate. Unlike a mother, the preschool teacher as a general rule has to subordinate her feelings and needs to the children's. Even while a preschool is helping its pupils mature, it remains more child-centered than any home could healthily be.

It would seem, in sum, that the central qualification of a preschool teacher is maturity, but a special form of maturity responsive to childhood and its magic. The preschool teacher can react appropriately to both sides of the growth ambivalence expressed by Stuart:

> Being big is the best, best thing, isn't it? . . . But sometimes I wish I didn't have to grow big. *NOW!* That's why you must take care of me and we will pretend I'm a little baby and have a long time to wait till I grow big.

Intelligence, Intelligence Tests, Intellectual Differences, and Intellectual Development

Now, when the child has moved out of the natural environment of the family into the seminatural habitat of the preschool and is on the threshold of formal school, seems an appropriate time to talk about intellectual diversity, the fact that some people are smarter or dumber than others. The fact of intellectual diversity is not to be disputed. The debate centers around the ever persistent nature-nurture controversy, where intellectual differences come from. This is an important issue in terms of practical action. One's willingness to invest large sums of money in school depends on how much faith one has that education can bring about important changes in cognitive functioning. One's attitudes toward racial integration depend the extent to which one accepts the debased social and intellectual status of Negroes—or of the poor in general—as a product of inferior biological endowment or of the degrading conditions in which they have been forced to live. A proper scholarly discussion of the nature-nurture issue would require a book in itself, and indeed has been the subject of several recent volumes, such as Hunt's.[29] We can only outline the course such an argument would take, referring the reader to the relevant literature, and put forth a few assertions which the reader can accept or reject—but, we hope, on the basis of careful consideration.

Let us say that we are in general agreement with the view that intellectual development represents an interaction between genetic and biological factors and experience, the physical and social settings and events with which a person grows up. But let us caution that we know very little about the biological side of this interaction. Apart from the organic pathologies that affect some 10 per cent of the population, very little is known about the constitutional correlates of intelligence. The only reasonably clear evidence about differences in brain function associated with differences in learning ability comes from studies of rats and mice, and here the most impressive evidence is on central nervous system differences that have been produced by differences in experience.[30] We are also coming to know something about differences in brain structure and function produced by dietary factors, as in the case of protein deficiency, and by the action of hormones. What is missing from our picture of the constitutional correlates of intelligence is the role of the genes in controlling intellectual development. All the evidence makes clear that there is no single gene for intelligence. Whatever the constitutional differences may be that make for differences in intellectual ability, they must be produced by the action of a multiplicity of genes. We must also be aware that intelligence expresses itself in a variety of ways, and the various forms of intelligence may represent the action of very different genes and gene combinations.

A full discussion of the matter would require an analysis of the instruments by which intelligence is assessed, the so-called intelligence tests. Most of the common instruments, like the Wechsler Intelligence Scale for Children, the Stanford-Binet, the Otis Self-Administering, or the Kuhlmann-Anderson, are described in textbooks on tests, measurements, and individual differences. The tests have been around for so long and have been used so widely that people have come to take them for granted as valid measuring instruments.

When one looks closely, however, as writers such as Hunt, Anastasi, Church, Fowler, Sigel, Spiker and McCandless, Stott and Ball, and Tyler[31] have done, the tests are almost pathetically flimsy tools with which to study an important topic like intellectual ability. They are open to both empirical and logical criticism on many grounds: lack of independent validation, inadequate standardization, cultural bias, conventionality of content, errors of mathematical logic, lack of any theory or even a good definition of what it is that they are supposed to measure, instability of individual performance from one testing to another, and untested assumptions about how intelligence is distributed. It is a curious bit of intellectual and cultural history that the tests have become as solidly entrenched as they have without the test-makers ever responding in any serious way to the damning criticisms that have been made. Particularly objectionable has been the indiscriminate use of tests for school placement, so that young children who score at different levels on the test are assigned to different educational tracks, which raises suspicions of self-fulfilling prophecies. This is particularly true of the use of simple, overall, summated test scores, like the IQ. Individual tests are nonetheless valuable instruments for trained observations of the cognitive processes, if only because each trained clinician has seen hundreds of children perform in this setting and can therefore readily recognize what is individual and diagnostic for understanding a child's ways of learning or note disturbances in his development.

For a complete discussion of intelligence and intellectual diversity, we should also have to examine the indirect evidence for a biological view of behavior. This evidence would include Tryon's selective breeding of maze-bright and maze-dull strains of rats;[32] comparisons of the intelligence of identical twins raised apart with the intelligence of identical twins raised together, of identical twins with fraternal twins and nontwin siblings; and comparisons of the correlations of intelligence in adopted children with that of their true parents and adoptive parents.[33]

The findings from all such studies support a hereditarian view of intelligence, but all have met with environmentalist criticism. For instance, Searle[34] has concluded that the difference between Tryon's two rat strains is a difference of temperament rather than intelligence (although the measurement of animal intelligence is as confused an undertaking as the measurement of human intelligence). We must note also that most animal studies have omitted the vital environmental control of cross-fostering. This technique swaps newborn litters between mothers of different genetic strains to insure that the behavior of the young is due to genetic causes rather than behavior learned through being raised by their own mothers (see page 214). When the data from the most famous of the twin studies, which compared identical twins raised apart, by Newman, Freeman, and Holzinger,[35] are regrouped, as we have done in Table 3, to take account of psychological dissimilarity between the physically separate environments in which the members of twin pairs were raised, it can be shown that environment did in fact exert an influence on the twins' intellectual development.

TABLE 3 / Comparison of identical twins in terms of differences in IQ and differences in educational and social advantages (DESA)

	Large DESA	Small DESA
IQ differences < 10	1, 4, 7	1, 1, 1, 2, 2, 5, 6, 8, 9
IQ differences > 10	10, 12, 12, 15, 17, 19, 24	—

Source: Adapted from Newman, H. H., Freeman, F. N., and Holzinger, K. J. *Twins.* Chicago: University of Chicago, 1937; and Johnson, R. C. Similarity in IQ of separated identical twins as related to length of time spent in same environment. *Child Development,* 1963, 34, 745–749.

Decreasing similarity in IQ's as we go from identical twins raised together to identical twins reared apart to fraternal twins to siblings in general can be seen to be associated with decreasingly similar environments. Even fraternal twins, because of their differing stimulus characteristics, can provoke quite different reactions from people around them and so in principle can inhabit very different psychological environments even while living in the same physical one. The critic has no ready answer to the finding that foster children often (although by no means invariably) are more like their real parents than their adoptive parents in measured intelligence, except to say that nobody has yet sufficiently studied the psychology of adoption and the possible problems of identification involved. In addition, those who are interested in possible environmental influences on intelligence point to positive evidence of the kind discussed in the next paragraph.

Most of our knowledge of environmental effects on intelligence comes from studies of infrahuman species, although Wellman conducted a still-controversial series of studies which seemed to indicate that nursery-school experience of the right sort could markedly raise a child's IQ, and we are beginning to get highly optimistic returns from studies of the effects of Head Start programs.[36] At the animal level, we have such studies as that by Forgays and Forgays[37] on the behavioral consequences of growing up in rich or dull environments, and analogous studies by C. J. Smith[38] on brain localization and by Bennett, Krech, Rosenzweig, *et al.,*[39] on brain biochemistry. The impaired intellectual functioning of institution-reared children could also be used to show the effects of environment, except that we have no possible way of knowing that such children would have been brighter had they grown up in more favorable circumstances. Skeels,[40] however, in a thirty-year follow-up study, found dramatic differences in the life histories of thirteen "retarded" children given enriched experience, by contrast with twelve others raised in a standard institutional environment. Sayegh and Dennis[41] found differences in institution children given only three weeks of supplementary experience. Those concerned with environmental influences would say further that we must also take account of the prenatal environment and its possible role in developing the person's intellectual ability. Wellman was widely attacked on statistical and logical grounds, but in general few psychologists nowadays uphold a strongly hereditarian view of intelligence (at least in public), and those who do, like Hirsch,[42] insist that they are interested only in population distributions rather than individuals.

It seems safe to conclude from the available evidence that we do not know much about the relative contributions of constitution and environment to intellectual development or how, concretely, they interact to produce a spread of intelligence. Pragmatically, our ignorance is not important, since we cannot do much to manipulate heredity anyway (although we do know how to overcome such hereditary defects as phenylketonuria and diabetes, and although there are those who claim that the hereditary strings are almost in our hands), and we do know that environment can have a large impact on intellectual development. There are two logical possibilities: One could, by particular educational arrangements, either squeeze almost everybody into a narrow range of high intelligence; or simply displace the present distribution curve upward as a whole, so that the new average IQ of 100 would correspond to a higher level than it now does. Either of these outcomes, it seems to the authors, would be socially desirable.

Nevertheless, it is unsatisfactory, if only because we want to advance our understanding, to be purely atheoretical and pragmatic in our thinking about intelligence. We believe that some of the confusion on this subject comes about because people have tended to localize intelligence in the organism, or even more narrowly in the central nervous system, as though it were some kind of mechanism or structure. Instead, following Stoddard,[43] we would like to propose abandoning the noun "intelligence," which invites reification, the translation of a convenient hypothetical construct into an entity, and substitute the adjective "intelligent" as a characteristic of organism-environment relations. In this view, it makes just as much sense to talk about more or less intelligent environments as about more or less intelligent people. Intellectual development in this view becomes the progressive discovery of reality, and the task of education to give the child an intelligent—differentiable, thinkable, manipulable—environment. Here we are returning to our somewhat modified version of Kurt Lewin's field theory (see page 187).

Our transactions with the environment—which includes, let us remember, the natural and man-made physical world, animals, people, things, institutions, and symbols, and all the meanings, sounds, odors, and demand qualities that emanate from them—are obviously conditioned on the way our environment appears to us, the way our personal life space is constituted. Out of our cultural learning and our personal experience we come to perceive the world in diverse ways, so that different individual life spaces have different organizations of what stands out as figure and what blends into the background, different possibilities for action and manipulation, different causal dynamics, and, in sum, different patterns of meaning. The unintelligent life space is the sphere of primitive experience into which we are all born and which is perceived egocentrically, dynamistically, phenomenalistically, and magicalistically, activated by psychic and spiritual forces of a kind unknown to science. The psychologically primitive environment permits full play to superstition and is populated with imagined beings and entities, from poltergeists to the miasma to "intelligence." Such an environment is phrased in tradition-bound formulas, platitudes, axioms, precepts, taboos, myths, and slogans. All action has a moral component and must be accompanied by the proper ritual observances lest it misfire. The primitive environment invites acceptance and submission and discourages invention and innovation. By contrast, the more intelligent life space is one in which primitive forces are subordinate to more orderly and manageable ones, as generally known in the educated parts of our society, so that magic gives way to science, we look beneath the surface of things to see what makes them tick, and we evolve sets of principles applicable to various domains of reality. We learn to distinguish between moral and morality-free spheres of action and to emphasize the pragmatic rather than the ritual. We invent new—and sometimes better—ways of doing things, we learn to exploit natural forces, we let machines do our work for us (including a certain amount of our thinking). In the arts, we experiment with novel combinations of light and sounds and words and meanings. We search for new, largely secular formulations of the meaning of it all. We invent new social doctrines. Most radically, we look for ways of altering and improving human nature, through child-rearing practices, education, drugs, surgery, and psychotherapy.

Let us note that even the most emancipated of us are still hobbled by superstitions, dogmas, irrational convictions and intuitions, rigidities, and some imperviousness to evidence, but we have moved away from the Stone Age and the Middle Ages, from witch trials and public executions, from mass manias and holy crusades. We still have a considerable way to go, as one can read in the headlines, but we have made a beginning. In this interplay of person and environment, the part that seems to remain most stubbornly as in the person is language and symbols, and the environment can be no more intelligent than the symbolic system with which the person can manipulate facts and relationships intellectually, in thought.

If, as we propose, we now consider education to be a process of giving the child an intelligent environment, one whose workings and possibilities and impossibilities he understands, we must take account of our society's profound ambivalence about intellectual development and education. For it is only some fraction of the community that has worked its way into the light of modern understanding, and that fraction is none too well represented in the seats of power. On the whole, many parents are more interested in whether the child is "doing well," in the sense of getting good marks, than in what and whether he is learning and whether he finds learning exciting. This duality is also expressed in the contradictory attitudes communicated implicitly to boys and to girls. Boys are expected to do well, but it is assumed that they will find intellectual activity unmanly and will dislike school. Girls are expected to be more docile and to accept the schooling process, but they are assumed not to be capable of serious intellectual achievement, which in any case is viewed as irrelevant and perhaps even inimical to their eventual feminine role. In fact, girls do learn better in school than boys, partly at least because the schools are run by women and offer an effeminate, prettified curriculum.

Equally important is the distinction that can be drawn between safe and unsafe areas of learning. We can see the various school subject matters as a spectrum running from the skill subjects (reading, writing, and arithmetic) through the physical sciences, the biological sciences, the social sciences, the arts and humanities, to philosophy and metaphysics. Branching off from this array are the applied fields: engineering, agriculture, medicine, social work, and so on. We encourage the child in mathematics and the natural sciences, particularly if he is a boy, just as we welcome new knowledge in these fields. We smile upon the learned technologies such as engineering and medicine, but as we move away from this region of the spectrum, learning and logic begin to clash both with established social doctrines and with our emphasis on what is practical, manly, and uncontroversial. Even the generally esteemed, not to say revered, field of medicine becomes controversial in such areas as birth control and surgical abortion. The applications of chemistry and biology in agriculture become controversial when they raise economically important questions about pollution of the natural environment. In biology itself, the hypothesis of evolution still arouses distrust and antagonism and its teaching is still outlawed in several of the United States. Sex education is taught in many school systems, but most courses stop short of the psychology, sociology, and ethics of sex. Conservatism and conventionality restrict thinking in many fields, and it is extremely easy for the child to acquire a conventional outlook, beginning in the preschool years. Even when young people realize that the adult world has not dealt with them honestly—as when adolescent disillusionment sets in—they lack the knowledge necessary to arrive at reasonable formulations of their own.

As educators, we have to bear in mind that intellect is not purely intellectual: We sometimes become so preoccupied with the symbolic tools of thought that we neglect the factual substance of knowledge, including the reaches of human virtue and evil, reason and stupidity, nobility and pettiness, plasticity and fixity, sensibility and opacity, passion and prejudice. As a rule, schools do not discuss the ethical demands of modern life. Since most children, prior to entering school, have grown up among adults who live in a twilight zone between primitive and sophisticated thought, some part of an intellectual education has to be devoted to dis-educating children of the errors they have learned, to divesting them of the clichés, the slogans, the platitudes, the dogmas, and the unspoken assumptions that dominate much of conventional thinking. A free and rich preschool education—whether in school or at home— which encourages questioning and deliberately avoids dogmatism seems to be a vital part of the total span of intellectual development.

Notice, however, that giving the child an intelligent life space also means giving him an intelligent view of himself. For every differentiation and higher-order integration of external reality implies a corresponding differentiation and integration of the person himself, a greater freedom to think, to act, to know himself, to become involved, to care, to be

357

committed, and to wonder. This, in sum, is what we mean by being intelligent.

REFERENCES / Chapter 7

[1] Verplanck, W. S. A glossary of some terms used in the objective science of behavior. *Psychological Review*, 1957, 64, Supplement 8, 42 pp.

[2] Bernstein, B. Elaborated and restricted codes: Their social origins and some consequences. *American Anthropologist*, 1964, no. 6, part 2, 55–69.

[3] Hess, R. D., and Shipman, V. C. Early experience and the socialization of cognitive modes in children. *Child Development*, 1965, 36, 869–886.

[4] Ortar, G. R. Classification of speech directed at children by mothers of different level of education and cultural background. Paper read at 18th International Congress of Psychology, 1966.

[5] Klüver, H. The study of personality and the method of equivalent and non-equivalent stimuli. *Character and Personality*, 1936, 5, 91–112.

[6] Kreezer, G., and Dallenbach, K. M. Learning the relation of opposition. *American Journal of Psychology*, 1929, 41, 432–441; Robinowitz, R. Learning the relation of opposition as related to scores on the Wechsler Intelligence Scale for Children. *Journal of Genetic Psychology*, 1956, 88, 25–30.

[7] Inhelder, B. Criteria of the stages of mental development. In Tanner, J. M., and Inhelder, B. *Discussions on Child Development*. New York: International Universities, 1953, I, 75–107.

[8] Robinson, H. B. An experimental examination of the size-weight illusion in young children. *Child Development*, 1964, 35, 91–107.

[9] Stevenson, H. W., and McBee, G. The learning of object and pattern discrimination by children. *Journal of Comparative and Physiological Psychology*, 1958, 51, 752–754.

[10] Ghent, L. Form and its orientation: A child's-eye view. *American Journal of Psychology*, 1961, 74, 177–190.

[11] Wohlwill, J. F., and Wiener, M. Discrimination of form orientation in young children. *Child Development*, 1964, 35, 1113–1125.

[12] Berens, A., and Church, J. Subcultural and age differences in performance on figure-completion tasks. Unpublished ms.

[13] Hunton, V. C. The recognition of inverted pictures by children. *Journal of Genetic Psychology*, 1955, 86, 281–288.

[14] Wohlwill, J. F. The perception of size and distance relationships in perspective drawings. Paper read at meetings of Eastern Psychological Association, 1962.

[15] Caldwell, B. M. *Preschool Inventory Manual*. The author, 1965.

[16] Inhelder, B., and Piaget, J. *The Early Growth of Logic in the Child*. New York: Harper & Row, 1964.

[17] Dennis, W. Animistic thinking among college and university students. *Scientific Monthly*, 1953, 76, 247–250.

[18] Michotte, A. *La Perception de la Causalité*. Louvain: Institut Supérieur de Philosophie, 1946.

[19] Olum, V. Developmental differences in the perception of causality. *American Journal of Psychology*, 1956, 69, 417–423.

[20] Heider, F., and Simmel, M. An experimental study of apparent behavior. *American Journal of Psychology*, 1944, 57, 243–259.

[21] Bateson, G., and Mead, M. *Balinese Character*. New York: New York Academy of Sciences, 1942, p. 5.

[22] Hall, E. T. *The Silent Language*. Garden City: Doubleday, 1959. (Also available in paperback.)

[23] Carpenter, E., Varley, F., and Flaherty, R. *Eskimo*. Toronto: University of Toronto, 1959.

[24] Maier, N. R. F. Reasoning in children. *Journal of Comparative Psychology*, 1936, 21, 357–366.

[25] Hochberg, J., and Brooks, V. Pictorial recognition as an unlearned ability: A study of one child's performance. *American Journal of Psychology*, 1962, 75, 624–628.

[26] Chesler, M. A. Ethnocentrism and attitudes toward the physically disabled. *Journal of Personality and Social Psychology*, 1965, 2, 877–882. See also Fiedler, M. F. *Deaf Children in a Hearing World*. New York: Ronald, 1952.

[27] Minuchin, P., and Biber, B. A child development approach to language in the preschool disadvantaged child. Paper read at meetings of the Society for Research in Child Development, 1967; Bereiter, C., and Engelmann, S. *Teaching Disadvantaged Children in the Preschool*. Englewood Cliffs: Prentice-Hall, 1966.

[28] Bruner, J. S. *The Process of Education*. Cambridge: Harvard, 1960.

[29] Hunt, J. McV. *Intelligence and Experience*. New York: Ronald, 1961.

[30] Bennett, E. L., Diamond, M. C., Krech, D., and Rosenzweig, M. R. Chemical and anatomical plasticity of brain. *Science*, 1964, 146, 610–618; Levine, S., and Mullins, R. F. Hormonal influences on brain organization in infant rats. *Science*, 1966, 152, 1585–1592; Smith, C. J. Mass action and early environment in the rat. *Journal of Comparative and Physiological Psychology*, 1959, 52, 154–156.

[31] Hunt, *op. cit.*, and Anastasi, A. Heredity, environment, and the question "How?" *Psychological Review*, 1958, 65, 197–208; Church, J. *Language and the Discovery of Reality*. New York: Random House, 1961, Chapter 7; Fowler, W. Cognitive learning in infancy and early childhood. *Psychological Bulletin*, 1962, 59, 116–152; Sigel, I. E. How intelligence tests limit understanding of intelligence. *Merrill-Palmer Quarterly of Behavior and Development*, 1963, 9, 39–56; Spiker, C. C., and McCandless, B. R. The concept of intelligence and the philosophy of science. *Psychological Review*, 1954, 61, 255–266; Stott, L. H., and Ball, R. S. Infant and preschool mental tests. *Monographs of the Society for Research in Child Development*, 1965, 30, no. 3; Tyler, L. E. *Tests and Measurements*. Englewood Cliffs: Prentice-Hall, 1963, Chapter 4. For a striking recent study of self-fulfilling prophecies, see Rosenthal, R. *Pygmalion in the Classroom*. New York: Holt, Rinehart & Winston, in press.

[32] Tryon, R. C. Genetic differences in maze-learning ability in rats. *Thirty-*

ninth Yearbook of the National Society for the Study of Education, 1940, 111–119.

[33] These studies are reviewed in Tyler, L. E. *The Psychology of Human Differences.* New York: Appleton-Century-Crofts, 1965, Chapters 17 and 18.

[34] Searle, L. V. The organization of hereditary maze-brightness and maze-dullness. *Genetic Psychology Monographs,* 1949, 39, 279–325.

[35] Newman, H. H., Freeman, F. N., and Holzinger, K. J. *Twins.* Chicago: University of Chicago, 1937; Johnson, R. C. Similarity in IQ of separated identical twins as related to length of time spent in same environment. *Child Development,* 1963, 34, 745–749.

[36] Crowell, D. C., Shiro, L. K., Cade, T. M., Landau, B., and Bennett, H. L. Progress report: Preschool readiness project. Honolulu: University of Hawaii, 1966 (Mimeographed); Kamii, C. K., Radin, N. L., and Weikart, D. P. A. A two-year preschool program for culturally disadvantaged children. Paper read at meetings of American Psychological Association, 1966; Gray, S. W., and Klaus, R. A. An experimental preschool program for culturally deprived children. *Child Development,* 1965, 36, 887–898.

[37] Forgays, D. G., and Forgays, J. W. The nature of the effect of free environmental experience in the rat. *Journal of Comparative and Physiological Psychology,* 1952, 45, 322–328.

[38] Smith, *op. cit.*

[39] Bennett, *et al., op. cit.*

[40] Skeels, H. M. Adult status of children with contrasting early life experiences. *Monographs of the Society for Research in Child Development.* 1966, 31, no. 3.

[41] Sayegh, Y., and Dennis, W. The effect of supplementary experiences upon the behavioral development of infants in institutions. *Child Development,* 1965, 36, 81–90.

[42] Hirsch, J. Behavior genetics and individuality understood. *Science,* 1963, 142, 1436–1442.

[43] Stoddard, G. D. *The Meaning of Intelligence.* New York: Macmillan, 1943.

8 The Middle Years of Childhood: 1

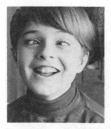

The period of life from age six to age twelve-plus is known by a number of labels, each pointing to important characteristics of development. To call it the *middle years* is to stress the relative tranquillity of this age between the turmoil of the preschool years and that of adolescence. To label it the *school years* is to point out that this is a time highly favorable to formal learning of the kind that should go on in schools. The designation of the *gang age* refers to the cardinal importance of affiliation with one's age mates—the gang. Psychoanalysts call this period *latency,* a time of sexual quiescence between the Oedipus complex and the upheavals of adolescence. The middle years begin with the loss of the first baby teeth and end at about the time the permanent teeth are all in, so that we can call this the *age of the loose tooth.* For some observers, this period is noteworthy for its *literalism* of thought, and for others for the strong *ritualism* to be found in children of this age.

An Overview of the Middle Years

The middle years are perhaps the age adults know least about. One reason is that children of this age turn their backs on adults and unite in a society of children. Parents, caught up in their own concerns, tend to be satisfied to let these newly competent children go their own way—which the children do, clustering into same-age and same-sex groups drawn from the pool of neighborhood and school acquaintances. At this age, the

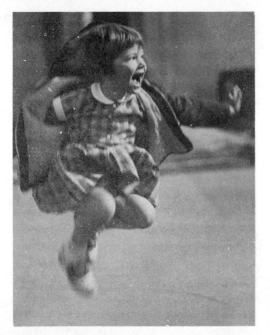

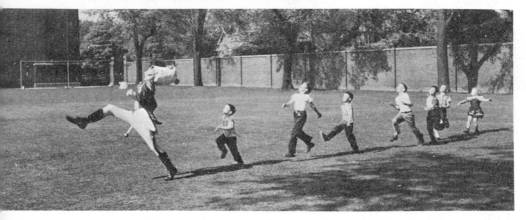

The "halcyon days of childhood."
(Left) W. L. Faust; (below) Alfred Eisenstaedt, LIFE Magazine © Time Inc.

values of one's peers become considerably more important than those handed down by adults. What is more, school-age children learn to keep their thoughts from adults. They stop thinking out loud and, besides, practice deliberate guile and deception. To fortify their sometimes hostile, sometimes bland taciturnity toward adults, together with their peer-group solidarity, they form secret societies. Although a given club may last no more than days or weeks, it may be protected by mortal oaths and covenants, binding for life and countersigned in blood (or perhaps red ink). Another factor in adult ignorance about the middle years is that adults take this age for granted, as though it had no secrets. Adults are concerned with how to civilize or educate their middle-years children, but it seldom occurs to them to wonder about what their children are like, what the children themselves think about and are concerned with.

Yet, when we stop to think about it, the middle years can be an open book to adults. It is at this age that people begin to have organized, continuous memories rather than the piecemeal, episodic ones of the preschool years. We learn some of life's most basic lessons as babies, but we cannot recall the events that taught us. We can bring back snatches of early childhood, but the special flavor of life is gone. But our school years are our own and can be evoked readily by the proper cues: the way one worked a loose tooth about with one's tongue, the reluctance to break the last thread that held it in place, putting the now-fallen tooth under one's pillow for the tooth-fairy to take in exchange for a gift; the pungent and unchanging smell of chalk dust and disinfectant in a schoolroom; the memory of the books one read; the recollection of the jokes, riddles, and rhymes of childhood; or, in the case of a Marcel Proust, the flavor of

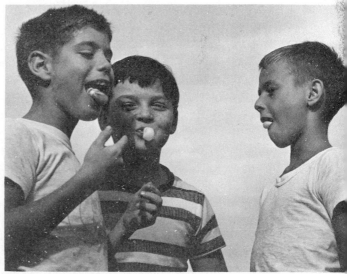

The school-age child spends as much of his time as possible in the company of his peers.
(Right) Bernheim/Rapho Guillumette; (below) Wayne Miller

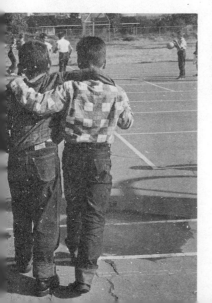

biscuit dipped in herb tea. When parents of older children reminisce, it is about their children's preschool years; but when adults harken back to their own childhoods, it is to their middle years.

The middle-years child himself recognizes the special qualities of this period. When asked what the best age is to be, preschool children and adolescents yearn either forward or back; the school-age child, by contrast, likes his own age period best. At no other age has he as much freedom and as few responsibilities. Middle-years children may aspire to be teen-agers, and in many respects today's middle-years children are the teen-agers of just a few years ago: They listen to rock-and-roll and folk-rock music, they wear their hair in the teen-age fashions, they emulate teen-age dress and slang, they do the more advanced dance steps, they watch teen-age programs on TV and go to teen-age movies, but they reject the heterosexual entanglements of adolescence and the worries and burdens of adulthood. Indeed, adult life seems incomprehensible to the middle-years child: He cannot understand why adults, with all their power and freedom, do not gorge themselves on ice cream and candy, or perpetually watch television, or otherwise exploit the good things of life instead of being the fretful, trouble-ridden creatures they are.

The school-age child spends as much of his time as possible in the company of his peers, from whom he learns at firsthand about social structures, about in-groups and out-groups, about leadership and fol-lowership, about justice and injustice, about loyalties and heroes and ideals. But even as he becomes a member of the distinct society of children, with its own roles and rules and folkways, he also, sometimes unwittingly and sometimes grudgingly, learns the ways and standards of adult society. It is possible that this dual social learning is the basis for many of the strains and conflicts that arise in adolescence, when the youngster is at war both with the adult world and with himself. Among his friends, the middle-years child lives in a special culture with its own traditional games, rhymes, riddles, tricks, superstitions, factual and mythical lore, and skills, transmitted virtually intact from one childhood generation to the next, sometimes over a period of centuries, with no help from adults and often in spite of them. The peer group corrupts the child's linguistic practices, and he learns to speak reasonably proper English (or whatever) at home and an agrammatical, scatology-laden jargon with his contemporaries. In the group, middle-years children jabber constantly, but they seem to have very little to say. There was a recent vogue for walkie-talkie radios, and the messages that came through the crackling static seemed to be exclusively of this order: "Can you read me? Over." "Yes, I read you loud and clear. Can you read me? Over." "Yes. I'm over in Charlie's yard. Can you still read me? Over."

As we shall reiterate, adult society and middle-years society intermix spatially, but with no more attention back and forth than between the sparrows and squirrels feeding side by side. Middle-years children are everywhere. They ride their bikes all over town, they explore woods and fields and ponds, or junk yards and construction sites, they scale fences and take shortcuts through yards and alleys, they play on the sidewalks and in the streets, they erect clubhouses in vacant lots and tree houses where they can, they set up refreshment stands and stage shows and hold exhibits. They congregate at all events and spectacles, shinnying lamp-

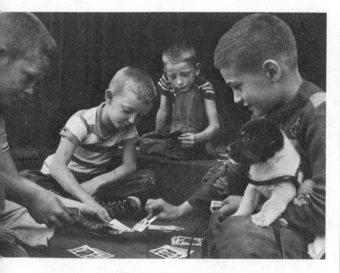 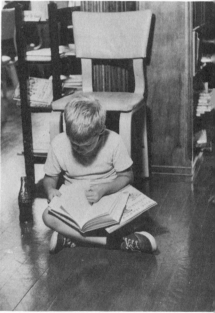

Middle-years children play games like poker and Monop-
oly, they toss a ball back and forth, and sometimes
they even do solitary things like reading.
(Above) Ken Heyman; (right and below) Ray Shaw

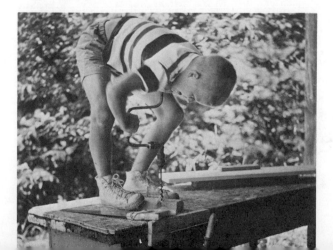

posts to see a parade, sitting on the edge of the platform during a political speech; they turn up at fires and smash-ups and to watch the drowned body brought ashore. They go to the movies in pairs or packs. They sprawl in front of the television set (and even television-watching becomes a social activity), consuming endless snacks. They play games like poker and Monopoly, they toss a ball back and forth, and sometimes they even do solitary things like reading or putting their stamp or baseball card collection in order.

As with other age periods, we have to point out that the middle years are not a single steplike unit. We find it convenient to distinguish three subdivisions of the middle years, corresponding roughly to the American school divisions of primary (grades 1 to 3, or six- to eight-year-olds), elementary (grades 4 to 6, or nine- to eleven-year-olds), and junior high school (grades 7 to 9, or twelve years plus). The six-year-old retains many babyish characteristics, including a taste for silliness and a tolerance of or even a desire for cuddling. He is likely to be but a fringe member of the gang, imitating its ways with literal dead seriousness and doing the bidding of the older children, and still likely to blab its secrets and activities to adults. He still, in these early school years, cries easily. By age nine, the child is sparing with his affections (particularly if he is a he and not a she), an active member of the gang, and skilled in its ways. He has learned to bear everyday buffetings and disappointments stoically, and if he has to cry he does it away from the gang. By age twelve, with exceptions and variations, he has developed a cocksure air, is controlled and competent (although his table manners may have deteriorated steadily throughout this period), scorns all things he considers childish, and is fiercely independent. Girls by age twelve have outgrown the long-legged, knobby gawkiness of the early school years and often merit the description of "womanly"—although they may be on the threshold of another awkward age.

Our scheme does not fit boys and girls equally well. Girls change much faster than boys during this period, and many sixth- and seventh-grade girls have entered puberty. It is at this point that one feels the shock of anomaly in watching a full-bosomed, perhaps lipsticked and permanented young woman playing tag or jumping rope. Class photographs of the seventh grade show how the young ladies tend to tower over their male classmates.

Children's rate of growth slows down during the middle years. They continue to grow, but at a slower pace than earlier and later. The average six-year-old is slightly over 3½ feet tall (107 cm.)—Oriental children are slightly smaller on the average than their Caucasian and Negro age mates, but are fast catching up. By the time he begins his adolescent growth spurt (average age eleven for girls, thirteen for boys), he is crowding the 5-foot mark (152 cm.). During this same period the child's weight doubles, from 40 to 80 pounds (18 kg. to 36 kg.). Most boys double in muscular strength during this period, while girls lag somewhat in this regard.

Striking changes come about in the child's physiognomy, the cast of his facial features. From birth until adolescence, the brain case takes the lead in growth over the face, so that babies and children have a small face crowned by a high forehead. In the neonatal period, facial features are indistinct and more typically neonatal than clearly individual. Fat pads fill out the baby's cheeks, giving him a round-cheeked, full face. The fat pads dwindle during toddlerhood, and by the later preschool years the child's face is comparatively lean. It is the successive losses of baby teeth and the appearance of permanent ones that distinguish the changing face of the middle years. The baby teeth go approximately in the order in which they came, beginning with the lower front teeth and moving symmetrically back. The six- to seven-year-old is noted for his gap-toothed grin. When permanent teeth come in to fill the gaps, they loom disproportionately large, and the eight-year-old is distinguished by his outsize, "tombstone" front teeth. It is only in adolescence, when the nose and jaw come into full flower, that the face at last catches up to the teeth in size. Later losses of baby teeth during the school years are not so conspicuous, since they occur farther back, but the shedding of old teeth and the eruption of permanent ones go on until age ten or twelve (the four so-called wisdom teeth may not grow out until late adolescence or early adulthood and sometimes fail to appear at all).

The middle years are the time for the acquisition of many major and minor motor skills, related to the climate and the culture. Although some children learn earlier or later, the typical (northern) American middle-years child learns to ride a two-wheeler, to swim and dive, to roller-skate and ice-skate, to hang by his knees and to skin-the-cat, to play baseball, football, or whatever other sports his culture favors, to cross his eyes, spin tops, jump rope (which is mainly a pastime for girls, but boys too jump rope when away from girls), snap his fingers, to wink one eye, and to whistle. Boys play mumblety-peg and girls jacks.

Boys and girls mature at different rates during the middle years, and, what is more, questions of masculinity and femininity become prominent. Boys associate more—and more ostentatiously—with boys, and girls with

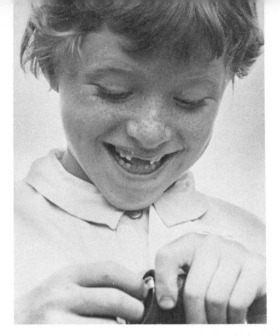

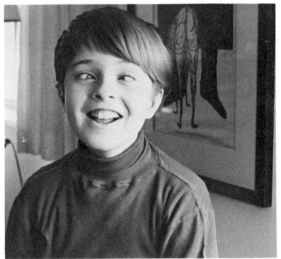

The faces of childhood.
(Left) W. L. Faust;
(below) Alexandria Church

girls, each sex pursuing its own separate interests and identities until communication is cut to a trickle. In adolescence, of course, the sexes will suddenly find new reasons to come together again, but this time in the new guises they have meanwhile assumed.

Having thus sketched in a picture of traditional childhood, let us qualify it. It is not that new research has revealed formerly hidden truths—in fact, there has been a dearth of recent research on the middle years—but that middle-class United States childhood itself seems to have changed somewhat. Urbanization and the space age have brought changes in the schools, and the children learn faster than they used to. Increased homework cuts down on the number of hours that children can spend in childish pursuits. Children are brighter than they used to be, not merely in the sense of learning more in school and scoring higher on intelligence tests, but in the sense of being more alert and sensitive to their surroundings and asking more logical and penetrating questions.

Children, if one can believe accounts like Joyce Cary's *House of Children*,[1] or the authors' own memories, used to drift through life in a misty, half-focused, dreamlike, dissociated state, but no more. The children of yesteryear used to harbor endless superstitions and beliefs, were prone to dread and terror, and were genuinely moved by ghost stories and horror movies. Today's children laugh at myths and superstitions, and horror movies have become satirical and farcical. Boys used to be dirt-streaked ragamuffins; many now choose and display their wardrobes with care, emulating teen-age grooming, though they may still dislike bathing and their clothing becomes easily disarrayed. Yesterday's twelve-year-olds used to hammer or rope together makeshift rafts which constantly threatened to disintegrate in midstream; today's twelve-year-old fits together a well-joined skiff, tightly caulked and waterproofed, and makes it work.

Through the mass media, children come to an early awareness of sex, and boys, in the words of one observer, learn to leer before they have learned to giggle. The schools, the mass media, the teen-age world, and commercial interests all exert tremendous pressures to precocity, and flat-chested little girls in the late middle years wear beginner bras and discuss questions of feminine hygiene; the commercial world offers children junior bridge, and boys are given junior dinner jackets. Children may dance the latest steps at mixed parties, which may also encourage crude ventures into necking and petting, and in some families they are served nonalcoholic cocktails before dinner.

Most generally, parents have moved in on child life, often with a wish to give their children every advantage but sometimes, we suspect, in an attempt to recapture their own childhood—ironically, at the cost of their children's. The result, for large numbers of children, is a highly organized and tightly scheduled round of music lessons, dance lessons, horseback-riding lessons, visits to the orthodontist, Little League and various other leagues, parties (at which many parents seek to outdo each other in lavishness, offering poolside parties, theater parties, bowling parties, skating parties, restaurant parties, and handing round lavish favors), and other activities—with the mother cast in the role of chauffeur—which, together with school and homework, quite effectively fill the child's day. Nowadays, especially if the mother works and so has to be out of the house for a good part of the day, many children spend their summers in summer school or at camp. Many camps, too, are no longer places where one swims or hikes or communes with nature, but have become either specialized schools, as in the case of music camps, or general academic ones in rustic settings. The plight of the contemporary middle-years child has been amusingly set forth in Robert Paul Smith's *"Where Did You Go?" "Out." "What Did You Do?" "Nothing."*[2] Smith makes the point that today's child no longer collects butterflies or rocks or sea shells, but buys collections already classified, mounted, and labeled. According to Smith, childhood lore no longer gets transmitted from child to child, to the point where Smith himself has felt impelled to write a book telling children all the things they used to tell each other.[3] We do not know how childhood is faring in other lands, and it certainly is not a wholly lost way of life in the United States, but the things we will have to say about this period must be interpreted in the light of the changing reality.

The Society of Children

It is only during the middle years, as we have said, that the child surrenders to and revels in his status as a child, aspiring neither backward to babyhood nor forward to adolescence and adulthood. Although the school child lives within adult society, he seems to pick his way through it, preoccupied with the concerns of childhood. One of the most striking characteristics of the middle years in our own and many other societies is that the children have a special, separate subculture with traditions, games, values, loyalties, and rules of its own. The culture of childhood shares many of the attributes of primitive cultures. It is handed down by word of mouth, it includes many rituals and magical formulas whose original meanings have been lost, it is hidebound and resistant to alien influences and to change.

In one sense, the immersion in being a child and the strong peer-group affiliation of the middle years seem like time out from the process of development. From another standpoint, though, they seem necessary and valuable in the process of finding an identity. The preschool child takes his identity from his parents. The middle-years child, with this much of a foundation, is now ready to begin the quest for an independent identity and existence. As he has grown in stature, he has become able to see his parents more realistically, to know their frailties and imperfections, and has begun to realize, however dimly, that he must find stability in himself. This "time out," then, represents an essential moving away from the parents toward a genuine separate sense of self.

But the school child differs from the preschooler in more than independence. He is also becoming less egocentric, more able to view himself with a certain detachment and objectivity. He begins to see himself in terms of the labels society applies to him—male or female, age six to twelve, white or colored, rich or poor, smart or dumb—and all that these connote. The gang, too, has its set of labels by which it knows the child and he knows himself. The gang is quick to seize on any idiosyncrasy of constitution, manner, skill, or whatever, and thereafter to treat the child in terms of this trait. The stereotype which the gang holds of the child is often expressed in his nickname: Skinny, Fatso, Four-eyes, Dopey, Professor, Limpy—the total frankness, especially of boys, often startles adults. Most children wear their nicknames proudly, even opprobrious ones, as a badge of their belonging, of having an identity for the group. Any recognition, even contempt or mockery, is preferable to being ignored. Even the outcast or scapegoat would rather have the gang persecute him than act as if he didn't exist, and even the label "Stinky" means that he has an identity. The child's sense of self comes largely from the way others, adults and children, treat him, but it also comes from actual accomplishment and a feeling of competence. As he gets older, it increasingly depends on knowing that he has a role to play, that there is a place for him in society, and particularly that there is a place in which he can do something useful. All this implies further that the child becomes able to criticize himself according to the standards of other people, and, increasingly, to measure himself against abstract standards, a set of ideals.

Child society is a proving ground where the child learns to function apart from adults, but it has its dangers as well. The child's declaration of independence is not merely a withdrawal from adults, it is also in some part a turning against them. But because the child cannot stand up to adults by himself, he is doubly dependent on the gang for support and reassurance. The child's independence may thus turn into a new slavery, complete subservience to the group.[4] (The conformity of this age is expressed in an eight-year-old's lament that "Everybody in my class has poison ivy except me!") Such subservience contains two dangers. The first and immediate one is that pressure from the gang may force him, against his own better judgment, into dangerous, foolish, or immoral deeds. We are not speaking here of such minor immoralities as trying out smoking, or stealing apples, or sexual exposure or sexual play, which, however adults may view them, are a normal part of gang activity and appear to have no ill effects on the child. Rather, we have in mind the serious acts of violence or degradation into which the mob spirit sometimes leads children's gangs, particularly boys' gangs.

The second, long-term danger of submission to the group is failure to grow out of it, to be able to think and judge and behave independently, even in the face of social pressures. This is not a hazard for most children, who, it should be remembered, are simultaneously learning several sets of cultural norms: the parents', the gang's, the school's, and perhaps those of a much larger culture as embodied in stories, poetry, and works of art and music. The child of highly educated parents, who may entertain values quite different from those of society in general, may have to juggle yet another conflict in reconciling what he has learned at home with what he encounters in his school classmates and their families. However, some children grow up to be people who feel threatened and disoriented if obliged to take a stand without knowing the "right" way of thinking as set by group opinion, and doubly so if they sense that their feelings run counter to the group's. It is perfectly normal to experience some discomfort or anxiety when one is ignorant of or in conflict with group standards, but a mature identity permits us to know what our opinions are and to stand by them confidently even in opposition to the group. Let us note a contrary danger. Some children, meeting persistent rejection by the gang, may too quickly take refuge in an inappropriate identification with adults. The "good boy" or the "good girl," who may appear to adults as a model for childhood, may be missing out on an important part of experience, with possible repercussions to come. Such a child's estrangement from his peers may be made worse by adult acceptance and approval, as he or she gets to be known as a "goody-goody," "Mama's boy" (or girl), or "teacher's pet." In sum, the tensions that go with the usual multiple identifications of the middle years, even though sometimes painful, are probably all to the good in the long run of development.

For the child does assimilate the several adult cultures to which he is exposed. He may argue against parental precepts one day and be overheard the next passing them along as his own convictions. Sometimes his conversion comes after the fact. In one case we know of, the girls in a fifth grade had ganged up on one of their members and were making her life a torment. When word reached the parents of one of the ringleaders, they commanded her, to the accompaniment of tears of resentment mixed with guilt, to be friendly toward the scapegoat and to invite her home to play the next day. In no time at all, the former victim had been reintegrated into the group and stood high in its esteem. As most adults realize, many of their preachments sound fatuous to the children they are meant to influence, but they ought not on that account to abandon their notions of conduct and morals. The way children continue to take on adult values even as they resist them implies also that little pitchers have big ears. Just as the child may seem deliberately deaf to parental strictures, so he may simulate casual deafness to things that are not really meant for his ears, and which parents believe they are keeping to themselves.

We should note that the gang spirit does not necessarily die out with childhood but may extend well into adulthood. The outlaw gangs of the horse opera show many of the same traits as children's gangs, as do rebel bands roaming whatever forest or jungle. Military units often have ganglike qualities, as do adult fraternal organizations, lodges, and clubs, especially those that live on rules and rituals, with content left largely undefined.

Later on, we shall talk more about children's contacts with adult society, how they resist it, take it in, and conflict with it. For the present, we want to look at middle childhood where it is purest, in the peer group: kids moving in packs and doing things in packs.

CHILDHOOD TRADITION

The children themselves form the society of children, but the beliefs they profess and the lore they practice are its culture. This culture is seen in the group codes of solidarity, stoicism, prowess, conformity, and the like, but shows forth perhaps most vividly in the ancient tribal rituals. We do not say "ancient" lightly. While historical research is impeded by the gulf between adult and child, and by childhood culture's being a spoken rather than a written one, it has been possible to trace many still-common games and chants back to the Middle Ages and beyond to Roman and Druid, and perhaps Sanskrit, sources. This body of culture has been handed down from generation to generation, but from generations of almost-adolescent elders to the generations of younger brothers and sisters whom they initiate. As we said, though, this chain of cultural transmission is being attenuated, and the culture itself is losing out to commercial and urban pressures as a living thing. We should therefore be grateful that the Opies have set down a large part of the vanishing heritage in their charming compendium, *The Lore and Language of School Children.*[5]

Adults, looking back, will realize that childhood culture is a world that closed behind them and which they do little or nothing to communicate to their children. Grownups may teach children their prayers, but children teach children counting-out rhymes. Adults may teach children baseball, but children teach children stickball and keep-away. To recall the games and chants and rituals of the middle years is, like the evocative loose tooth, another effective passport to our own childhoods. And when, comparing recollections, somebody offers a minor variation in the wording of a rhyme, we feel a thrill of indignation at this intolerable unorthodoxy. Such indignation is a further clue to the relative fixity of this culture and to the unthinking way we learn it as given. To add one more accent to the feat of transmitting a culture virtually intact down through the ages, we might point out that it takes only three or four adult generations to span a century, but there are perhaps fifteen childhood generations per century. This remarkable cultural durability depends in large part on children's love of ritual for its own sake and on their (mostly unspoken) sense of magical power in the literal repetition of forms having the character of rites and incantations and spells. Hence, any violation of the strict formula is felt to nullify its potency, or implies that one is tempting fate.

Games and Chants. Brueghel's sixteenth-century "Children's Games" and a 400-year older Chinese painting, "100 Children at Play," show children at already venerable pastimes, yet much like those one can see on any contemporary American playground, centuries, languages, and nations away. Among the more durable of children's games are hide-and-seek, marbles, tag, hopscotch (observable in India as in Indiana and called *Klassike* in its Russian version), blindman's buff (often rendered "bluff" and now played mostly by adult prescription at the birthday parties of young school-age children), Red Rover, dodge-ball, jacks, London Bridge (along with ring-around-a-rosy, increasingly the province of preschool children)—the reader is invited to supply his own favorites. London Bridge is believed to date back to the medieval custom of entombing someone alive in the foundations of a bridge to propitiate the river spirits, just as the bottle of champagne smashed against the prow of a new ship is a libation offered to Neptune. Many children's traditions preserve early forms of adult culture. The metal forms used in jacks are derived from the knucklebones or vertebrae used in a similar game in Roman times. Notice here that we are talking only about games, which do not cover the full range of children's activities. Such other pastimes as playing catch, making snowmen, swimming, bicycle riding, and kite flying are widely engaged in but do not qualify as games with stable sets of rules.

Many games go on to the accompaniment of ritual chants, like those that go with London Bridge and ring-around-a-rosy, with skipping rope ("Mabel, Mabel, set the table"), and with ball-bouncing ("One, two, three, a nation"). Closely allied are the counting-out rhymes: "Eeny, meeny, miney, mo," "One-potato," and so forth. There are rhymed guessing games: "Buck, buck, you lousy muck, How many fists have I got up, One, two, or none?" This particular specimen has been traced back to Nero's day: *Bucca, bucca, quot sunt hic?* One decides who will go first by "Junk and a po," the outcome being decided in terms of paper, stone, and scissors. Some chants are reserved for special occasions: "Ladybird, ladybird, fly away home," "Last one in is a rotten egg," "I scream, you scream, we all scream for ice cream," "It's raining, it's pouring, The old man is snoring," "No more spelling, no more books, No more teacher's dirty looks" (this last is still a compulsory recital even by children who love school and their teachers). Some are magical incantations: "Rain, rain, go away." Others are taunts: "Susie's mad, and I'm glad, And I know what will please her," "Roses are red, violets are blue, If I had your mug, I'd join the zoo." Many favorite chants are burlesques on standard songs ("Here comes the bride, Big, fat, and wide") and may or may not be attached to specific occasions.

Even though the words of children's sayings are often empty of literal meaning for the child, the charm of saying them and the need to say them accurately are there. Much of the charm seems to stem from the sense of participation in group ways and from satisfaction that one is in the know, that one has the key. The sense of fraternitylike membership is well demonstrated when two children catch themselves saying the same thing at the same time and instantly fall into the ritual of hooking their little fingers together, making a silent wish, and then exchanging the prescribed phrases before they break the hold with a ceremonial flourish and remain mute until a third person speaks to one of them and so breaks the spell. If they forget and speak without this release, the wish is lost. All the other children are aware of their role in the rite and of their power to enforce silence until they choose to free the main participants. The point is the shared character of such rituals, and the obligation on each person to play the required part. One assumption of the game is that the principals should not be liberated too quickly, and if anyone speaks too soon, this is felt as a gratuitous and offensive destruction of a magical moment, to be greeted by the indignant and almost equally ritual cry of "No fair!"

Young school children play their games, just as they recite their sayings and perform their rituals, according to ironclad formulas that permit of no variation. Later in the school years, this initial absolutism mellows somewhat in favor of a degree of relativism. Piaget,[6] in his investigation of children's concepts of rules and morals, found definite changes with age in the way rules are conceived. Early in the school years, they are accepted as *given*: timeless, immutable, and inherent in the game itself. If it is pointed out that children in the next county, say, follow slightly different rules, this departure from The Right Way may be viewed as pitiably ignorant or verging on the sacrilegious. When a child enters a new community, he is often made to feel somewhat ashamed of the incorrect rules he used to follow. When, in the middle of the middle years, the child begins to realize that the rules come from somewhere, he may conceive of them as the work of some obscure Rule-maker who fixed them for all time. Still later, minor changes in the rules are permitted, provided everyone agrees—there arise what adults would call local ground rules. Finally, late in the school years, children can grasp the fact that rules are arrived at by consensus and serve merely to define the conduct and purpose of the game in an orderly way.

It should be noted that this development in the conception of rules runs parallel to a change in the kind of games children play. Increasingly, during the middle years, children engage in competitive games which do not simply run their course like London Bridge or farmer in the dell, but have an outcome, a score. Nevertheless, ritual predominates for most of the school years, in the compelling nature of rules, in the self-contained quality of games, in the inflexibility of sayings, and in the conservatism of children's attitudes.

Other Childhood Rites. In addition to communal rituals, there are solitary ones which are nevertheless defined by the child culture and carry strong group sanctions. Among these are the superstitious observances (not walking under a ladder, turning back if a black cat crosses the path ahead); obsessive humming and counting (including counting repeated things, like freight cars, counting by fives or by tens, and counting backward); avoiding or stepping on sidewalk cracks; touching every lamppost, and so on without end. Many children invent private rituals as well. One adult recalls how he had to be in bed and under the covers before the door swung shut, or else the (imaginary) mice under the bed would bite his toes. A woman recalls how she had to get upstairs before the basement toilet stopped flushing lest she be captured by some obscure bogey; it is interesting to note that this ritual was taken over, in modified form, by each of her two younger siblings in turn. In general, such rituals serve to ward off some threat, nameless or specific.

There are yet other forms of behavior in the middle years which, though less ritualistic than those we have described, are still closely bound up with traditional childhood culture. There are the ever-recurring *jokes and riddles,* which seem wholly threadbare to adults but which come as revelations to each new wave of children and are for them the essence of sophisticated wit: "Why do firemen wear red suspenders?"; "Waiter, there's a fly in my soup." Some of these are standard, but others may come and go in cycles, which seems to be the case with the Knock-knock jokes and the little moron stories, while others, like the recent elephant jokes and sick jokes, may have a brief vogue and then vanish forever. Traditional children's humor is still with us, but is being fortified with adult-manufactured humor of the kind found in *Mad* magazine, TV cartoons (which nowadays tend to the satirical), and in the person of various culture heroes such as TV and rock-'n'-roll figures, and in slogan-bearing buttons.

There are the *stunts,* the tricks one learns to do with one's own body, control of which is extremely important at this age and which has so many peculiar and unexpected potentialities. School-age children learn to make themselves cross-eyed, to see double, to contort their faces into horrendous shapes, to rub their bellies while patting their heads, to snap their fingers, to whistle, to turn somersaults, to skin the cat, to perform exercises in double-jointedness, to cross their arms and clasp their hands and be perplexed as to which finger is which. Late in this period, a fortunate gifted few will be able to wiggle their ears. Children learn to slide needles through the upper layer of skin without hurting themselves. They ink themselves with mock tattoos. A verbal counterpart of stunts is found in the perennial *tongue-twisters.* The learning of body stunts goes along with learning such *physical skills* as jumping and vaulting over barriers, swimming and diving, skating, playing ball, and all the rest. Some skills involve the manipulation of external agencies, as in riding a horse or sailing a boat. And, of course, the child's practical competences feed into his total sense of identity.

Still another characteristically ritualized way of dealing with reality at this age is the making of *collections.* In the early school years, at least, collections should more properly be called aggregations: pocketfuls and drawerfuls of the incredible and often unspeakable miscellany that every mother of a school-age child has to cope with. Later in the school years, collections tend to become more homogeneous and orderly: stamps ranged neatly on the pages of an album, dolls propped neatly on a shelf. But no matter how disorderly or even repulsive the child's accumulations appear to adults, to the child every length of twine, every scrap of cheap jewelry, every broken model, every thumb-eared comic book, every faded sea shell deserves the designation of "very valuable." Often, in fact, the objects that the child collects take on highly charged magical or talismanic properties.

The child masters the magic of reading, writing, and arithmetic, and then goes on in the middle-middle years to *coded talk and writing*. The child's codes, ciphers, and secret languages emphasize both communication with the in-group and exclusion of the out-group. Again, their function is largely ritual—the child who has mastered a code is hard put to think of anything to say in it. They contain a touch of the magic found in the special priestly language of many societies, and even the most commonplace message takes on a mystical tinge when couched in Pig Latin or Op, or laboriously transcribed into code or cipher.

The world of the middle-years child is highly differentiated but it is far from being integrated into a coherent whole. This time of life is full of joy and abandon, of delightful discoveries and surprises, of wonder and amusement, but it is likewise full of dreads, terrors, anxieties, uncertainties, and worry. The child is touched with a sense of his essential human isolation in a vast, powerful, unpredictable, and largely uncontrollable world. His childhood culture as expressed in shared group activity gives him the emotional strength to carry on. His culture as expressed in skills and rituals and collections give him a magical dominion over an otherwise unmanageable reality. Without the devices of his culture the regressive components in his perpetual growth ambivalence might overwhelm him. But, as we have said, the culture of childhood is a crutch to help him through a stage of development, and if he does not gradually free himself of it, it becomes a millstone.

THE PEER GROUP

Having looked at the highly formalized traditions in the culture of childhood society, it is now time to look at the actual society of children, at children functioning in groups, how such groups are organized, what they do, and what their activities tell us about children of this age. The gang may have many degrees of organization, from a loose cluster of children playing in the schoolyard or the street, to well-defined pairs or groups of friends, to clubs for the sake of having clubs, to special-purpose clubs such as ball teams or delinquent gangs. It seems to be the case that children can play in pairs or bunches, but not in threes. When three children play, two of them almost inevitably band together against the third.

Let us stress the psychological separateness of the world of kids and the world of adults. It is fascinating to walk down a city block—ideally, after the evening meal in summertime—and to observe the child and adult societies carrying on their activities in and around each other but reciprocally oblivious except when they collide. Children step aside for cars without breaking the rhythm of their game. The driver of the car slows down for the kids, but without really noticing what they are doing. Strolling adults are unaware that they walk through a game of stickball at a crucial moment, while the children barely pause to let the invaders pass. The conversations and greetings of the adults mingle in the observer's ear with the shouts, chants, and jeers of the children, but the two sets of sounds do not interpenetrate each other. And along the shifting boundaries between these two societies are strung the younger children, the toddlers and young preschoolers the responsibility of the adults, the older preschool and young middle-years children the province of older brothers and sisters, who keep watch on them with a bored but remarkably efficient eye. Some of the children on the fringes are making the transition to the gang. Instead of hanging back and keeping out of the way, they begin to move in around the edges, watching, listening, taking in, imitating doggedly, and participating when allowed to, gratefully accepting whatever roles or crumbs of attention that come their way. For children in the early middle years, somewhat older children are invested with enormous authority and prestige. In many ways, the children who have arrived in gang society appear more grown-up and knowledgeable to them than do adults. By age eight or nine, the transfer of affiliation and loyalty from the adults to the gang is nearly complete.

Parents are often distressed to find that their erstwhile loving child now seems to have lost his affectionate and confiding nature and become a stranger to his family. He is likely to be taciturn, sullen, and insolent. He affects odd mannerisms, gaits, and postures. When he does speak, his speech is likely to be slurred and careless. He uses the special, restricted language of the gang. He praises things with "keen," "swell," "cool," "a fun thing," "neatsy." Currently popular pejoratives are "junk" and "queer." The child uses the scatology of the streets liberally, partly to shock his parents and partly to demonstrate his sophistication. The argot of the middle years is often the teen-age slang of yesterday.

The group-oriented child seems to live only for the moment when he can tear from the house and join the other kids, leaving, if he can get away with it, chores and lessons undone. Parents, seeing their child draw away from them, may be moved to become more demonstrative or possessive, to quiz the child about what is ailing him, or to storm at him for lack of filial devotion. Such measures are more likely to drive the child deeper into the gang than to win him back to the family. The child is taking a necessary step on the road to maturity, he is filing his private Declaration of Independence—an independence, let us remember, that is in fact merely submission to a new set of controls. Furthermore, we cannot take the child's behavior at face value. Much of his behavior is role playing, doing what is expected of him, and this applies to all the kids in the gang. If the child turns strongly against his family, it is probably a measure of the strength of the bonds that tie him to it and have to be overcome. If he is all bravado and self-assertion, it is because he has to cover up his doubts and anxieties.

It is not from his parents alone but from the adult world in general that the child declares his independence. On the lips of school-age children, "the grownups" is a term of derogation. The teacher who invites the children to identify some miscreant will meet a wall of silence which masks outrage that the children should be asked to violate the code against snitching. In schools where adult policies and conduct give the children little to resent, it sometimes seems that the children will invent issues just to test themselves against adult authority. In such cases, of course, some of the children may half-humorously half-recognize that they are inflating a trivial matter out of all proportion. Commonly, the child invokes gang authority to counterweight parental authority: "Gee, Mom, all the other kids . . ." (are going on a particular outing, have later bedtimes, get permanent waves, watch a forbidden television show). Sometimes gangs, especially of boys, do things that seem expressly designed to arouse adult retaliation just so that they can outrun or outwit it. It is a lot more fun to steal apples from an orchard or a pushcart if you are seen and chased. Adults who view such behavior either disapprovingly or indulgently ("Boys will be boys") may be missing the psychological point: I can stand up to adults and survive.

The extremism of the child's declaration of independence reflects the fact that every middle-years child is more or less in the position of what Margaret Mead[7] has called the "immigrant personality." The child of immigrant parents in the United States typically finds himself ashamed of his parents' foreign, old-fashioned ways and strives feverishly to be as unlike them and as like members of the host culture as possible. So it is with the school-age child, whether or not the child of immigrants. In his case, of course, the host culture is the subculture of childhood. And his parents, no matter how solidly American, are no longer the source of all wisdom and power. Indeed, they may appear all too contemptibly weak and mundane and merely human. By this age, the child has overheard too many parental quarrels, witnessed too many episodes of worry and panic, been too often the butt of arbitrary adult authority, ever again to believe in the omniscience and omnipotence of adults. This is the age at which some children spin "foundling fantasies," suspicions, often reaching the point of profound conviction, that the child is of exalted birth and by some dreadful mischance has fallen into the hands of base-born foster parents.

In our society, the attitudes of both immigrant and native-born parents abet the immigrant-personality syndrome in their children. In the case of immigrants, no matter how firmly they cling to the old-country customs and values, parents are likely to feel ashamed of their ignorance and differentness and to take pride in their children's successful Americanization. Even native American parents share with their children the assumption that the younger generation will outstrip the older in both attainment and wisdom. As Mead has pointed out, parents are aware that the world their children are growing up in is in fact radically different from the one they knew as children and will be still more radically different by the time their children have grown up, so that many of the established precedents are becoming outmoded. The children know this, too, and feel that their parents belong to an alien era, just as the children of immigrants feel that their parents belong to an alien place. Children have always retorted that "Times have changed" when parents launched upon a lecture beginning "When I was a boy" (or girl). In times past, though, the parents have always felt secure in the belief that there were eternal verities transcending the fads and foibles of the moment. Now, by contrast, they realize that the eternal verities have been left behind by the political, economic, moral, social, scientific, technological, and philosophical revolutions of the century. Unfortunately, this realization has tended to weaken the parents' confidence in their own authority. How prescribe for life in a world transformed beyond recognition? As we shall see later, parents must somehow continue to find the strength to be parents, but meanwhile let us return to the child and his gang.

381

We have already pointed out that social organization changes during the school years. Probably the first real coalition of young school children consists in the sharing of a secret and the formation of best-friend attachments—which may change from day to day, and which may inspire the announcement, "You know what? I have four best friends!" Genuine affiliation and stable group membership, and the climax of love for the secret society, are found in the middle middle years. By the later middle years, clubs and gangs are less likely to exist primarily for the sake of belongingness or for the formal rites they practice, and are more likely to be organized around particular kinds of activities and functions. The older school child is likely to be involved in and handle easily (although not without conflicts) multiple memberships and affiliations. The fact that he is moving closer to adult society and its distinctions and discriminations is also evident in the composition of the groups and cliques to which he belongs. Within a given sixth grade, there is likely to be a clearcut social hierarchy (or two hierarchies, one for boys and one for girls) with very little contact between adjacent strata. The patterning of social organization during the middle years reveals the same principles of differentiation and functional subordination as other aspects of development. For instance, the gang spirit differentiates out of the totality of fellow feeling and at first is valuable in its own right, so that just being with the gang is satisfaction enough. Later, the value lies in the things the increasingly better integrated gang does.

Depending on the number of children available, the neighborhood play group, with its unannounced but regular meetings before and after supper, may either include a variety of kids playing together or break down into subgroups divided by age and sex. In some areas, there is direct continuity between early childhood play groups and adolescent street-corner society, or even adult-sponsored delinquent gangs. Some urban delinquent gangs maintain their organizational identities intact while successive generations of youngsters pass through them. In rural areas, and to some extent in the suburbs, children's friendships depend on family friendships and contacts made in school. Play groups are likely to include perforce a wider range of ages, although boys and girls tend to play separately. In cities, affiliations are usually made within the home block. Outside "our block," one is in alien or even hostile territory. Notice that possessiveness toward and readiness to defend the home "turf" have much in common with the territoriality of many infrahuman species, observed in birds most strongly during the mating season.[8]

Since geographical divisions in many American communities correspond very closely to ethnic and economic divisions, neighborhood affiliations may help perpetuate in children's society the same segregation and prejudices that prevail in adult society. (Needless to say, specific indoctrination in prejudice also plays its part.) However, children's groupings along geographical lines in the cities are partly counteracted by other influences: schools that draw children from several neighborhoods (although "ability" groupings within the school may simply mirror neighborhood groupings), adult-fostered visiting relationships, the chance to meet children in formal after-school programs and at summer camp, the common experience provided by the mass media, and the telephone, which is fast becoming as important a medium for school-age kids as it is for adolescents. (The younger school child transacts his business and hangs up; older children hold protracted, often whispered and furtive exchanges.) In the suburbs, the school, adult-organized activities, the family car, and considerations of which friendships are socially advantageous for "my child" become powerful determinants of affiliation patterns.

Certain individual children—usually the best-looking, the biggest, the strongest, the most physically mature, in some circles the brightest, the most energetic, the wittiest—acquire a great deal of popularity and, with it, some power of leadership. However, children of this age are in many respects hard-headed pragmatists, and when it comes to engaging in particular activities—a game of baseball, say, or staging a play—they look for leadership to those children competent in that activity.[9] Popularity may weigh heavily in choice of activity, but once the decision has been made, practical considerations take over. The technique of sociometry (see page 218) reveals how leadership shifts from one undertaking to another.

Let us repeat and emphasize that group membership has two faces: belongingness and exclusion. Just as six-year-olds love simultaneously to share a secret and to define its secretness by keeping it from someone else, ten-year-olds, in forming a club, can experience a sense of "we"-ness only by leaving out "them." Something of the flavor of a school-age club, apart from the ceremonial aspects, is well conveyed in the following quotation from *The New Yorker:*

> The rules of a secret society of nine- and ten-year-old girls in a certain community on Long Island that shall here be nameless are as follows:

1. Do not tell a white lie unless necessary.
2. Do not hurt anyone in any way.
3. Do not hit anyone except Ronny.
4. Do not tell a black lie.
5. Do not use words worse than "brat."
6. Do not curse at all.
7. Do not make faces except at Ronny.
8. Do not be selfish.
9. Do not make a hog or a pig of yourself.
10. Do not tattle except on Ronny.
11. Do not steal except from Ronny.
12. Do not destroy other people's property, except Ronny's.
13. Do not be a sneak.
14. Do not be grumpy except to Ronny.
15. Do not answer back except to Ronny.*

Usually, a number of children are left out and they in turn form an equally exclusive club of their own. Notice that such clubs commonly have an overabundance of officers, codified rules, ceremonies, oaths, and vague but portentous secrets. The members enunciate ambitious if ambiguous goals, but the underlying, unspoken motivation seems always to be to formalize and solidify belongingness. Sometimes, however, a child gets left out or is deliberately excluded from all memberships. Such children often are cast in the role of scapegoats on whom children higher in the pecking order can vent all their hostility and antipathy. Rejection by the entire group points to the despotic nature of majority rule: The minority of one experiences a strong, if perhaps temporary, inner conviction that the group must be right and that there must be something wrong with him. Herein lies the tragedy for the permanently or repeatedly excluded individual, whether the exclusion be on personal or ethnic grounds.

Every child who comes into a new neighborhood is at first a minority group member as he faces the bristling outside of in-group feeling. We can be thankful that middle-years group organization is unstable, offering, during periods of reorganization, openings through which the excluded individual can slip inside—provided, of course, that his exclusion was not on ethnic grounds. Notice that ethnic and racial prejudices work both ways: It comes as a shock to many white Americans that their skin is a signal for dislike. A fascinating series of studies by Sherif and associates[10] has shown how one can produce and undo prejudice experi-

* By permission, copyright, 1954, The New Yorker Magazine, Inc., September 18, 1954.

mentally by varying group composition and goals and by putting goals in a competitive or cooperative framework.

THE SEX CLEAVAGE, SEX ROLES, AND SEX DIFFERENCES

The tendency for the sexes to go their separate ways begins in the late preschool years and reaches a peak at about age ten. First- and second-graders invite both boys and girls to their birthday parties (or whatever other occasions are thus celebrated), but by age eight the idea of including the opposite sex in any kind of formal social arrangement becomes unthinkable (or so it used to be). This cleavage of the sexes is partly a matter of different interests and activities, but at a more basic level it is built into the childhood culture, probably a vestige of ancient adult cultural views on the inferiority of the second sex. Girls continue to play house and games like hopscotch and jacks, while boys roam farther, play rougher, wrestle, and learn baseball. The institutionalization of the sex cleavage, such that one must actively profess disdain of the opposite sex, suggests that here, as in declaring one's independence of adults, one must go to extremes to assert one's boyness or girlness.

Virtually all boys go through a period when they reject the female sex (with the possible exception of their mothers), loudly announcing vows of total, permanent celibacy. Notice that the knightly ideal, which found its ultimate expression in the cult of the Virgin, depicts womankind both as a fragile vessel to be placed on a pedestal and worshiped from afar and as a Delilah who, given half a chance, will castrate the male and drain him of his manhood. The knightly idea is perpetuated in the rhetoric that surrounds Mother's Day (Father's Day is a pallid afterthought), in the teaching given to athletes and military personnel, and in the standard cowboy movie, which no longer gets filmed but which nonetheless haunts late-evening television. Middle-years boys experience a mixture of puzzlement, outrage, and contempt when they see their just-older heroes, who until now have shared, and perhaps even taught them, their misogyny, beginning to tolerate and even seek out the company of girls.

Girls, by contrast, although expressing a complementary disdain for boys, nevertheless carry along a romantic vision of domesticity in which they picture themselves as brides and even as mothers and housewives, but mated to misty figures bearing no resemblance to the grubby, uncouth boys they know in real life. In the same vein, girls of this age may enjoy "love" movies, whereas boys are volubly disgusted by them. It should be stressed that many mature young women enter marriage in the spirit of the young girl's daydreams, with almost any presentable male cast in the role of groom, and with the focus on an elaborate nuptial ceremony and reception, with what comes later left in the vague realm of "happily ever after." It is also worth stressing that the mothers of girls may begin playing the marriage game when their daughters are hardly out of the cradle, arranging circumstances and encounters that will guarantee the girl an early and socially satisfactory marriage. Such mothers may themselves be thoroughly disenchanted with the institution of marriage, but they have not been able to shake loose from the idea that marriage is the ideal state for women. The women's suffrage movement early in the century aimed to win for women the right to vote, and, in addition, sought to emancipate women from the bonds of matrimony. In the 1940's and 1950's, a reaction set in, expressed in what Betty Friedan[11] has scathingly described as *The Feminine Mystique,* and the homemaker role for women was actively glorified. Now, perhaps as a product of increased education, women are once again seeking to define a new role and a new image for themselves, in which love, sex, marriage, and parenthood can each be considered in its own right rather than as part of a package deal in which one cannot have one without all the others.

The sex cleavage shows up too in attitudes toward pets. Boys and girls both love animals, but with a difference. Girls typically love puppies and kittens, which some would interpret as an expression of a maternal instinct, and such relatively inert creatures as guinea pigs, rabbits, fish (the heroic measures some girls will take to keep guppies from eating their young are a wonder to behold), and parrots in all their varieties. Boys, by contrast, like dogs, who can serve as companions and stunt artists. Boys used to like horses, perhaps in identification with cowboy heroes, but seem to have transferred their affections to motorcycles and motorcars. Girls, on the other hand, love horses to the point of mania, collecting pictures and figurines and begging for riding lessons. Girls have been known to select a college because it had its own stables. Some psychoanalysts have interpreted the girl's affection for horses as an expression of the masculine protest and an accompanying penis envy (see page 168). In this view, control over such a powerful creature would be a symbolic subordination (and perhaps castration) of the male.

The sex cleavage is not, however, absolute. Brothers and sisters sometimes play together, especially when there are no other playmates available. If there are few children in the neighborhood, boys and girls intermingle. Late in the middle years, boys engage in sham-hostile invasions of girls' play groups, girls stand around making fun of the boys at play, and in the neighborhood play group, games of tag, catching, and mock-wrestling go on between the sexes, signaling the breaking down of the barriers in anticipation of adolescence. With the approach of puberty, though, girls are likely to turn their attention to older boys—and sometimes to develop crushes on older women or men—rather than to make peace with their male contemporaries.

Whether they play apart or together, boys and girls do many of the same things. Nonetheless, there is a distinct bifurcation of tastes, interests, and activities during the middle years, some areas of play being entirely feminine and others almost entirely masculine—a few girls are likely to participate in predominantly male pursuits, but practically no boys ever openly engage in what are thought of as purely female ones. However, as our culture changes, and as girls get bigger and stronger and thus able to compete with boys on a more nearly equal physical basis, it seems likely that the interests of the two sexes will become more similar. Unfortunately, there are no up-to-date findings on sex differences, and the older research is unreliable both because children have changed and because they engage in a different array of activities nowadays. In fact, the older lists of games contain entries like Salvation Army, Pound the Back, and Halma, that the authors are at a loss to recognize.

In general, boys tend to be doers and girls talkers. Boys tend to be oriented to things, with a special emphasis on things mechanical, and girls to people and social relations. Girls engage in sports (including touch football), but boys in addition read about them, idolizing the heroes and clustering in search of autographs around the hotel where the visiting team is staying. Girls like to ride bicycles, but boys also enjoy taking bicycles apart and putting them back together. In school, girls perform better than boys in the early years but gradually slip back into second place.

Girls think about love whereas boys are curious about sex—and, in the gang, exchange endless sex lore and sometimes engage in sexual experiments, including simultaneous masturbation, reciprocal masturbation, or even fellatio and other sexual acts. Obviously, many a school-age girl and boy have engaged in reciprocal sexual inspection ("I'll show you mine if you'll show me yours"), but heterosexual exploration at this age, to the best of the authors' knowledge, rarely goes beyond this. Apparently it does not spontaneously occur to middle-years boys and girls that they can stimulate each other's genitals other than by coitus, and their occasional clumsy attempts at intercourse are almost certain to meet with frustration, if only for reasons of anatomy and mechanics. Middle-years girls may have powerful sexual fantasies, but they apparently engage in homosexual activities only when these are initiated by an older woman, such as a tutor or governess. It is possible that boys' homosexual experience in the gang arouses or expresses a streak of latent homosexuality in American males (as the widespread homosexuality in the British public schools seems to produce a great deal of practicing homosexuality in upper-class male adults; as one observer put it, "It is more than the old school tie that binds the Establishment together"), which might help account for the adult American male's ambivalence toward women, his liking for all-male activities, and his sometimes frantic assertions of masculinity, as when he projects an image of himself as the fearless, two-fisted frontiersman or makes a great compensatory display of sexual prowess.

Boys generally identify more strongly with the gang and peer culture than do girls, who remain parent-oriented even while identifying with their peers. Indeed, the male peer culture is very different from and in many instances at odds with the standards of adult culture, while the female peer culture, although distinct from that of adults, is very much like it. Not all boy groups, of course, are preoccupied with physical action. Some, perhaps the more bookish, like to relive the Robin Hood or King Arthur legends, or invent private countries or planets or historic events which they can draw or write about or stage in makeshift but no less heroic dramatizations.

The differing interests and activities and attitudes of boys and girls can be thought of as expressions of their sex roles, their assumptions, spoken or tacit, about what it means to be a girl or a boy. Since conceptions of sex roles differ greatly from culture to culture, it seems safe to conclude that sex roles are in some part learned. Some explicit teaching of sex roles ("Big boys don't cry," "It's not ladylike to sit that way") is done by adults, older children, and age mates. A considerable portion of the learning of sex roles, however, takes place after the manner of operant conditioning, by virtue of the rewards and punishments—the feedback—one gets for acting in appropriate or inappropriate ways (as defined by the culture). Then, too, a certain amount comes to pass as a result of deliberate or unconscious imitation of the models, real and fictional, that one is exposed to and who exemplify masculine and feminine styles of life. One can speak of a sex role as a set of social expectations, the way people expect other people of a given anatomical sort to behave. The ways sex roles are taught and learned are called collectively *sex-typing*. In the learning of sex roles, there seems to be a learning set, or snowball, effect. Thus, once the child has taken on certain aspects of the masculine or feminine role, he or she is then more open to the incorporation of further aspects of that role, so that masculinity breeds further masculinity and femininity femininity.

The anthropologist Ruth Benedict[12] has written of cultural differences in *continuity of sex roles*. In our society, sex-role continuity seems to be greater for girls than for boys. If we assume that the female adult role is that of wife, parent, homemaker, and participant in local school and community affairs, then we can see how even the childhood culture of the girl prepares her for such a role. By contrast, the boy's childhood culture teaches him to be a hunter, woodsman, warrior, roustabout, and free-swinging playboy, which is quite at variance with the life he faces as husband, father, citizen, and good provider who will earn his living at desk or workbench. (Let us note that there are occupations more or less continuous with boyhood culture, like being a forest ranger, but only a few of these, such as the military and the construction industry, employ large numbers of people; and even if the boy grows up to enter such an occupation, it is usually combined with a domesticity for which boyhood has prepared him hardly at all.) The girl's role continuity is further enhanced by the fact that child-rearing, at home and at school, is largely in the hands of women. In one respect, though, we feel that there is some disadvantage for girls as well as for boys in having so much of their upbringing taken care of by women: Just as boys may lack male models to identify with at firsthand, so may girls lack males to relate to. A further complication is that women are looking for a new image of themselves, and there are very few models to tell them what this new image might be. The girl's female preceptors expect her to be like them, or at least like the ideal selves that they aspire to.

The situation for boys is also difficult but in a different way. The boy's female preceptors expect him to meet their standards of decorum, yet if he fails to exhibit a certain amount of rebellious spirit, of aggressiveness, of boisterousness, and even of ruthlessness, adults—women and men—become perturbed and feel that "something is missing." The role expectation for boys includes the parts of both Little Lord Fauntleroy and Tom Sawyer. The boy is taught obedience, generosity, and kindness, but if he does not stand up for his rights he is scorned as a sissy. Besides meeting adult role expectations, of course, the boy has to measure up to the rather different role expectations of the gang. Conflicts apart, boys are expected, perhaps in anticipation of their later responsibilities, to be ambitious and to strive for tangible achievement. Let us remember, however, that adults do not realize they are teaching their children to play sex roles but believe, rather, that they are simply witnessing, now with trepidation and now with satisfaction, the natural unfolding of male and female development.

The accomplishment-oriented role expectations for boys, plus the conflicts in expectations, plus the lack of adequate models, may account for the fact that boys are consistently more prone than girls to minor and major emotional, scholastic, and behavior problems (although mortality statistics suggest that boys may be biologically more vulnerable than girls). Boys are more likely than girls to stutter, to have reading disabilities, to wet the bed, to develop tics, to be rowdy and undisciplined, to become schizophrenic, and to run afoul of the authorities. The most central male difficulty seems to be control of aggression, and it is in this area that role expectations are most ambiguous, with conflicting and subtle pressures to act out one's feelings in some circumstances and to restrain them in others. But the incidence of misbehavior in the two sexes is not simply a matter of what children do; it is also a matter of how adults judge what children do. Research has shown that girls' misbehavior is judged more leniently than boys'—partly because boys, with greater available energy, make more noise in the course of misbehaving—which suggests that the greater frequency of misdeeds by boys may be an artifact of greater adult sensitivity to its occurrence.[13] A similar tendency

The role expectation for boys includes the parts of both Little Lord Fauntleroy and Tom Sawyer.

Wayne Miller

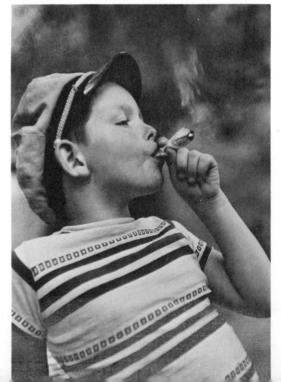

may be at work in the fact that girls get better grades in school, whereas boys score higher on academic aptitude and achievement tests. And we must not forget that the people who judge behavior and give school marks are very often women.

The long-term effect of education and of a sophisticated culture in which there is less demand on sheer muscle is to make males more feminine and females more masculine. Historically, as the level of education rises, men become capable of greater tenderness, take an interest in domestic affairs, consider women their partners rather than their chattels, and take an interest in esthetic matters. At the same time, women become less flighty and capricious, become more analytical and logical, assert their right to sexual equality, and enter traditionally masculine occupational fields. These changed patterns are transmitted culturally in the educated classes, whereas the children of uneducated parents move in this direction as they rise through the educational system. This is not to say that in the future all sex differences will be abolished. It does imply

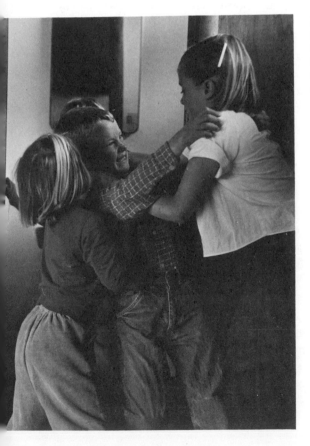

If siblings are fairly close in age and are all within the middle-years age band, their contacts at home are likely to be marked by baiting, bantering, bickering, battling, belittling, and bedlam . . .

Wayne Miller

that, as parents, teachers, and social engineers, we can see through the artificiality and even perniciousness of some of our sex-role expectations. We brutalize boys when we expect them to be cave men living in a technological, educated, humane society, and we brutalize girls when we expect little from them in the way of intellect and creativity, and when, on the other hand, we expect them to be passive, docile, accepting, and cast in traditional roles. In Freudian terms, we cultivate the boy's id and superego, we cultivate the girl's superego, and neglect the ego development of boys and girls alike.

Home and Family

In order to make various features of the child's behavior stand out, we have to exaggerate them, and in the process we tend to distort and caricature them. Thus, both the child and the authors overdo his declaration of independence from the family. In fact, home and family continue to be an important emotional refuge and source of learning, entertainment, and companionship throughout these years. To begin with, some of peer-group life is lived within the home. Singly or in small groups, children visit each other's abodes, becoming involved in kite- or model-building projects, sometimes grandiose in conception and hurried in execution, in jewelry-making or embroidery, in writing and staging plays, in table games, in drawing pictures, in sharing marathon feasts in front of the television screen, sprawled in remarkable postures which may indeed be genuinely restful but are at the same time part of middle-years role playing.

But the child has siblings as well as friends, and we should take a moment to look at his dealings with his brothers and sisters. Granted that every family and every relationship is unique, we can still risk some generalizations. If siblings are fairly close in age and are all within the middle-years age band, their contacts at home are likely to be marked by baiting, bantering, bickering, battling, belittling, and bedlam, interspersed with some joint activities, some comparing of notes on school, people, activities, tastes and preferences, and, lest we overlook it, some more or less harmonious sharing in whole-family enterprises and in chores. (We should observe that many poor families have no all-family activities, not even whole-family meals.) If there are two siblings of the same sex and fairly close in age, the older often takes the role of mentor to the younger: Sometimes this is welcomed and accepted, sometimes not. When sibs are in different periods of development, as when a school child has preschool or adolescent brothers or sisters, the gulf is likely to seem unbridgeable. The postpubertal elder is inclined to be particularly critical of the grubby, noisy, ill-mannered, sassy younger child. He sometimes expresses this in open rage, occasionally through slaps and blows, and sometimes in elaborately haughty doubts as to their common parentage. The school-ager, in turn, shrewdly hacks or picks away at the adolescent's new and precarious dignity. A preschool brother or sister, on the other hand, is seen by the middle-years child as constantly underfoot or tagging along, disturbing and wrecking his property, and receiving favors and indulgences from the parents such as he was certainly never granted in the long bygone days (and since parents tend to be more indulgent with successive children, he may be right). The elder child is highly jealous of the hard-won prerogatives of his age, while the younger resents them as preferential. If the younger child is much younger, an infant or a toddler or young preschooler, and so not in competition with the middle-years child, he is likely to be treated affectionately and indulgently—if sometimes as a nuisance. Occasionally, a new baby comes into the family after the first crop of children has reached adolescence. In such cases, the adolescents often seem to pitch into the role of assistant parents with great zeal.

Parents, all too aware of the turbulent aspects of sibling relations at home, are often thoroughly startled to learn how the children close ranks in family solidarity outside the home when one of them is threatened or abused. The terms "kid brother" and "big sister" may be used disparagingly, but they also carry considerable affection, which is supposed to be masked from the gang. It should further be pointed out that lower-class middle-years children, rather more often than middle-class ones, are likely to be put in charge of their younger brothers and sisters, who play on the edges of the group while the games go forward. It should be noted, too, that this responsibility for the younger kids is usually coupled with real authority over them. It is possible that the wielding of such authority is intrinsically satisfying in its own right, fits in well with the child's drive for independence, and enhances identification with the parents and their segment of society. Such responsibility is very common in many other cultures.

For all their insistence on freedom and privacy from adults, for all their sassiness and rebelliousness, and for all the fault they find with their parents and parental ways, children do not suddenly stop loving their parents. Indeed, as in displays of sibling solidarity, the same children who criticize their parents freely will not tolerate the slightest slur on them from outside the family. Parents cannot hope to remain high on a pedestal, but if they can bring themselves to climb down gracefully, they will find that there are other bases on which to be parents. And let us stress that there is no sight more pathetic than a father or mother trying to be a "pal" to son or daughter (not that there is any lack of things that they can enjoy doing together). There are plenty of peers around to serve as pals, and the child needs his parents as parents, which means as adults and not as pseudochildren. He needs them to turn to when he feels cut off from the gang in one of its periodic realignments, when he is sick or at other vulnerable moments, he needs them as consultants on ethical and moral problems, and simply at times when he wants to be a member of his family, trading news and jokes and confidences, asking for information and advice and help with homework. At bedtime, he is likely to welcome a frolic, being read to (even though he is a perfectly proficient reader), and cuddling (those boys who have been taught that demonstrations of affection are unmanly may reject cuddling, but we suspect that they crave it nonetheless).

The child boasts of his parents' achievements to the gang, perhaps partly in hopes of gaining prestige but also because he is identifying with his parents, no matter how grudgingly. The child's conscious models are the gang and the gang's heroes: cowboys, nurses, athletes, movie and television stars, and other glamorous luminaries. It is mostly when one's father happens to be in an interesting and visible occupation—plumber, fisherman, garbage collector, fireman—that direct and conscious identification takes place. The case is more difficult for mothers, whose domestic activities form so accustomed a background of the child's life as to be all but invisible, or, when the child has to help out, are experienced as drudgery pure and simple. (In emergencies, such as a maternal illness, the children may pitch in with real enthusiasm.) Even if she has a career, it is unlikely to meet the double specifications of glamor and visibility.

Whatever the manner of the child's identification, he continues to need regulation. He may need parental backing to maintain his own values in the face of group pressure. Just as he expects privileges—a growing allowance, later bedtime, more freedom to roam, as he passes various developmental milestones—in keeping with increasing maturity, so is he able to accept increasing responsibility. When the child shares in family prosperity or hard times, in its triumphs and disasters, when he contributes by picking up his room at age six, by making his bed and doing dishes and hanging up laundry at age ten, by shoveling the driveway or raking the yard at age twelve, when he has an appropriate part in family decisions—whether to acquire a pet, where to spend a vacation—he is becoming aware of the bonds of reciprocity that tie together a family, and, eventually, the world. It is worth noting that the democratic privileges accorded to children are still limited and subject to adult authority. Children in the school years are not usually ready for full democratic self-determination. But sound authority, even when it hurts them the most, is on their side and is aimed at producing sane, rational, sensitive, humane adults.

Even though adults must be strong, their authority, with children of this age, cannot be absolute. Parents have to recognize children's commitment to the peer-group mores and understand the importance of the group for the child's growth toward independence. Obviously, adults have to combat the gang's more pernicious teachings, but in full awareness of the constructive functions of group affiliation. The peer culture is a mixed blessing, but we do not know of any substitute for it or shortcut to the benefits it brings. Here, as at all ages, parents must be prepared to let the child try out some enterprises that the parents know to be foredoomed, to let him make some mistakes and, we hope, to learn from making them. And it is the job of parents to support the child through the pain of failure and to help him learn the lessons it teaches—without rubbing it in.

Sexual Latency and Growth Latency

Earlier, we defined Freud's concept of *latency* as a hiatus in sexual interest and activity beginning with the resolution and repression of the Oedipus complex and ending with the urgent reawakening of sexual desires associated with puberty. In Freudian terms, the sex cleavage of the middle years, accompanied by a lavish show of indifference and even animosity toward the opposite sex, would be a reaction formation, a going to the opposite extreme, in order to keep sexual impulses repressed. The upsurge of intellectual curiosity observed in school children would be a sublimation, a transformation of repressed sexual energies, and also a disguised sexual curiosity. The child's rituals, chants, and rigid adherence to rules and formulas would be viewed as magical devices for controlling impulses and feelings, including the anxieties and hostilities brought on by the traumatic climax of the Oedipal drama.

In point of fact, the collective and individual rituals of school-age children bear a marked resemblance to the behavior of adults burdened with what psychiatrists call an *obsessive-compulsive* neurosis. Obsessions, which do not always accompany compulsions, consist of the thoughts one cannot get rid of, like the snatches of melody that run unwanted, mindlessly and maddeningly, through consciousness. Obsessive humming, recitation, and counting are common in the school years. Adult compulsions are an irresistible need to perform some useless act: to wash one's hands repeatedly, to check the door locks over and over again before leaving the house, an incessant taking stock and tallying of things and arrangements, arranging one's work materials neatly over and over again before starting work, and other senseless but obligatory rituals, such as rubbing one's hands together three times, that precede any action and that sometimes become so protracted that the action itself is never begun.

There are two ways of looking at compulsions, and perhaps two types of compulsions, both relevant to behavior in the middle years. The first sees compulsive rituals as a way of giving order, meaning, and manageability to a world in flux, and so of finding security and certainty. Compulsive preparatory rituals are a way of making sure that everything is in place so that one can safely act, or perhaps even a device for postponing indefinitely a secretly undesired action. The second perspective on, or type of, compulsive behavior is as a disguised, symbolic enactment of an impulse or past event that is too strong to be wholly repressed but too threatening to be admitted directly to awareness or acted on. Thus, compulsive handwashing might be interpreted as expressing feelings of uncleanliness generated by one's unacknowledged "dirty" cravings. Analogously, the child's rituals may be seen as a partial expression of imperfectly repressed Oedipal urges.

However, Freud's original notion of latency as an asexual time-out has had to be modified in the light of what we now know about sexuality in the middle years. Sexual interest and play are not snuffed out, but are simply hidden from adult attention. It is worth noting that whereas Freud had to combat the popular belief that there was no infantile sexuality to become latent, the post-Freudians have to combat Freud's idea that there is a gap in the chain of overt psychosexual development. A possible reconciliation, not inconsistent with psychoanalytic theory, is that it is only attraction to the parent of the opposite sex that is repressed, making possible attention to other sexual objects.

Children, regardless of any theory, are eager to acquire forbidden information and to pass it on to other children. We have already mentioned some of the actual sexual behavior that goes on during these years. By the middle school years, there is a steady traffic among children in off-color stories, which may be poorly comprehended but are sure to elicit titters and giggles. Children likewise giggle together over the dictionary in which they look up words referring to sexual or excretory functions, or over the Bible in which they look up references to fornication. The doctor's child is guaranteed popularity by allowing his friends to consult the plates in medical texts. One outcome of the child's researches is his discovery that sex is a general human phenomenon, and not just something peculiar to him and his group. Notice also that sex and toilet functions are poorly differentiated at this age. We should also note the sexual component in the teasing and tussling between boys and girls of this age, and in the bodily discovery and mastery underlying the physical skills and stunts the child practices.

It is not always easy to tell, of course, the extent to which the child's sexual behavior is motivated by real, internal lusts and cravings, and to what extent by simple curiosity, especially curiosity about the unknown and forbidden. It is our guess, however, that spontaneous lust rarely arises much before the end of this period, and that sexual feelings have to be externally stimulated or, once the child has learned about the possibility, self-stimulated. But whatever the motivational basis of their sexual curiosity and behavior, children know that such things are frowned on by adults and the mere mention of them will meet with explicit threats (some of our children are still being told that masturbation will stunt their growth, or cause mental deficiency or insanity, or cause disease, or cause the penis to drop off), reproaches, or, at best, a strained reserve and a sense that one is in taboo territory. As a result, most children experience some anxiety and guilt in connection with their sexual investigations.

SEX EDUCATION

Children are further made aware of adult ambivalence about sex and of the ambiguity of taboos, including adult violations of taboos. Indeed, in this area as in such others as honesty in money matters (including income tax and traffic fines), generosity, telling the truth, levels of competence and importance, adult hypocrisy becomes plainly evident to children of this age. The parents themselves, who grew up under even more restrictive conditions, can be pardoned if they feel that sex is a highly sensitive topic about which it is hard to talk to children. Yet most parents feel that they want their children to know the facts of sex, to understand them, and to grow up to enjoy sex wisely and thoroughly. Their first problem is to know for themselves what the morally and psychologically relevant standards are for the conduct of adult sexuality. This is something that they have to decide for themselves, since the culture today provides answers ranging all the way from total sexual license, whereby it would be rude and selfish to refuse just about any prospective partner, to a harsh puritanism which says that sex should be enjoyed minimally, and then only in the narrow context of procreation, disarranging one's nightclothes as little as possible.

The second problem for parents is to know what to tell children and how and when. To take the last question, that of timing, first, the school-age child, with his greater wariness about expressing his feelings and his awareness of adult taboos, is less likely than the preschool child to cue his parents with specific questions. All the same, the parents can be sure that the child is picking up information and misinformation—and attitudes—from his contemporaries, and if the parents wish priority for their views, they should begin giving information sooner rather than later. As with the preschool child—to move to the what and how part of the problem—this is never done once and for all; it must be taught and retaught at increasingly complex and concrete levels. Certainly in dealing with children in the later middle years, there is no reason a girl should be left to experience her first menstruation as a shocking and perhaps terrifying surprise, as so many girls still do, or why boys, for that matter, should not have some factual knowledge of the menstrual cycle instead of deep ignorance or a dim awareness, fed by Biblical or other sources, of some great, dark female secret. The principle of early timing applies not only to anticipating events or rival information, but is important also in giving information while it is still primarily of informational interest, before it gets mixed up with the emotional storms of adolescence.

The question of how to impart knowledge may also be one of who imparts it. Frank discussion of sexual matters between parent and child may imply an intimacy that both find very trying, and it is possible that somebody else should do the job. As one insightful ten-year-old observed to her teacher, "My parents are very understanding and all that, but there are some things it's easier to talk about with other people." The "somebody else" may be a book designed for young readers, of which there are several excellent ones available.[14] It may be an uncle or an aunt, a family friend, a physician, a clergyman, a recreation group leader, or a teacher, although none of these positions guarantees that the person has the requisite knowledge, skill, sensitivity, and wisdom for the task.

The teacher who sets out to impart sex information must feel secure herself, must have already won the confidence and respect of the children, must have some sort of understanding with the children's parents (some proportion of parents simply do not want their children to know about sex, although how they can keep them from finding out that there is such a thing eludes us), and must deal with small enough groups of children so that she can discuss rather than lecture, maintaining a one-to-one relationship with each child (the tittering bystander changes the whole tone of the situation). Under such optimal conditions, the teacher can deal with mixed groups of boys and girls. However, if she—or he—makes tactful opportunities for it, she is more likely to be approached by individuals or by small same-sex groups seeking enlightenment.

The what of sex education has to include more than where babies come from, and cannot leave children with the sense that sex is one more pleasant activity along with eating sweets, watching television, playing children's games, and going for outings with the family. It is not enough to say that sex is beautiful or that it occurs in a context of love. The parent or other instructor has to convey, preferably before the upheavals of adolescence begin, some idea of the urgency of sex drives, of the ecstatic pleasure of erotic experience, sex differences in sexuality, the varieties of sexual experience and stimulation, and, more subtly, of the place of sex in temporary as well as in more profound and lasting relationships between people. From this point of view, we consider it desirable, when parents are comfortable in communication, for the boy to get some sex truths and views from his mother and the girl from her father—if only inside warning of the wiles and ploys of the other sex. The parent who has been frank in these respects will find it easier, as the need requires, to convey the role of sex in mature love, and the desirability, in terms of such later relationships, in terms of one's own feelings of personal integrity, and in terms of enjoying sex in all its fullness, of accepting restraints on and postponements of gratification.

The authors are not prepared to say when the right moment comes for which kinds of sexual experience. It is clear that many school-age children are seduced into one kind of sexual activity or another, by other children, by adolescents, or by adults of their own sex or the opposite sex, for the most part without apparent harm. The ultimate meaning of childhood sexual experience has to be judged in terms of how it influences the individual's self-image relative to other people, and this, in turn, has to be judged in the context of the values and disvalues assigned by the culture to various forms of interpersonal relations. We strongly suspect, however, that the child's sexual taste and discrimination will be learned less from parental admonition than from the concrete behavior of the adult world. Above all, it is the child's parents who provide a model of adult love and affection.

GROWTH LATENCY

While the notion of sexual latency seems to be at least partially contradicted by the facts, there is another sense in which the concept of latency is quite applicable to the middle years. We have chosen to call this *growth latency*, referring to the slower pace of physical development than in the periods preceding and following the middle years. The school-age child is on a plateau of growth between the first spurt of infancy and the one that introduces puberty. Physical growth and reorganization continue during these years, but at a slower pace, without the abrupt emergences of earlier and later phases. A number of workers, including Bayer and Bayley, Flory, Krogman, Olson and Hughes, Sontag and Reynolds, Stolz and Stolz, Tanner, and Todd,[15] have developed the notion of *growth ages*, providing separate measures for the various asynchronous aspects of growth. Thus, the child's chronological age can be compared with his Mental Age, Reading Age, Height Age, Weight Age, Grip Age (the strength of his grip), Dental Age, Carpal Age (bone ossification as determined by x-rays of the hand and wrist), and so forth, yielding various "indexes" of growth. (Such research relies heavily on the use of x-ray studies of the interior of the body, and has become much less common as people have become aware of the perils of exposure to ionizing radiation.)

Within the general framework of the growth latency pattern, any number of individual growth patterns are possible. Some of the more characteristic growth pathways are represented in the so-called Wetzel grid, on which an individual's growth indicators can be entered to see if he conforms to any of the standard growth patterns. If he does, fairly accurate predictions can be made of ultimate growth status. Such predictions may bring realistic reevaluation both to the shrimp who feels that he is forever doomed to be dwarfed among giants and to the erstwhile giant whose growth has slowed down and who sees the former shrimps shooting past him. However, so many factors of health, diet, exercise, and endocrine function enter into physical growth that individual predictions have to be made with considerable caution.

Growth latency may be the physiological counterpart of the psychological phenomenon of the middle years as a period distinct from all the rest. It is the psychological stability of these years, between two periods of turbulence, that make them seem, at least in retrospect which may be misguided, the "halcyon days of childhood" which many adults look back on with nostalgic longing.

REFERENCES / Chapter 8

[1] Cary, Joyce. *A House of Children*. New York: Harper, 1955.

[2] Smith, R. P. *"Where Did You Go?" "Out." "What Did You Do?" "Nothing."* New York: Norton, 1957. (Also available in paperback.)

[3] Smith, R. P. *How to Do Nothing with Nobody, All Alone by Yourself.* New York: Norton, 1958.

[4] Asch, S. E. Studies in the principles of judgments and attitudes: II. Determination of judgments by group and ego standards. *Journal of Social Psychology*, 1940, 12, 433–465; Harvey, O. J., and Consalvi, C. Status and conformity to pressures in informal groups. *Journal of Abnormal and Social Psychology*, 1960, 60, 182–187; Patel, A. S., and Gordon, J. E. Some personal and situational determinants of yielding to influence. *Journal of Abnormal and Social Psychology*, 1960, 61, 411–418; Walters, R. H., Marshall, W. E., and Shooter, J. R. Anxiety, isolation, and susceptibility to social influence. *Journal of Personality*, 1960, 28, 518–529; Wilson, R. S. Personality patterns, source attractiveness, and conformity. *Journal of Personality*, 1960, 28, 186–199; A study of the "Asch effect" in children is reported by Berenda, R. W., *The Influence of the Group on the Judgments of Children*. New York: King's Crown Press, 1950.

[5] Opie, I., and Opie, P. *The Lore and Language of School Children*. Oxford: Clarendon, 1959. See also Withers, C., *A Rocket in My Pocket*. New York: Holt, 1948.

[6] Piaget, J. *The Moral Judgment of the Child*. Glencoe: Free Press, 1948 (originally published in 1932); Kohlberg, L. Development of moral character and moral ideology. In Hoffman, M. L., and Hoffman, L. W. (eds.) *Review of Child Development Research*. New York: Russell Sage Foundation, 1964, I, 383–431.

[7] Mead, M. *And Keep Your Powder Dry*. New York: Morrow, 1942.

[8] Scott, J. P. *Animal Behavior*. Chicago: University of Chicago, 1958. (Also available in paperback.); Ardrey, R. *The Territorial Imperative*. New York: Atheneum, 1966.

[9] Hendry, C. E., Lippitt, R., and Zander, A. *Reality Practice as Educational Method*. New York: Beacon House, 1944.

[10] Sherif, M., Harvey, O. J., White, B. J., Hood, W. R., and Sherif, C. W. *Intergroup Conflict and Cooperation: The Robbers Cave Experiment*. Norman, Okla.: University Book Exchange, 1961.

[11] Friedan, B. *The Feminine Mystique*. New York: Norton, 1963.

[12] Benedict, R. Continuities and discontinuities in cultural conditioning. *Psychiatry*, 1938, 1, 161–167.

[13] McClelland, D. C. *The Achieving Society*. Princeton: Van Nostrand, 1961.

[14] "Recommended reading on sex education," a pamphlet describing books and booklets for both parents and children, is available from the Publications

Office, Child Study Association of America, 9 East 89th Street, New York, N. Y. 10028. One popular paperback, prepared by the Child Study Association, is *Parents' Guide to Facts of Life for Children*. New York: Maco, 1965.

[15] Bayer, L. M., and Bayley, N. *Growth Diagnosis*. Chicago: University of Chicago, 1959; Flory, C. D. Osseous development in the hand as an index of skeletal development. *Monographs of the Society for Research in Child Development*, 1936, 1, no. 3; Krogman, W. M. The physical growth of children. *Monographs of the Society for Research in Child Development*, 1955, 20, no. 1; Olson, W. C., and Hughes, B. O. The concept of organismic age. *Journal of Educational Research*, 1942, 36, 525–527; Sontag, L. W., and Reynolds, E. L. The Fels composite sheet: I. A practical method for analyzing growth progress. *Journal of Pediatrics*, 1945, 26, 327–335; Stolz, H. R., and Stolz, L. M. *Somatic Development of Adolescent Boys*. New York: Macmillan, 1951; Tanner, J. M. *Education and Physical Growth*. London: University of London, 1961; Todd, T. W. The roentgenographic appraisement of skeletal differentiation. *Child Development*, 1930, 1, 298–310.

9 The Middle Years of Childhood: 2

Cognitive Functioning in Middle-Years Children

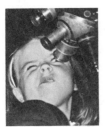

In speaking of the middle years, thus far we have referred only in passing to the fact that the school-age child goes to school. In developmental terms, going to school is a singularly appropriate thing for him to be doing—however much a boy might feel called upon to deny it. Actually, boys' protests against school seem to be a vestigial rite perpetuated by the peer culture. Two things seem to have happened over the past decade to change the way boys feel about school. First, the child-development approach to education has taken fairly firm roots in American schools, and school is a much more pleasant place to be than it used to. Second, even where the schools have not changed, or have used child-development principles erroneously, getting an education (or at least earning diplomas) has become the thing to do—indeed, the lament of the Negro boy is likely to be that he wants more education than he is getting. In the gang, in conversations at home, in their reading, and in schools that stimulate rather than deaden curiosity, children of this age are gluttonous learners.

Somewhere around the beginning of the school years, a major shift in cognitive functioning seems to take place, expressed in various general and specific learning readinesses—general school readiness, reading readiness, number readiness, and so forth. It used to be assumed that learning readiness was largely a matter of physical maturation, but we have come to know too much about the effects of early enrichment and privation on school learning to accept so simple a view. There may indeed be maturational differences between those who learn easily and those who do not, but we do not know what they are or to what extent they are the product of differences in emotional and cognitive stimulation. To complicate the matter further, let us remember that diet, hygiene, and medical care or its lack all play their part in maturation, beginning with the zygote.

Assuming conditions favorable to the development of learning readiness, we see that the middle-years child characteristically turns his attention away from family involvements and outward toward the world at large. He begins to substitute a naturalistic view for a magicalistic one. He learns to appraise human behavior objectively as well as affectively. He learns—slowly—to try to take other people's points of view. He comes to turn away from an exclusive preoccupation with human affairs (in which we would have to include the child's dealings with domestic animals) toward the analysis of the living and inert nonhuman sphere. He becomes able to think about things distant in time and space. He wants to know about the mechanics of things, how they work and how they are made. Make-believe is no longer blended hit-or-miss with his reality. He has not abandoned magic and make-believe, but they are more private than before, and the line between being and pretending is sharply drawn. He is learning, however imperfectly, to think systematically, in terms of organizing schemes and principles like the taxonomies of biology and the characteristics of numbers. But above all else, he wants to know.

He wants both knowledge and know-how. He wants information (although, at this age, he does not discriminate well between information and misinformation) and he wants to catch on to the skills and tricks and competences and procedures that are the mark of the initiate. Many kindergarten children seem to have the half-formulated belief that simple enrollment in first grade will magically confer such skills and membership. Even at a slightly higher level of understanding, abilities like reading or playing the piano seem to the child to be a matter of knowing the right trick—one reason why practicing palls when the trick is not immediately forthcoming. Thus, the same forces that move him to embrace the rituals of childhood partly govern his approach to school learning and give to it some of the other's ritual flavor. Even late in the school years, the child may consider it an achievement to memorize the Gettysburg Address, even though he knows little or nothing about its occasion. At the same time he asks, "You know the Gettysburg Address? 1270 Elm Street, Gettysburg, Pennsylvania."

SYMBOLS

At the heart of the school child's cognitive status is his increasing mastery of symbols. The preschool child is caught in word realism, such that words and statements are as real as anything else and are easily confused with the things they stand for. Notice that word realism is never outgrown. It is this attitude toward words that makes some topics unspeakable, that drives people to euphemism, whereby an unlovely subject is given a safe name; to hints and allusions, whereby people never really say what it is they are talking about; and to circumlocution, whereby they define a topic by talking all around it without giving it a name. Part of the job of educators and writers is to put into words things that their students and readers cannot or dare not say for themselves. We have rather often heard from lecture audiences that the views we have expressed on values, divorce laws, abortion, and other touchy topics, were things that they had always thought but had never put into words. Needless to say, we have also received some abuse for daring to say such things. It is verbal realism, too, that enables one to participate vicariously in stories, to respond to oratory and to poetic evocation.

Nevertheless, the school child has begun to sense that words and the concrete things or actions or attributes they may refer to belong to distinct orders of reality. This differentiation of levels gives the child greater freedom to manipulate symbols, as seen in the delight he takes in playing with symbols and meanings. Middle-class middle-years children typically are fascinated by rhymes, alliteration, anagrams, codes and ciphers, foreign words and phrases, onomatopoeia, and puns (including double-entendre—but not yet metaphors). They like to play with the ambiguities of language, as in "I simply can't bear it. It's much too heavy," or "You want me to take my vitamins? O.K., I'll take them to my room." They play with negatives, as in the poem about "The Little Man Who Wasn't There." That symbols have not been completely differentiated from the rest of reality is shown, however, by children's literalism: their unquestioning acceptance of the words of chants and rituals without wondering what they refer to, and their inability to detect sarcasm or irony, where one often says the opposite of what one means.

They do comprehend broad travesty and burlesque, and a favorite occupation is to compose playlets satirizing television commercials. Sometimes they make the connection between words used in a variety of senses, as in *bear-bear,* or to tell a *lie-lie* down, and sometimes they do not. Asch and Nerlove[1] report that children may understand the meaning of *a sweet person,* but deny any connection with the sweetness of sugar.

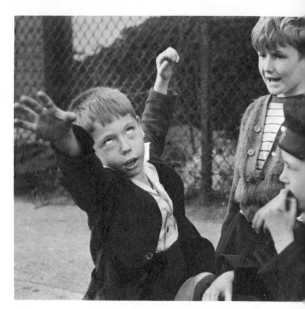

School children do comprehend broad travesty and burlesque.
Ruth Orkin

They love big words and use them globally, without really knowing their meaning. Werner and Kaplan[2] carried out an experiment to study age differences in ability to deduce the meaning of a word from its use in various contexts. The child would be given a series of sentences containing the same made-up word and asked to guess the word's meaning. Some characteristic responses were that the word means the whole sentence (the response to the word "bordicks" in the sentence "People talk about the bordicks of others and don't like to talk about their own" was "People talk about other people and don't talk about themselves, that's what bordick means"); that the word means itself (that "contavish" means "You know, like contavish"); or that the word stands for some condensation of the sentence (the response to "bordick" in the sentence "If you are smart and work hard your work will not have a bordick" was "Bordick means smart so you won't get a D").

Indeed, for many young school children, language seems to be only partially differentiated into single words, which may be a factor in beginning reading difficulties, since the divisions of words on a page may not correspond to the sound groupings the child hears and uses. (Even among college students, we find such undifferentiated terms as *anotherwords, infact, alot, alittle, inspite, outloud, otherhand, motorability.*) In reading, the child may have further difficulty with the analysis of words into phonetic elements, and some number of children read at first simply by memorizing the words that go with certain letter combinations. Notice that initially this process goes only in one direction: The child knows that c-a-t on the page in front of him spells *cat,* but he himself cannot yet spell *cat.* Traces of immature language persist throughout this period, as in difficulty with the past tenses of irregular verbs ("Harriet baby-sitted with us over the weekend"). In general, however, children of this age become increasingly able to dominate language, to make it do their bidding, and, as at other points of near-mastery, they practice their skills indefatigably.

Among the particular symbolic skills that appear early in the middle years—given the proper stimulation now and at earlier ages—are the ability to define words, to supply antonyms on demand, to find similarities between related things (that is, to make explicit the nature of equivalences), to detect and specify absurdities and incongruities in pictures and stories (as when the child is presented with sentences like "They looked out and saw that the sun was shining, so they took their raincoats with them"), to count indefinitely, to count by twos, fives, and tens, to count backward (although even four-year-olds nowadays learn from television the refrain, "10, 9, 8 . . . zero, blast off!"), and to add and subtract (like many primitive peoples, some children find it hard to grasp that one can use the same number system to tally qualitatively different things).

Such skills do not emerge full-blown, but develop over a period of a year or two in a fairly regular progression. When it comes to defining concrete nouns, for instance, the child may at first give a partial definition in terms of a single characteristic or function, which, while accurate enough, is insufficient to describe the class of things under consideration. Thus, *bicycle* may be defined as "It's got pedals" or "You ride on it." At a slightly later stage, a bicycle becomes "Something that you ride on [for want of the word *vehicle*], and it's got two wheels, and these pedals that you push, and handlebars to steer with." Notice that this sort of definition is far less egocentric than the earlier ones in that it supplies the information necessary for understanding. Observe, too, that the more advanced style of definition implies a detached, gamelike, abstract attitude to the task, since the child knows that the examiner knows what a bicycle is and that the examiner is asking the child not for the sake of the information gained but to see how well the child can convey information.

A somewhat similar pattern of development can be seen in the way a child attacks the task of finding similarities. The five- or six-year-old may misconstrue the task and, asked in what way a cat and a mouse are alike, reply simply that "The cat chases the mouse." At a more advanced stage, he seizes on peripheral, nondefining characteristics of the two things, as when he says that a cat and a mouse "Both have whiskers," or "Both have four legs," or that an apple and a peach are alike "Because you eat them both." At a still more advanced stage, the child is able to name the class of things to which the two specimens belong, and can make explicit that cats and mice are animals, that apples and peaches are fruits, and that bicycles and cars are both means of transportation. Notice that the ability to define words or to give similarities is not some generalized mental mechanism that develops in the child: His level of competence depends very much on the characteristics of the materials he has to deal with. It is easier to define concrete nouns than abstract ones like *justice*, and it is easier to define nouns than adjectives like *proud*. It is easier to say how a bicycle and motorcar are alike than to specify the similarity between *salt* and *water*, 25 and 36, or *first* and *last*, so that the child who can say that an apple and a peach are both fruits may still respond to the pairing of *salt* and *water* with "They make salt water," or to the pairing of *coal* and *paper* with "Paper is white and coal is black," or "You can write on paper with a piece of coal." The child may have special difficulty dealing with the similarity between opposites like *first* and *last*; it requires considerable sophistication to appreciate that, in order to be opposite, things must belong to a common domain.

One way of finding out what words mean to the child is to ask him to define them. Another is to infer the meanings of component words from the way he interprets whole statements such as common proverbs.[3] It is only late in the middle years, as we have suggested, that the child begins to sense the metaphorical meanings of many proverbs. When he does begin, he fails to see the need for any logical parallels between the proverb itself and the more general idea it is meant to express. As a result, his first attempts at a metaphorical interpretation reveal the physiognomic, global way in which he apprehends the proverb. For example, a nine-year-old boy defined *An ounce of prevention is worth a pound of cure* as "Well, if something is too heavy for an old person, you could help him carry it"; an eleven-year-old girl defined *Every cloud has a silver lining*: "There's a blue cloud in the sky." Some interpretations, however, show common misunderstandings of particular words. A nine-year-old defines *Absence makes the heart grow fonder* as "It makes your heart grow weaker, I guess." Now the primary misunderstanding here is not of the word "fonder," but of "absence," which to this child, as to many others, means "sick," by a process of you're-absent-from-school-because-you're-sick.

Sometimes emotional associations or moral considerations distort the child's understanding. Many middle-years children are taken aback by *Revenge is sweet,* and may even refuse to try to define it. When they do try, children are likely to change the meaning of the statement, even to the extent of forcing words out of shape, as in "You don't revenge too hard" or even "It means the same thing as 'forgive.'" We can see the way personal, subjective matters intrude on the thinking of children in a typical nine-year-old interpretation of *A stitch in time saves nine*: "Like if you had a broken hand, you stitch it, like if someone got hurt, say, like a nine-year-old, he needed stitches."

Two well-known techniques, the *word association test* and the misnamed *semantic differential,* seek to get at the feeling tones associated with words rather than at their content. The word association test requires the subject to say the first thing that occurs to him in response to each of a series of stimulus words. Although originally meant as a device for locating sensitive areas of a person's experience, the word association test has proven at least as useful for studying systematic developmental changes in the organization of associations. The young middle-years child is likely to respond with concrete, contextual associations drawn from everyday life, as in *dog*—"barks" or *mother*—"cooks." (Notice the analogy to such similarities responses as "The cat chases the mouse.") Some young children give rhyming responses, as in *table*—"Mabel," or *Klang* responses, where the response word bears a global phonetic resemblance to the stimulus word, as in *baggage*—"language." With increasing age there is a shift from contextually related responses to formally, logically related ones such as synonyms, antonyms, and logical coordinates (*chair* —"couch") or subordinates (*gem*—"diamond"). Studies by Koff and by Jenkins and associates indicate that the patterning of children's word associations has changed in the last half century,[4] with today's eight- to twelve-year-old children giving far more formal and fewer contextual responses than their counterparts of yesteryear. While these findings may indicate that today's children are more mature than children of an earlier day, a secondary finding is that the modern groups agreed more in their responses than the early samples, which may imply a lessening of diversity over the years. The semantic differential scales (which elicit only a small part of the semantic content) require the subject to rate "concepts," words or phrases such as *mother* or *wild strawberries,* on antonymic dimensions such as hot-cold or strong-weak. The scales as they now exist have numerous logical deficiencies,[5] and they have been little used with children,[6] but they offer some promise as a research tool in understanding the meanings words have for children.

Later in the school years, the child becomes capable of such advanced symbolic manipulations as multiplication and division, and translating back and forth between words and numbers. Indeed, we consider the one almost unqualified success among recent attempts at curricular reform in the grades to be the introduction of New or Modern Mathematics, which begins with the logic of numerical relationships and brings the child early to such algebraic operations as finding unknowns, generalized formulas, factoring, and finding roots and exponentials. The chief reservation we have about the New Math is in its teaching: The derivation of shortcut methods of calculation is too long delayed in most schools, leaving the child to solve problems by perfectly logical but unnecessarily cumbersome roundabout techniques.

Children also learn to make and use maps and the special concepts of geographers. Middle-class urban and suburban children do not, however, characteristically orient themselves to the points of the compass in the way children living in the country learn to do. In the same way, children learn to understand charts, graphs, and diagrams, and can translate simple blueprints into material objects. Notice, too, that the world is full of diverse symbols (some of which are better described as *signs*, conditioned signals for particular reactions): The policeman symbolizes authority, the expensive new car symbolizes high status, the trademark symbolizes the company or the product, money symbolizes work and buying power, the flag symbolizes the social or political group, and so forth. There has been little formal study of the way children come to react to such signs and symbols.

GENERAL INFORMATION

In his transition from an egocentric, personalized, subjective orientation to an objective, relativistic view of the world (which, obviously, is never complete), the child builds up a framework of expectations. It is this framework, which must be constantly revised, that enables him to marvel, to wonder, to be curious, and to organize—however primitively—the facts he accumulates. He locates himself in time (although his early years have been largely erased from memory) and recognizes, if with little personal conviction, that the world existed before he entered it and that it will survive his passing. He meditates upon what it means to be age ten or twelve or twenty. He ponders the mysteries of life, birth, and death. He becomes aware of the processes of his own body, respiration, circulation, digestion, the senses, of the hiatus of sleep. He learns about germs and viruses and disease and may have bouts of hypochondria. When the city child first learns where meat comes from, this may be quite disturbing, and a number of children go through a period of partial or total vegetarianism. The child is interested in causal sequences to the extent that he wants to know how to do things, but he remains largely phenomenalistic and realistic, and hence fatalistic, in his outlook. Nonetheless, his framework of regularities makes some new relationships stand out for him: He sees the burst of the fireworks display and notes that it takes a second or so for the sound to reach him. The concept of gravity comes to him with the force of revelation, and the idea of weightlessness becomes a new field of fantasy. Children are fascinated by space travel and space exploration and, more recently, have discovered the world

Children are fascinated by space travel, space exploration, and astronomy.

P. W. Freeland/The Franklin Institute

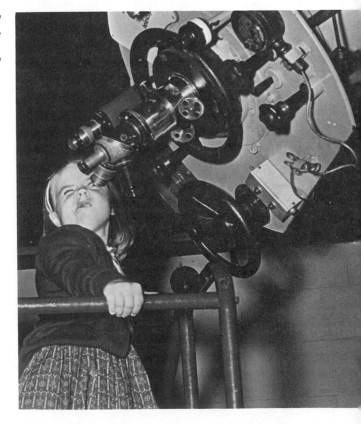

beneath the sea through snorkeling, scuba diving, and the underseas adventures of Cousteau.

As times change, children seem to be increasingly pragmatic and decreasingly romantic. As they read more and travel more, they are less impressed by the glamor of the frontier, of American Indians, of warfare, of exotic climes and people, and more concerned with careers, domesticity, and human relations. And, as we have said, the movies and television shows they prefer stress the sardonic and the satirical even when dealing with traditional themes like mystery and adventure and cowboys and Indians. Like yesterday's children, today's are very much moved by questions of justice and injustice, especially with regard to themselves. The child, with his magicalism and artificialism, finds it hard to accept that it is the accident of rainfall or competing parental obligations that cause him to miss out on some treat, and instead looks for some malevolent agency to account for the injustice. Increasingly, though, children seem able to deal with general principles of justice and to see how these apply to problems like poverty and racial integration. We will have to wait to see whether today's middle-years generation will grow up better able than their parents to view things in planetary perspective, to take it as axiomatic that no man and no society can be an island unto itself.

The middle-years child's growing objectivity and skepticism have other consequences than in the realm of factual knowledge. The child becomes able to judge his own performances by stable, external standards, enabling him to comment, "Isn't this a junk drawing?" or to compare his athletic skills with those of his classmates. Middle-class children come to feel at home with the "objective" test, whether of how far one can throw a ball as compared to others of the same age and sex, of ability, or of achievement, and they take their scores on such measures as seriously as do adults. Another by-product of the child's new detachment, his new ability to stand off from things and eye them critically, is that he turns the tables on adults. Previously, he was a transparent object of adult appraisal. Now, he can return the adults' scrutiny and do his own appraising, a gift that they may find unsettling.

THINKING AND REASONING

As we have said, the middle-years child's growing mastery of symbols and his ever-broadening fund of general knowledge permit him to think in ways that come to approximate those of adults. Indeed, in some areas, the child may know a great deal more than his less educated parents and so be able to think more rationally than they—parents typically complain that their children's homework demands more knowledge than they the parents can muster. But however adroitly he can deal with certain circumscribed topics like doing proportions, batting averages, interplanetary travel, and the habits of starfish, his everyday thinking on matters of personal concern is likely to be muddled by emotionalism, confusion of levels of discourse, magicalism, facts invented *ad hoc* to substantiate his point of view, *non sequiturs*, superstition, misinformation, and the murk of ignorance. To the best of our knowledge, no one has ever applied a systematic logical analysis to the spontaneous reasonings of school children, but it seems likely to us that children are abundantly guilty of every logical fallacy known to philosophers.

One common form of thought in children and adults is scapegoating, the venting of one's frustrations and resentments on some convenient person, animal, or thing, sometimes explicitly putting the blame for one's misfortunes on the scapegoat. When the child puts the blame for some disappointment on his parents or the Almighty, he is scapegoating. In general, it is very hard to convince children (and many adults) that some events just happen, that no one is to blame, or that an action or a state of affairs can be multiply determined, with no single person or agency responsible. But scapegoating seems to be only one form of a more general process by which one seeks out an object on which to fasten one's feelings. Many school-age children suffer a certain amount of diffuse anxiety or even dread, and the child has to find something to be frightened of—he seeks a fear-goat, so to speak, for his fears. In general, children of this age attach their fears to real things—animals, kidnappers, burglars, and the rest—but fears of imaginary entities—ghosts, witches, punitive forces—persist throughout. And even when the child is afraid of real things, he fears them out of all proportion to their actual menace. We can see further analogies to scapegoating and fear-goating in the love-goating of the older middle-years child's crushes and hero worship and in the adolescent's eager search for someone to fall in love with. This general process seems to work both as a means of handling feelings and also as a way of identifying and giving shape to otherwise elusive feelings. Notice, too, that such emotion-goating has much in common with the private, compulsive rituals we talked about earlier.

Moral Judgments. The child's logic, as we have said, is colored by his knowledge and ignorance and by his emotions. One special dimension of his feelings about things is the moral meanings he attaches to them.

The preschool child has a conscience, but in terms of responsibility for his acts he must be thought of as amoral, a view shared by most theologians (with due provision for the cleansing away of Original Sin). The middle-years child, by contrast, is moralistic. He learns and applies the rules of right and wrong in a harsh, rigid, absolutistic way that, early in this period, makes no allowance for good intentions and extenuating circumstances. Having been told that he lives in a free country, he cannot understand why he cannot always do just as he wishes. The battle cry "It's not fair!" (nowadays often phrased as "It's cheat!") expresses the child's detection of a departure from the rules as he construes them. Piaget[7] has proposed that the two main characteristics of the child's moral judgments are *moral realism,* the assumption that moral rules have an existence in their own right, analogous to the conception of Natural Law, and *immanent justice,* the sense that misdeeds carry within them the seeds of their own punishment. Milton Senn[8] gives an interesting example of immanent justice in a twelve-year-old boy who violated hospital rules to sneak in and visit a relative who had a broken leg, then himself was in an accident in which he broke his leg, and was profoundly convinced that his injury was a punishment for his transgression. In this case, the boy's sense of immanent justice was exacerbated and compounded by a nurse who told him that if he did not cease his cries of woe, the doctors would be obliged to cut off his ailing leg. Not too surprisingly, the boy screamed harder and more persistently than ever.

Children judge each other much more stringently than would adults, and are likely to suggest summary execution or a session on the rack as appropriate remedies for minor infractions. We suspect that such harshness—as in the Freudian reasoning about the compulsive traits of latency—represents the child's concern about keeping his own impulses in check. It may also be an attempt to give order to shifting reality by putting the world into rigid compartments, with the result that any injustice or untruth threatens the still-precarious stability of the universe. It may appear to adults that children flout every established moral tenet, but when we look closer, we see that children are regulated by codes (especially those they impose on each other in the gang) more binding than adults could tolerate.

Obviously, children do violate their codes, and, like adults, they find devices for avoiding guilt. They become masters of denial (which often seems to include actual loss of memory for the misdeed), rationalization, and self-justification. In general, the defense mechanisms against guilt consist in using the magic of words to change the meanings of an act so as to make it fit the person's conception of right and wrong. This process is greatly facilitated by the child's literal-mindedness: The letter of the rule is more important than its spirit. He will argue legalistically and litigiously for the narrowest possible interpretation, so that his behavior falls outside the letter of the law: "You said not to run. I was galloping." Later in the school years, children relinquish much of their absolutism in favor of tolerance, flexibility, and relativism, just as they learn to be more dispassionate about the gang's codes and the eternal fixity of the rules of games. Adults, too, find themselves coming in for censure: A casual expletive, such as the child himself would delight in using in the gang, on the lips of an adult may provoke real moral indignation.

Philosophers have wrestled for centuries with the meanings of *good* and *bad,* and almost all agree that the moral dimension of *virtue-evil* is relevant. Other dimensions on which people pretty regularly evaluate things are the esthetic, or *beautiful-ugly,* the pragmatic, or *useful-injurious,* the *rational-irrational* dimension, and the dimension of emotionally *pleasant-unpleasant.* It seems to be characteristic of school-age children that their evaluative judgments confuse these dimensions, so that to denounce something as "queer" or "crazy" is also to question its morality, beauty, utility, and emotional qualities.

Middle-years children do learn to echo adult judgments of sunsets, vistas, and works of art or music as "beautiful," but this seems to be more a learning of which objects fall in the esthetic realm than any ability to make autonomous esthetic judgments. Formal studies of children's evaluations of works of art are still in their beginnings,[9] but everyday observation of which things children own and treasure, and the things they aspire to own, not to mention their preferences in food and music, suggests that their taste is at best vulgar and at worst atrocious. It probably does little good to try to cultivate the "right" tastes in a child, since the end result is likely to be simply a narrowing of enjoyment to the conventionally accepted finer things in life. The child who, in time, develops his own tastes is likely to arrive at sounder, more meaningful esthetic evaluations, and to be more receptive to esthetic innovations, than the child who has learned to accept and reject on the basis of ordinary standards.

Eidetic Imagery. As far as we can tell, children at first think and remember in images, which may be so vivid as to compete with reality itself. Such naturalistic, hallucinatory images, which may be auditory, tactual, olfactory, gustatory, and proprioceptive as well as visual, are called *eidetic* images (something like what is popularly referred to as a "photographic memory"). The sometimes fantastic memory of the pre-school child seems to reside in a capacity for evoking eidetic images. Some people retain their eidetic capacity throughout life, being able to recall effortlessly and with uncanny accuracy such details as the contents of a drugstore window or the costumes at a fancy-dress ball. Eidetic imagery seems to be important for specialized talents like drawing, music, and arithmetic, and many musicians report that they can look at a score and hear the music being played. Eidetic imagery is more than mere memorization, since the eidetic subject can spell out from an imaged street sign long foreign words which he cannot even pronounce, or "read off" in any sequence numbers from, say, a five-by-five arrange-ment of twenty-five digits which he has examined briefly. Most of us retain only a weakened, faded capacity for eidetic imaging, which gets submerged, with experience, in the abstract gist, the symbolic essentials of experience, rather than the lifelike totality. Except for special purposes, eidetic images are cumbersome tools of thought, and it is probably just as well for the child's cognitive development that eidetic imagery is sub-ordinated during the school years to more abstract, manipulable symbolic thinking.

All told then, the world of the middle-years child includes isolated domains or segments of experience which are logically organized and about which the child can reason in a mature fashion. However, the world as a whole has not yet come to be a coherent, integrated system, and clouds of magicalism surround and sometimes invade the more orderly realms of thought. It is obviously the work of education to make the world comprehensible, manageable, and manipulable in thought, with the ambiguities and paradoxes and controversies made plain, and it is the topic of schooling to which we turn in the section that follows. The reader is asked to bear in mind, however, that schooling is not always educational, and that education goes on not only in school but also in the family, in newspapers and magazines, on the playground, in the bushes, and in the gutter.

A School for the School Child

We now want to discuss those formal institutions which our society provides for the indoctrination of its school-age young. Foremost among these, of course, is school, but the scout troop, the recreation center, and similar agencies serve many school-like functions, and much of what we have to say applies to them as well. Also, although we are talking about grade schools, our discussion applies in some measure to secondary schools and colleges. In what follows, we want to take account of what the schools are, what they conceive their goals to be, what they actually do, the problems they face, and how they can supply what we consider to be the optimal conditions for sound psychological development.

In the past decade, the United States has been struggling, at the federal, state, and local levels, with the backing of various autonomous authorities like the curricular research groups and to the jeers and catcalls of critics, to overhaul its educational system, while gearing it to deal with a vastly enlarged population, with a mixed record of successes and setbacks. Great numbers of additional people have been drawn into teaching, new schools have been built, new books have been published, new curricula have been drawn up in mathematics, earth sciences, biology, and so forth, and new techniques and technologies have been devised: ungraded classes, team teaching, assistant teachers, programed instruction, teaching via television, language laboratories, greater use of audio-visual aids, until one may have trouble finding the child (or the teacher) in the gadget jungle. Colleges of education are being rehabilitated into liberal arts colleges, sometimes simply by fiat, sometimes in fact; the requirements for teacher certification are being changed to require more emphasis on subject matter and less on "methods" in the teacher's own education; and national figures have taken the time to philosophize and psychologize about the process of education. Preschool education for poor children has come into being—still spasmodically and uncertainly—on a national scale, with sometimes bewildering and friction-generating speed. Probably most gratifying is that children are less likely to dread school, but like it and learn better than ever before. Supplying the textbooks, chairs, chalk, and apparatus of education has become a huge business.

Ten years ago (in the first edition of this volume), the authors wrote a criticism of American schools that in some respects now seems very much out of date. It is true now as then that taxpayers still lament the cost of education, although as more and more funding comes from federal and statewide sources and less and less from local real estate taxes, the cries of pain grow muted. It is true that some school superintendents and principals are tyrants. It is true that some teachers cannot stand the childishness of children (one teacher impatiently asked her class, "Why do you keep having to go to the toilet? *I* only have to go once a day"). It is true that some children continue to find school work an

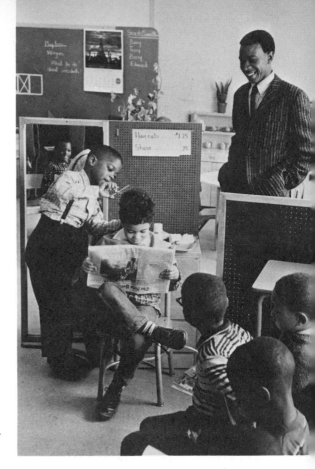

A school for the school child.
Leonard McCombe, LIFE Magazine
© Time Inc.

impenetrable mass of irrelevancy that blunts their enthusiasm and curiosity. But by and large, these problems lie behind us in principle if not in actuality. And still we are unhappy.

Our dissatisfaction resides in the fact that vast educational reforms and expenditures have taken place within the same framework of assumptions and values that produced the dreary schools of yesteryear. No matter how fervently we talk about the virtues of education, and back up our talk with money, we have not, as a society, shaken loose from our distrust of the intellectual. Let it be noted that not all intelligent people or people who do intellectual work such as writing, teaching, or the professions qualify as intellectuals. The intellectual is to be recognized by his skepticism, his tendency to criticize, his impatience with traditional solutions, and his moral concern—in Socrates' term, the intellectual is a gadfly. In his role of gadfly or thorn in the flesh, the intellectual makes life unhappy for all the people who do not want to be bothered with social problems like education, sex, poverty, prejudice, pollution, war,

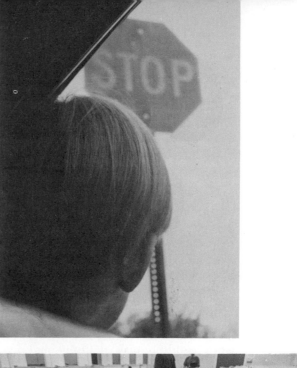

(Right) *The child learns to read not only from books but from cereal packages, television commercials, traffic signs, and other features of a symbol-laden environment.*

Theodor H. Nelson

(Bottom) *Electronic teaching: The machine stimulates the student and responds to the student's responses.*

Ralph Crane, LIFE Magazine © Time Inc.

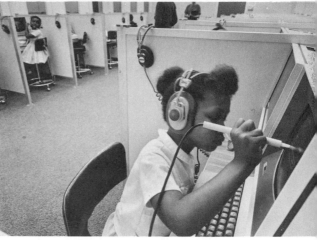

and overpopulation. And so, as we have said, we go about the business of education ambivalently, teaching well the safe subjects with obvious practical applications, but dealing out banalities and platitudes in areas of controversy.

The child quickly picks up conventional attitudes to sensitive subjects and he conspires gladly in the game of seeming to teach and learn something without ever saying anything about it. The lower-class child may smell the falsity of it all, but he lacks the words with which to combat it. For the middle-class child, the teachings of the school in the areas of biology and sociology are not so much patently false as ambiguous. Middle-class parents, some because they themselves began life in the slums, others because they have really forgotten about the humanity of poor people, especially poor people of a different race, manage to bring up their children in a middle-class capsule buffered against the bitter realities of poverty. The middle-class child knows about social problems such as poverty and war, but without the immediacy of firsthand experience. He could summon up the words to argue with his textbooks, but he lacks solid knowledge of the facts.

The teacher feels—and not without reason—that he or she should stick to the syllabus and the textbook, and not go venturing forth into untrodden realms. In general, the teacher is not thought of as someone who communicates his own life experience to children; he is simply the mediator between child and prescribed curriculum. Thus, a considerable part of the educational process becomes gamesmanship at which middle-class children play skillfully and lower-class children less so. If one continues to play the game skillfully for sixteen years, one is rewarded with a degree which entitles one to marry a handsome, well-bred spouse, get a good job, live in a nice house in a nice neighborhood, have nice friends, join the country club, and bear healthy children who will then repeat the cycle.

The school as an educational device is competing with the gang, the television set, and extracurricular literature, and it is small wonder if the pallid fantasies taught as social studies and literature lose out to the bloodstained fantasies of fiction and the real world. It is our contention that schools as educational devices will begin to work only, as Bruner[10] has said, when they are prepared to tell the truth—and, we might add, to tell it truthfully, without hiding or playing down the emotions and values involved. The subject matter of social studies, people are often startled to realize, is the world, how it is, how it got to be the way it is, the economic, political, ideological, and psychological forces that keep things moving and changing, and what if anything people can do individually and collectively to make the world humanly habitable. In staying silent on the burning issues and controversies, the schools are communicating attitudes of timidity and impotent acquiescence. If the schools want to engage in liberal—and liberating—education as well as vocational training, they have to be prepared to talk about life and death, sex and love and hate, fanaticism, superstition, corruption, motives, power, propaganda, bigotry, communism and capitalism, and the causes people kill and die for. The schools have to be prepared to deal with issues frankly, critically, and analytically, and with constant appeals to the evidence.

Obviously, this view of the educational process assumes teachers possessing a wealth of knowledge and understanding as well as independence and commitment. In fact, of course, our teachers are products of the same sorts of schools in which they themselves are teaching, and it is unlikely that the schooling of most of them has prepared them to undertake the kind of education we are talking about. Fortunately, the vicious circle of education is not quite a circle, so that each generation of teachers is better educated and brighter than the one before. In addition, of course, the teacher's educational opportunities are no more confined to the classroom than are the children's, and quite a few teachers manage to learn a great deal in the great outside world. The problem is to convey to teachers the notion of *personal knowledge* (a term coined by the philosopher Polanyi),[11] the idea that knowledge is not something external to oneself but something to be absorbed and incorporated into one's own world view.[12]

But the approach to teaching we have suggested requires not only a substantive change in what the teacher is capable of but also in the teacher's image of himself, and in the community's and school hierarchy's role expectations and image of the teacher. The teacher must be, and be accepted as, autonomous (which does not mean irresponsible), free to adapt and experiment and respond, to digress, and to be as creative as he knows how. The teacher has a responsibility to parents and the community to impart certain conventional skills and key facts. He may choose to do his teaching within the framework of a standard syllabus. But he needs to have some freedom to choose. He also needs time and latitude to invent and to vary and to deal with individual children. He has to be free to teach both convergent thinking, which leads to a verifiably correct solution, and divergent thinking, which is concerned with possibilities rather than testable conclusions.[13] For his first responsibility is to the children, to give them—or help them acquire—skills and knowledge and principles that will be useful to them in understanding the world and where they do or can fit in. He can help them develop zest and spirit and curiosity and imagination and originality. But he has to be trusted as a professional who knows his job and his children and who comprehends the ethical restraints that go with dealing intimately with immature—but maturing—human beings.

This means freedom from bureaucratic control and endless petty regulations. It also means freedom from endless chores, paper work, clerical duties, and nonprofessional assignments like playground duty and corridor duty. It means a humane working schedule so that education can go on at a pace suited to the child's capacity to absorb things and mull them over. The hectic tempo of the average teacher's day is one that no assembly-line worker would tolerate. Teachers need time not only to teach, to prepare lessons, to read and think, but also to go to the bathroom, to have a relaxed lunch with colleagues, and to participate in the planning and thinking of the school as a whole.[14] The teacher needs time to take courses, attend lectures, take part in professional meetings, and do whatever else enhances his professional competence. Somehow, education has become infected with the business ideal of efficiency, and the teacher is expected to perform accordingly. Some teaching and learning can be efficient, and it is our hope that children will not go on very long painfully deciphering each printed word or toiling laboriously over every simple calculation. But thoughtful, serious learning in the substantive fields takes time, and time is a commodity in short supply for teachers and pupils.

THE LIBERAL SCHOOL

Three main approaches to education have dominated the United States schools. Classical, traditional education, modeled on British and Continental practices, has been found in some of our most prestigeful private schools. Such schools characteristically place heavy emphasis on classical languages, French, mathematics, history, and sports, with rather less attention given to natural sciences, social sciences, and such languages as Spanish, Russian, Japanese, and Mandarin. Another segment of our private schools has been in the forefront of the progressive education movement in all its varieties. The progressive schools have tended to be child centered rather than subject-matter centered, stressing good mental health and emotional development as salient goals of education. Their approach to teaching at the elementary level typically is less concerned with the usual separation of disciplines, and aims at integrated education, with facts and skills learned incidentally as subordinate parts of projects and themes. Art, music, and poetry, with the children being urged to be active in these fields, loom large in the usual progressive curriculum. We can see that traditionalism differs from progressivism in what is considered the important content of education and in methods of instruction, with the traditional schools emphasizing the magisterial role of the teacher and the progressive schools emphasizing the discoverer role of the pupil. Strands of traditionalism and progressivism can be found in the public schools, but in general public education has been dominated by the "basic education" approach, which emphasizes fundamental skills like the three R's and training for life's practical problems.

Historically, the basic education approach seems to have had its origins in the need to Americanize our polyglot population and to guarantee a minimal level of literacy to everyone. The basic education approach found its empirical and philosophical justification in the work of Thorndike and his associates from 1900 on.[15] Thorndike denounced the doctrine of "mental discipline" which was invoked by traditional educators in support of the study of German, Latin, mathematics, and other subjects that were supposed to teach students a generalized logic. Thorndike conducted a series of studies from which he concluded that there was no generalized transfer effect or that such transfer as was found occurred only between highly similar skills (the reader will recall the principle of "identical elements" in perceiving equivalences, page 176). The lack of a transfer effect and the futility of mental discipline were duly recorded in psychology textbooks and have been interpreted by educational theorists to mean that the schools should concern themselves with teaching specific, useful skills. In this view, teaching was subordinated to training, on the analogy of the way one trains animals.

It is interesting, in a grisly sort of way, that the doctrine of skill training took the ascendancy despite a good deal of contrary evidence, almost as though it met some culturally given psychic need. Indeed, one can see in Thorndike's work the formalization and glorification of American anti-intellectualism. Harlow's work on learning sets, which imply the transfer of principles rather than of specific elements, even at the infrahuman level (as when the animal applies the principle of oddity from having learned to choose the odd color to choosing the odd shape or size), goes against Thorndike's conclusions. But the most telling argument against Thorndike's position comes from Thorndike's own work. For in fact Thorndike found a transfer effect, even after elaborate statistical manipulations designed to minimize it. It is true that the transfer effects were small, but they were measures of change over only one year. If we consider that similar effects could be gained year by year over a period of eight or twelve or sixteen or twenty years of schooling, they would add up to a very impressive total effect. In any case, it is perhaps more important that the literature on the transfer effect, both pro and con, is pathetically naïve and can hardly be taken seriously by anyone concerned with advanced intellectual functioning. (The studies in this area concerned themselves, for instance, with whether a skill learned with the left hand transferred to the right, ability to memorize nonsense syllables, learning to hit a submerged target with a BB gun, paired associate learning, and so forth.)

These three views of education can be summarized by saying that the traditional approach is subject-matter centered, the progressive approach is child centered, and the skills-training approach is social-utility centered. In our own thinking about the design for a "liberal" or "modern" school, we want to embrace all three views, at the same time giving to each a somewhat different meaning. Our approach is child centered in that we favor giving the child an education that will be personally relevant and that will contribute to his full development as a person. One of us has summed up the goals of personal education as:

> . . . multiplying our perspectives on reality; by informing us about a far greater range of phenomena than we ever can know from personal experience; by teaching us the sets of principles according to which different realms of knowledge cohere; by teaching us techniques of logical, psychological, and stylistic analysis; and, most centrally, by equipping us with the symbolic systems—verbal, mathematical, diagrammatical, representational, expressive—by which we master reality conceptually and shape new realities in imagination.[16]

Our approach is not child centered in the sense, sometimes encountered, of education being a continuous process of individual or group psychotherapy, or in the romantic-naturalist sense that the child should be sheltered against instruction and left to find his own way. Our approach is, however, child centered in the sense that we have to take account of how children think and learn, and of the individual child's style of thinking and learning. There is a common subject matter—the world—for all children, but this does not imply that they all have to learn the same things at the same time and in the same way. Thus, we are subject-matter centered in the sense that the child's ego and feelings of self-worth are not at stake, that he is free to pay attention to the demands of the learning task without being distracted by irrelevant emotions. This is not to say that learning should be emotion-free, but that the emotions should originate in the subject matter and the child's feelings about it and not in his feelings about himself. There is also an obligation on the school to teach the world as the best modern minds view it in the light of the best available empirical evidence. We want to teach the actualities of economics rather than the dreams of economists. Here we should bear in mind Bruner's notion of the "spiral curriculum,"[17] which says that children can learn at their own level any subject matter at any age, that we can settle for incomplete, intuitive understanding at intermediate stages of learning, and that full knowledge and understanding come with repeated attacks, at ever more mature levels, on the same topics. It is obviously not enough to teach the substance of a subject matter; in addition, one must teach its logic, its organizing principles and the deductions these will or will not permit. Finally, our thinking about education is centered not in utility for society, but in terms of how one can build a more rational, more humane society than the one we know at present.

Discipline and Authority. Thus, the questions of teaching methods, techniques, and materials become subordinate to how one defines, and with what evidence, what is good for the child, in terms of his present and future intellectual competence and in terms of those personal qualities that will enable him or her to be effective as friend, lover, spouse, parent, breadwinner, citizen, and sometimes solitary searcher after goals and meanings. There are times when good order in the classroom is meaningful, when the children should be listening to the teacher or to the child who is making a report, when only one child at a time is allowed to raise a question or make a comment. But there are other occasions when good order rightly gets lost in the play of ideas, in construction projects, in the search for information in dictionary, encyclopedia, reference book, field, or laboratory, as children go questing individually or in small groups.

A modern school in which children are active participants in their own education has to tolerate a reasonable amount of noise and confusion. The teacher must retain authority, but he uses it judiciously, balancing group and individual interests and educational values. The teacher provides as much leadership and allows the children as much initiative as seems educationally wise. But the children's respect has to be based on the teacher's qualities as a person, on his command of knowledge, and on the sense that, even at his most authoritative, he is on the children's side.

The traditional view of school discipline has been that the children would erupt into chaos if adult controls were even momentarily relaxed, and proponents of this view could point to the actual behavior of children to support it. What they failed to see, of course, was that the restraints they imposed built up the very tensions and hostilities that caused the children to explode. They likewise failed to grasp that the traditional subject matter traditionally presented often induced a boredom and a craving for change and activity that were almost irresistible. By contrast, the more doctrinaire progressive educators wanted to remove all restraints and demands on the child, who, they assumed, left to his own devices and provided with abundant learning materials, would flower naturally into knowledge, wisdom, and humane fellow-feeling. This approach is summed up in the plaint of the cartoon child, "Do we have to do what we want to do again today?" Here we have the contrast drawn by Kurt Lewin and his collaborators[18] in the 1930's between *authoritarian,* adult-dominated, rigidly controlled styles of leadership, and the *laissez-faire* style in which the adult renounced virtually all control. What we propose, again following Lewin, is a *democratic* style in which the adult retains authority but uses it flexibly, with due respect to the wishes, needs, and inspirations of the children.

The liberal school as a whole is organized, and is perceived by the children, as an institution that helps children learn the truth. This means that it trusts its children who, like their teachers, are free from endless petty regulations and procedures. In too many schools, colleges, and universities, one gets the impression that the school belongs to the administration and is run for their comfort and convenience. The administrative machinery of a school is supposed, rather, to relieve teachers and students of administrative cares and thus facilitate the process of teaching and learning. But all too often, the administrators become the policy-makers, decision-makers, and authorities, who set standards for hiring, admission, promotion (of both teachers and pupils), leaves of absence, and discharge or suspension. The student's record folder tends to turn into a dossier, so that many parents and children come to fear the permanent consequences of "getting a black mark on your record." A student's performance has to be evaluated for the information of his parents, for his own guidance, and for the guidance of his successive teachers. But in general a school that respects its pupils will release to an agency outside the school only such information as is authorized by the parents. The form of the evaluation—grades or grades plus comments or detailed evaluations—can probably be left to the individual teacher, who may choose a variety of systems to suit individual pupils. As much as it may horrify administrators, it really is possible to live without a standardized system of evaluation. When it comes time for the child to move on to another school, it proves quite easy to extract a summary of his achievement, in general and in particular areas.

If the school has done its work well, we should expect a high level of achievement by all its pupils. For people are likely to think of a poor grade as a judgment on the child and, through him, on his parents. We are liable to forget that a poor grade reflects on the teacher and the school and their ability to communicate an essentially simple subject matter to children. The insights of the great scientists and philosophers were, in their day, remarkable accomplishments. But, once formulated, the great ideas become obvious and can be assimilated by anyone who is not markedly defective. The problem is one of communication, and often highly individualized communication, and it is here that the genius of the school and the teacher is put to the test. We may some day discover the one right and universal way of presenting the world so as to guarantee comprehension, retention, and the power of generalization to new instances, but until that day teachers are going to have to improvise, diagnose, analyze, and intuit to find ways to open each individual's senses and understanding to the marvels of reality. Since adult understanding is far from perfect, we also have to bear in mind that sometimes the children's discoveries and insights will outrun our own, and we have to be prepared to listen carefully and to learn from the children themselves.

The Practices of Liberal Schools. All this implies that a liberal school needs small classes, and if the idea of liberal schooling takes hold in public education, it means that we are going to have to spend still vaster sums of money on more classrooms, more books and equipment, and more teachers—and, in all probability, more administrators. We can easily afford to do it. Whether we do it depends on where the values and priorities lie. If we do support education on the scale it deserves, we should do so in full awareness of the power of knowledge and ideas to subvert traditional beliefs and practices and lead to fundamental social changes.

Let it be said that the authors speak here as observers. Neither of us has ever been responsible for a classroom of children except preschoolers and college students. We do claim to know something about children, however; we have sat in on (and filmed) a great many classes, we make some inferences from the behavior of college students about what their earlier educational experience must have been like, we have talked to a great many teachers and principals, and we think we have some perspective on society as a whole. What is more, we have seen some approximations of the liberal school at work and working. The best of the slum schools, and some good classes in some dreadful schools, follow modern-school principles. Whatever the chances in political terms for a liberal-school orientation in the public schools, we are confident that the modern school can accomplish the task of education, which is, after all, the single most vital collective task of a society.

In stating as we have that children in the middle years are alive with curiosity about every conceivable subject (with the possible exception, in the case of boys, of romantic love), we are ranging ourselves with those who feel that education can be meaningful and interesting and need not, in general, be forced. By the same token, we are not substituting carrots for sticks, singing piously of praise versus reproof, advocating gold stars, irrelevant rewards, or sugar-coating. We favor, rather, keeping the acquisition of skills and knowledge intrinsically rewarding, sometimes on an immediate and sometimes on a long-range basis. In short, we believe that the child himself should be enlisted as much as possible in the learning process; that he should not be seen as a receptacle at the far end of a pipeline through which the teacher pours her accumulated wisdom; that the teacher should stand beside or behind the child, guiding him toward a reality that exists independent of them both; and that the emphasis should be on learning and acquiring skills for finding knowledge as well as on teaching.

The more seasoned and successful of the liberal schools, private and public, assume and build on the eagerness and desire for knowledge we have spoken of; the early need for concrete, inductive experience; and growth toward pleasure in and ability to handle abstractions. Such schools free the child of arbitrary and unnecessary restraints—folded hands, no whispering—and of deadly and deadening routines—thirty-five children in turn reading aloud the same passage from the same book. They do not, however, tolerate the enforced anarchy that sometimes reigned in the early progressive schools. They provide scope for group and individual projects and research, and go as far as possible in the direction of original problem-setting, direct experience with subject matter, and the use of first sources rather than canned, diluted ones.

In the early grades, they know that effective learning can be built on the child's drive toward reality, his need to know what the world is all about, to understand how things are done, how they are put together, where they come from, and his desire to master tricks of the adult trade such as the magic of the written word and using numbers. They give him time and encouragement to figure things out for himself, to see things in action, to formulate and record his ideas; to read not only from textbooks but from charts, from accounts of exciting activities and events he himself has taken part in, and from "real" books; to put his thoughts into words and to communicate them to other people, sometimes by dictating stories and articles before he himself is able to master the mechanics of writing; to experience the satisfaction of achievement, to drill and memorize multiplication tables, spellings, and so forth, as these become needed and their value is apparent to him. By the time he is in the third grade, the

428

child is learning about other, perhaps more distant people, sharing their experience vicariously so that he will have some feeling for them as living people, rather than merely acquiring some notion of their strange and perhaps subhuman differences. At the same time, he is laying the groundwork for his coming interest in viewpoints and attitudes. In later grades, such schools rely more exclusively on the child's developing ability to grasp experience through symbols, without the same need as before for concreteness. At all times, the child is kept informed about the relationship of what he is doing to what he has been doing and is going to be doing.

In teaching the child, such schools, knowing his delight in exercising and working hard at what is his own, make sure he is kept learning at a pace that stretches his thinking apparatus without overwhelming him or making his task look hopeless. They adapt their teaching and demands to the child's ability, urging him on when he falters but recognizing and accepting that everyone does his share of backsliding, that everyone has spells of barrenness and vacancy. They likewise accept children's occasional need to rebel, being able to cope with insurrections without becoming disorganized and without surrendering. They know that children cannot always manage the entire job of self-control and are prepared to clamp down when it is in the child's and the group's best interests. They know that children sometimes are lazy and need some prodding. They know that children are sometimes impatient and would rather reach a goal in one magical leap, bypassing all the intervening steps, and they are prepared to insist on first things first. They know that the child is bound up in the values of his group of childhood society, but that he will outgrow his slavish conformity and that meanwhile, no matter how oblivious he seems, he is absorbing an education. Indeed, they encourage affiliation with and loyalty to the gang as a valuable part of the learning process, intervening only when the children's absolutism and intolerance threaten harm, or when the gang takes on an antisocial aspect.

Where the traditional school, in attempting to give children responsibility, alienates the "monitor" from his group by artificially investing him with adult powers, the liberal school allows groups to plan and function together, and, without pitting children against each other, on occasion lets the able speller help the poor one, or the child skilled in arithmetic coach the less skilled. They know that as children develop, they become more self-critical and work to improve past performances, competing with themselves. (A certain amount of competition among the children themselves is probably inevitable and perhaps even beneficial if kept within bounds; the children also like to compete individually against national norms, although here the danger is that instruction will be distorted into "teaching the tests.") Children also make demands on themselves and accept rigorous demands from the teacher, including extra assignments and homework. On the other hand, liberal educators know that children, like adults, often grade their own achievements unrealistically high (or low) and need a critical, hard-headed evaluation of their efforts. Throughout, the child is kept working not for the sake of grades or "rewards" but for the intrinsic satisfaction of moving step by step in his own understanding, completing tasks, and meeting and mastering new ideas.

The liberal school, unlike the ordinary compromise school, does not march forward under the banner of "adjustment." It allows for vigorous, outspoken individuality. It recognizes as its goal for the child not adjustment, with its risks of submissive conformity, but becoming an interested and interesting person. It knows that much important development—even social development—takes place in solitary imaginings rather than in social groups, that one of the chief avenues to good social relationships is developing interests which are not necessarily social but which can be shared, and that a sound social sense is not to be measured by counting the number of social "contacts" a person makes.

The liberal school, needless to say, shares with all schools certain of the problems of our society. The factor of increasing urbanization brings other problems in its wake. It means, for one thing, that children have little play space, except in the city streets. As a result, the school is often given the responsibility of providing after-hours recreation and hobby facilities for its pupils. Urban living further means, especially for the middle and upper classes, that family friendship patterns, church affiliations, and other community contacts may correspond but poorly to neighborhood distributions, so that the family in times of crisis, major or minor, turns increasingly to the school for help.

What with one factor or another, the school is being forced to assume functions—ranging from guarding the child's mental health to making sure he knows how to swim, to giving him an opportunity to roam through a forest, to providing sex education, and so on—that formerly belonged to the family, the neighborhood, and the family's spiritual and medical advisors. Whether or not this trend is inevitable, we regard it as deplorable. We believe the child's family has the primary responsibility and privilege of raising him, and the more this function is turned over to some outside agency, the more the family's enjoyment and sense of competence is depleted and the more it loses the richness of shared experience, a loss that cannot be compensated by "helping" children with their homework. We further believe that this multiplicity of functions dissipates the school's energies and further contributes to the need for a complex, interlocking bureaucracy. While it is true that the school must educate the whole child—no matter how hard it might try, it could not do anything else—it should not have to undertake the whole education of the whole child on a full-time basis. We applaud the use of school facilities for recreation, community meetings, adult education, and so forth, provided these functions are administered separately from, and do not interfere with, the school's primary function of educating children.

OTHER PROGRAMS FOR MIDDLE-YEARS CHILDREN

What we have said about teachers and teaching applies almost *in toto* to other adult-led childhood enterprises such as recreation groups, scouting, or the rehabilitation of delinquent gangs. While different kinds of preparation may be necessary or sufficient for leaders in these situations, it is still imperative that a leader have a genuine zest for the activity, a thorough understanding of children, a knowledge of the individual children he is dealing with and of their individual needs, an awareness of the forces governing adult society, and how to make his ideas and purposes relevant to those of the children. One can force a child to attend school, at least in body, but the leader of voluntary activities must attune his program to the needs and values of children or else the program will deteriorate or the children go elsewhere. The adult working with delinquents or in a high-delinquency neighborhood must likewise understand that he is not dealing with children who are simply wicked, or who only need to have their time filled with wholesome pursuits to keep them out of mischief, but with children facing real and terrible problems who seek magical solutions and ready reassurance through identification with the gang. The defense of the home turf by the block gang is only a miniature of the psychopathology of nations. The values of the gang may seem far more meaningful than those of the respectable, alien, teacherlike middle class. But even when dealing with middle-class children, the group leader has to take account of the child's own motives and wants, and of the gang's mores, or the program will evaporate in a cloud of boredom or fisticuffs.

Too many adult-sponsored programs are like child or adult clubs in which the fact of organization takes precedence over actual goals, leaving the membership floundering, or providing ersatz functions, once the ceremonial activities have been unrolled. Part of the trouble, as we have suggested, is that adults do not sufficiently trust children to be able to manage their own free time, and so invent a plethora of time-killing boondoggles. Perhaps it would be better if the kids just watched TV.

REFERENCES / Chapter 9

1 Asch, S. E., and Nerlove, H. The development of double function terms in children: An exploratory investigation. In Kaplan, B., and Wapner, S. (eds.) *Perspectives in Psychological Theory.* New York: International Universities, 1960, pp. 47–60.
2 Werner, H., and Kaplan, E. The acquisition of word meanings. *Monographs of the Society for Research in Child Development,* 1950, 25, no. 1.
3 Richardson, C., and Church, J. A developmental analysis of proverb interpretations. *Journal of Genetic Psychology,* 1959, 94, 169–179.
4 Koff, R. H. Systematic changes in children's word-association norms 1916–63. *Child Development,* 1965, 36, 299–305; Jenkins, J. J., and Russell, W. A. Systematic changes in word association norms: 1910–1952. *Journal of Abnormal and Social Psychology,* 1960, 60, 293–304; Palermo, D. S., and Jenkins, J. J. Changes in word associations of fourth- and fifth-grade children from 1916 to 1961. *Journal of Verbal Learning and Verbal Behavior,* 1965, 4, 180–187; Jenkins, J. J., and Palermo, D. S. Further changes in word association norms. *Journal of Personality and Social Psychology,* 1965, 1, 303–309.
5 Weinreich, U. Travels through semantic space. *Word,* 1958, 14, 346–366.
6 An exception is an interesting study by Maltz, H. E. Ontogenetic changes in the meaning of concepts as measured by the semantic differential. *Child Development,* 1963, 34, 667–674.
7 Piaget, J. *The Moral Judgment of the Child.* Glencoe: Free Press, 1948 (originally published in 1932).
8 Senn, M. J. E. Personal communication.
9 Machotka, P. The development of esthetic criteria in childhood: I. Justifications of preference. *Child Development,* 1966, 37, 877–885; Shesh, D. B. Measurement of aesthetic sense of children. *Psychologia,* 1966, 9, 236–238.
10 Bruner, J. S. After John Dewey, what? *Bank Street College of Education Publications,* 1961, no. 54 (originally published in *Saturday Review,* June 17, 1961).
11 Polanyi, M. *Personal Knowledge.* Chicago: University of Chicago, 1958.
12 Ashton-Warner, S. *Teacher.* New York: Simon & Schuster, 1963.
13 Crabtree, C. A. Effects of structuring on productiveness of children's thinking. *Dissertation Abstracts,* 1962, 23, 161. Reprinted in Gordon, I. J. (ed.) *Human Development.* Chicago: Scott, Foresman, 1965, pp. 249–250; Biber, B. Premature structuring as a deterrent to creativity. *Bank Street College of Education Publications,* n.d., no. 67 (originally published in *American Journal of Orthopsychiatry,* 1959, 29, no. 2).

14 Kreutter, M. The teacher in the brown paper bag. *Urban Review*, May, 1966.

15 For a survey of the relevant literature see Grose, R. F., and Birney, R. C. (eds.) *Transfer of Learning*. Princeton: Van Nostrand, 1963.

16 Church, J. Innovations, excellence, and children's learning. *Bank Street College of Education Publications*, 1962 (originally published in *School and Society*, 1962, 90, 401–404).

17 Bruner, J. S. *The Process of Education*. Cambridge: Harvard, 1960.

18 Lewin, K., Lippitt, R., and White, R. K. Patterns of aggressive behavior in experimentally created "social climates." *Journal of Social Psychology*, 1939, 10, 271–299; White, R. K., and Lippitt, R. O. *Autocracy and Democracy*. New York: Harper, 1960.

10   *Adolescence: 1*

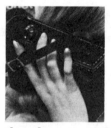

It used to be, as we have said, that the middle years were a time in which the child was content with his lot, whereas adolescence was a period that he entered reluctantly and left as soon as people would allow. Nowadays, by contrast, middle-years children often aspire to be teen-agers, and the teen-agers themselves seem to feel (much of the time) that they have found the ultimate mode of existence. This belief seems to be shared by many adults who adopt teen-age styles of coiffure, dress, dancing, recreation, and slang. Currently, and not alone in the United States, adolescence has been institutionalized and is glorified in television programs, periodicals, the world of radio,[1] and merchandise aimed at the teen-age market.[2] Even those adults who neither join nor exploit the cult of adolescence may conspire to propagate it, as though to live it vicariously. Teen-agers have cars and seemingly endless resources of cash and credit with which to amass sports equipment, guitars, records, cosmetics, clothes, and accessories. They flock to adults-only movies and to spy thrillers and in general are bombarded with subtle and not-so-subtle pro-sexual propaganda. They talk a great deal about sex, but all the indications are that few practice it, and then only in special circumstances.

We despair of knowing accurately the social extent or the personal pervasiveness of the teen-age style. If teen-agers are very much with us, it is partly because there are so many of them, some 24 million in the thirteen-to-nineteen age range, the largest seven-year segment of our population. They are the product of the post-World War II baby boom, and as they grow older they will swell different portions of the population curve. It seems safe to say, though, that certain features of adolescent life endure through the surface changes, the fashions and fads.

Physical and Psychological Adolescence

Writers on the subject of adolescence—beginning, as far as formal psychology is concerned, with G. Stanley Hall[3]—have been struck by the adolescent's agonies of self-consciousness, his preoccupation with who he is and where he belongs. They have noted his proneness to idealism, religious conversion, moodiness and changes of mood, to feelings that life is futile, and to rebellion and iconoclasm. Adolescence has come to be known as a time of inner turmoil, as a period of *Sturm und Drang,* of "storm and stress." Needless to say, this inner turmoil finds external expression, and the adults who have to deal with adolescents come in for their share of turmoil, too. Many writers have attributed the turbulence of this age to the physiological upheaval associated with puberty, and, by implication, to the discrepancy between the adolescent's sexual maturity and mental immaturity.

It now seems obvious that this explanation will not do. For one thing, there are societies, and sections of our own society, in which adolescence is not a time of *Sturm und Drang,* so that although all young people go through the physical changes of adolescence, only those in particular cultural settings show the behavior we take to be characteristic of this age. Furthermore, careful observation shows that the psychological crises of adolescence do not ordinarily begin until a year or more after the period of most rapid physical change; for some individuals, there seems to be virtually no relation between physical changes and typically adolescent behavior. For these reasons, we are obliged to view adolescence as a cultural phenomenon derived from the way people in our society (and similar societies) interpret the fact of physical maturing. Adults and the peer group both define roles for the adolescent to play, and in assuming these roles he takes on his adolescent identity.

The distinction between physical maturing and culturally defined roles makes it necessary to separate their two vocabularies. There are three terms which we should begin by making clear: pubescence, puberty, and adolescence.

Pubescence refers to the period of about two years immediately before puberty, and to the physical changes during that period which culminate in puberty. The beginning of pubescence is marked by an increase in the rate of physical growth, the onset of the *prepubertal growth spurt,* and the end of growth latency. Along with the growth spurt come changes in facial and body proportions, the maturing of primary and secondary sex traits, and an assortment of other physical changes which we shall describe later. (Some writers refer to the period of pubescence as "preadolescence." Psychologically, to be sure, the pubescent youngster is in many respects more of a middle-years child than an adolescent. However, preadolescence is a confusing term because yet other writers use it synonymously with the middle years.)

Puberty is the point in life at which sexual maturity begins, marked in girls by the *menarche,* the first menstrual flow, and in boys by a number of signs, the most reliable one probably being the presence of spermatozoa in the urine (detectable under the microscope). In fact, the borderline of puberty is not altogether clearcut for either girls or boys. Menstruation at first is likely to be skimpy and irregular, sometimes with months intervening between flows. Boys may feel strong phallic urges and discover that female propinquity is a potent stimulus to erection, but still be unable to ejaculate. In law, twelve is commonly designated as the age of puberty for girls, and fourteen for boys. There are, however, such wide individual and group differences, possibly associated with nutrition, health conditions, and any number of possible unknown factors, including, perhaps, exposure to sexual stimulation, that any statement about averages becomes meaningless. It is clear, though, that boys tend to lag about two years behind girls in reaching puberty. There seems to be a comparable lag in boys' social development, making for certain dislocations which we shall discuss later.

Adolescence is used in two somewhat different senses. In terms of physical development, it refers to the age span that begins with the prepubertal growth spurt and ends with the attainment of full physical maturity. This statement is more ambiguous than it may seem, since "full physical maturity" is hard to define. In the physical sense, adolescence is a universal manifestation. In psychological terms, adolescence refers to a state of mind, a mode of existence that begins roughly with puberty and ends—but we prefer for the time being to evade this question and say provisionally that psychological adolescence ends with full social maturity. It is the main business of this chapter and the next to define adolescence as a state of mind. But psychological adolescence, unlike physical adolescence, appears only in certain cultures. It should be clear from the context when we are talking about maturational adolescence and when about psychological.

Like all the other age periods we have talked about, adolescence is a time of continuing change, and we shall find it necessary to draw a distinction between "early" and "late." Early adolescence, as we use it, refers to the period from the beginning of pubescence (which in the individual case is known only in retrospect) until about a year after puberty, when the youngster's new physiological patterns have fairly well stabilized. Late adolescence, of course, is the remainder of the period up to adulthood.

The central theme of adolescence is that of *identity*, coming to know who one is, what one believes in and values, what one wants to accomplish and get out of life. The adolescent has to come to terms with a new kind of body with new potentialities for feeling and acting, and to rearrange his or her self-image accordingly. Corresponding to changes in his body there emerges a whole new constellation of meanings in the life space. For many adolescents, the world becomes libidinized, sexualized, so that the most innocuous objects and events take on erotic implications. The adolescent's new and often confused self-awareness—manifested largely as self-consciousness—involves a new push for independence.

In early adolescence, the youngster seeks independence in new areas like religious beliefs or dating, but very much in the same way as when he was younger: He wants more privileges, more freedom from adult supervision and restraint so that he can follow the dictates of the gang (which he now probably calls the "crowd"), but with little sense of responsibility for the consequences of his own actions. The young adolescent, perhaps even more than during the middle years, is concerned about his status with his immediate peers; he strives to be as much like the others as possible, perhaps because he feels so much out of step with them. For, almost against his own volition, he is becoming ever more of an individual, with ideas and values that may not match the essentially conservative code of the gang, but his own only half-understood uniqueness is not completely welcome.

The older adolescent shares the younger one's concerns but is, in addition, confronted by the problem of where he stands with respect to the entire adult world of independence and responsibility—sex, marriage, jobs, military service, politics, parenthood—and must face the chilling prospect of being on his own, without the material support of his family or the moral support of the peer group. It is part of our social ethic that the person—specifically, but not exclusively so, the male—who maintains dependent status after he reaches adulthood has something wrong with him, and this is felt as acutely by the individual as by his family and neighbors. We can say that the young adolescent is concerned about who and what he is, whereas the older adolescent has to be concerned, in addition, about what he is going to do with himself for the rest of his life.

In these chapters, then, we shall first consider the peculiarly European phenomenon of adolescence as an aspect of culture. (Notice that European, in this sense, includes non-European countries settled by Europeans or s⁺ ɔngly influenced by Europe: Latin and North America, the Asian sections of the Soviet Union, Australia and New Zealand, Japan, and the emerging middle class in whatever part of the world. Adolescence, along with concern about mental health and creativity, and along with waste and pollution, seems to be a luxury that only reasonably well-to-do societies can afford.) This description will include the classical symptoms of adolescence and the newer manifestations to be observed on the current scene. It seems to us that the individual psychology of adolescence can only be grasped against the sociology and social psychology of this age. Therefore, we shall begin with a description of adolescence as a social phenomenon: adolescence as a cultural invention, the adolescent subculture, family relations, and typical adolescent activities. In the next chapter, we shall examine the adolescent himself, his developing body and awakening sexuality, his attitudes, values, aspirations, and ambitions. Then, in Chapter 12, we shall return to adult society and the provisions it makes and fails to make for welcoming the adolescent into maturity. In this context, we shall say something about conceptions of what it means to be psychologically mature.

Psychological Adolescence as a Cultural Phenomenon

In primitive societies, there is no equivalent for our concept of adolescence. In some primitive societies, the transition from childhood to adulthood is so smooth that no particular note is taken of the process. More usually, we find that the young person on the threshold of maturity goes through a ceremonial adolescence. The rituals by which adulthood is conferred are variously called *puberty rites, rites de passage,* and *initiation ceremonies.* They may be carefully timed to coincide with puberty, children of various ages may be rounded up and initiated, or it may be left to the child himself to decide when he is ready to assume the rights and cares of adulthood or when he feels able to endure what may be a rigorous procedure.

At their simplest, initiation rites may consist of nothing more than a haircut or a change of clothes. More complex rituals may involve elaborate tattooing, periods of isolation or fasting, or a search for a vision or revelation. Some ceremonies are ordeals which serve at least partly as tests of character: circumcision with a sharpened stick, surgical removal of the clitoris, having one's teeth filed to a point, the ability to take torture without crying out, the infliction of lesions which will leave scars considered a mark of beauty. Young men may have to demonstrate their manhood in mortal combat, and the scalp at the belt or feasting on the heart and genitals of the man you have slain may be the ultimate measure. Such *rites de passage* seldom last more than a few weeks (admittedly, these may be highly vivid weeks), and even the longest of them are negligible compared to the approximately seven years that we take for granted as a transition period. Once the puberty rite is successfully at an end, the young person has attained full adult status and apparently assumes it without any lingering sense of ambiguity. The demands and prerogatives of his new role are perfectly clear and other people take it for granted that he will play the role correctly. In most primitive societies, adultlike obligations are gradually imposed on the child, and he and his peers practice the prerogatives, such as sex, on their own, often with adult approval, so that childhood tends to flow continuously into adulthood, with only the ceremonial punctuation of the puberty rite to break the continuity.

It is tempting to go beyond these generalizations about other societies and to detail the diverse ways in which the seal of maturity is bestowed. It would also be interesting to discuss the meanings attached to various practices, and how the young people themselves view them. So detailed an account would take us deeper into anthropology than is appropriate, and we refer the curious reader to his local library, where he will find the relevant literature in locked cases. The essential fact that emerges from a comparison of our culture with others is that psychological adolescence is not a necessary corollary of physical adolescence, but a cultural phenomenon produced by a delay in the assumption of adult roles. That is, the more we prolong the period of subadult status, the more elaborate become the rules that govern behavior. Sometimes the role demands come into being unconsciously or on a wave of social contagion. More and more, adults and adolescents alike are taking thought with regard to the adolescent condition and giving explicit voice to what they understand its role characteristics to be. It is adolescents taking stock of adolescence, sometimes in response to adult teachings, who have proclaimed doctrines of sexual freedom or the glories of marijuana. On the other hand, it is the shrewd poll-takers and promoters who have set forth the notion of the teen-age charge account or credit card, and it is the image-makers who have conveyed that cigarette-smoking and motorcycle ownership are essential ingredients of the adolescent role.

As we shall discuss later in more detail, it would appear that as societies become industrialized, the total period of apprenticeship is lengthened, the taking on of adult roles is deferred, and the interval between sexual maturity and adult status gets longer. Indeed, a long adolescence is a relatively recent phenomenon in our own society. It is worth noting that such ceremonies as the Christian confirmation, which requires the individual, once he has reached the "age of discretion," to confirm on his own the religious beliefs he has been taught, and the Jewish Bar Mitzvah, both held at about age thirteen, probably began as puberty rites. We might also recall that Shakespeare's tragic heroine Juliet was only fourteen, and that in colonial times marriages often took place in the early teens. On the law books of many states today, the marriageable age is still twelve for girls and fourteen for boys, although it becomes a matter of momentary nationwide interest when youngsters of this age actually assert their legal prerogatives. Nowadays, in our aristocratic social strata the girl "comes out"—implicitly into the marriage market—at age eighteen. In the more plebeian segments of society, the girl makes her debut somewhat earlier, at a "Sweet Sixteen" birthday party. (The idea of a debut is alien to members of some ethnic groups in which marriages are arranged between families by a marriage broker or go-between; and in the middle class, dating provides the way to get to know prospective mates.) The important point here is that the former symbols of adulthood—financial independence from the parents, completing school (not only does one need more education in order to work in a technologically advanced economy, but in recent years the graduate schools have become favored shelters against the biting winds of the draft)—are being postponed to ever later ages. Also, in our society there is no one event or criterion that marks off immaturity from maturity. The adult world gives the adolescent ambiguous information about his status, reinforcing his own ambiguity about himself.

Our culture contains numerous micro–*rites de passage*, some written into law and others simply part of the folkways, but no single one a true indicator of adulthood. Indeed, as we have suggested, these micro-rites may be in conflict with each other. Even the law is inconsistent, from state to state and from one area of functioning to another. The age of consent for girls may be anywhere from age twelve to age eighteen—but while the law specifies the age at which sexual intercourse without marriage may take place, in most states and localities it prohibits or penalizes extramarital sexual intercourse. (Although we ordinarily think of statutory rape as applying to girls, the laws have sometimes been invoked against older women who seduced boys who had not reached the age of consent. There is a further instance of a group of seventeen-year-old boys being charged with statutory rape for having relations with a prostitute just below the statutory age of eighteen.)[4] Depending on which state he lives in, the individual may be allowed to drive a car at fourteen or not until he is eighteen. Up to age twenty-five, the male must pay an extra premium on his car insurance. Employers must pay a higher rate for accident insurance if they employ minors, further complicating the already difficult picture for the would-be adolescent worker.

The adolescent suffers from two kinds of technological unemployment. First, automation reduces the need for production workers. Second, the conditions of our society reduce the need for unskilled workers. A third consideration is that adolescents are reluctant to enter occupations which are accorded low status in our value system, even though there may be plenty of openings and even though the actual work may be highly useful: barbering, plumbing, nursing (for both males and females), auto repairing, and so on. (It is interesting that the craft unions, like the medical profession, conspire to keep workers in short supply in order to enhance their market value.) The child labor laws, while serving the perfectly admirable purpose of keeping children (all except newsboys and farm workers) from being exploited economically, may incidentally deny adolescents the chance to get practical experience and, with it, a sense of growth, accomplishment, and independence.

The age at which the young person can buy alcoholic beverages may be set at eighteen, nineteen, twenty, or twenty-one, which makes for very real problems as in the case of New York, which permits drinking at age eighteen, so that adolescents from adjoining states drive in, tank up, and then drive drunkenly in the direction of home. Quite a number never make it. Seventeen-year-olds may enlist in the military, and eighteen-year-olds can be drafted. But while teen-agers are considered old enough to kill and be killed, they may not be considered old enough to drink or vote, and at various times people get very agitated about making the boys' military surroundings more homelike, both to ease the shock of transition and to provide a wholesome moral atmosphere—in other words, draftees should still be treated like children. The platoon sergeant is cast in the dual role of Fagan and house mother. Again, the right to vote may come at age eighteen or at age twenty-one. If one is a Negro, of course, the opportunity to exercise that right may never come. In general, we try to keep Negroes in a perpetual childhood, and then are shocked if they behave childishly.

In the past, our society's views of when one should stop being a child and become an adult have been very much influenced by transitory conditions. During the great depression of the 1930's, for instance, there was considerable pressure to keep young people out of the overcrowded labor market. They were urged to stay in school, and those out of school were organized into "youth groups," many of whose members were fully mature people, if not middle-aged. When World War II came along and reversed the manpower picture, the pressure on young people was to get into the armed forces or the production and distribution of war goods.

Now, when we have an oversupply of young people, there is an almost automatic channeling of young men into higher education, with the assumption of later careers as entrepreneurs, managers, or professionals; into miscellaneous jobs; into cannon-fodder; and into the garbage heap of chronic unemployment or underemployment, with implications of criminality and psychopathology. But the fact that society has developed fairly stable selective mechanisms that decide the young person's future does not mean that these correspond to the young person's psychological needs. None of the pathways open to him may offer a meaningful solution to the puzzle of his identity as a person.

Childhood is certainly being increasingly prolonged in the sense of financial dependence on parents. In other areas, though, adulthood is coming earlier than before. The age of marriage is going back down, although it does not promise ever again to coincide with puberty. This trend was accelerated during a period when marriage brought with it exemption from the draft, but has probably returned approximately to its former rate. An appreciable number of marriages take place prior to full financial independence, with parental subsidies. Several states have lowered the voting age to eighteen.

Perhaps most striking is the change in dating patterns. Although young boys and girls have always gone to shows and parties together, the members of each sex were likely to cluster together, with little or no pairing off of boy and girl. The real "date" used to be considered proper only for later adolescence. Currently, dating at age thirteen or fourteen is not uncommon and, in spite of some adult resistance, is becoming increasingly widespread. We keep hearing reports of dating prior to the teens. This produces some anomalies, as in the case of a thirteen-year-old boy about to meet a girl at the movies for his first date, who asked his mother, "Do you suppose I could tell her to meet me inside? That way I wouldn't have to pay for her ticket." Thirteen- and fourteen-year-olds are also said to "go steady," although this term no longer seems to mean an informal betrothal, but rather that the pair enter into a contract, sometimes for a specified period, and almost always with an understanding that it is temporary, that guarantees both of them a partner on whatever dating occasions arise.

The same earlier maturing appears in the increasing frequency with which young adolescents work part time, whether at baby-sitting, doing the neighbors' chores (some enterprising youngsters borrow or save capital with which to buy a power mower or snowplow), or even founding a business such as a neighborhood newspaper or a truck garden. There are a number of minor milestones (which may appear anything but minor to the adolescent) which are now passed at ever lower ages: the age at which a girl gets her first permanent, or is allowed to wear lipstick, or raised heels, or acquires her first formal gown. Over the years, the age at which the boy gets his first long trousers (formerly quite a ceremonious affair, with the boy feeling embarrassed and pleased) has been moved down almost to the cradle, and "knickers" have vanished from the scene. Now the pressure is for a dinner jacket, which may come as early as age eight; the junior dinner jackets we have seen come in paisley, plaid, or pareu or tapa print, and are only a touch more flamboyant than those worn by adult males. The age at which the boy gets a razor of his own is, of course, probably too closely tied to physical maturation to be lowered greatly. But the razor too is a token of progress toward adulthood, one of the many tokens which in our society replace the single initiation ceremony of more primitive ones. With such tokens, adults nudge the youngster toward maturity, and ambivalently toward sexual maturity.

To some extent, this pushing of milestones toward the beginning of the time scale seems to be an upward diffusion of lower-class practices into the middle and upper classes. In general, mature status is granted relatively early in the lower classes, and children higher in the socioeconomic scheme of things (especially boys) have always envied the freedom of their lower-class counterparts. Upper-class parents used to resist their children's clamor for various privileges with the argument that certain things were "vulgar" or that "there's plenty of time yet for that." Now, with the extensive homogenization of our culture (including a certain amount of affluence even among those who on other measures might be called plebeian), vulgarity is much less of an issue. As for time, parents nowadays are inclined to share the adolescent's feeling that time is running out and that he must hurry to taste life's pleasures before the world goes smash or, an equally dread alternative, his capacity for enjoyment is vitiated by adulthood. Also, psychologically, time does slip away from children and adolescents faster than it used to, because we fill their days with so many demands and activities, and filled time passes much more quickly than empty time. On the other hand, filled time is later recalled more vividly than empty time, which may be one reason that adults who have had an active adolescence look back so fondly, whereas those who were bored as adolescents are glad to have left this period behind.

Although adolescence seems to have arisen almost by accident out of the evolving pattern of our society, it has become solidly institutionalized as a period when the individual is no longer a child but is not yet an adult, and it has been bound about with rationalizations. Our key rationalization is that the manifestations of adolescence are natural and inevitable, that adolescent behavior is rooted in the adolescent's incomplete maturity. We should like to make the point, anticipating later discussion, that the immaturity of adolescents is largely a product of the way we treat them, that interactions between the adult world and the adolescent world too often form a vicious circle, a positive feedback loop in which every reaction produces a more intense counterreaction, bringing out the worst in everybody. It is our contention that much of the strife between adolescents and adults is useless and destructive and could be eliminated to everybody's benefit. Some conflict between the generations may be inevitable, and some kinds of conflict may be beneficial, but much of it is simply the reciprocal discharge of frustrations. There is no denying that the complexities of adult life in our society demand an extended apprenticeship, but, as Nixon[5] points out, this does not mean enforced immaturity, and there is reason to question whether the apprenticeship we provide is the most effective one possible.

The Adolescent and His Parents

If the adolescent's central problem is to define an identity independent of the authority and support of his parents, it follows that he has to break innumerable ties to his family based on authority, affection, responsibility, respect, intimacy, money and material goods, immaturity, possessiveness, and force of habit. In this section, we shall deal primarily with how the adolescent and his family work toward and at the same time resist this painful series of ruptures, and the stresses engendered in the process. Here again, we lean to the side of exaggeration and caricature (although reality sometimes defies caricature) to make the important features salient.

We should begin by saying that adolescents and their parents spend some part of their time getting along with each other very nicely, sharing discoveries and fresh looks at experience, exchanging banter, talking over plans and problems, and simply enjoying each other's company. It is also important to note that some adolescents grow up with essentially no conflict with their families beyond the frictions that go with living together. Such adolescents, who are more likely to be girls than boys, show an early and thorough identification with the family's values of whatever kind, whether upper-class or lower-class hedonism, the super-respectability of the static lower middle class, prosperous middle-class self-satisfaction, upwardly mobile ambition and acquisitiveness, or the values that go with living by thievery.

The family of such adolescents lets go easily, confident they will continue to be emotionally close and that the youngster "has got the right stuff in him" to enable him to make his way. The general rule, however, seems to be that the adolescent grows away from his family, both in spirit and in body, until home sometimes seems little more than a rooming house where he eats, sleeps, drops his clothes to be picked up and laundered, looks at the sport pages (or, if a girl, at the advice columns) and comics, watches television, and makes and receives phone calls. Chores are likely to be executed in a straw-boss–convict relationship rather than as a shared work experience, which deprives them of most of their value. The adolescent's own room, if he has one, or the privacy of a hotly contested bathroom, serves as a refuge where he can study and register his own growth, where before the mirror he can experiment with, practice, and perfect the masks he wears, the styles and images he wants to project. Mealtimes, in those families which eat together, are perhaps the only remaining opportunity for real exchanges with his family. And although the dinner table may serve as a forum, it can also become an arena. A substantial part of the time the adolescent spends with his family is likely to be colored by feelings—on both sides—of frustration, outrage, humiliation, sullenness, resentment, and dramatic (or melodramatic) despair.

Underlying a great many conflicts are the allied states of ambiguity and ambivalence. Ambiguity haunts the young adolescent especially with regard to his own body, such that he is not sure whether he should be acting like a child or an adult. He tends to repudiate his childish self, but hardly with assurance or without regrets. He feels perfectly self-confident up to the moment that he confronts the task of demonstrating his competence. He demands privileges but views their corresponding responsibilities as onerous. From the parents' point of view, of course, the ability to bear responsibility is as much a mark of maturity as is having privileges. To the child, by contrast, responsibilities are imposed by adults and so are degrading tokens of his inferior status. The parents do not share the young adolescent's ambiguity about where he stands. He is clearly still a child, but a child big enough to help out.

It is with reference to the older adolescent that parents experience amibiguity, uncertainty about where he stands and how he should be treated. The older adolescent looks very much like an adult and sometimes even acts like one, but his occasional slips and even blunders betray the child who lurks inside. The older adolescent feels little ambiguity about his grown-up status. His probem is growth ambivalence, an urge to take the final step into adulthood coupled with a sense that to do so is to step into the void. His growth ambivalence, morever, is shared by his parents, leading to an intensification of the pattern of *dual ambivalence* whereby parents and child are at war with each other about his status and each side is at war with itself. To complicate the pattern further, father and mother may have somewhat different patterns of ambivalence, which can set them at war with each other. Further, there may be a triangle of back-and-forth emotional ambivalence in which love and devotion war with resentment and hostility.

One source of the older adolescent's growth ambivalence is the fear of failure. Every time he reaches for adulthood, he puts himself on trial. Consciously, of course, the adolescent refuses to acknowledge the possibility of failure, but it repeatedly crops up as a chilly, threatening presence. Another source of growth ambivalence for the young person is that adult privileges themselves hold half-sensed terrors. The adolescent is by no means sure that he wants to liberate and indulge the new forces at work within himself. He has not yet learned to sense these forces as truly his own, he has not yet integrated them into his self-schema, and he is not sure whether he can control them once they are turned loose.

Thus, protest and grumble though he may, he sometimes feels a secret relief when his parents add the weight of their authority to his own uncertain controls. Into the bargain, it is likely that the vehemence of his protests is in direct proportion to the anxiety he feels, and the protests are partly against his own uncertainty. Even if his parents did not already share his growth ambivalence, it would still put them into what Bateson[6] calls a double-bind situation, so that they are damned if they do and damned if they don't, and so cannot win. For if the parents exercise control, they are snoopy and domineering; if they let the youngster decide for himself, they are neglectful and uncaring. An early version of the adolescent's dual attitude is seen in a composition by a high school sophomore who says, "The parents should make it their job to see to it that their children do their homework" (which, it is promised, will ensure "less juvenile delinquencies") and, in the next breath, "Parents should treat boys of fifteen years of age as grownups and not children."[7]

This parental double-bind does not mean that what parents do is of no importance. Parents still have to provide limits and guidelines and values, and if the child fights them, this has its developmental importance, too. For if the young person is going to find a set of durable values that he can call his own, he will probably have to begin by contesting the established values of his parents. And parents, if they expect the youngster to listen, have to react with something better than moral indignation.

Parents, of course, are eager to have their children grow up. Indeed, when parents criticize an adolescent it is likely to be on the grounds that he is acting childishly. But although parents urge the young person toward adulthood, they often act as though his reaching the adult state is still in the comfortably far-off future. It is said that readiness for adulthood comes about two years later than the adolescent claims, and about two years before his parents will admit. As often as not, parents, without knowing it, retard development, even though they may show no open regret over losing "my baby." There seem to be several possible roots for parents' unwillingness to let the child grow up. For one thing, they know their own child too well and are all too aware of his weaknesses and inadequacies. They are overaware, also, of the perils and pitfalls of the great outside world. They fail to see, however, that the only way the youngster can overcome his weaknesses and cope with the problems of an independent life is by actually moving into the world. No one is ever fully prepared in advance for adult life, and every developmental step has its risks—letting the child walk by himself, cross the street alone, sending him off to school, letting him run with the gang, letting him go out unchaperoned, letting him use the family car—each requires a fear-provoking wrench that has to come.

At a more hidden motivational level, the youngster's growing up may be threatening to his parents. By a process of reverse identification of parent with child, it may reawaken the unresolved fears and conflicts of their own adolescent pasts. It may bring home to them with new and frightening force how the years and dreams have slipped away, leaving them members of an aging generation. It may even breed a species of jealousy over the pleasures that still await the adolescent, perhaps tempered by a wry recognition that youth is wasted on the young. It may simply coincide with or it may provoke the later crisis of identity that many adults go through, women at age thirty-five to forty and men at forty-five to fifty (see page 512). It may imply the end of the parents' usefulness, that their mission in life is at an end, or it may spell a lonely life in a house that has suddenly become too big. Parental resistance to the child's growing up may stem from unwillingness to relinquish authority built up over a decade and a half.

Parental resistance may be greatest for a firstborn child, who in this area as in so many others has to break trail for the other siblings. In general, parents, like everybody else, resist change, they are unwilling to surrender old habits and adopt new ones, to let go. As we have said, the growth ambivalence of parents dates back at least to late infancy, and if the adolescent is not so well prepared for adulthood as he might be, it may be because of an intermittent, if loving and well-intentioned, sabotage of his autonomy by parents over the years.

With dual ambivalence as the background, conflicts between the adolescent and his parents can arise on almost any subject. Much of the passion attendant on these conflicts is probably generated by both parties' need to drown out their own feelings that contradict what they are expressing. Among the favorite topics of dispute are dating, friendships, dress, time schedules, chores and duties, money, automobiles, school marks, future schooling, morals and manners, access to the telephone, religious observances and beliefs, politics and economics—not necessarily in this order of prominence or importance. In all these matters, the adolescent wants to be free and unconfined, but at the same time he is coming to realize that he is enmeshed in a network of reciprocity that inevitably restricts his freedom of action. Often, indeed, it is this very inevitability which he is fighting, rather than the specific restriction he is made to observe.

It is worth pointing out that the inescapability of reciprocal responsibilities may add another dimension to the adult's ambivalence as well. When the parent rages to the child about responsibilities, his wrath may be in direct proportion to his own secret wish that he could repair to a tropical isle, slough off his duties, and live a life of anarchic selfishness.

No matter how well adults—particularly males—have adapted to a life based on social reciprocity, they cannot restrain a twinge of sympathy for those who refuse to yield—in the adolescent's term, "to sell out to the system." The adolescent is often shrewd enough to detect this source of ambivalence and to be outspokenly aware of his parents' departures from their own professed standards. It is quite common to hear adolescents call their parents "hypocrites." While this allegation may have some truth, some part of parental hypocrisy may be an attempt to help the adolescent make a better life for himself than the parents'. Parents often try to give their youngsters the "benefit of their experience," to teach the lessons which they had to learn the hard way, from life itself, sometimes too late for it to do them any good. But it seems to be the case that the adolescent cannot learn these lessons. He simply does not know enough about the workings of the world for the lessons to make sense, he is too much wrapped up in his immediate personal concerns, and he feels that his parents are fundamentally ignorant of his situation and are living in the past. Again, let us remember, both generations agree that times have changed.

Let us look at some exceptions to this pattern of dual ambivalence. We have already said that many young people identify early and thoroughly with their parents' ways and values, and slip easily into the roles for which they have been preparing. In upwardly mobile families, parents and children may work hard and cooperatively to launch each child in turn toward a level of achievement beyond that of the parents. In the lower classes, the pressures are rather consistently on the side of rapid maturing and early assumption of adult roles. There may be conflicts, but they are not the conflicts of dual ambivalence. While the lower-class child is more likely than his middle-class or upper-class counterpart to leave school early and get a job, there may be pressure from his family to stay at home and contribute his earnings to the family. Here, too, then, we often find friction about freedom and money. The situation is further complicated when the family belongs to an immigrant or other minority group, with traditions of strong parental authority, entailing additional problems in identification and conflicts between mores. For many young males nowadays, the possibility of being conscripted adds one more complication. It is also a fact of our times that many young people leave school, are rejected for military service, and cannot find work.

On farms and ranches, where the youngster's life is necessarily centered in the home and home place (although fast cars and private airplanes and helicopters have done much to break down the former isolation of country people), and where he participates directly in a relatively self-sufficient family economy, there tends to be less of a gap between the generations. In the present era of factory farming, the parents are even likely to be college-educated. The parents are likely to welcome and accept the child's growing up, and he in turn finds it easy to demonstrate his competence in the terms by which they measure maturity. It is largely in a market economy of specialized services centered outside the home that conflicts are most likely to arise. It has always been said that farm children learn the facts of life early, from watching the animals, but we know of no evidence showing that farm children have either more or fewer problems than city children in coming to terms with their own sexuality.

Let us note that lack of visible conflict is not necessarily a sign that all is well. One way to achieve a seemingly idyllic order of peace is through authoritarian and repressive methods of child-rearing. The effects of an authoritarian upbringing can be seen in a composition written by a fifteen-year-old girl:

> I'm glad my parents are people who know what is best for us to do and know how to go about making us do it. There are many parents today who do not know how to handle their children. As a result of this the children become too independend [sic]. Then the parents wonder why they do not get good marks in school. . . . When [my mother and dad] say no once there is no use asking a second time, because they will not change their minds. Mom says she wants us to grow up and get a good job and be respected by other people, if nothing else. . . . It makes me proud and happy when I think about how my parents have protected me from becoming a junvenile [sic] delinquent.[8]

We can see that the writer's parents have accomplished their goal of indoctrinating her with their values. Paradoxically enough, however, one can produce the same sort of dogmatic authoritarianism by following the opposite course of giving the child a minimum of direction. The child who is left to find his own values is very likely to seize upon the most conservative, traditional, orthodox ways of doing things, probably because the lack of guidance makes him so insecure that he is forced to grab for the obvious. Thus, one is obliged—assuming that one wants to produce a child who can truly think for himself—to steer a middle course, not in some abstract pursuit of the Golden Mean, but because it is what works.

Democratic-minded parents also want to impart values to their young. But they distinguish between basic, humane values and superficial, merely conventional ones, and between moral and moral-free spheres of action. They know that the way to teach values is not in terms of external, rigid rules of behavior, but by getting the child to think about the consequences of his action. They know that there is room for differences of opinion about how values are translated into behavior, that in real life one sometimes has to choose between values, and so do not try to map out in detail a "correct" way of thinking for children.

One can produce authoritarianism by browbeating the child or by leaving him to his own moral devices. But one can also obtain essentially the same result by various more subtle manipulations. One can, without saying a word, teach values by operant conditioning methods, simply in terms of the emotional feedback one supplies to the youngster's deeds and utterances. One can "explain" with sweet reasonableness why one course of action is better than another, and that by clinging to his own wishes or convictions the child is willfully hurting the parent. Since the adolescent's feelings are often ill-formed and elusive, one can even convince him that he really wants something quite different from what he thinks he wants. The adult, with his greater command of logic, can stack the cards to persuade the young person that he is behaving irrationally— if violence attends a student demonstration or an attempt to register Negro voters, it is somehow made to appear that it is the students or Negroes who are engaging in violent means of protest. In sum, the adult can manipulate the child into reaching the parents' point of view as though it were his own. But an adolescent so manipulated is even more helpless than the browbeaten one. He no longer knows what he really feels or wants or believes in, he always is vaguely at odds with himself and senses an uneasy and irrational guilt no matter how he acts.

If parents use these various techniques of indoctrination, it is perhaps because they have long since stopped thinking about the issues involved. But we cannot take values for granted, especially if, as in our society, we espouse two—or more—sets of conflicting values. It would seem to follow that reasonable parents, who do think seriously about values, would have no trouble communicating them to their offspring. This, however, is not the case. The young person, with his limited experience, simply cannot share the perspectives of those who have been around twenty-five or thirty years longer than he has. In times that change as rapidly as ours, there is bound to be a gap between the generations, exemplified in the remark of a young teen-age girl who, preparing blissfully for her first formal dance, turned to her helpful mother and asked, "Did they have parties like this when you were alive?"

The Adolescent's Activities and Associates

Like the school-age child, the adolescent shuttles back and forth between two cultures, that of adults and that of his peers. Now, however, the situation has changed radically. For the adolescent peer group no longer, as in middle childhood, thinks of itself as a childhood society, but as a new kind of adult society, the wave of the future. To this end, there is a conspiracy of silence among adolescents about their own and each other's pasts. The very thought of their recent immaturities is too agonizing to bear, and they firmly block out any possibility that such immaturity could still be part of their nature. This emphasis on being grown-up—"sophisticated"—does not, of course, lessen friction with the world of chronological grownups. It is only the occasional adult who represents an ideal, or the one who, like the athletic coach, flatters the adolescent by treating him bluntly and without reserve, who the adolescent feels is an exception to the alienness of the adult world.

It used to be that adolescents hurried toward adulthood, with a view to bringing into being their own version of Utopia. Nowadays, they are held back by various forces. The idealistic ones suspect that, far from taking over and transforming the system, they will become its slaves.[9] Many adolescents shy away from the involvements and responsibilities of adult life. The adolescent culture, both spontaneous and insinuated from without, and epitomized by the cult of the electric guitar (or whatever talisman succeeds it), has become so powerfully institutionalized that for many adolescents it has come to seem a permanent way of life—indeed, the middle-aged ski bums, surf bums, and beatniks that we see give the impression of perpetual adolescence.

As larger numbers of adolescents discover that they can have such benefits of adulthood as sex and money without the annoying clutter of careers, spouses, children, mortgage payments, and the responsibilities of citizenship, adolescence seems an increasingly attractive way of life. In Greenwich Village the young people used to support themselves by operating trucking businesses or by doing odd jobs; nowadays they stand on the street corner and cadge dimes and quarters from passersby. It is reported that some number of teen-age girls in the Village support themselves by casual prostitution. In the surfing communities, some young men get money from girls who either hold regular jobs or work as prostitutes. Suburban youth can count on generous allowances to finance their acquisitions and activities. This side of the fringe, the stable teen culture—which is now apparently assumed to embrace everybody from eleven to twenty-five—is a communal and community-minded culture. There is great emphasis on popularity, conformity, and being "in" or "with it."

There are loners, male and female, but most adolescents seek the safety, warm companionship, and reciprocal reinforcement of the group. Some are kept in the group by pressure from the contemporaries or even from misguided parents or guidance counselors who worry unduly about the boy or girl who "doesn't have enough friends." During adolescence, the cliques into which young people form become ever more homogeneous and stratified by social class and academic achievement level. Increasingly, individual friendships are based on common tastes and interests. As adolescents become more mobile—by age sixteen or seventeen many of them have, or have access to, a car—they can maintain friendships over an ever wider geographical range.

Let us point out that adolescents are diverse individuals so that our generalizations about them, and about what we see as the chief styles of being adolescent, do not apply to all adolescents equally, and to some hardly at all. Also, much of what we say applies only to outward behavior, and may not do justice to the adolescent's actual feelings—indeed, in later sections, we shall see how inner feelings may be very much at variance with what outward behavior would lead us to believe.

As we have seen, the adolescent spends less and less time at home, and very little of the time he spends there may be family-oriented. He may even do his homework at a friend's house, or he may prefer to spend his evenings at the public library, where he can study among his friends or, in nice weather, hang around on the library steps smoking and chatting. A major portion of the adolescent's time, at least until the minimum legal school-leaving age and probably well beyond, is spent in school. It seems safe to say that, for most adolescents, the academic side of school and college seems merely the price one has to pay in dull drudgery for the privilege of being an adolescent. And, to anticipate future discussion, let us say that what we know of most school and college programs leads us to feel that the young people are all too often right.

Most adolescents—and most schools—are anti-intellectual, and even those who find their studies attractive are inclined to conceal the fact, lest they gain fatal reputations as grinds. It is socially acceptable to get good grades, since otherwise one cannot get into the right colleges where one makes the right contacts and acquires the credentials needed for the right jobs, but it is taken for granted by school and student that the most the adolescent gets from his education is a few socially and vocationally useful skills and a veneer of culture.

But even if the education the school offers is only a purgatory to be endured, school is still important as the source of friends and even as the site of certain shared activities—dances, athletic contests, plays, and special-interest clubs. The primary social life of the school is that which erupts when the bell rings and the teacher's authority lapses. In high-school corridors, the commotion is enormous, partly as an explosion of pent-up exuberance and partly for display—it is important for both sexes that they are noticed. The boys show themselves at their most masculine—many adults mistakenly conclude that the foppish attire and long hair currently in vogue among adolescent males are a badge of emasculation, but a stallion's heart can beat as well beneath an embroidered waistcoat and a frilled shirt as beneath a black leather jacket. The girls are at their most feminine, extravagantly vivacious and alluring. And no matter how interested in their own group the clusters of boys and girls seem to be, they are really proclaiming and radiating how interesting they are—it makes a considerable difference in their behavior whether anyone worth-while is watching. Here we see the first symptoms of what has been called "Hollywood eye" or "cocktail-party eye": the repeated glances to see if anybody important has entered the room. There is some pairing off of steadies and best friends. A few boys may slip into a secluded corner for a cigarette, less because they want it than because it is the sophisti-cated thing to do. There is a constant exchange of greetings, much making of plans and dates, loud outcries of elation or despair at examina-tion results, much comparing of notes and trading of gossip. The school's wheelers and dealers may be busy politicking and making time, but so is everybody else. In a sense, they are all running for office, for the esteem and acclaim and recognition that will tell them where they stand.

The pattern is more subdued in college, but essentially the same strands are there. There may be more talk of careers and jobs, more conversation about topics raised in the classroom, more talk of books, plays, concerts, and exhibitions, more plans for weekends out of town, but the fundamental theme is still that of making time, seeking recogni-tion and status, and finding an identity as a member of the group.

While it is true that the adolescent wants to be popular, and while he tends to court important figures and shun lesser ones, he is becoming selective on a number of counts. Some American high schools, of course, are highly homogeneous in their make-up, but most are sufficiently variegated to allow a predictable social hierarchy to emerge. In most schools, the chief social division is into *sets,* the major blocs into which the students distribute themselves. Sets may be based on orientations to the future, social background, ethnic background, or personality type, or on some combination of these. Thus, the rich kids form a set, the youngsters from a particular poor neighborhood form a set, the church-goers may form a set, the college-bound form a set, those active in school affairs form a set (or perhaps a subset of the college-oriented), and so do the playboys and playgirls. Since sets form spontaneously and not by decree, they defy systematic classification. The important thing is that they are psychologically real, and the adolescents know to which set they and other people belong, even though in a large school some people in the same set may not know each other. A set's members may have in common only that they have been rejected by everybody else, and such social rejects (referred to as "nobody") may draw together to form a company of lepers. The other important fact about sets is that they overlap virtually not at all. Even though, technically, one might qualify for several sets, one is assigned (and usually accepts the assignment) to the one set that seems most suitable. Within a given set, distinct, rather exclusive friendship groups—"crowds" or "cliques"—take shape, usually on the basis of common tastes, interests, and styles.

Only rarely do cliques form across the boundaries that separate sets. Personal friendships of the one-to-one variety usually develop within a clique, although a shared consuming interest—in amateur radio, in hot rods, in writing, in chess—can draw together people from several cliques or even sets. Some individualists cannot be assigned to sets and refuse or are unable to align themselves with cliques, and may have a lonely time of it within the standard school structure. Where the middle-years child's peer group was peopled with friends, best friends, and faceless strangers, the adolescent has a wide circle of casual acquaintances as well. One of the adult social skills he is acquiring is the ability to exchange flip, breezy greetings with people he knows only slightly, and the number of such exchanges is a measure for himself and others of how near he is to his goal of popularity.

Thus, the pattern of teen-age associations is quite intricate, based as it is on group (set and crowd) identification, arbitrary class lines, personal likes and dislikes, tastes and interests, and keen attention to the overall popularity hierarchy within the school. In thinking about joining a club, the adolescent may be far less concerned about the club's theme and program—travel, photography, dance, art, hiking—than with who its members are and where he stands in relation to them, or where he wants to stand. Status motivation is strong, since status determines dating patterns, whom you hang around with in and outside school, whom you emulate and whom you despise, and the adolescent keeps checking his status by other people's responses to him and to the rest of the group.

In many schools and colleges the hierarchy of cliques is even more sharply formalized in fraternities and sororities. Although the situation has softened slightly in recent years with regard to racial, ethnic, and religious discrimination, fraternity membership is still a way of defining "our kind of people" and excluding "the wrong sort." Notice that fraternities continue the pattern of middle-years clubs, except that the standards for belonging now become more sharply delineated. Candidates for membership are screened through a ruthless selection process that subjects them to crude, uninhibited, searching, and sometimes brutal personality analyses. A successful candidacy produces a feeling of total triumph; rejection one of total, abysmal loss.

The irony in the whole system of judging oneself by the company one is allowed to keep is that everybody is in the same boat. The mask of self-assurance worn by the campus leader is as false as the mask of independent aloofness worn by the outcast, and the poses and postures fool everybody except the one who assumes them. Adolescents are too self-involved to be able to see deep into other people's feelings. They see that adults, who play a somewhat different game by different rules, hide behind a facade, but they do not know what it is they are hiding. But when dealing with their contemporaries, whose opinions are so all-important, they do not even recognize the false faces as false.

Now let us take a moment to trace the development of this pattern of adolescent social organization. In the junior high school, as we have said, there is a spectacular mismatching of the sexes. The average junior high school is populated by young ladies and male children, with most of the girls well launched into adolescence and most of the boys still in the middle years. This works some hardships on the girls, who are ready for male companionship, but hardly of the kind to be had from their classmates, and who find it almost impossible to penetrate the social order of the high school. They are usually forced to make do with the materials at hand, and a school dance is likely to be characterized by the young ladies towering over and dragging around grudging and grubby escorts who would rather be playing baseball. The junior high school years are a kind of limbo for many girls. Around the sophomore year of high school, boys begin to catch up to girls in maturity, and the interests of the two sexes, while not identical, now better complement each other. Boys give up their bicycles and, for the most part, the neighborhood games, and become increasingly oriented to social relations at the verbal level, with physical activity taking second place. Boys and girls begin playing the game of status, with the assumption that status determines dating and mating and that dating also helps decide status. With status the key, the football game itself is less important than whom you go with and how you conduct yourself while there.

The school, however, is only one focus of adolescent social life. Another is the *hangout*, the gathering place. It is permissible to go to the hangout alone, but it is preferable to go with a few other people of one's own sex, hoping and expecting to meet and mingle with a bunch of the other sex, without the formalities or financial responsibilities of a date (a recent sidewalk poll of relatively affluent teen-agers indicates that a regular date costs the male from five to twenty-five dollars, while the female may spend as much as ten or fifteen dollars having her gown cleaned and her hair done). Steadies, of course, may meet at the hangout by prearrangement. Some community centers serve as hangouts, occasionally as deliberate substitutes for unsavory commercial establishments. The ones that succeed best are those which reproduce most clearly the atmosphere of the neighborhood hangouts and allow the youngsters to feel comfortable in their clumsy amorousness. More commonly, though, the deliciously dangerous—but outwardly blasé—encounters between sexes take place on the premises of those drug stores, candy stores, diners, shopping centers, drive-in restaurants, dime stores, or, in warm weather, on favored stretches of beach, which the kids view as hospitable. In the case of the drug store or sweet shop, being hospitable to adolescents means sacrificing the magazine display and, usually, adult patronage.

Adolescent social life goes on around as well as within the hangout. Boys cluster near the entrance, appraising and commenting on the clusters of girls who stroll casually by and then back again, ostensibly bound on some errand or absorbed in shop-window displays, but tinglingly aware that they are being scrutinized. The frankness of the mating calls and the amount of wolf-whistling and hip-twitching are governed by class differences, but the basic phenomena remain the same. Notice that, unlike school, where sets and crowds are mixed together in the same building (although they may segregate themselves by patterns of course elections), the hangout usually caters only to a single set.

Car ownership by adolescents has altered the physical structure of their society. The kind of car one owns is a symbol of status, although the relationships are by no means simple. Sports cars, old or new, are high in status but low in convenience, although there may be a special merit in packing six people into a two-seater. Old touring cars carry much cachet, especially when the hood conceals a supercharged engine. Family sedans are for squares, and probably the most successful combination of assets is the mock sports car which combines racy lines and high performance with commodious and comfortable seating. But any car is better than no car, and, failing a car, a motorcycle or motor scooter is better than walking or being dependent on the charity of others or, most humiliating, having to ride the bus. In some circles, of course, the motorcycle is the key to social organization, and status is correlated with size, power, and gleaming complexity—motorcycles are groomed with the care once lavished on horses. To introduce a note of irony, there is a strong negative correlation between car ownership and school marks, such that honor students rarely own cars, and car owners rarely become honor students.

In their cars, adolescents go to drive-in movies, sometimes on dates (often, to bolster their courage, on double and triple dates), sometimes in same-sex herds which jockey from space to space looking for a car loaded with an opposite-sex herd with which to intermingle. Sometimes they prowl through the entertainment district looking for action. If a group of boys can gather a like number of girls, they may go drinking and dancing, or they may seek out a lover's lane in which to pet. The drive-in theater itself may be a petting ground, but wandering security officers keep the expressions of passion in check. The car is thought of as a setting for sexual intercourse, but again surveillance by highway policemen may make such an outcome unlikely—one may, of course, wonder about possible motives of voyeurism and sadism that impel policemen to sneak up on parked cars and suddenly shine a bright flashlight into the interior. Sometimes cars are used in drag racing, sometimes in chicken racing, and often just as transportation.

The most usual pattern is just riding around, headed nowhere in particular, sometimes at high speed but often at a leisurely pace, watching the scenery go by, shouting and whistling at girls, and just idly talking—the adolescent conversations to which we have been privy seem like monuments of aimless banality and almost wholly devoid of content. It is only in special conditions of emotion or intimacy that one finds shared convictions and concern with such profundities as life, death, human nature, religion, war and peace, and the meaning of it all. We should point out that the enormous prestige that attaches to cars, plus the pleasures of riding around in them, accounts for some 90 per cent of car thefts—the youngster (or, more often, a bunch of youngsters) simply rides around for a few hours, parks the car, and walks away. It should further be noted that motor vehicles are the greatest single cause of death between the preschool years and adulthood, and that motor vehicle accidents account for almost two-thirds of deaths among eighteen- to nineteen-year-old boys. Motorcycles are especially lethal.

Herd life sometimes takes youngsters to big dances, although, in early adolescence, dances are really "big" only for girls. Rather often, girls arrive at the prom in their most elegant formal gowns, accompanied by boys wearing their studiously casual daytime attire. But except for the annual prom, the formal dance seems largely a thing of the past. Nowadays, there is a great deal more spur-of-the-moment dancing, to records or to local rock-and-roll singing groups, at the recreation center, at the hangout, at the beach, or in somebody's house or back yard (the currently popular free form and astonishingly contact-free dance steps do not require a polished dance floor).

Sometimes the herd goes to church socials, sometimes on hay rides, on bus trips to the big city, sometimes on outings to the seashore or ski slope or just hiking. Perhaps the most important part of herd life, however, takes place when the herd is dispersed to its various homes and the telephone is brought into play. On the phone, friends can have intense, confidential discussions impossible in the public eye of the herd itself. It is worth noting that the protracted phone calls that drive parents to a frenzy—and have driven many families into becoming two- and three-telephone families—are usually between members of the same sex, especially girls. The opposite sex is still pretty much of an enigma to the adolescent, and although the youngster may yearn toward it, chaff with it, neck and pet and perhaps even have coitus with it, talking with it comes almost as hard as talking with a speaker of an alien language. At least until late adolescence, phone conversations between a boy and a girl are likely to be brief and to the point—indeed, almost curt and abrupt. Superficially, talking seems like the simplest and most innocuous form of human communication. In psychological fact, however, to talk to somebody means to let down one's guard and be prepared to reveal oneself, and the telephone does not permit one to do much besides talk. With the herd, one fills up time with scuffling, catch-phrases, comments, wisecracks, banter, snatches of song, a few chords on the guitar or the blast of a record player, a sip of soda or a drag on a cigarette, a dance step, all devices that replace saying something, but which are only the incidental stuff of telephonic communication.

Our description of herd life has elements of caricature, but it is essentially true. However, as we have said, it is not equally true for all adolescents. Some youngsters participate very little in herd life, some because they have overriding interests and some because the various herds will not let them. Sometimes both forces are at work: Because the herd has rejected him, the adolescent casts about for a hobby or interest. Solitude is not the only alternative to herd life, however. Some young people dislike the mindlessness of herd activity and prefer more direct, individualized friendships. The youngster who does his homework conscientiously has very little time for herd life except during holidays. Some adolescents alternate periods of intense study with periods of group life, but few can combine them. Some youngsters like to read a great deal, or take solitary walks and daydream. Some have parents who strictly limit group participation. Poor youngsters have a group life, but it cannot range as freely as do the more affluent hordes. It is lived more on the streets, since there is nowhere else to go in the slums. Finally, a fair number of adolescents nowadays use their free time to make money, perhaps by tending counter in the hangout.

POPULARITY AND CONFORMITY

The dependence of the adolescent on peer-group standards and values is, if anything, even more slavish than that of the middle-years child. The greater the wall between adolescents and adults, the more elaborate the peer culture becomes and the more the adolescent has to turn to it for support and identity. He seizes upon and displays all the trademarks of his kind, so that nobody can possibly miss them. Rigid conformity is the rule, extending to matters of dress, adornment, hair styles, hair color (the streaky blond color of the surfer's hair is much admired—even the surfer helps along the bleaching action of sun and salt

Much of the middle-class adolescent's social life is lived via telephone.
Rita Freed

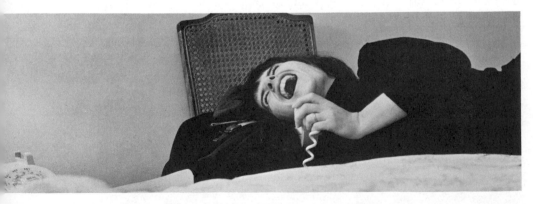

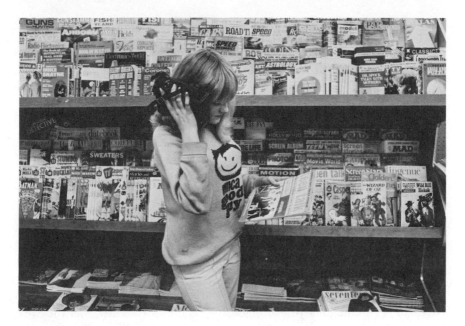

Teen-agers live partly in a world of images, symbols, styles, and ideals created for them by the mass media of communication.
Fred Schnell

water with peroxide or lemon juice), tastes in foods and music, posture, vocabulary, and intonation. The individual and his crowd are ever eager for innovations, but the kind of innovations that fit the established framework of teen culture.

When an adolescent wishes to assert his individuality, he is likely to do so by carrying whatever fad is prevalent one more step toward its ultimate utterness. Partly because he wants to stand out, and partly to reassure himself of the solidity of his new culture, he is always striving for vividness and extremes, as in his slang. Note, however, the forced, strained, artificial quality of much adolescent behavior—even when he plays the role of hip teen-ager well enough to fool his fellows, adults can sense the synthetic character of his performance. Fads and crazes propagate rapidly among teen-agers, so that we have the fascinating spectacle of very rapid change within a highly conservative framework. We shall talk in a moment about some real changes that seem to have occurred in adolescence in recent years, but the basic traits of adolescent culture yield slowly to social pressures.

As we have said, much of adolescent culture originates in the fertile brains of adults—magazine and newspaper columnists and the publishers of teen-age periodicals, composers and musicians and music publishers, clothing manufacturers, the makers of novelties—who skillfully gauge the adolescent *Zeitgeist* with the help of opinion polls and informants and panels, and who plant or pass along ideas for new fashions in dress and decoration, new kinds of parties, new turns of speech, new recording stars, and so forth. The teen-age market has come to be recognized for the potent force it is, and we have evolved a whole new subeconomy catering to the tastes of adolescents. Resort hotels and cruise ships have parallel programs of entertainment for adults and for their teen-age children. One day's program at a Catskill resort included the following activities for teen-agers: ice skating, a ping-pong tournament, a choice of dance lessons or a coed volleyball game, a shuffleboard contest, a splash party, a swimming meet, a joint teen-age and adult cocktail party, and finally, at 10 P.M., a "Coke-tail" party. Thus, adults connive with young people in the construction of a separate culture, even though they may bemoan its existence and influence. But while teen-age doings may strike adults as inanely or perniciously juvenile, to adolescents they are part of the swinging new adulthood that will replace the drab one of the oldsters. And since so much of the time the adolescent does not have a great deal that he wants to do (he craves action and excitement, but is vague about where to find it), cannot have the things he wants the most, and isn't sure that he really wants them anyway, he uses passing fancies to fill up the vacancy of waiting and to preserve group solidarity until the days of waiting are over.

The young person's dependence on group belongingness to tell him who he is, and his submissive conformity to group ways to guarantee that he belongs, can produce highly injurious results. In the street gang, the youngster (male or female) may have to prove himself in combat or by taking part in a murderous assault on some arbitrarily chosen victim. Characteristically, young people arrested for violent assault claim, in a convincing sort of way, that they did not want to take part but felt that they had to lest they be thought "chicken." The chicken race (for example, racing two cars to the edge of a cliff) by which adolescents tested their manhood seems to have gone out of fashion, but it is far from inconceivable that it will reemerge, particularly in the bloody times we live in. The girl may be forced by group pressures into promiscuity, and in some cases into sex acts before an audience. It is not enough to say that young people should have sufficient moral character to resist group pressures; failure to conform can produce feelings of guilt and inadequacy as severe as going against one's own conscience. Thus, the group can place the adolescent in a double-bind situation such that either of the courses open to him will lead to painful consequences. What is interesting is that a single strong leader can sway the group to act against its own better feelings, but in some cases no leader is needed; that is, each individual in the group can be opposed to a course of action and yet sense a group demand so strongly that he follows the course anyway.

The dependence of the adolescent on group approval is so severe that it has been labeled the "popularity neurosis" (to which American adults are not always immune). It is only late in adolescence that some young people define abstract standards of virtue against which to measure their own behavior. Meanwhile the adolescent acts primarily in ways that he thinks will make people like him. His concern about having a "good personality" is often less a search for inner strength than for the tricks that will win acceptance by others—being an athletic star, playing a musical instrument, developing a sense of humor, augmenting his vocabulary, being active in things. The devices are legion, and again the adult commercial world has moved in with stories and articles on how to be popular: what to say on a date, how to refuse a boy's advances without antagonizing him, how to obey one's parents without losing face, how to get rid of or conceal the blemishes that make one feel a pariah. And for those who cannot buy popularity at any price, there is an abundant literature providing fulfillment in fantasy.

The need for popularity stems in large part from the lessons parents teach their children: It is important to get along with people, to have people like you, to be well-adjusted, to harken to the voice of public opinion. But it becomes particularly acute in terms of the intermediate stage of the adolescent's self-knowledge. The adolescent cannot be satisfied with what he thinks about himself; he needs someone out there to tell him that he is all right. Nor can he judge his own worth in terms of what he produces—jokes, observations on events and people, the product of a special talent, the physical appearance he creates—unless it meets with special acclaim. And the louder the acclaim, the better. The adolescent is not one for subtleties (except his own, which he treasures), and unless his audience is noisily appreciative, he may doubt the sincerity of its applause. But again we come full circle to the consideration that the vigor with which one adolescent applauds another may itself express a seeking for the applauded adolescent's approval. The self-involved adolescent usually fails to recognize that everybody else feels out of step. Ironically, the occasional adolescent who is indifferent to popularity and goes his own way may find that his peers flock round him as a tower of strength. The adolescent's parents are as anxious as he is for him to be popular, but they are likely to disapprove of the particular people he courts. This is because they are blind to the group standards of whom it is important to be in with and whom it is better to keep at a distance. To parents, almost every adolescent other than their own looks like a potentially bad influence; parents want their youngsters to be popular, but they may be hard put to say with whom.

Social Class Differences

We have already said that adolescence may be very different for lower-class youngsters from what it is for those from the middle and upper classes. Before we go on to point to some of these differences, one thing should be made clear. The recent rediscovery of poverty in the United States has made us keenly aware of the social and economic injustices that have been perpetrated on Negroes, to the point where many people come to assume that all Negroes are poor and that all poor people are Negroes, neither of which is true. A larger proportion of Negroes than whites is poor, but there are a goodly number of well-to-do and rich Negroes. Because they are usually forced to live in segregated communities, many white people are unaware of their existence or numbers. There are also a great many poor white people packed into urban slums or dispersed through rural ones. We should also bear in mind that there is some socioeconomic spread among American Indians, Americans from the Latin countries, Polynesians, Orientals, Micronesians, and Eskimos. The interesting, if perhaps depressing, thing is that people of racial minorities take on middle-class ways of thinking as they rise financially, and, while not forgetting the hardships of their former existence, lose all sense of identity with their origins.

One point of difference between the classes is that lower-class adolescents may be systematically excluded from participation in middle-class activities. They are treated as second-class citizens by teachers (who may themselves be in the process of escaping from a lower level of society and overidentifying with the middle class), employers, the police, the courts (the middle-class transgressor may be let off with forfeited bail, a fine, or a rebuke, whereas the lower-class one may go off to jail), welfare agencies, housing authorities, and middle-class contemporaries. Tied in with second-class treatment is psychological exclusion, so that even those areas of participation that are theoretically open to all comers—school, school-sponsored clubs and activities—are cast so strongly in middle-class terms that they are meaningless or even repellent to lower-class youngsters. Here we have the vicious circle of the self-fulfilling prophecy: Like any out-group member, the lower-class adolescent may come to accept the in-group's view of himself and in so doing conform to the middle-class stereotype of the lower-class personality. Thus, he both "justifies" middle-class rejection and increases his own alienation from the majority society. It is only the extraordinary lower-class adolescent—the athlete, scholar, or artistically gifted, the extremely ambitious or ruthless one—who can move into the middle class. Notice that the change from lower-class to middle-class status involves more than a change of financial circumstances: It means, as *Pygmalion* (and *My Fair Lady*) have indicated, a change of speech patterns, of personal attire, or tastes, attitudes, and style of life.

Although there are obvious disadvantages to being a lower-classs adolescent, it has its compensations. Lower-class parents are more willing than middle-class ones to acknowledge and accept their children's adulthood. The lower-class youngster may be spared the stress on academic and material achievement that bears constantly on the middle-class one (although some upwardly mobile parents bring strong pressures to bear on their children for the good school grades that will give them a better life). In a limited sense, sexuality is taken more freely for granted in the lower classes, especially for males.[10] Indeed, many middle-class youngsters may envy the lower classes their greater apparent freedom, and envy may lead to emulation. We usually think of culture as spreading downward in society, but in fact there is a steady upward spread of culture from lower to middle classes, largely by way of adolescents. The middle-class boy may date a lower-class girl in hopes of finding her sexually compliant, or he may join a crowd of lower-class boys in order to share in their sexual adventures. Middle-class youngsters may romanticize the lower classes, as eighteenth- and nineteenth-century painters romanticized peasants and milkmaids, and adopt the externals of their way of life. The Mod look in clothing, jazz and rock-and-roll, and a great deal of slang began in the lower classes. When middle-class youngsters take over lower-class slang, they often do so in response to qualities of toughness, vividness, and daring, but without any exact understanding of the rich and often scatological metaphors involved. It is interesting to note that members of racial or ethnic minorities, particularly in low-tension areas, are often accepted on their own merits by their adolescent contemporaries—as long as they are in school. Outside school, where the in-group members feel themselves exposed to adult eyes, they are likely to become cool and distant. We should note that all the impediments to assimilation of ethnic and lower-class out-groups do not come from the middle-class white North European Protestants. Out-group members themselves form strong group identifications to which they may cling tenaciously.

A Taxonomy of Adolescence

Even among middle-class adolescents, however, one can recognize a number of styles, and it is now our task to try to specify some of the chief variants of the breed. Tentatively, we distinguish four main types, with a number of subvarieties: *conventionalists, idealists, transitory hedonists,* and *psychopaths.* These categories are not as mutually exclusive as strict logic demands, but they provide a convenient framework for discussion.

The *conventionalists* are, to judge by a test of values to be described in a minute, probably the most numerous group. They are the ones who have never seriously questioned adult values and whose main goal in life is to fit in and get along with society as it exists. They may aspire to rise above their parents or wish simply to repeat the pattern of their parents' lives, but they have no misgivings about the established order and consider it their job to find out how best to adjust to things as they are. This group produces the bulk of the early marriages, the precocious and often premature reaching out for standard adult roles. We have given a series of incomplete sentences to a great many college students and asked them to supply their own endings. The five sentences are: "I like children who . . . ," "I dislike children who . . . ," "When I was a child I liked adults who . . . ," "The most important thing for a child to learn . . . ," "I wish my parents had. . . ."[11] The responses to all five questions are interesting, but the key statement is the one dealing with what it is most important for children to learn. Overwhelmingly, students say that children must learn to accept authority, to obey, to be good, to have nice manners, to be well adjusted, to accommodate, to get along, and similar themes. A fair number stress love as an essential of human existence, and quite a few emphasize independence, but seemingly less in the sense of being able to think for oneself than of not being a burden to others. Relatively rare are such themes as originality, creativity, self-knowledge, and autonomy. Religious beliefs and practices are seldom mentioned, although most of our subjects profess some creed. A limitation of our findings is that our subjects have been predominantly female, and it seems to be males (for the most part) who stress deviant or defiant styles. The conventionalists may go through the motions of teen-age culture—they believe strongly in "having fun"—but they never feel really shut off from the adult world. The conventionalists, and to a lesser degree the idealists, supply most of the volunteers who work on hospital wards, teach retarded children, and provide companionship for the aged, infirm, and emotionally disturbed. They are likely to be active in junior-grade social, civic, and business organizations.

The *idealists*, obviously, are those who express profound dissatisfaction with the state of the world and either work hard to change things or simply withdraw into a private world centered upon personal satisfaction. The idealistic adolescent corresponds most closely to the classical image of the iconoclastic, moody, romantic rebel portrayed by Goethe, Mann, Joyce, Alain-Fournier, Salinger, and other novelists.[12] There seem to be three main ways in which idealism is manifested by today's young people.

First, we have the reformers, exemplified by the civil rights and peace movements and the campus protest and political movements. As Paul Goodman has pointed out, the campus group includes both radicals and conservatives.[13] The unifying theme seems to be populism, faith in ordinary people and distrust in government and authority, with an almost anarchistic belief in freedom of individual self-determination. There are, however, fundamental and important differences. Young conservative reformers view human nature as fixed, and social differences as biologically (and perhaps divinely) determined. In the conservative scheme of things, fixed human nature tends to be vile, selfish, and competitive, but the pursuit of selfish ends will "naturally," through the workings of a fully competitive free enterprise system, produce the good of the whole. But without the spur of economic want, people will stop working and relapse into animality. The conservatives have great faith in tradition and believe that we have simply wandered from the right, natural path and need only to return to it. For all our shortcomings, the evidence of our national prosperity shows that we are still God's chosen and should feel free to coerce and subjugate inferior people in the interests of keeping the system going, which is ultimately for their own good. They believe that the disorder and unpredictability of capitalism are a creative ferment which leads to an orderly, harmonious society. Those who fail to benefit from the system are the victims of their own defective character, but large-scale social disorders are produced by interfering with the free workings of the system and will disappear automatically when we return the system to its natural state. The progressive adolescent reformers, by contrast, see the present state of society as the predictable outcome of capitalism, which in their view intrinsically moves toward monopoly, vested interests, and a powerful establishment which manipulates and exploits ordinary people. From this standpoint, tradition tells us what not to do, what dreadful errors to avoid, and that what is needed is new, creative solutions to our problems. This view assumes a plastic, morally neutral human nature and says that the way society is now organized brings out man's most brutal, rapacious, inhumane potentialities. The progressive adolescents believe that a rearrangement of society in which economic and political considerations were subordinated to humane ones would enable people to develop the capacity to love, to cooperate, to explore the full range of human feelings, and to find meaning and satisfaction in useful work which is done for its own sake rather than just for the sake of making money. They believe in self-sacrifice for the common good, but they are by no means antihedonistic. For them, however, apart from the intrinsic pleasures of useful work, pleasure is to be found in human contact and shared experiencing rather than in the possession of material pleasure-stimulants.

The second main type of idealist is exemplified by the Peace Corps or VISTA volunteer, the young person who actively works directly, in contact with people, to redeem mankind. The first kind of idealist resonates sympathetically or empathically to the motivations of the second, but questions whether it makes any sense to remold people without at the same time reshaping the framework of the society which impoverished and brutalized them in the first place.

The third kind of idealist is typified by the beatnik or hippy or digger, the quester after personal fulfillment in esthetic experience, sex, drugs, and all forms of communion and communication, regardless of the suicidal tendencies of society at large. This group differs from type one in that it withdraws instead of working to redeem. It has in common with type one its stress on freedom, openness, disregard of constraining conventions (such as personal cleanliness), humanness, and savage nobility. Such concerns may be phrased in quasi-religious terms, and many beatniks embrace forms of Zen Buddhism or other faiths. It is interesting that some proportion of surfers have viewed their art as a pursuit of sanctity akin to the beatniks', but have tended to preach asceticism, as opposed to indulgence, as part of their code.

The *transitory hedonists* play the role of teen-agers to the hilt and make it their life style. They feel alienated from the adult world but, instead of combating it, simply want to leave it behind, confident that when their generation comes to power, they will set the tone for the new

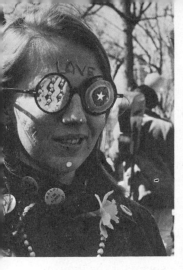

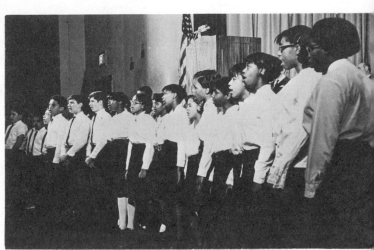

Aspects of adolescence.

(Top left, top right, and middle)
© 1967 by Fred W. McDarrah;
(below) © 1965 by Fred W. Mc-
Darrah

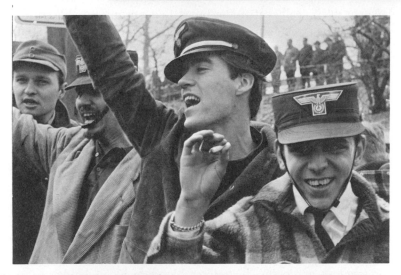

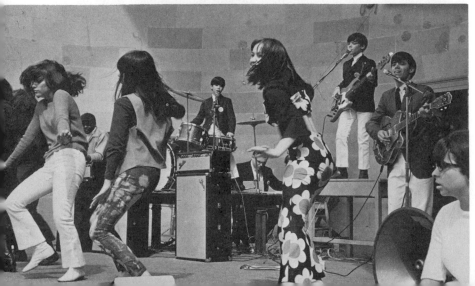

society. This group produces early marriages, too, but of a different kind from that of the conventionalists. For the transitory hedonist, early marriage is simply a convenient way of incorporating sexuality and freedom from adult supervision into the rock-and-roll culture. The domestic life of such couples looks like an awkward game of "playing house"—the family shopping basket is piled high with chocolate milk, soft drinks, frankfurters, potato chips, bread, cupcakes, and sugar-coated cereals. Parenthood may come as a rude surprise, although they may enjoy having a live doll for their house play. There is some reason to think that this group increasingly experiments with sex outside of marriage, and that relatively free sex, or sex with one's steady of the moment, is on its way to becoming a cultural given. But no matter how seemingly imbued with the spirit of the teen age, these young people quickly settle down into more or less conventional adult roles. Work, however, is not seen as intrinsically satisfying but is taken as inescapable drudgery which has as its goal the acquisition of money to buy necessities, luxuries, status symbols, and the leisure, freedom, alcohol, and social standing that will enable them to continue the pursuit of pleasure. Whereas the conventionalists look back on youth as a lost age of innocence, this group looks back on youth as a lost time of splendor and gaiety and perpetual fun and games.

(There are *permanent hedonists* who differ from the transitory kind in that their estrangement from society is more deliberate, more a matter of personal conviction, and perhaps life long. Life is a search for kicks, often centered around surf or ski slope, but with generous helpings of alcohol, drugs, sex, travel, or whatever else holds the promise of thrills. They support themselves by begging, petty thievery, casual homosexual or heterosexual prostitution [they may sometimes attach themselves to a wealthy older person], as beach boys or ski instructors or sidewalk artists or strolling musicians, by selling blood to blood banks, or even, when times are tight, by odd jobs. They have their gathering places around the world, largely the spas and pleasure spots frequented by the idle rich, movie stars, and homosexuals. Some permanent hedonists are young people of good education and good looks, with nice manners and a kindly outlook on their fellow man, and they seem to have little trouble maintaining themselves and finding sources of kicks.)

Outwardly, the *psychopaths* (a small but highly visible group) have much in common with the permanent hedonists, but they are more cold-blooded and brutal in their exploitation of other people, and may even find in brutality a major source of kicks. The hedonist really seems to enjoy life, while the psychopath is a restless, dissatisfied grasper after pleasure. The kicks never come through with full pungency, the laughter is always a little hollow, the sexual partners are never as beautiful and responsive as one thought, people are never quite intimidated enough by one's appearance, one's motorcycle reaches top speed just below the threshold of ecstasy. The periodic resort riots are probably started by transitory hedonists on a group spree, but the riots turn nasty when the psychopaths get involved and cut loose. Characteristically, the psycho-path lacks humor. Although he lives outside society, or leaves ordinary society behind as soon as he can shed his working clothes and don his uniform—sometimes literally the uniform, as of American Nazi groups— he is thoroughly conventional in his thinking and will tolerate no slur on Motherhood, Capitalism, and the American Way of Life. Indeed, the psychopaths have aligned themselves with their traditional enemies, the police, to practice violence against idealists who criticize the system. One of the more bemusing paradoxes of our day is to hear right-wing spokesmen extolling the sterling virtues of the black-leather-jacket con-tingent, virtues which, a few years back, they might have found it hard to define. Also, reports from the San Francisco Bay area suggest a com-mingling, although perhaps not a stable one, of psychopaths, permanent hedonists, and idealists. Again, notice that many individuals who live the psychopathic life may not themselves be psychopathic personalities, but are seizing on a culture that offers them an identity they could not find on their own. We assume that it is the psychopaths who are the participants in and spectators at romps like those described in this advertisement:

WANTED
YOUNG MEN NOT AFRAID TO DIE!

If you think you have lots of guts, plenty of nerve and can stand the pressure both mental and physical of crashing and wrecking auto-mobiles deliberately, then you are the man we want. The require-ments are simple: you must have a valid driver's license and supply a car that will be demolished—with you in it. You must be prepared to risk life and limb, as you will be part of a

100 CAR DEMOLITION DERBY.

Since no system of categories that we can think of is going to capture all adolescents in all their wondrous variety, we ought to mention those who seem to have no peer-group affiliation. There are those whose shyness keeps them apart, who feel more comfortable with younger children or with adults, and who watch the antics of their contemporaries

471

with a certain amount of envy without knowing how to become a part of the herd. There are those youngsters who go through adolescence in a state of bewilderment, who seem to have no idea of who or where they are or of where they are going or why. There are the solitary romantics, who read novels and drink in the glories of nature and write poetry and contemplate suicide and dream of heroic adventures and form crushes on older people—again, much as in the images of "classical" adolescence. But even those who rejoice in the clamor of Babylon keep listening for the final blast.

REFERENCES / Chapter 10

1 Adler, R. Onward and upward with the arts: The new sound. *The New Yorker,* February 20, 1965, pp. 63–105.
2 MacDonald, D. Profile of Eugene Gilbert. *The New Yorker,* November 22, 1958, pp. 57 ff., and November 29, 1958, pp. 57 ff.
3 Hall, G. S. *Adolescence.* New York: Appleton: 1904, 2 vols.
4 Sherwin, R. V. The law and sexual relationships. *Journal of Social Issues,* 1966, 22, 109–122.
5 Nixon, R. E. *The Art of Growing.* New York: Random House, 1962, PP 23.
6 Bateson, G., Jackson, D., Haley, J., and Weakland, J. Toward a theory of schizophrenia. *Behavioral Science,* 1956, 1, 251–264.
7 This is from one of a group of essays by high school students on the theme of "My Parents," collected by L. Joseph Stone.
8 *Ibid.*
9 Friedenberg, E. Z. *The Vanishing Adolescent.* Boston: Beacon, 1959.
10 Rainwater, L. Some aspects of lower class sexual behavior. *Journal of Social Issues,* 1966, 22, 96–108.
11 This technique was originally suggested by Mary Langmuir Essex.
12 Goethe, J. W. v. *Leiden des jungen Werthers,* 1795; Mann, T. *Stories of Three Decades.* New York: Knopf, 1936; Joyce, J. *A Portrait of the Artist as a Young Man.* New York: Modern Library, 1928 (originally published in 1917, also available in paperback); Alain-Fournier, H. *The Wanderer.* New York: New Directions, 1946 (originally *Le Grand Meaulnes,* 1913); Salinger, J. D. *The Catcher in the Rye.* Boston: Little, Brown, 1951.
13 Goodman, P. Moral youth in an immoral society. In Time, Inc., *The Young Americans.* New York: Time-Life Books, 1966, pp. 18–19, 110–111.

11   *Adolescence: 2*

Pubescence, Puberty, and Physical Development

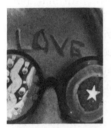 It is now time to look in somewhat more detail at the physical changes of adolescence, with puberty as the physical climax. Let us once again caution the reader that the ages and sizes we cite are at best approximate, since the research on which they are based was done some years ago on healthy, well-fed youngsters of the kind who keep getting bigger at ever earlier ages. Over a forty-year period, fifteen- to sixteen-year-old boys have shown an average gain of almost 2 inches in height and 10 pounds in weight over their forebears; girls have gained better than ½ inch and 1¼ pounds. Interestingly enough, seventeen- to nineteen-year-old girls are about 3 pounds lighter than their counterparts of forty years ago, reflecting changes both in diet and in concepts of beauty.

With due allowance for these trends and for group and individual differences, we may state that, in general, youngsters shoot up in the two years before puberty, and especially in the year just before, which is known as the *maximum growth age* (MGA), with puberty marking the *apex* of the growth-rate curve. Thereafter, the rate of increase slows down, with girls reaching their full height at about nineteen and boys at twenty-one or twenty-two—nobody really knows just when growth stops, and changes in body proportions go on lifelong. During physical adolescence, the child's height increases by about 25 per cent and his weight doubles—obviously, weight is less strictly determined than height. During the latency period, children gain a little more than 2 inches (5 cm.) a year in height and between 4½ and 5 pounds (2+ kg.) in weight. At the peak of adolescent growth, girls grow about 3½ inches in a year (9 cm.) and gain about 11 pounds (5 kg.), while boys grow 4 or 5 inches (11 cm.) in a year and put on 12 or 14 pounds (6+ kg.). But let us note that there are early maturers and late maturers, and an almost infinite number of individual growth patterns. Boys are somewhat bigger than girls except between the ages of eleven and fourteen, when the earlier maturing of girls sends them sprouting past their male coevals.

The maturational changes of adolescence, including changes both in size and in physiological patterns, are governed by stepped-up activity in the pituitary "master" gland, an endocrine organ recessed in the base of the brain and producing a number of different hormones. Secretions from the pituitary regulate other growth-governing endocrines, notably the thyroid, adrenals, and gonads (the testes and ovaries). The functioning of the endocrine glands during adolescent growth provides a nice example of feedback control. Pituitary hormones stimulate adrenal hormones which stimulate gonadal hormones which then inhibit the pituitary. But as the pituitary slows down, the pituitary-inhibiting secretions of the gonads also slow down, and the pituitary once again becomes active. Note, however, that we have no way of accounting for the increase in pituitary activity except to say that it is part of the genetically programed pattern of normal maturation.

In both sexes, the extremities and neck grow faster than the head and trunk during pubescence, which gives youngsters of this age their long-legged, gawky, coltish look. In boys, there is a marked broadening of the shoulders. In girls, the pelvis enlarges—an artist can draw middle-years boys and girls with essentially the same proportions, but as they mature he must take account of very different configurations. Facial proportions also change as the nose and chin become more prominent. Girls more than boys develop a layer of subcutaneous fat that rounds and softens the contours of face and body, whereas boys develop a leaner, more angular and more muscular appearance than girls.

On the surface of the body, the development of the secondary sex characteristics expresses changes in underlying physiology. Both boys and girls develop pubic hair, at first as a downy tuft on the forward face of the pubic mound, and axillary (armpit) hair. Facial hair and chest hair appear in boys, and are considered a mark of manhood. Girls, too, may develop a slight mustache and a sprinkling of facial hair and hair around the nipples, which in no way contradicts their femininity. The pubic hair, or pubes, appears first, whence the name "pubescence." The pubic hair spreads until it surrounds the genital area, becoming in the process darker, longer, coarser, and kinkier. In boys, facial hair comes earlier than axillary hair, appearing first as a darkish shadow on the upper lip. Chest hair—to the despair of the young adolescent boys—appears only in late adolescence and continues growing well into manhood, which fact may have given it its special status as a badge of virility—even though the boy may by then be past the peak of sexual prowess. In boys and girls alike, the skin becomes coarser, with larger pores, and the sebaceous glands become more active, producing an oily secretion. As a result, young people become more subject to blackheads and acne. The composition of sweat is altered, and it becomes much stronger in odor. Much adolescent self-consciousness is caused by awareness of the odors of sweat and menstruation, and adolescents are a special target of advertising for deodorants and skin ointments.

The shift in physiological organization is further refle′ u in blood pressure, in basal metabolic rate (BMR: the rate at which the body in a basal—resting—state consumes oxygen), and in pulse rate, all of which show a rise at about the time of puberty. BMR relative to body size and pulse rate thereafter decline, with girls continuing to have a higher pulse rate and a lower BMR than boys. Prior to puberty, blood pressure is higher in girls than in boys, but after puberty the reverse is true.

The girl's external genitalia enlarge but otherwise change very little, whereas the boy's external genitalia change markedly. To begin with, there is a considerable increase in size. One of the signs of pubescence in the boy is the enlargement of the testicles. As the testes and scrotum grow in size, they become pendulous. Since sperm cells need a fairly constant temperature (below normal body temperature) to survive, an effective thermostat is built into the testicular structures: When the surrounding temperature goes down, the testes are drawn closer to the groin as a source of body heat, and vice versa. The shaft of the penis becomes longer and thicker, the glans (the head of the penis) grows until, in some cases, it emerges completely from the foreskin, and the penis as a whole also becomes pendulous. The penis is capable of erection from birth on, but until pubescence erection is likely to be in response to local stimulation or irritation and carries little sense of sexual urgency. Around the time of puberty, the penis begins to tumesce very readily, either spontaneously or in response to sexually provocative sights, sounds, smells, language, or whatever—as we have said, the male adolescent inhabits a libidinized life space where almost anything can take on sexual meaning. Now tumescence is accompanied by strong, unequivocal urges to ejaculate.

The literature suggests that close to 100 per cent of male adolescents masturbate more or less regularly, although lower-class culture dictates that masturbation is unmanly and lower-class boys are likely on that account to take less pleasure in the act. In a sample of forty-eight male college students, unfavorable ratings of masturbation effectively canceled out favorable ones, yielding an average rating just below neutrality. Boys may also have "wet dreams" (technically, *nocturnal emissions*), ejaculation during sleep, perhaps to the accompaniment of erotic dreams. Perhaps the publicly most noticeable secondary sex trait in boys is the "change of voice" brought about by enlargement of the larynx, the voice box. (In an earlier day, boy sopranos were kept permanently so by castration; without the gonadal contribution to growth, the larynx remained immature.) Most boys go through a period when their resonantly baritone voices shift treacherously and instantaneously to a squealing falsetto. Girls, too, have a change of voice, but it is less marked than in boys. Girls' voices become slightly deeper and considerably fuller.

Apart from the growth spurt, the first sign of pubescence in girls may be either the appearance of pubic hair or enlargement of the breasts, or both developments may coincide. The areolas grow larger, become elevated and conical in form, and take on a darker pigmentation. We do not know at what age the nipples become capable of erection. The breasts usually reach almost full size prior to the menarche, the beginning of menstruation. Some boys show a slight and temporary enlargement of one or both breasts during pubescence. There is still a great deal of debate, largely among anthropologists, about the concept of "adolescent sterility," the idea that girls cannot conceive for several years after puberty. In some societies, such as Samoa, the postpubertal years are a tacitly acknowledged period of experimental promiscuity for girls. (Since the explicit culture decrees virginity until marriage, chicken blood is dabbed on the nuptial couch to represent the ruptured hymen, or maidenhead.) It is clear that, in our own society, menstruation is skimpy and irregular for the first few years, and the rate of spontaneous abortion and of fetal and neonatal deaths is decidedly higher for sixteen- to nineteen-year-old mothers than for those in the twenty to twenty-nine age group. However, enough teen-age pregnancies and parturitions occur to make adolescent sterility less than safe as a method of birth control. Even less is known about when actual fertility begins for boys, since spermatozoa need to be present in considerable quantity for impregnation to take place.

One of the typical features of pubescent physical development is *asynchrony*, which we defined earlier as the way the body's various organs and subsystems grow at different rates and at different times. Asynchrony, or "split growth," is especially evident during pubescence, when arms, legs, nose, and chin may seem suddenly to sprout individually, with no regard for overall proportions and harmony. Indeed, the left and right sides of the body may grow at different rates, although by puberty the various body parts have come back into approximate balance. (Needless to say, people at all ages have some left-right asymmetry, as becomes evident when we piece together a photograph made of two lefts or two rights, with one reversed.[1])

One of the characteristics of adolescence is a feeling of being out of step, and asynchrony may enhance this feeling. Moreover, any deviation from the group average is likely to make the child feel out of step. The early-ripening girl probably feels out of place among her unripe classmates, and the late-maturing girl is a lost soul among the hips and bosoms that surround her. The early-maturing boy, by contrast, is likely to be at a social advantage, although he may suffer the pangs of dethronement as the others catch up and even surpass him. The late-maturing boy may suffer the most of all. The late-maturing girl may be neglected to the point of ostracism, but the late-maturing boy is likely to be made a butt, a scapegoat, and an object of scorn and ridicule.[2] Interestingly enough, as Mary Cover Jones[3] has shown, personality differences between early- and late-maturing males persist well into adult life. Following up in their forties a group of men who had been classified in their teens as early- or late-maturers, Jones found that the early-maturers were poised, responsible, successful, and conventional, and the late-maturers were active, exploratory, insightful, independent, and impulsive—all with due allowance for individual differences. There are growth tables from which one can make fairly good predictions of eventual adult stature, and adolescents might derive some comfort from these and the reassurance they give that most people sooner or later end up, by definition, in the normal range.

Now that we have seen some of the major changes that take place in the adolescent's body, it is time to consider how these changes fit into his changing view of himself.

The Adolescent Self

As we have said, the central theme of adolescence is finding an identity, a sense of self in relation to the world at large. The adolescent's self-awareness is in great part expressed in self-consciousness, a concern about how well he measures up. The adolescent worries about where he stands on a number of measures—how much money he has to spend, how good-looking and attractive he is, how intelligent he is, how witty and how daring, whether he can meet the demands of his moral conscience. His key concern, however, is with his progress toward physical maturity.

To the adult, it seems that the physical changes of adolescence go on at a rapid pace, from which we might conclude that the main problem of adolescence is having to come to terms with his successive incarnations. This is partly true. Certainly the fast-growing young adolescent often seems not to know what to do with his gangling arms and legs, new internal stirrings and impulses may take him unawares, and boys find it hard to control the vagaries of their voices and are panic-stricken lest a suddenly taut phallus be visible through their clothes. It is not for nothing that this has been called the "awkward age." It is equally true, however, that growth is almost always subjectively experienced as excruciatingly slow, no matter how objectively fast or slow, early or late, it may be. The boy may daily fondle the fuzz on his lip or cheek, wondering if it is yet time to shave it off, or he may watch anxiously the slow growth of a hair on his chest. Having learned about ejaculation, he may masturbate furiously, wondering if he can yet make it happen. The girl may measure her height or her bust once a week, anticipating the time when she will reach some magical ideal—as she approaches it, of course, she begins to worry about when and whether she will stop, or instead shoot on to a new record. She may hopefully lay in an anticipatory supply of bras, or, at a later age, eye shadow, false eyelashes, and hair spray. Or she may equally well resist acknowledging the changes that have come over her body.

Whether maturing takes place too fast or too slowly, it can be a source of agonized self-consciousness. The simple awareness of new and still-elusive potentialities for feeling, acting, and being acted upon can be unsettling. Equally important is the way physical changes and their psychological implications get reflected back from the environment. This mirroring happens at all levels: The tightness of his clothing tells the youngster that his body has grown; the realization, especially in girls, that her style of dress is no longer appropriate; the way adults tease boys about the change of voice, about how often they have to shave, and about taking an interest in girls—an imputation the pubescent boy may welcome but vehemently deny; a girl's becoming aware of the appraising stares men direct at her—or they may even approach her; the realization that one has outgrown certain playmates, or been left behind by others, not only physically but in terms of interests; the new meanings that emerge in what people say and do, or simply in the way things look and taste and smell and sound.

This is a time of painful sensitivity, when one's fragile self is raw and bleeds easily. Girls may feel that they cannot bear to be looked at. They may adopt a hunched or cringing posture to minimize their height or their breasts. They may wear voluminous and somewhat bizarre clothing to conceal their bodies. They may be prone to fits of seemingly unprovoked weeping. Girls may have several quite different attitudes toward their menstrual periods: Some feel a warm, quiet satisfaction at this manifestation of mature femininity, some feel polluted, some are frightened by it, and some take it matter-of-factly.

Boys are traditionally less modest about their bodies than are girls, but at this time they may find all manner of excuses and devices not to expose themselves in the school locker room or shower room, for fear their development differs grossly from that of their fellows. By the same token, the adolescent boy snatches furtive glimpses of his mates' anatomy in search of standards of normality (such checking up should not be thought of as homosexual leanings). Obviously, these body awarenesses are closely tied to sexual feelings, which we shall treat separately in the next section. Here we want to stress the out-of-stepness, the need to check up on oneself relative to one's contemporaries. Let us remember that markedly early or late maturing, of which we spoke above, has both practical social consequences for how the child fits in, and psychological consequences for how he views himself, objectively as measured against age mates, and intersubjectively in terms of how he perceives their perception of him.

But self-awareness is only in part a matter of body-awareness. And body-awareness is only partly a matter of maturational status. It is also a matter of having a male body or a female body, of a sickly or healthy or strong or weak body, a beautiful or plain or ugly body—and such self-judgments are often a hopeless mélange of objective and subjective. That is, a person who in other people's eyes is altogether comely can nevertheless experience himself as homely or physically loathsome, he can accept the odors he radiates as normal or intolerable, he can ignore facial blemishes or regard them as total disfigurement. Beyond body awareness is awareness of self as a person at various levels of competence, virtue, self-direction and self-control, importance, and orientation in time. Some young people acquire a sense of going somewhere while others drift aimlessly or flounder in agitated despair. Some feel that their best years lie behind them and live on past triumphs, while others feel trapped by past disasters. Some people learn to experience themselves as possessing an immortal soul which will survive the death of the body and go on to a new life in other realms.

This differentiation of layers of self, and, with good fortune, their eventual integration into an identity, develops out of a sense of ambiguity. The ambiguity of early adolescence is beautifully expressed in Phyllis McGinley's "Portrait of Girl with Comic Book":

> Thirteen's no age at all. Thirteen is nothing.
> It is not wit, or powder on the face,
> Or Wednesday matinées, or misses' clothing,
> Or intellect, or grace.
> Twelve has its tribal customs. But thirteen
> Is neither boys in battered cars nor dolls,
> Not *Sara Crewe*, or movie magazine,
> Or pennants on the wall.
>
> Thirteen keeps diaries and tropical fish
> (A month, at most); scorns jumpropes in the spring;
> Could not, would fortune grant it, name its wish;
> Wants nothing, everything;
> Has secrets from itself, friends it despises;
> Admits none to the terrors that it feels;
> Owns half a hundred masks but no disguises;
> And walks upon its heels.
>
> Thirteen's anomalous—not that, not this:
> Not folded bud, or wave that laps a shore,
> Or moth proverbial from the chrysalis.
> Is the one age defeats the metaphor.
> Is not a town, like childhood, strongly walled
> But easily surrounded; is no city.
> Nor, quitted once, can it be quite recalled—
> Not even with pity.[4]

The perspicacity of McGinley's observation is borne out by interviews with thirteen-year-old girls and with their parents. The case of early adolescent boys is less clearcut. They certainly seem subject to ambiguity, but they seem able to function with less emotional waste motion than girls. It is possible that the adult world and the peer group are more accepting of the boy's burgeoning sexuality than of the girl's, allowing him to be more at ease about it. Also, the adult role of the male is more sharply defined than that of the female, so that the signs of becoming adult do not raise quite so many questions. The boy seems to encounter more ambiguity later in adolescence when it comes time to match concrete competences with the role demands of adulthood.

Filled as they are with ambivalences, few adolescents feel really in control. They tend to be trapped between impulses that are not really a part of themselves and what often seem like unreasonable or capricious adult constraints. But lack of control also carries the hidden blessing of lack of responsibility, and adolescents become masters at the mechanisms of defense. They learn to rationalize their behavior with all the guile of an expert lawyer. They project blame either onto motives beyond their control or onto an environment that does not understand the real, interior adolescent. (One teen-age girl to another: "So I said to him, 'How do you know this is the real me you're talking to?'") They play tricks of memory, prettifying and justifying their own role in past events and downgrading that of others. The younger adolescent spends hours before the mirror trying desperately to read off from his own features the secret of who he is, and, incidentally, of what he looks like to other people—which for him, at the moment, is more or less the same thing. The older adolescent spends hours before the mirror trying on hair arrangements and facial expressions and postures, worrying a pimple on his chin, trying to gauge how best to achieve maximum effect—that is, to reveal his True Self. It should be noted that the perpetual solitary self-appraisal of the adolescent is more emotional than objective. He (or she) is able to see himself only through the haze of an ideal image. An unhappy adolescent will focus on the ways in which he fails to meet this ideal, and appear to be quite unaware of his assets. Another adolescent, less prone to self-disparagement, will equally unrealistically blot out of consciousness any unsightly features (as opposed to blemishes), lingering intently over any that seem promising.

We have stressed how the adolescent escapes from the adult world into the peer society. We can now see how he is also escaping from himself, how the roles the peer culture offers him are a refuge from the doubts, ambiguities, and ambivalences that confront him in solitude. The peer group, of course, is not a perfect refuge. It makes demands, too, and these demands may violate the adolescent's self-image. Just as we maintain a zone of sensitivity around our material bodies, so that we leave a margin for error in our adjustment to space, so do we maintain a zone of personal privacy. This zone is not uniform around all regions of the body: We shake hands freely, but an embrace is more special; the girl may tolerate the boy's hand on her arm, or his arm across her shoulder, or even a slap on her buttocks, but his hand on her breast or thigh may be an encroachment on the zone of privacy. Group life entails endless invasions of privacy, and there may be powerful pressures to act contrary to conscience. But the group does offer an identity, in terms both of acceptance and of the roles it defines. Many authors speak of "finding one's identity," but it is as much a matter of constructing an identity as of discovering who one already is. Perhaps one reason that adolescents avoid self-knowledge even as they seek it is a vague sense that once one acknowledges traits and motives, they crystallize as permanent features and so obstruct the formation of a superior self.

In his role playing, then, the adolescent can be seen as trying on ready-made identities to see how well they suit him. Some of these roles are modeled on particular people, movie and television stars and heroes of the day, others are based on fictional characters from literature or the mass media (the female karate expert and sex-kitten seems to be a popular image nowadays), and some are based on culturally defined "types": the tough guy, the sweet young thing, the gay young thing, woman of the world, the man's man, the bored sophisticate, the esthete, the clown, the beatnik. Those youngsters who are actually moving toward particular careers begin to play the roles, to affect the mannerisms, associated with occupational types—the role playing of young people aiming toward medical careers is a marvel to behold, and so is that of young Marines or of youngsters who have identified with business careers, journalism, the law, teaching, whatever. We take the adolescent search for identity so much for granted that we tend to forget that it is peculiar to cultures in which there is a fair amount of social and economic mobility. In societies where the adolescent has no choice but to fit into a predetermined niche (which is coming to be the case in our own society as it stabilizes and ossifies, so that the offspring of public servants go into government, movie actors' children grow up to be actors, and psychologists' children—those who make it—grow up to be psychologists), the problems are different.

It can be seen that the adolescent, like the preschool child playing cowboy, tends to seize on the externals of a role and may miss its essence. This concern with outward appearance sometimes verges on the magical, as when the adolescent chooses a new name to be known by. The choice is made with earnest care, and only after much weighing of alternatives, since it must express in pure form the very innermost ideal self, it must project the perfect image. A similar force seems to lie behind the new and ornate handwritings many adolescents adopt, especially girls. The adolescent is seeking to capture the style of his role portrayals, a style conveying one whole approach to life which he can sense forcefully but not put into words. He is discovering what various styles of life feel like to him and also what sorts of reactions they produce in others. These reactions have to come mainly from peers, in early adolescence from peers of the same sex, and increasingly in later adolescence from peers of the opposite sex. Teachers may sometimes play along with adolescent role playing, but parents make a most unsatisfactory audience. When, in the course of quick changes of role, the adolescent girl decides to try out a new hair style or color, or to speak in a lazy, insolent drawl, or to wear a saintly appearance, or when the boy decides to wear his shirt casually unbuttoned to the waist, or to greet with a cynical, sneering grunt whatever people say, or assumes an air of unaccustomed humility and submissiveness, parents are likely to respond by asking, "Who are you being today?" The adolescent is taken aback when adults fail to recognize that the new self now on display is the true and final one. The adolescent easily forgets that earlier role incarnations were equally valid at the time, and when reminded of them he repudiates them wholly and contemptuously: "That was ages ago! I was only a baby then!" Indeed, he may be guarding against the realization that his present self is as ephemeral as past ones, and so cannot tolerate any reminders of what he once was. To have his baby pictures shown—above all to his peers—brings him to the depths of mortification.

In short, every new personality is assumed totally and cannot be questioned—this week—and every old one is remorselessly buried. But even here there is a hint of ambivalence. The adolescent, adrift as he is, may have a private urge to recapture the continuity of his life and may secretly welcome reminders (in private) of his forgotten past. By late adolescence, the young person may, with luck, be able to reintegrate the various selves he knows—his body, his public personality, and the private core of feeling that is the "real me," his past, his present, and an image of the future—into a single functioning schema that he can take for granted without endless embarrassment, introspection, and anxious reading off of other people's reactions.

Adolescent Sexuality

A major part of adolescent self-awareness involves the further sexual awakening that comes with the approach of biological maturity. In Freudian terms, pubescence spells the end of latency and the beginning of adult genitality. The task of this age, according to the psychoanalysts, is to master (to inhibit, control, and direct) sexuality in the service of mature love, and to sublimate surplus sexual energies into productive work. As Freud pointed out, sexuality affects and is affected by behavior in every sphere of activity. Even if one does not accept Freud's thesis that sex drive is the basis for all constructive action, it is still necessary to acknowledge its pervasiveness and importance, particularly in adolescent behavior.

The first point to be made is that sexuality is not the same for adolescent boys and girls. In boys, sexual desire is highly specific and is clearly centered in the penis. It can be easily aroused by a variety of external stimuli, by words, pictures, random thoughts and associations, or it may be deliberately sought by self-stimulation or by seeking external stimulants. Sexual desire in boys is urgent and aims toward rapid discharge of tension in orgasm (even so-called oral and anal erotics finally seek orgasm).

Among girls, there is a much wider range of normal individual differences. Some girls experience desire in much the way boys do, and a few are so avid for constant sexual experience as to fit the clinical picture of nymphomania. Many others may not know direct sexual urges until later in life, and some apparently never do (although Freudians would want to know the reason). It is interesting that many a twenty-year-old girl can talk about sex as though it had nothing to do with her. College instructors are sometimes amazed at the bland "sophistication" with which female students can discuss erotic literature. What the instructor may not realize is that such literature may simply have no libidinal impact on such students. For most adolescent girls, however, "desire" or "lust" is not the correct description, and we might do better to speak of "sexual stirrings." These, unlike male desire, are diffuse and not as clearly differentiated from other feelings: romantic yearnings, maternal cravings, mild intoxication, enthusiasm, pity, sensual feelings such as come from having one's back rubbed or one's hair combed, or even such emotions as anger and fear. Many girls find, in fact, that sexual arousal occurs only in the midst of a general state of tension, excitement, or agitation. Ordinarily, specifically sexual arousal in girls must be brought about by direct stimulation of the body, particularly of the erogenous zones. Female sexual arousal seems to be less climax-oriented than male desire—that is, it is experienced more as a state to be maintained indefinitely than as the prelude to orgasm (although there is every reason to believe that most girls are capable of orgasm).

The lower intensity and specificity of sexual feelings in girls than in boys may be related to several factors. It may derive from the double standard which says that girls are supposed to be less highly sexed than boys, and that manifestations of female sexuality are to be met with disapproval and repression. If this is the case, females should become more like males in the nature of their sexual cravings as the climate of values shifts toward greater permissiveness. The difference may correspond to the lesser degree of anatomical differentiation of the female genitalia. Even the fact that the girl's genitals are less visible to her than the boy's to him may reduce the clarity of genital sensations.

In addition to differences between boys and girls in the nature and strength of sexual feelings, there are important differences in developmental timing.[5] For boys, the peak of sexuality—measured by the frequency with which orgasm is sought—comes a year or two after puberty, at sixteen or seventeen, after which there is a slow but steady decline. In girls, the peak comes much later, often not until age thirty or beyond—the actual timing seems to depend a great deal on the amount of sexual experience. Again, as exposure to sexual stimulation through advertising, literature, movies, and television becomes more common, it is possible that girls will be moved to a full sexual awakening at ever earlier ages.

Simply because sexual desire in boys is a distinctive state, unlikely to be confused with other feelings, we should not assume that it is uncomplicated by other feelings. It becomes involved, first of all, with the universal adolescent fear of embarrassment. We have already mentioned that the boy may be alarmed lest an erection be noticed by others. He may furthermore be afraid that he will let slip some of the illicit thoughts that are so often with him. Because of the many conflicting ideas about sex that he has picked up, he may be unsure about how he should act. A special source of confusion is his ignorance of how girls feel about sex— the folklore, after all, paints them as both monuments of purity and Jezebels. Notice that girls themselves embody this duality: They expose their bodies, paint themselves alluringly, sing siren songs, sit, walk, and writhe lasciviously, and lash out viperlike when boys "go too far." European males in the United States find American girls very confusing, since they seem to be inviting coitus but in fact are saying only that males should find them interesting and attractive. The boy may have doubts about his own sexual adequacy, from questioning his appeal to girls, to worrying about premature ejaculation, to wondering if he simply wouldn't wither at a crucial moment. He may have been told that sexual indulgence weakens men—athletes are still warned that girls will undermine their manliness. Sex may appear dangerous merely because it entails such violent feelings. The boy may have been frightened by descriptions of venereal disease—some of the anti-V.D. instruction given by the military perhaps unwittingly makes girls a conditioned stimulus for loathing; this in addition to religious training that may tell the boy that sex is sinful and unclean. American boys take it for granted that their first sexual experience should be with girls their own age or slightly younger, whereas in European societies it is assumed that an older woman will initiate him into the mysteries. In well-to-do families, a maid is often hired with this tacit assumption in mind. It is considered uncouth for a young man to enter marriage without the knowledge necessary to instruct his bride. Notice that this kind of cultural arrangement is rather more congruent with what we knew about sexual development than is the American one.

For boys, sexual cravings are initially quite separate from notions of love. Although a boy, when aroused, would prefer a sexual partner of his own age and of his own or higher social class, he may not be too discriminating and may be willing to settle for masturbation or a prostitute. The homosexuality of middle-years childhood goes underground in adolescence except for occasional adventures instigated by older homosexuals, and except for those adolescents who seem committed to the path of homosexuality. But when a girl does invite a boy's favors, even though she yields herself only up to a sharply defined point, he finds it very easy to fall in love with her. Many male adolescents carry about a free-floating amorousness that settles readily on a convenient love-goat. But this love is quite different from what he will feel as a husband and a father. It is more an amplified form of the affection he feels for his male friends and seems to be compounded of delight in shared intimacy, the freedom to let down one's guard, and the glow that comes from being accepted, all in the heated atmosphere of sexual desire. Needless to say, he attributes to his love-goat those qualities he hopes to find, regardless of what she may actually possess. Love-goating works the other way, of course, with females falling in childish love with convenient males, but the purely sexual components may be muted, diffuse, or missing. Mature love, we presume, includes a measure of objectivity in viewing the beloved object, which makes for rather less disillusionment as the relationship evolves.

For girls, love takes a decided priority over sexuality. The love-goating of girls comes in part from the adolescent cultural climate, which says that falling in love is the thing to do. But it also seems to be motivated by some notion that attachment to a male is the way to an identity. It seems that the passivity built into females by the larger culture may impede identity formation by requiring a merger with someone stronger. This may mean, to both the girl and her partner, sexual surrender, but its more basic origin seems to be the need for identity. This may be why girls are attracted to physically powerful males (much to the despair of the less powerful). If the girl vacillates about surrender, it is perhaps in part because surrender both promises an identity and threatens its loss. For the point of belonging to a male is really to possess him, to make him a more potent extension of the self. This notion is a vestige of the knightly ideal, that the man becomes a slave to the love of the empedestaled virgin, who remains virginal in spirit even after she has rewarded the man with her favors. By the judicious manipulation of her favors and favor, she can make the man her puppet.

We can see how, in girls, romantic feelings centered about a possessive surrender point straight to domesticity. Partial surrender becomes a highly effective device for keeping the male's motivation at fever pitch. Total surrender risks "losing the man's respect" and thus the man himself. Sometimes total surrender permits the girl to manipulate the male by playing on guilt feelings, but this is obviously less satisfactory than the manipulation of sexual drive. When the game is played right, the young man comes to accept that marriage is the price he has to pay for sex with a "nice" girl. Lower-class girls are more likely to yield than middle-class ones, partly because the lower-class ethic is less stringent, partly because lower-class living conditions make sex a fairly public matter and increase the probability that the girl will have an early introduction to sex, and partly because sexual compliance wins friendship, affection, and sometimes material rewards. The lower-class girl is more likely than the middle-class one to have an illegitimate baby or to end up with a husband won by bribery or coercion. We should repeat that middle-class mothers encourage their daughters to play the game of husband-catching, and are fairly explicit about the rules—"Never go all the way." They begin early in the game a painstaking cultivation of the mothers of eligible boys. In sum, when adolescent girls become "boy crazy," it is evident that sexuality may play only an indirect and minor role in this phenomenon.

We should note that while our culture's attitudes toward sex are often ambiguous and inconsistent, they are more liberal than those of some other cultures. For instance, in a study of values by Church and Insko[6] in Hawaii, Caucasian-American undergraduates showed significantly more favorable attitudes to items dealing with aspects of sex than did Japanese-American subjects, and males gave significantly more favorable ratings than females. A subsample of Chinese-American female subjects gave slightly more favorable ratings than Caucasian-American females. The contrast among groups shows up clearly if we consider the number of subjects who gave a favorable rating to premarital sex: 18 out of 24 Caucasian-American males, 9 out of 24 Japanese-American males; 8 out of 24 Caucasian-American females, and 1 out of 24 Japanese-American females. We have made some personal observations that tend to confirm these findings; it appears that in marriage Japanese and Japanese-American women submit obediently to the wishes of the male, but with only simulated pleasure. There were cultural differences, too, in which aspects of sex were favored or disfavored. Masturbation had the highest rank among items for Japanese-American females, and tied for first place with petting for Chinese-American females, whereas it ranked third or fourth with the other groups. It is possible that masturbation may not be for the sake of sexual stimulation and discharge, but instead serve as a technique of self-soothing.

Intellectual curiosity about sex continues to be a component of adolescent sexuality. Boys and girls are voracious seekers after sexual information and get it from whatever sources they can. Part of the frustrations of this age comes from not even having a vocabulary with which to talk about these vital matters. The youngsters know all the four-letter words, but to use them in a serious conversation cheapens the topic. Curiosity in adolescence, of course, goes way beyond a craving for anatomical and physiological knowledge and extends to "What do you do?" "What is it like?" "Does it hurt?" "What happens when?" and "Is it all right if you . . . ?" One of the difficulties is the sense that there must be something more that one does not know about. Even adolescents with a fair amount of sexual experience are likely to feel vaguely baffled and cheated. Their experience somehow never quite measures up to the promise of the erotic episodes they read about in books or see in motion pictures. Many adolescent discussions of sex, and much reading of erotic literature, have as their unspoken theme the search for the "something else" that presumably lies beyond. Young people's craving for knowledge is not merely a desire to find out what sex does or should feel like to them but equally what it is like for the opposite sex. Girls understand the potency of male urges, but unless the girl has equivalent feelings, their special sexual quality is likely to elude her. Male ignorance about female sexuality is amazingly great. Males may project their own sexuality onto women, they may see women as essentially frigid, indifferent or hostile to sex, or they may see them as emasculating Delilahs. Boys are uncertain which, if any, version of female sexuality to believe.

From what we have been able to learn by talking to young people, they feel profoundly ambivalent about sex, and even those who practice it regularly may get little satisfaction from it. On the male side, the pleasure of orgasm is, as one young man put it, like using a woman to masturbate with. The chief pleasure sex seems to bring young men is the satisfaction of triumph, of being able to boast of his conquests to his fellows, or of describing the unusual circumstances of a liaison (like deep in the icy water of a lake). But even these pleasures are marred by the sense of being cheated, by guilt, by fear of pregnancy (young men report that they do not use contraceptives because it would seem disrespectful of the girl), by worry about venereal disease, and by doubts whether a girl who would sleep with him is worth sleeping with. Since most male adolescents are not masters of the art of love (and it is likely that the girl would reject the practices involved as "unnatural," "abnormal," or "dirty"), the girl may be denied even the simple fleshly pleasures. In addition, the fear of pregnancy, for obvious reasons, is considerably greater than for the boy. Since many males feel strongly that the woman they marry must be chaste, the girl who gives in knows that she is reducing her value on the marriage market. She also knows that if she is found out, censure will fall more heavily on her than on the boy, who is expected to sow his wild oats pretty much where he can. Indeed, the girl in a rape case or a paternity suit can expect to find herself portrayed in court as a slut or a whore.[7]

The authors are frequently asked what the revolution in sexual attitudes is doing to the morals of young people. It seems to us a prior question to ask whether there is a sexual revolution. If there is, it is much more pronounced among adults than among adolescents. It is adults, after all, who invented mate-swapping and group sex. If California is the harbinger of the American future with regard to sex as with regard to so many other things, a juvenile sexual revolution may be on its way, but it has not yet arrived. As Freedman[8] points out, the main change that has come over college women is a willingness to talk frankly and without embarrassment about sex. He says that any actual increase in sexual activity is attributable to a new willingness to sleep with the man you are going to marry, but only after the betrothal vows have been pledged. (Notice that in Okinawan society the young man moves in with his fiancée immediately the engagement has been announced.[9] Scandinavian society is not too different.) Girls are the key of any sexual revolution, since, if we can believe the data, most boys are ready to engage in sex at every opportunity—if ambivalently. There are boys who seem not to experience strong urges, and others who observe a single standard that says that males as well as females must remain pure before marriage, but both these are a decided minority. Some of the social-class differences noted by Kinsey[10] still seem to apply: Lower-class boys are less likely than middle-class ones to practice masturbation, are more likely to engage in homosexual practices (but without becoming committed full-time homosexuals), and, as we have said, have easier access to hetero-sexual intercourse.

While the American culture's proclaimed sexual values are rapidly disintegrating, this does not mean such values are useless. Increasingly, though, values are going to have to be individualized to suit persons and situations. It seems to the authors that sex is most meaningful and satis-factory when one has reached a stable degree of emotional and social maturity. It seems to us that the young woman ought to beware of impulsive sex, generated in a moment of unthinking passion, because, when the passion is past, she is liable to feel disgust and self-disgust. It may seem cold-blooded and antisexual to say that one should enter a sexual relationship open-eyed and clearheaded and after a certain amount of deliberation, but the alternative is likely to be psychologically damaging. Sex at its best is too marvelous a thing to be attained casually and indiscriminately. It requires full openness and intimate fusion be-tween two persons, and one does not want to be that intimate with just anybody. But without the intimacy and openness, sex becomes a matter of sensations which can be induced as well by self-stimulation as by contact between bodies. It is our contention that it is this intimacy which constitutes the "something else" that adolescents find missing from sex. And in general, still-unformed adolescents simply do not have this capacity for opening themselves freely to another person. The campus clamor for "free sex" overlooks that the restraints on free sexual expres-sion lie as much in the immaturities of adolescents as in adult controls. And the proclamation that "sex is beautiful" is more likely in adolescence to be an article of faith than a statement of verified fact. Thus, without invoking any of the traditional moralities, one can find good psychological reasons for going slow and waiting for adulthood—if not necessarily marriage—before looking for sexual fulfillment.

However, if girls are going to exercise restraint, they may have to learn to stop provoking males to lust by tricks of dress (or undress), gait, manner, voice, and partial surrender that promise more than the girl is willing to deliver. Girls early acquire an elaborate provocativeness that probably has little to do with sexual feelings. In preschool or middle-years girls, provocative behavior often resembles the ritual mating patterns of infrahuman species, semi-instinctual movements that appear in the right releasing circumstances and which, stimulated by the proper reciprocal behavior in the male, culminate in sexual receptivity. Such evolutionary remnants probably enter into the sexual dances of many societies, which are so effective that they can bring the participants up to and even into climax.[11] It is conceivable that Americans could return to tribal sexual patterns, but it seems more likely that, as part of the burden of civilization, we will move on to the cultivation of a highly developed eroticism based on a special relationship between two persons. As it is, American girls behave—in many cases unconsciously—in ways as sexually stimulating as those of the Tahitian maiden, but they don't really mean it. In terms of playing the marriage game, such promising and then backing off works to lure the male into the trap, but we cannot help questioning whether this is a psychologically sound approach to a mature relationship between a man and a woman.

It seems to us that people can get to know each other, fall in love, decide to have sexual relations, to live together, to get married and raise a family, without the maneuvering and manipulation that go into the marriage game. But it may be Utopian to think that men and women can learn to treat each other as human beings who can talk openly and honestly and who can get to know each other before embarking on a sexual adventure. It seems sad that it is only in the marriage bed that many men and women find that they do not really like each other so very much after all. But, in principle at least, a new understanding and the end of exploitation between the sexes may lead to a discovery of the glories of real sexual fulfillment.[12]

Adolescent Idealism

Like the preschool child, the adolescent is full of contradictions. These contradictions, however, seem to be simply diverse expressions of the central theme of finding and constructing an identity. Since much adolescent behavior strikes adults as offensive, infantile, and even bizarre, they may find it hard to see that, underneath the superficial manifestations of fads, costumes, slang, wisecracks, and poses, posturing, and role playing, a thread of idealism runs through much of his behavior. (Idealism, as we shall see, is found in all varieties of adolescents to some degree, and not just in those we have labeled as *idealists* in an earlier section.)

In this section, we want to emphasize the side of the adolescent that we do not see when he is with groups of his peers and which he may conceal from all but his closest friends. Indeed, when he complains that his parents do not understand him, he is often saying that they fail to see this side of him. The adolescent is busy losing old illusions and building new ones to take their place. At times, he becomes convinced of the hopelessness of all illusions and lapses into cynicism or despair, no less genuine for the melodramatic display he makes of them. The air of bored sophistication he sometimes affects is meant to say that he has seen through the flimsy pretensions of the world around him and feels above its pettiness and corruption. His occasional apathy and lack of involvement express feelings of futility about the state of the world. But even though his disillusionment is often grist to his histrionic mill, it means at heart that he is really searching for an ideal and decent world for his ideal and decent self to respond to. When he lashes out at adults, it is often in protest against the sick society to which they acquiesce and in punishment for its lack of idealism. Needless to add, his idealism is often at odds with his own animalism, the sordid cravings and weaknesses that threaten to undermine his purity from below. Adolescent boys, especially, may be quite poignantly conscious of and troubled by a sense of duality, a split between their carnal and spiritual natures. And through it all, of course, the adolescent tends to enjoy his suffering for the romantic picture it gives him of himself and for the emotional workout it affords.

A great part of the adolescent's idealism probably stems from his resistance to growing up. Particularly in early adolescence, he wants to enjoy his new powers in total freedom uncontaminated by the practical demands of life. Furthermore, very little that he sees around him matches the glory he senses in his new powers. By comparison, the world of everyday adult activities, the world of political machinations that he reads about in the papers, looks tainted and shopworn. The young adolescent, viewing himself largely from the inside, experiences himself (when he is not embarrassed, despondent, or self-accusing) as pure spirit, and the only worthy external counterparts of this experience are to be found in the majesties and austerities of religion, in the beauties of nature, in certain idealized public or fictional personalities, in poetry or music, in political abstractions—in short, in reality seen from a great distance.

As long as the adolescent is less than totally disillusioned, as long as he can hold on to the conviction that virtue and decency are possible, that there exist external counterparts to his ideal self, he can keep going, often on a plane of high elation. But when, perhaps in response to some minor personal setback such as being refused permission to use the family car, or having been stood up on a date, or having been forbidden to wear one's new bikini, the adolescent feels alone and helpless in a vast, unresponsive, hostile world, he is prone to depressions of the sort that the Germans have aptly named *Weltschmerz*—world pain. It was this phenomenon that most impressed early European writers on the subject and which we find memorialized in the writings of Goethe, and perpetuated in the quest for sincerity and good faith of Huckleberry Finn and Salinger's Holden Caulfield. It is when enveloped in *Weltschmerz* that the adolescent takes long, solitary nocturnal walks (preferably in the rain), composes long, melancholy poems, or toys with the idea of suicide—a special kind of suicide following which the disembodied adolescent can still stand by and witness and savor the remorse that people will feel "after I'm gone." It is in times of *Weltschmerz*, too, that the adolescent may first become attuned to the miseries of the world's downtrodden and the social ills, inequities, injustices, anomalies, and absurdities that generate great quantities of misery. Needless to say, those adolescents who have grown up in conditions of misery have known about them all along, but adolescence may bring a planetary awareness of and identification with other people who share a similar fate. The social concerns of the adolescent may mark a new stage of fellow-feeling for humanity at large, to the point of advocating instant revolution.

Some adolescents find the answer to their idealism in religion, embracing it seriously for the first time, intensifying the beliefs they have always held, or converting to another, more promising faith. For some number of adolescents, religion as it is practiced exemplifies the worst in hypocrisy and corruption, and religious belief the most debased of superstition, and these idealistically leave their faith, often with great difficulty, as depicted by James Joyce. Different religions may appeal to the adolescent in different ways. He may be enthralled by the ornate pageantry and symbolism of one, by the puristic austerity of another, by the militancy of another, or by the castigations of yet another. Whatever religion he chooses is a vehicle by which he can project himself beyond mundane reality and into the heady realm of the ideal absolute. His concern with religion is, of course, part and parcel of his concern with the nature of the world into which he is moving; and the nature and existence of God, and the need for and the possibility of faith are among the topics endlessly debated in adolescent bull sessions—which, incidentally, provide adolescents with one of their best opportunities to find out how other people feel and to try out their own opinions. For some adolescents, faith is a source of comfort and gives assurance that their individual lives have some meaning. For some, it provides order in a disorderly world. For some, faith provides an escape from concern about the state of the world, since everything by definition is for the best and particular events are only the working out of the inscrutable divine will. Some faiths promise an apocalyptic resolution of human vice and stupidity, which many adolescents find a grimly appealing prospect. A number of adolescents, while rejecting organized religion and established faiths, espouse a diffuse, generalized belief in some vague divinity. Some adolescents see in the promise of an afterlife a reward for whatever torments they may have to suffer in this world.

It is important to understand that even delinquent and destructive behavior can be an expression of a disappointed idealism. We may wish that all disillusioned young people would join the Peace Corps or VISTA, and we may sympathize with civil rights workers and protest demonstrators as idealists on the march, but we must remember that some portion of young people are in basic revolt against all the assumptions and doctrines and ideologies and values of our society, and that some of these know of no other way to express their loathing except through acts of destruction and violence. The adolescent conventionalist may feel that the world as it exists is already an approximation of the ideal and so is unaware of any basic contradiction in becoming a part of it. The conventionalist may express his idealism in volunteer work for worthy causes. Even the psychopath, as we have said, subscribes to conventional ideals, and may furthermore experience his psychopathic life style as conforming to the knightly ideal—notice the names that street gangs assume: the Dukes, the Barons, the Black Knights, the Dragons—of chivalry and valor.

A few youngsters carry their idealism beyond adolescence and find careers which give it some practical expression: political organization, work with civil rights groups and peace groups, the arts, a religious vocation, teaching, social work, work with the handicapped or deprived, scientific research, and so forth—although it should not be assumed that everyone working in these fields is an idealist. Most youngsters, however, by late adolescence have pretty well come to terms with things as they are—in the words of the idealists, they have "sold out"—and have given up on working any major changes in the social, political, or economic structure (although in later years they will contribute a certain amount of time to "good causes" and crusades for "better schools"), or in the culture's value system, and are trying to find their place in society as it is given to them. This is the time when they have to weigh the advantages of further education against the appeal of getting directly to work and settling down, when they have to balance their actual skills and capacities against their often grandiose ambitions, and their preparation and ambitions against the economic realities. On this and other adolescent themes, see the research reported by Douvan and Adelson.[13]

This is often a stressful time for the adolescent on two counts, omitting the stress of abandoning idealism. First, the variety of possible occupations has become so large as to be bewildering. Indeed, despite the almost total vocational and geographical mobility theoretically open to the young person, the choice of a career is usually settled by accident: whom one knows or whom one's family knows, what one happens to hear about or stumble upon, what is available locally. Second, the thought of having to measure up, on his own, to the rigorous standards of commercial competition is likely to provoke one more upsurge of ambiguity and ambivalence amounting to panic. All his life the child is asked, "What are you going to *be* when you grow up?" Now the question suddenly and alarmingly becomes, "What are you going to *do* after you finish school?" Nowadays, of course, the choice is often, for the moment, between school and military service, which does not relieve the panic, and the youngster who hopes to dodge the draft by getting married and siring a child while still in school may find that he has put himself in an extra financial bind. The young person's panic may obliterate his dreams, ideals, and ambitions and send him rushing into the best job he can find in a hurry, giving up on sailing to the South Seas or painting in Paris or regenerating the world. The pressures and seductions are many, and it is a rare and admirable young person who can hold fast to his ideals in this turbulent transition.

REFERENCES / Chapter 11

[1] Wolff, W. *The Expression of Personality*. New York: Harper, 1943.
[2] Faust, M. S. Developmental maturity as a determinant in prestige of adolescent girls. *Child Development*, 1960, 31, 173–184; Weatherly, D. Self-perceived rate of physical maturation and personality in late adolescence. *Child Development*, 1964, 35, 1197–1210.
[3] Jones, M. C. Psychological correlates of somatic development. *Child Development*, 1965, 36, 899–911.
[4] McGinley, P. *The Love Letters of Phyllis McGinley*. New York: Viking, 1954.
[5] Kinsey, A. C., and associates. *Sexual Behavior in the Human Male*. Philadelphia: Saunders, 1948, p. 219; *id., Sexual Behavior in the Human Female*, 1953, p. 353.
[6] Church, J., and Insko, C. A. Ethnic and sex differences in sexual values. *Psychologia*, 1965, 8, 153–157.
[7] Sherwin, R. V. The law and sexual relationships. *Journal of Social Issues*, 1966, 22, 109–122.
[8] Freedman, M. B. As older sexual codes crumble on campus, a newer honesty takes their place. In Time, Inc. *The Young Americans*. New York: Time-Life Books, 1966, pp. 98–99.
[9] Maretzki, T. W., and Maretzki, H. *Taira: An Okinawan Village*. New York: Wiley, 1966.
[10] Kinsey, *et al., Sexual Behavior in the Human Male*, pp. 335–363; Rainwater, L. Some aspects of lower class sexual behavior. *Journal of Social Issues*, 1966, 22, 96–108.
[11] Danielsson, B. *Love in the South Seas*. London: George Allen & Unwin, 1956.
[12] Kirkendall, L. A., and Libby, R. W. Interpersonal relationships—crux of the sexual renaissance. *Journal of Social Issues*, 1966, 22, 45–59.
[13] Douvan, E., and Adelson, J. *The Adolescent Experience*. New York: Wiley, 1966.

12 *Becoming Mature*

Helping the Adolescent into Adulthood

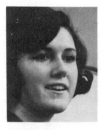 The quantities of knowledge that a person needs to make his way in a complex civilization like ours is reason enough for the long apprenticeship that we call adolescence. But we may question whether the apprenticeship we provide is the best one for adolescents and for society as a whole. At best, we prepare adolescents to go on living in a world that is a forward projection of the present one, and at worst, to live in a long-vanished phantom environment. Since we know that the world will either have to change radically or go smash, and since it is out of the question that the direction of change can be toward a bucolic "good old days," we obviously are teaching adolescents wrong.[1] They have their own answer, of course, in the perpetuation of teen-age culture into adulthood, but inasmuch as the teen-age culture is inadequate even to the needs of adolescents, we can doubt whether it will work for adults.

We cannot achieve preparation for adulthood in adolescence alone. It must begin in infancy. But it is in late adolescence that the preparation reaches its culmination, when the ambivalences must be resolved in favor of growing up into independence. We have so far left open, just as our society does, the answer to the critical question of when adolescence ends and adulthood begins. The young person passes many milestones, but there is no single marker that tells him that he has left childhood behind. The best we can say, then, is that the individual is grown up when his society tells him that he is—that is, when adults, other than his parents, begin more or less consistently to treat him as one of themselves. Parents may be the last to detect and acknowledge the adolescent's changed status.

It is in the behavior of teachers, parental friends, uncles and aunts, employers, and especially strangers such as waiters, taxi drivers, and barbers that the young person can read his adulthood. These people, less biased than his parents, will be reacting to something in his appearance and manner that betoken maturity. As we suggested earlier, there is a strong element of circular reinforcement, of positive feedback, in this process. The sooner people begin to take the young person's adulthood for granted, the sooner and more easily he assumes the role, and the easier it is for others to react to him as adult. Early in the process, there may be some irony on the part of adults, and some self-consciousness on the side of the adolescent (it may be a long time before the young person can refer to himself or herself without awkwardness as "Mister" or "Miss"), but even as a semiformal game, recognized as such by both parties, it serves the adolescent as a way into adulthood. The interesting thing is that the adolescent, for all his straining for acceptance, usually passes into adulthood without immediately being aware of the fact. At some point, he realizes that he no longer half-expects people to challenge his adulthood, that he himself is no longer bluffing or merely playing a role, and, looking back, that he has already crossed the threshold that he has still been half-anticipating.

The basic theme of this section is that, in addition to providing a rational society for him to grow up to, adults can best help the adolescent into adulthood by treating him, at least in public, as much as possible like an adult without, however, throwing him so completely on his own that he is overwhelmed by anxiety. In elaborating this theme, we have to remain on a level of some generality to allow for all the diversity that exists among families and individuals. In the things we say to parents, the underlying principles of parent-child relations are the same ones that we have outlined all through these pages, with the changes of emphasis made necessary by the special character of adolescence.

PARENTS

Parents find it hard to be consistent in their treatment of adolescent offspring. One day they may acknowledge the youngster's maturity, responsibility, and independence, and the next day express impassioned doubts that he or she will ever make the grade. And acknowledgments of maturity are often coupled with a reproach, a command, or a stricture which automatically negates the young person's maturity: "*Since* you are grown up, I expect that . . ." or "I'm surprised that . . ." Adolescents, whatever their individual differences, unanimously bristle when parents offer adulthood with one hand and take it away with the other. Parents, obviously, want to teach their children lessons, at the levels of fact, principle, and ethics. What they may not realize is that, by late adolescence, the time for such teaching is past, that from now on the young person is going to learn his explicit lessons elsewhere, from books, contemporaries, teachers and other perceptors, employers and bosses, and in meditation. However, there remain many implicit lessons that the adolescent can derive from his ventures into independent action, sometimes directly from the consequences of action and sometimes indirectly, from the way his parents react to the consequences. But even when parents are reacting with dismay or anguish or anger, they can still convey a basic respect for the adolescent, for his sometimes fragile dignity, and for his need to preserve his self-esteem. Parents can thus play an important role in encouraging and restricting independence and in mediating between the youngster and the results of what he does. Sometimes parental respect will be tinged with amusement, but it is probably not a good idea to let it show. On the other hand, it often helps if the adolescent can laugh at himself.

The key lesson for parents to learn is how and when to let go and not to let go. But adolescence is too late to begin to learn this lesson. From toddlerhood on, children and parents have to practice letting go of each other; like other kinds of weaning, this one is better done gradually. Prior to late adolescence, however, the child has needed the assurance that he was not letting go for good. Adolescence, by contrast, is an exercise in really letting go and a preparation for a new kind of relationship between parent and child based on reciprocal respect between older and younger adults. Parents generally feel, and sometimes announce, that they would gladly sacrifice themselves for their child. Come late adolescence, they have to make good; but it may come as a shock to discover that the sacrifice consists not in giving themselves up but in giving up their child. Furthermore, considering the adolescent's own ambivalence, they must likewise help him give them up. This two-sided giving up may be especially difficult when the adolescent is a girl. We take it as normal that a young man, even though single, may find a job and go out on his own. The girl, by contrast, may find that marriage is the expected escape route from the nest. Until marriage, even though she may be working and perhaps having affairs, there are internal and external pressures to remain at home in a grown-up little girl sort of status.

One of the advantages of partial independence is that it permits the young person to make mistakes. Obviously, parents have to stand firm against clearly disastrous courses of action, but the young person is going to try things that his parents do not know about in advance, and there will be various ambiguously risky enterprises where his parents will simply have to hope for the best. Even if the young person lands in jail or the hospital, finds himself stranded penniless on some remote shore, or finds himself in danger of becoming a father, or if she discovers that she is pregnant, or when he or she finds it impossible to cope with debts, parents have to help salvage the situation and try, in genuine cooperation with the young person, to analyze what went wrong. Obviously, if one reads the newspapers, a certain proportion of young people are doomed. However, we must beware of self-righteous moralizing, of "I told you so," and of giving up too readily.

Even in less consequential matters, such as letting the adolescent choose his own costume or observing a family curfew, too many parents are likely to rescind a privilege the first time the adolescent abuses it, intentionally or mistakenly. We have to expect occasional regressions and blunders as part of the developmental process, and the adolescent cannot be penalized every time he goes astray. In adult life, major mistakes carry their own major penalties, but in adolescence the young person's feelings of guilt, shame, embarrassment, and inadequacy may be sufficient corrective penalty, without his necessarily having to take lifelong consequences for foolish acts. As things now stand, of course, the fewer the family's financial resources and the less its influence in the community, the more likely it is that the young person can get himself into a permanent bind with a single rash deed. The poor family is less likely than the well-to-do one to know what community resources are available to help in times of crisis. Fortunately, though, most adolescents do not get into major trouble, even though parents may feel constantly threatened by the possibility. If they can have faith in their child's basic soundness, they can be truly on the side of growth and freedom and can ride out whatever crises arise.

The most reasonable of adolescents will sometimes lash out and rail and rage. Parents have to be able to discern the issue and to know whether it is a real issue, on which they have to stand firm, or a sham issue that simply needs clarifying or that represents a psychological rather than a practical need. Sometimes the adolescent demands freedom of self-determination because he really feels ready for it, and sometimes as a way of finding out whether indeed he is ready. Parents have to exercise judgment, knowing that in some cases to give the adolescent what he insistently claims he wants (drowning out his own doubts and misgivings) may drive him to renounce it forever. Furthermore, no matter how perverse it seems, the adolescent may feel that his parents have betrayed their responsibility to him when they yield to his demands.

In times of anger, the adolescent may denounce or belittle his parents, but such denunciations need not be taken literally. In the heat of the moment, the adolescent means them with all his heart, and wants them to hurt. But they spring less from a sweeping rejection of his parents than from a need to assert himself as autonomously individual. In some ways they resemble the toddler's negativism and the preschool child's "I hate you!" Neither the preschool child nor the adolescent expects his parents to take such outbursts as a final statement of how he

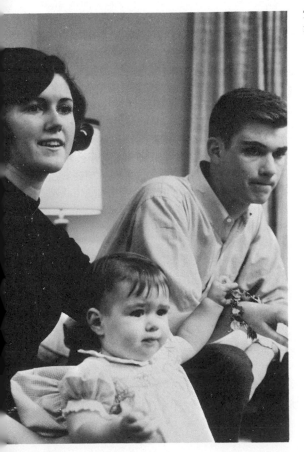

Teen-age marriage.
Leviton-Atlanta

feels. Also, in the language of adolescent ambivalence, "I hate you" may mean "I'm afraid I love you too much." Such attacks do not call for retaliation, nor need they trigger lectures on the ingratitude and insolence of today's children. If an adolescent wants to be independent of his parents, it is because they have taught him autonomy as a value, no matter how hard they find it to let go. The conscious gratitude comes later, when the young person has achieved a certain amount of stability and perspective and can appreciate that his parents did a better job of preparing him for life than he realized at the time. Or it may not come until the adolescent, now grown up, has children of his own and can share a parental view of things.

Some writers have suggested that conflicts between the generations are not only inescapable but essential to the process of growing up. Without necessarily espousing this view, we feel that a complete lack of conflict may indicate that the adolescent is in a bad way. He (or she) may have evolved fancy techniques for lulling parental concern, and outside the home does exactly what suits him. If such a youngster gets into trouble, the results are likely to be especially devastating. On the other hand, there are adolescents who have been beaten, cowed, or brainwashed into abject submission to the dictates of their parents and who seem wholly unable to think for themselves. On a scale of authority which runs from complete lack of adult control through ineffective or erratic control to absolute control, we can locate a point where the final decisions are up to the adult but the youngster has wide latitude to try things out and make mistakes.

Adults must be willing to mean it when they invite the adolescent to make his own decisions and not feel betrayed or snatch back the freedom if the decision is not the one they would have made. This is particularly important in the domain of ideas and ideologies. If the young person is to be someone who can think and act for himself, who defines his own code of values, then he needs an opportunity to try on and oppose all sorts of doctrines and convictions. Adults who try to suppress deviant patterns of thinking in young people may be troubled by misgivings about how well their own assumptions would stand up in the marketplace of ideas. It is a proper function of parenthood to challenge the youngster's more wild-eyed notions—although the odds are very much against his ever trying to put them into practice—but on a plane of tough-minded fact and reason, treating the youngster's discoveries and inventions as something worth discussing seriously and respectfully. An adult can find ways to demolish a child's line of argument without demolishing the child. Sometimes, of course, the child's hare-brained notions happen to be correct, whether or not he can defend them rationally, and parents have to be ready to lose a few debates.

One thing that parents might be aware of is the hidden topics in many debates. That is, the ostensible issue may be politics or economics or continuing in school, but beneath the surface may be raging unresolved issues left over from earlier years. The young person may still, for instance, be fighting the battle of basic trust, or autonomy, or feelings of guilt about his body and its functions, he may have met social rejection in the middle years, or he may secretly be worried about his parents' relations with each other. Parents, too, as we suggested earlier, may be fighting battles that have little to do with the issues at hand: their own lost youth and idealism, ambivalence about their own sexuality, feelings of inadequacy related to work or community standing. Sometimes the adolescent's behavior breaks down in response to the pattern of pressures and weak spots, and professional intervention may be called for. For the most part, however, crises have to be worked out the hard way, in the crucible of the everyday world. What happened when the child was two or five or ten cannot be undone when he is fourteen or seventeen or twenty, but must be dealt with in terms of the new person he has become. Short of the near-redoing of intensive psychotherapy—about whose efficacy we have little assurance—his problems can be solved only at their new levels and in their new forms. To recognize their buried sources, however, is to understand them better and to avoid the trap of taking immediate issues too literally.

Sexual attitudes and behavior are the key to many conflicts between the generations. In the matter of sex education, as in other areas, parents must build on earlier foundations. Factual education about sexual matters should be virtually complete before puberty. During adolescence, sex education must be addressed to the meaning of sexuality, to the meaning of the youngster's own body experiences, to answering his doubts and allaying his anxieties. In spite of all their knowledge, many children feel that they are sexually abnormal in some respect, and the only way of reassuring them about this is to let them know what people in general are like. The sexuality of boys is taken for granted, even though parents may find it disagreeable to contemplate in detail. But what is overlooked is that both boys, with their high level of overt sexuality, and girls, with their high level of latent sexuality, need instruction to make sense of these matters. They need to know about the differences between the sexes, and especially about the greater diversity of sexual responsiveness in adolescent girls than in boys. They need to learn that sexual activity does not automatically imply pleasure or satisfaction, that conquest in itself is meaningless except insofar as the girl can truly participate or the young man can truly reveal to her the delights of full expression; they need to know that masturbation is neither morally wrong nor a mark of depravity, nor yet the equivalent of full sexuality; they must realize that intermediate forms of gratification are possible and acceptable.

Both young men and young women should understand that social pressures to make the girl acquiesce in sexual intercourse contrary to her own feelings are psychologically harmful, and that a girl who lacks strong urges during adolescence is not on that account frigid. On the other hand, the girl who finds sex repugnant, rather than merely uninteresting or dangerous, may have more general problems of openness and intimacy. The Freudian enlightenment has had one unfortunate consequence in that a great many people have come to believe that sex is or should be the *summum bonum* in life, and young people need to learn that, whatever its joys, sex is only one strand in the fabric of life. Sex is not something to be exalted, almost like a new deity, any more than it is something to be locked up in the dungeons of the unconscious. The pursuit of the orgasm has become almost a way of life for some women, an elusive Holy Grail or Bluebird of Ecstasy, to the point where the woman who has never known orgasm, or who experiences it only occasionally, feels both biologically inadequate and cheated by her lovers.

We have to accept the fact of sexual urgency in some individuals, male and female, and we also have to accept with equanimity the fact that some people lack urgent drives and are largely unresponsive to sexual stimulation. The unresponsive ones should be free to try, but they should not be made to feel guilty if it does not work. Pro-sexual moralism is as foolish as antisexual moralism. But the answer to moralism is knowledge, and young people cannot bring sex into functional subordination to a total scheme of life unless they understand its diverse workings.

We must also bear in mind that a number of people, male and female, learn to exploit sex as a way of dominating and exploiting other people. Sex used in this way is incompatible with true maturity. True sexual morality is not to be instilled with threats and warnings. It is learned in day-to-day living with one's family. And a family in which the adolescent learns that the opposite sex is to be regarded as prey or as a natural enemy is not going to teach morality. Hence, as in other areas, morality arises from a sense of self-respect and respect for other people, and it is this that parents can impart to their adolescent children.

Throughout, of course, sex is confounded with love. Love is what the adolescent thinks he or she is in, or has just been in, or wants to be in, and which parents view as premature. In fact, adolescent attachments are only provisionally permanent, and the adolescent's feeling that they are eternally enduring is premature. But the adolescent's falling in and out of love is a vital preparation for mature love, for generously giving and receiving affection and for being able to live with a member of the opposite sex in a spirit of understanding and cooperation in a context of good communication. Thus, either to combat the adolescent's falling in love or to encourage it as a charming example of "puppy love" is irrelevant. And it is both irrelevant and injurious to try to relive one's own adolescence through the affairs of the heart of one's children.

Although parents may be favorably inclined to the idea of their child's falling in love, he almost always seems to them to fall in love with the wrong person. In fact, as we have suggested, the adolescent falls in love primarily with himself, projecting his romantic idealism onto almost anyone who offers the slightest encouragement, real or fancied. Needless to say, parental apprehensions about love between adolescents are based on fear of sexual involvements. However, love and sex are usually quite separate until late adolescence, and even then may converge only in a setting of anticipated marriage. For the adolescent boy, love is idealized, and he feels his sexuality as almost antagonistic to love. For the girl, her still diffuse sexuality is decidedly secondary to love. Falling in love may increase the probability of her yielding to a boy's advances, but reciprocal love is likely to reduce, at first, the intensity of the boy's advances. However, a goodly proportion of unwed mothers, or girls who are forced to marry because they are pregnant, are "nice girls" who yielded in the throes of adolescent love—the promiscuous girl ordinarily takes precautions. The bulk of unwed mothers, of course, are lower-class girls who acquiesce not out of pleasure or desire but as a response to social pressures and need for acceptance, and who know little about the facts of procreation and even less about how to prevent it; in some groups, of course, marriage is not expected or by custom follows getting pregnant.

Unless they are dealing with an overly docile child, parents will find that they can make little headway in either cultivating or suppressing a particular attachment. They can try to expose their child to what they consider suitable love objects, and they can speak frankly about what they consider unsuitable ones. The very rich can ship a son or daughter to a distant clime to "forget," but in general to try to forbid contact is worse than vain, since it will only increase the strength of the feelings, and to keep a child locked up ("grounded," in the current term), away from school or work or the hangout, is impossible for any length of time. If parents can think back to their own adolescent pasts, they can at least recognize and sympathize with the youngster's feelings, whatever they may think of the objects to which these feelings get attached. The time to talk such matters over is in the interludes between attachments. It is in such quiescent periods that one can best try to make clear the differences in the way the two sexes fall in love.

But since parental influence in actually shaping the child's character at this late date is limited, it may be appropriate to examine some of the provisions society makes or might make to help the adolescent over the threshold, beginning with schools.

SCHOOL AND SOCIETY

Nowhere are the shortcomings of our educational system more flagrantly apparent than in the secondary schools. Part of the difficulty is that the high schools have tried to be all things to all young people, to offer programs tailored to whatever kind or level of interest or ability the young person brings with him. Each program—various vocational training courses, Family Life Education, college preparatory—is compartmentalized from all the others, sometimes in a separate school. There is little concern for *personal education,* for deepening and enriching the person's understanding of himself and the world he lives in. The student in a primarily vocational program may miss out on the arts and sciences, and the student in an academic program may miss out on anything having to do with real people. While the schools tacitly acknowledge that the young person is on the verge of gainful employment, marriage and parenthood, or military service, he is still of too tender an age to be exposed to social controversy. Class work is isolated from adolescent interests and social life. Most adolescents consider schooling a form of penal servitude, and pointless except as an initiation ceremony. The teachers sense the pointlessness, too. Many of them do not really understand their own subject matters or have any good idea of why the student should learn what they have to teach. It is simply their job to make the student learn it. Even when a school tries to do a better, more meaningful job of education, it may find itself in the middle of a problem of infinite regress: Just as colleges have to repair the deficiencies of high school preparation, teaching remedial reading and mathematics, high schools have to remedy the defects of grade school education, and the grade schools have to make up for all the things the parents failed to do.

While we profess to believe in universal education, in practice we act as though liberal (and liberating) education is the privilege of only a select few. It seems to us that the educational system will not come into focus until we realize that there is a body of knowledge and skills and understanding that everybody needs—and not all of it vocational or narrowly practical. We have to acknowledge that there is a small proportion of young people who seem incapable of comprehending many of the essentials of life and who will have to settle for less than an ideal education. We also know that a certain number of young people are so caught up in neurotic or psychotic disturbances as to be temporarily or permanently inaccessible to instruction.

Having assumed that perhaps some 15 to 25 per cent of the adolescent population needs special educational arrangements, we still have to think about the remaining 75 to 85 per cent, without major organic or emotional handicaps. Experience tells us that only a few of these will perform brilliantly in the academic sphere. On the side of the young person, there is likely to be a distinct lack of academic motivation. On the side of the school, there is reluctance to leave off the pattern of academic gamesmanship and make a serious effort to communicate with the youngster, to make subject matter meaningful and interesting and personally relevant. It is, after all, in the best literature, with its power of enlisting strong identifications, that we learn the profoundest lessons about human relations and social structures. In principle, motion pictures could be used as supplements to literature, but most of the commercial films we know about would be usable mostly as horrid examples of how to falsify the human condition. But the schools should not be afraid of experimental literature, art, music, films, and multimedia concoctions. Scientists and philosophers as well as novelists and poets have been grappling for years with exactly the same cosmic problems that fascinate and frighten the adolescent, and it does not debase the wisdom of the ages to take time to find its relevance for the adolescent and his concerns. Such relevance is most likely to emerge when the adolescent is allowed to do his share of the talking, both to the teacher and back and forth with his fellows. It would probably be more fruitful to spend a semester in careful analysis of one significant novel that deals with real and burning problems than in slipshod reading of any number of dull "classics." If the point of instruction is to show that literature contains vital insights, to teach the student how to squeeze all the meaning out of a text, and to inspire him to read on his own, most high schools (and many colleges) fail. Indeed, the youngster is more likely to read a crib book, which tells him how to answer examination questions on a given work, than he is to read the work itself. The flowering of such cribs as the way to pass literature courses is one more example of academic gamesmanship at work.

But if one can get the full benefit of a work of literature only by reading the work itself, this is not true in science and philosophy. Some people may take pleasure in reading Isaac Newton or Immanuel Kant, but Newton's laws of motion and the idea of the categorical imperative are independent of their literary expression, just as one need know little about Bach to enjoy his music. If the student's long-dead interest, curiosity, and enthusiasm are to be reawakened, the classroom will have to become more like the bull session, but with a knowing, sympathetic adult to guide the discussion and supply needed information or a likely source. The school has a lot of suspicion, disdain, and even hostility to overcome, but it may be able to make a beginning if it can see its central task as communicating enlightenment to bored, defiant, alienated, muddled, groping young people, not with a view to breaking them to the harness, but with a view to giving them the means to understand themselves and use their energies constructively.

School, of course, is not the only service society provides for the adolescent, but the other resources are far too few. The adolescent often needs sources outside school and family that he can turn to for information and advice, for personal and vocational counseling. Counseling is now for the most part the responsibility of the already overburdened school, and it might be better to center it elsewhere, as in a special agency or in recreation centers. If counseling functions are left in the school, they should be understood as distinct from the educational process itself, with a separate organizational structure and budget. The young adolescent may need someone he can turn to who can tell him what is happening to him in terms of physical, emotional, and social growth, what course it will follow, what is expected of him, and what he can do about it—many parents simply do not know enough about these matters to be of help to the young person. The adolescent may want advice on family problems, and parents themselves may need someone they can consult. The older adolescent often needs vocational guidance, not merely in terms of what he is fit for but also in terms of the variety and scope of existing occupations—including areas the adolescent may never have heard of—what their future prospects are, what new specialties are likely to emerge, and what preparation is needed. He needs help in planning both imaginatively and realistically.

Girls need help in breaking out of the clerk-stenographer-teacher-nurse-housewife circle of choices they often seem confined to—some fair employment practices acts forbid discrimination on the basis of sex, and women are working in just about every occupation known to the Census Bureau. Good counseling can help a girl, if she so desires, find ways to divide herself between parenthood and further education or between parenthood and a career, timing things so that she can be with her children at the points where they need her most. For instance, a fairly common pattern is for a woman to take a medical degree, then have children, and, when the children have reached a stage of self-sufficiency, return to take her internship or residency. Another solution to being both a doctor and a mother has been found in shared practice, which permits the physician to work part time and guarantees certain hours of the day for her family. Obviously, too, if working is going to be the standard pattern for women, employers will have to find ways to be flexible, particularly with part-time and with maternity leave arrangements, and in letting a female employee do her work at home.

The community, whether through school activities, after-school activities, recreation centers, grange halls, or whatever, needs to help fill the vacuum that the adolescent years so often are. And it must, moreover, help fill it in ways meaningful to adolescents. Plenty of community centers stand empty, while the kids hang around in the streets, simply because the activities they offer have no appeal for their intended clientele. Since the adolescent is not yet a full-time worker, since he probably is not involved in raising a family, since he periodically wants to escape from home, and since he needs to find friends of both sexes, there have to be places for him to go and things for him to do. Not all youngsters need communal support, but a number see no alternative to boredom or vandalism and delinquency. Although adolescence came into being more or less by accident, it cannot be abolished, and we need conscious social planning to help young people make the most of it. So far, society has done little except to cry death to the dope-pushers, deplore the sad state of the younger generation, and threaten to punish parents or to ship the young men off to war. (Commercial exploitation of the teen-age market has not helped adolescents either.) The neighborhood center needs more than athletic facilities, games, a juke box, and soft drinks. It may also need a library, places to study, a study counselor, and perhaps a continuing forum under believable and uncondescending adult leadership on such topics as sex, marriage, religion, war, economics, careers, and values.

But community provisions for young people can make sense only if we revise our conceptions of adolescence. In general, we have been too much inclined to take problems—drugs, sex, delinquency, education, alienation—one by one, without seeing their psychological interconnectedness. We have to make concessions to the adolescent's physical maturity, particularly the sexual maturity of the male; we have to be willing to let adolescents try things out and make some mistakes, and it must be faced that some proportion of these mistakes will be lethal; and we must always be on the side of knowledge and understanding, even when the truth is wildly and sickeningly at odds with standard beliefs.

We have to recognize that adolescence is a distinct developmental period in our culture, neither childhood nor adulthood, with needs and capabilities of its own. The phenomenon of teen-agerism as a style of life represents young people's attempts to find a special adolescent identity, but one that is alienated from adult doings. The task, it seems to us, is to find meaningful and useful roles for the adolescent within society. But this means that adult society must be prepared to change so as to accommodate the needs and competences of the adolescent. Being a student, of course, is one adolescent role, but even if schooling were really addressed to enlightenment, it would still occupy only a portion of the adolescent's hours and energies, nor is school plus recreation enough. A real apprenticeship in preparation for adulthood includes an introduction to constructive work whereby the adolescent can gain experience, learn skills, have a sense of real accomplishment, and earn money of his own. The commercial job market will always absorb a certain number of adolescents, but probably not enough, especially of young people with interrupted or incomplete educations. The government can invent, finance, and organize youth programs and projects, but this does not strike us as the best way.

The key to a meaningful role for adolescents within society, it seems to us, lies in a return by adults to a sense of community, a feeling of belonging to, participation in, and responsibility for the larger social unit—the block, the neighborhood, the school district, and so on up to the nation and the world. A sense of community implies a cooperative attack on problems lying outside the purely commercial and economic sphere, and it is in attacking such problems that the ideas and energies of youngsters can be utilized to their and the community's advantage.

Indeed, we have prototypes right now for the kinds of roles adolescents can play in a community-minded society: working as hospital aides, teacher's aides, caretakers for the handicapped or infirm, recreation leaders, and tutors; working together in political action movements, in projects to improve schools or medical care, to convert vacant lots into parks, to clean up the streets and to plant trees and flowers, to make empty stores into nursery schools and recreation centers, and to secure basic human rights. The civil rights movement, at least in its early, idealistic phase, beautifully exemplified a spirit of community, with youth often taking the lead.

It would be nice to have public money available for community enterprises, but we believe that such enterprises work best when they originate within the community, either spontaneously or on the model of what is happening in other communities. Notice how young people and adults can work together in community action, with reciprocal consultation, counsel, and respect, and with a meaningful division of labor and responsibilities. But all this requires that the adults stop living and thinking in isolated units without any sense of common purpose. It seems to us that community participation is the most promising escape from the boredom and futility that often afflict young people, and the most promising alternative to the escapes of teen-agerism, kick-seeking, and violence.

A Definition of Maturity

Development does not stop when one reaches adulthood. One can even recognize such developmental periods as young maturity, middle age, old age, and senescence. While such periods are fairly well defined physically, in terms of stamina and vigor, sexual potency (which declines in the male even as desire increases in the female), sensory acuity, speed of reactions, loss of head hair in the male, the graying of hair in both sexes, a tendency for the waistline to bulge and the shoulders to hunch, creases and puckers in the skin, their psychological meaning is by no means as clearcut. There is, obviously, a progressive change of roles, whether one is moving up the ladder of success or is on the skids. One becomes, in turn, spouse, parent, grandparent, and oldster. Even if one's life appears to be at a standstill, the changes that are happening in other people mean that one's position relative to them changes, too. Friendship patterns change, recreational tastes change, and the life space is repeatedly transformed.

Many young people, and not a few adults, see adulthood as a slipping away of all that is dear, a series of renunciations, an exercise in loss and doing without, in resignation. In fact, our culture almost guarantees such a pattern. Young parenthood is often a time of mature delight, but for many it is only adult doll play and for still others it is a time of considerable resentment caused by the constant and inescapable burdens of child care. For some young people it may mean giving up youthful freedom for dreary responsibilities. Many young males become preoccupied with the pursuit of success or embittered by its elusiveness or unattainability, in either case to the neglect of the joys of fatherhood, husbandhood, and domesticity, the last being regarded as the preserve of bored young females.

Both men and women have a crisis of middle age, like that of adolescence probably largely unrelated to physical changes. If a young woman marries at age twenty-two, has one child when she is twenty-three and another, final one at twenty-five, by age thirty-five her most intensive maternal functions are largely over, the routines of housekeeping are easily disposed of, her husband is busy outside the home, and massive boredom may set in. It is bored women in the thirty to forty-five age group who become alcoholics, turn promiscuous, "take courses," go into psychoanalysis, engage in Good Works, or become chronic shoppers. Age forty-five to fifty and the menopause may bring life to a climax of boredom and frantic pleasure-seeking. While many women meet the crisis of middle age quietly or constructively, some of the prosperous ones of this age travel around the world, endlessly shopping for bargains in Hong Kong or Marrakech, lavishing money and favors on gigolos and beach boys. The less affluent shop at home and visit the neighbors, seizing on newcomers and spilling their medical or psychiatric autobiographies to anyone who will listen—usually to another woman in similar circumstances, who will reply in kind. The chronic players of bridge, Mah Jongg, solitaire, and similar time-killers (including beauty-parlor going) are prominent in this age group.

The crisis of middle age comes somewhat later for men, characteristically in association with—and with the awareness of—the physical changes of ages forty to fifty (the French call it *la crise de la quarantaine*): graying and balding, gaining weight, presbyopia, and so forth. In both men and women, middle age may bring on severe depression, sometimes called *involutional melancholia* from the involution, or regression, of the womb (the changes of middle age are called the *climacteric,* including the female menopause, but just as the female menopause need not mean the end of sexual enjoyment, so the male climacteric need not mean the end of potency). Fear of loss of potency may be a factor in the middle-age crisis of a number of men, leading to an extravagant pursuit of sexuality as though either to deny the decline or to harvest as much pleasure as possible before the end. Equally often, though, the crisis centers on work: High hopes may have turned to ashes, early resignation to mediocrity may have become bitterness, the postponement of achievement may have gone on too long until it now seems too late to begin. For some men, disillusionment comes with the discovery that they can succeed in work but in nothing else—that they have failed as husbands, lovers, friends, fathers, community leaders, and founts of wisdom. Ironically, the man who has attained success may in middle age feel a need to work even harder, as though to prove to himself and others that his powers are not flagging. However, it appears to be increasingly the case that men of forty-five to fifty who have laid by some wealth are willing to retire, or go into semiretirement, and devote themselves to the pursuit of pleasure, sometimes in company with their wives and families, sometimes not.

Old people are generally regarded by themselves and their families as a useless burden, to be filed away in a retirement colony or nursing home until the liberation of death. Even well-to-do old people may prefer the secure limbo of a retirement home to an active life in the community. Those who have done research in colonies for the aged report that the inhabitants typically cut off contact with and interest in the outside world and preoccupy themselves with the minutiae of everyday life.[2] They both let go and give up with a vengeance. As Kalish[3] points out, we exercise more options than we usually recognize, suicide and homicide apart, about death: where, when, how, in whose company, and even whether, since medical care is rationed. In some societies, of course, a "no work, no eat" philosophy prevails, and those who are too old to earn their keep are simply let starve. We, by contrast, tend to keep our old people alive, but grudgingly and on tiny pittances, and the physical and psychological isolation of the aged seems to hasten their decline and demise.

It is our thesis that maturity—all of postadolescence—can and should be a time of fulfillment, of continued growth and repeated discoveries and insights, of ever-renewed enthusiasms, of fresh understanding and solid wisdom. One has a choice: He can spend maturity and old age looking wistfully back on the good old lost days or he can, more than at any other period, relish the joys of the moment, savor the zest of things, and look forward to the excitements of the future. He (or she) can keep physically fit and vigorous, or he can strive foolishly to preserve the powers of youth, or he can cave in and go to seed; he can choose to spend old age as either a fossil (or a vegetable) or a sage. We want to try to describe the kind of maturity that represents a culmination rather than a downgrade, in which curiosity and the capacity to learn continue undiminished and even grow long after the body's tissues have begun to fail. Maturity in this sense does not come to everybody, and we know of no way to guarantee that it will, but we personally know enough exemplars of true maturity to feel confident that it is possible.

Many models and goals for maturity have been offered. The authors are not happy about most of them, and have some feeling that it is hopeless even to try to define this special kind of maturity. Nevertheless, they are inclined to go ahead, in full recognition of the risks. The first risk is of committing the "psychologist's error," which is a variety of ethnocentrism: Most psychologists—even, paradoxically enough, reductionists—have a strongly human-centered, individual-centered orientation and attach great value to verbal skills, social skills, social consciousness, intellectual attainments, and scientific and artistic creativity. They are inclined to overlook other styles and areas of achievement. They may praise the mechanic's craftsmanship, the clerk's conscientious thoroughness, the businessman's acumen, the athlete's strength and agility, but their ultimate ideal generally turns out to be Socrates or Einstein. A second danger is found in the fact that many models for maturity seem to be largely reflections of their authors' own idealized personalities, saying in effect, "See how wonderful I am" or "This is what I wish I could be." A third risk is that criteria for maturity may degenerate into a set of pious preachments which clothe in toplofty sentiments moralistic imperatives addressed to lesser men. Finally, standards for maturity are all too likely to seem to force everybody into a single, narrow mold, doing violence to the diversity that we have been talking about and extolling throughout this book.

The authors will try to avoid these pitfalls and offer a description of versions of maturity that takes into account man's frailties and imperfections and the variety of individual tastes and traits and endowments. Our procedure has been, first, to think of and to generalize about persons, historical and contemporary, who, in our view, have gone furthest toward effective functioning in all spheres of life—at work and at play, in relations with the world at large, with neighbors, co-workers, superiors, subordinates, with friends and families, and with themselves. (While some of these individuals might agree that we did well to select them, we have not consulted them and we feel sure that those still living would prefer to remain anonymous.) Second, we have borrowed selectively from those authors who have dealt with the nature of maturity, relying especially on the work of Maslow.[4] The result inevitably will reflect the authors' personal tastes and philosophies. In point of fact, however, there seems to be a good deal of agreement on this subject among various writers, whether theologians, psychologists, healers, or philosophers.

If an individual is going to grow toward the kind of maturity we are talking about, he will find it helpful to have secure developmental, preadult underpinnings—he should not have to deflect his energies into refighting childhood battles or nursing old hurts. Maturity can only be built on sound foundations. Unless the child has been able to establish basic trust, his world is quicksand. Without basic trust, he cannot establish autonomy, the trust in himself that enables him, by successive stages, to separate his identity from his parents and then from his contemporaries and stand on his own two feet as an integrated—both internally and to society—individual. The starting point of maturity is reached when, without rupturing his basic emotional ties to the environment, the individual is nevertheless free to move about within the framework they provide, when he no longer has at every moment to question his own identity, his own wishes and aspirations, when his freedom is no longer something to strive for but something to count on and to use responsibly. It is necessary to point out, however, that many people do survive and recover from developmental setbacks along the way, sometimes with therapeutic help and sometimes on their own. But they must somehow get beyond their childhood conflicts. While the task of maturity is made harder for such people, they occasionally do especially good, if delayed, jobs of growing up. Adversity, although hardly to be recommended, does sometimes seem to have a strengthening effect. We should make clear that growing out of childhood does not mean abolishing one's past. Apart from the pleasure that childhood recollections can bring, or the relief one feels in looking back at a closed chapter of turmoil, having sound foundations means that one can carry into adulthood those childhood qualities of freshness, enthusiasm, and emotional involvement that stand a person in good stead throughout life.

When a person can live with his past without being bogged down in it, he remains adaptable, *capable of continued change*. It is important to specify, however, what kinds of further change are and are not possible in adulthood. At birth, the individual, subject to constitutional limitations, is capable of following a great many developmental paths. Psychologically, at least, he could equally well become a Kaffir, an Eskimo, a Japanese, or a proper Bostonian. By the end of infancy, however, he is already irrevocably committed to a particular line (still, however, with many possible branchings) of development. If he has started off as an American, he can never go completely back and get a fresh start as a Samoan. While he might successfully live in Samoa, he could never think and feel and act exactly as a Samoan does. Similarly, as the effects and acquisitions of each stage of development are consolidated during childhood, certain doors are closed behind the individual, and new vistas open up ahead. The only way the individual can "go back" is via a pathological regression, and this does not mean a return to early plasticity. By the time he has reached adulthood, the individual's choices are strictly limited by his past experience, but they are nevertheless incredibly rich in terms of the new varieties of experience that will become available to him. It is important to note, too, that as the individual matures he has an increasingly greater say in what further lines of development he chooses to follow. His early development depended on an accident of birth and the play of circumstances, but as he moves toward personality integration he develops a species of *self-determination*. He becomes able to accept or refuse the choices offered to him, and, what is more, to invent new lines of development independent of immediate circumstances. He becomes, within certain inescapable limits, the master of his own destiny.

Another characteristic of becoming mature is the development of *wisdom*. The individual does not merely know things, but is able to apply his knowledge. He does not learn as voraciously as he did earlier, but this is due less to a decline in capacity than to greater discrimination about what is worth knowing. Also, he learns at a level of increasing generality and decreasing specificity. However, he becomes more aware of gaps in his knowledge, and is better able to define his own ignorance and learn what he needs to. His accumulated experience gives him new insight, sensitivity, understanding, and tolerance. Out of his experience, he builds up a broad perspective which permits him to see his own and other people's problems in a larger context. His emotions become more stable, and, while remaining strong, are tempered, controlled, and integrated. His enthusiasms are more focused and less volatile, so that he can plan and act in long-range terms. As he loses in primitive plasticity, he gains in mature flexibility. He has habits in the sense of automatic responses to the mechanical demands of life, but he is not bound by habitual ways of thinking. He is always willing to take a fresh look, to consider new evidence, and to have his assumptions challenged. He can change with the times, and shed values and principles made obsolete by the march of history. If he remains enthusiastic, it is certainly not always about the same things. He outgrows his old tastes and interests, he may even outgrow friendships and careers. He can make such changes and still hold fast to such fundamental values as esteem for human feelings and integrity.

We should not give the impression that wisdom always means assuming the role of philosopher—or at least not of the contemplative philosopher. The mature individual can be ribald or genteel, sweet or acid, jolly or glum. The important point is that he be alive, with vigorous interests that make him interesting to be with. But no matter what his tempo or temperament, it will probably find some of its expression in *humor*. This is not the same as being good-natured. The individual on his way to maturity can be a curmudgeon or a pessimist, and his humor can be bitter, sardonic, or ironic as well as frolicsome, earthy, or subtle. In any event, one of the stigmata of the maturity-bound person is that he both enjoys wit and is able to give his own original twists to his observations of the human comedy.

An important characteristic of the individual who becomes mature is that he is *at home with reality*. This does not mean that all mature people see reality in the same way. They will share a common body of facts governed by more or less fixed principles, but they will differ as to which facts are most important, what meaning to attach to them, and what opinions to hold about them. Being in touch with reality has two sides, being at home with oneself, and being at home with conditions in the outside world. The individual has to accept the stubborn reality of things as they are, without retreating from them or being overwhelmed by them. Obviously, he doesn't like everything that he sees, and he certainly need not leave well enough alone. Because he cares about the state of the world and its inhabitants, and because he wants to have some say in what happens to him and his fellows, he wants to act on reality. But he acts within the limits imposed by practical principles, and does not try to transform reality by magic or wishful thinking, and he acts within the framework of respect for other people's integrity and of awareness of his own fallibility, so that he is unlikely to use force except in self-defense— and not in anticipatory self-defense against some imagined future aggression. Knowing the limits on his own powers and the inertia that dwells in reality, he is not impatient for all change to take place right now, even though certain crucial situations may call for emergency measures. And he does not get so involved in trying to influence his surroundings that he

517

has no time for the simple but fundamental pleasures of life—love, conversation, food and drink, sunshine, exercise, catching up on chores, or pursuing hobbies and crotchets. And even while he is strongly committed to a set of values, he can remain sufficiently detached to maintain perspective, to see alternative points of view, to keep from suffering a personal destruction every time his values encounter a setback, and to be able to laugh at himself when necessary. The more in touch he is with reality, the more he becomes aware that it is full of rampant ambiguities, questions to which there seem to be no fixed and easy answers, and he has to learn to tolerate such ambiguities without taking refuge in dogmatism.

But, as we know, the individual cannot look outer reality in the face unless he is prepared to look himself in the face, too. He is *at home with himself.* He knows his own weaknesses and limitations, and, while he would like to change them for the better, he can tolerate them as well as he does the shortcomings of outer reality—and, as we have suggested, he can laugh at his own foibles. Perhaps even more important is his ability to acknowledge and accept his inner needs, cravings, and impulses. The individual must bring his feelings to consciousness and give them explicit shape before he can master and control them. The alternative is repression. The distinction between modulated control and rigid repression corresponds to the distinction between relaxed spontaneity and unpredictable impulsiveness. The person who has made his feelings truly his own does not have to be on constant guard against them—he knows where they are and what they are doing—and can act freely without being afraid that some hidden force will take possession of him. The person who tries to avoid or deny his own feelings must, by contrast, perpetually keep watch lest they spring out unexpectedly. This vigilance not only restricts his freedom to act but, what is more, is often in vain. While he is patrolling his defenses in one area, the caged enemy is liable to erupt as an uncontrolled impulse some place else. The integrated person can without dismay entertain notions which, if translated into action, would land him in prison or a mental hospital. Such eventualities might serve to restrain him from acting on his fantasies, but the really important deterrent lies in his knowledge that to carry out his more primitive impulses would probably bring harm to somebody else. Because he is human, it costs him something to keep his thoughts to himself, but far less than the person who has to fight with unknown forces. Being used to his own feelings, the individual is better able to recognize and formulate creative insights when they occur. Most important, a knowledge of his own feelings gives him insight into the feelings of others, and is in addition the surest guarantee we know of against projecting his own feelings onto the environment. It should be made clear that the person headed for maturity is not immune to guilt and anxiety. But he can keep them within bounds, accept them as part of his human nature, and even utilize their motive power instead of harboring them as free-floating energies.

It follows that the mature individual has to be able to live comfortably with his own body, whether it be strong or weak, handsome or ugly, healthy or failing. This does not mean that he fails to groom it or to tend to its ills, but that he can be at ease about it, not wasting his time in futile laments or hypochondria. He can use it as his means of contact with the world, as the vehicle of his feeling and sensation. And just as the individual can never wholly separate himself from his concrete standpoint in time and space and society, so he is always to some extent the captive of his own body. This means that he experiences it both from the inside and the outside, that it is both his and an organism with an existence of its own, that his self-knowledge can never be absolute but contains the same ambiguities as his experience of outer reality. The individual who would become mature has to learn to tolerate ambiguity in himself as well as in the outside world, not in a spirit of futility but in one of forging ahead regardless.

If the individual's growth toward maturity is rooted in the positive emotional bonds of early infancy, *human relationships* are going to have a high priority for him. In his own life, he may be concerned either with the people closest to him or with people en masse, or even with the fate of unborn generations, but he cannot help having a sense of affiliation with humanity at large. He feels this way in full recognition of human stupidity, perversity, weakness, and evil. Indeed, knowing his own nature as he does, he is likely to know that human beings are a mixed lot but, all in all, worth bothering about. Needless to say, he will not esteem all people equally, and recognizes gradations of affiliation, from profound involvement with those closest to him through less acute fellow-feeling for those at a distance to real hostility for those who threaten humane principles. But whether his existence is centered in family life or not, he needs and seeks close human attachments. He will be able to give and receive affection freely, without embarrassment or fear for his own integrity. He learns to adapt to various kinds of human relationships and roles: of lover to lover, of spouse to spouse, of parent to child, of man to woman or woman to man, of friend to friend, of student or of teacher, of employer and employee. He will find out that close personal involvements cost something in emotional wear and tear, in responsibility for those he is involved with, in loss of freedom, but he gladly pays the price. Most important, in his relations with people he will become better able to react to the people themselves, and not to some image of them formed out of his own needs and character. Similarly, he will want to be close to them for the sake of what they are, and not merely for the sake of the way they reflect him back to himself. When he can truly perceive people and be aware of their awarenesses, he will learn a respect for their integrity—or a compassion for their lack of it—that will forever restrain him from frivolous or selfish meddling with other people's lives. He will not have to go looking for affection. Because he is at ease with himself, because he is open to experience, because he has opinions and enthusiasm, people will want to be with him, to share in his excitement of life. Because he respects himself and other people, other people will respect him.

The person equipped with the human sensitivities that make for maturity will usually have a powerful *concern with social problems* and ways of alleviating them. This does not, however, necessarily imply that he engages directly in working for a new order on either a collective or individual scale. There are other approaches to advancing human welfare than working in the field of social reform or education or mental health, or than performing the functions of a "good citizen," such as voting, or joining the P.T.A., if his temperament inclines him away from these particular activities. One of the most effective forms of good citizenship is to be a sound person, part of a sound family, a good neighbor, and an influence for human charity on the level of personal dealings. An honest businessman—or an effective craftsman—can often accomplish as much, simply by being what he is, as a host of petition-circulators. Or he may function both ways.

For all his social-mindedness, for all his savoring of human relationships, the maturing individual is not dependent on always having company. Typically, he not only is able to tolerate but requires a certain amount of *solitude* in which to think his own thoughts and enjoy his own company. Furthermore, he likes to devote a certain amount of time to unsocial activities: reading, listening to music, gardening—whatever his tastes dictate. This capacity for entertaining himself, for drawing on his own resources, in fact contributes to his social life. It means that he has something to offer people. His wit, his freedom from pretense, even his occasional idiosyncratic crankiness, all the qualities that make him good company are the reflections of the qualities that enable him to be self-sufficient.

The kind of person we are talking about, with his sensitivity to other people's feelings and his respect for other people's integrity, is almost inevitably committed to a *democratic code of ethics*. But he is democratic in a deeply personal sense, and not merely ideologically. He has a sense of humility balanced by self-esteem, and he knows that there are satisfactions to be gained and things to be learned from almost everybody. One of the things that make him interesting to other people is the fact that he is himself interested in what others have to say. And these other people are not only the accepted authorities and pundits. The person headed for maturity is not going to be impressed by high estate or repelled by a low one. Neither, however, will he automatically and perversely disdain the high and espouse the low. Just as the small child judges people less by their station in life than by their emotional warmth, so our subject judges people by their vitality, their strength, their flexibility, their emotional richness, and their honesty—in short, by the virtues he himself strives for—rather than by their objective attainments and social position. Indeed, his own social position may be rather humble—enough admirable people have lived in slums and slave cabins to demonstrate that maturity is not a prerogative of the privileged few.

It is apparent that the person who is becoming mature *does not accept values ready-made*. He is likely to be quite unconventional in his opinions, or to hold them for unconventional reasons or in unconventional combinations. He is looking for a rational, consistent, humane, and realistic system of values, and is not likely to be happy with codes that represent the accretion of habits, traditions, superstitions, or prejudices, of outworn assumptions about human nature and the structure of reality. To look for a set of values of his own means, in effect, to try to extricate himself from his own culture. This can be done only to a limited extent, of course. If the mature American finds fault with American values, beliefs, and practices, he does it in an American sort of way. He may become an internationalist, but he can never wholly become psychologically an Englishman or a Swiss. Even people who live abroad and come to feel completely at home in their new surroundings present to the natives no problem in recognition as outlanders. Nevertheless, the mature individual may be able to bring a fresh view to standards and assumptions that other people take for granted, and in any case he will be willing to challenge the obvious. And a liberation of this sort is an important part of mature flexibility, creativeness, and humor that make life worth living.

On the other hand, his original ideas about values are likely to bring the individual into conflict with his society. Most mature individuals want to live within society, even when its goals conflict with theirs. They do not feel it necessary to advertise their emancipated views by going barefoot in the city streets or by refusing to pay their taxes. The individual has to learn when to conform and when not to conform, when to speak out and when to remain silent. His values must be so structured and scaled that he can distinguish between what is central and inviolable and what is peripheral and expendable—or at least postponable. He has to balance his beliefs against his natural wish to lead a quiet, comfortable life, doing his work and enjoying his family and friends. Mostly, of course, among one's friends one can freely express opinions which, stated in print, might look dangerous and subversive. This is because friends see the individual's opinions in the context of their own awareness of his sincerity, decency, humor, balance, and humaneness. Nevertheless, there is always the possibility that the person who tries to think for himself will run seriously afoul of public opinion and be forced to choose between recanting or suffering the consequences of his folly. Since the individualistic individual finds life pleasant, he will not enter upon martyrdom lightly. Nevertheless, he will by definition be committed to certain principles—religious, political, intellectual, ethical, or whatever—that take precedence over his own existence. Obviously, if he can live and struggle for his principles, he would rather do so, but if there is no choice but to abandon them or perish, he may well be willing to die for them. Mature people, in their everyday affairs, are probably brave and timid in about the same proportion as everybody else, but they generally have in common a streak of stubborn moral courage that appears when the chips are down.

To live realistically (which by no means forbids the conscious exploitation and enjoyment of fantasy) means to live in *consciousness of one's own mortality*. If this becomes a morbid preoccupation, it is no better than pretending that one will live forever. But held in perspective, the ability to face the certain expectation of death, of a final limit to one's period of achievement, lends a valuable urgency and importance to what one does, and helps keep one's values in focus and proportion. The older one gets, the greater the likelihood that people to whom one feels close will die. Bereavement brings with it special trials, and the mature person must learn to endure bereavement without repressing or otherwise blurring its impact. In general, the mature person has a healthy respect for danger, without being panicked into fleeing from commitments and involvements.

Obviously, we have not been painting a design for happiness, or at least happiness in the sense of surcease from turmoil and travail. There are built-in pains and penalties in becoming mature, a few of which we have already mentioned. The individual knows that certain things lie beyond his power of decision or influence, and that he simply has to tolerate them. But as an active person, he would prefer to make decisions wherever he can, instead of merely letting things happen. Because he wants to weigh the evidence and the outcomes, he may find some decisions hard to make—which can be trying for other people as well as for himself. Nevertheless, he knows that he has to go on choosing between alternatives, that each alternative costs him something, and there are things he will never be able to do and experience. He also knows that there are things he will never be able to do again, that he can never recapture his youth or relive his first encounters with certain experiences. He knows that his integrity is continually threatened by practical demands, by seductive temptations, by concessions and compromises, by conflicting values, and can only be preserved at the cost of some psychic strain. If his ideas are too much out of joint with the temper of the times, he may feel lonely and cut off from companionship.

In spite of these drawbacks, he knows that the only real rewards of life come with continued growth, and that there is no room in the one material life he has for major regrets. As Solon pointed out, one can only judge whether a man is happy when he dies. Too many people come to the end of the line with a sense of "Wait! Not yet! I was just going to begin!" The individual who has approached maturity can know that he has loved and been loved, has done his work, has made his mark on people, and, although he wishes there were more time, that he has made the most of what there was.

In sum, the adult with a capacity for true maturity is one who has grown out of childhood without losing childhood's best traits. He has retained the basic emotional strengths of infancy, the stubborn autonomy of toddlerhood, the capacity for wonder and pleasure and playfulness of the preschool years, the capacity for affiliation and the intellectual curiosity of the school years, and the idealism and passion of adolescence. He has incorporated these into a new pattern of simplicity dominated by adult stability, wisdom, knowledge, sensitivity to other people, responsibility, strength, and purposiveness.

REFERENCES / Chapter 12

[1] Platt, J. R. The step to man. *Science*, 1965, 149, 607–613. We should like to commend this brief document as one of the most moving and revolutionary statements of our time.

[2] Bennett, R., and Nahemov, L. Institutional totality and criteria of social adjustment in residences for the aged. *Journal of Social Issues*, 1965, 21, 44–78.

[3] Kalish, R. A. The aged and the dying process: The inevitable decisions. *Journal of Social Issues*, 1965, 21, 87–96.

[4] Maslow, A. H. Self-actualizing people: A study of psychological health. *Personality Symposia*, 1950, 1, 11–34. The concept of "self-actualization" or "self-realization" is also discussed in Goldstein, K., *The Organism*. New York: American Book Company, 1939.

13 Disturbances in Development

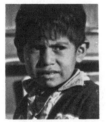

This book is about normal psychological development, the way people with reasonably sound constitutions grow up in reasonably favorable environments, including the normal "problems" that large numbers of parents and children have to face. Sometimes, however, the developmental process goes seriously awry, and this book would be incomplete if we failed to mention some of the major aberrations that occur in childhood, along with what we know about their causes and remedies. The study of abnormal development is important for practical purposes, in hopes of relieving human misery, and also for theoretical reasons, again in hopes that our theories will lead us to increased understanding of normal as well as disturbed development. It is in abnormal development that one can often see most vividly the subtle interplay of constitutional and social-environmental forces, sometimes to the point of total indistinguishability.

A Conception of Abnormality

In discussing deviant patterns of development, we shall follow the same chronological formula adhered to throughout this book. It is our general view that most psychological abnormality can be understood as a failure of identification. As we have seen, normal development involves a series of identifications: with parents, with peers, with adults outside the family, with society in general, with institutions, with principles and values, with styles, and with humankind at large. Identifications at each age set the stage for those to follow. Notice that some identifications may seem undesirable: A pattern of paternal brutality toward sons may be handed down through the generations, just as may primitive ways of thinking. But if the alternative is no identification, then even quasi-pathological ones become desirable. Defective identification may be rooted in organic impairments which interfere with the full apprehension and orderly schematization of reality, including identification figures and their behavior, in the lack of appropriate models and stimulus conditions, and, often enough, in the back-and-forth interaction of such conditions. For instance, parents may react to a child's being a cripple in a way that breeds intellectual retardation or neurotic self-loathing, even where neither is a necessary outcome of the child's condition.

Speaking broadly, we can say that defective identification is expressed in either defective functioning, such as general retardation or more specific blocks to learning, or emotional disturbance—even though intellectual functioning may be normal or superior—severe enough to interfere with normal living. Let us make explicit that we are skeptical of the "trauma theory" of psychological disorder. In our view, sustained privations and deprivations seem to be the key, with traumatic episodes becoming seriously traumatic when there are no compensating influences in the child's life. But in many cases we are at a loss to understand the causal history, the *etiology*. Even where we can demonstrate organic brain damage, animal studies suggest that it can be effect as well as cause (see page 112).

Most troubled or inadequate children show aberrant functioning most prominently in some one particular area, although closer examination usually reveals that other areas are involved as well. Thus, neither diagnosis nor treatment can properly be focused on a single symptom, although parents' (and other adults') worries are often phrased in terms of a single problem—bed-wetting, thumb-sucking, stealing, tantrums—and "what to do about" it. As we have seen, at every stage of development there are ways of behaving which may seem odd or ominous to adults but which are perfectly normal at that age. Indeed, any adult who acted in the way a child does would be a prime candidate for the mental hospital or the lock-up. But in this chapter we shall not elaborate further on such behavior, confining ourselves rather to those manifestations of genuine disturbance which parents or teachers may become aware of and which they have good reason to be troubled about.

We cannot hope, within the compass of a short chapter, to cover the whole field of behavior pathology in childhood, and those who wish to explore further are referred to more inclusive sources such as Kessler's recent excellent treatise.[1] We shall point out only a few of the more common or most intensively studied conditions that arise during childhood and adolescence. We shall deal only summarily with treatment procedures, partly for lack of space, partly for lack of expert qualifications, and partly because there are still so many unknowns.

The Neonatal Period and Infancy

A number of abnormal physical conditions are apparent or detectable at birth. The reader is reminded of the *Apgar Index* (page 46) as a useful means of detecting congenital disorders. Certain of these congenital conditions have clearly hereditary origins. For instance, *phenylketonuria*, described in Chapter 1, is the inherited absence of an important enzyme which, if the proper dietary measures are not taken, can lead to brain damage and mental deficiency through the accumulation of abnormal metabolites in the central nervous system. There are also a variety of inherited patterns of mental deficiency, some of which are signaled by characteristic physical stigmata.

Other conditions are thought to be associated with chromosomal anomalies produced by the action of viruses or radiation on the ovum while it is still unripe. One such condition is *Down's syndrome*, or *mongolism*, caused by the presence of a forty-seventh chromosome. Mongolism was originally named for one of its more conspicuous stigmata, an extra fold of skin over the eyelid similar to that seen in Asian peoples, but in fact it is an affliction of the total organism with a whole pattern of related somatic abnormalities. (It should not be necessary to say that the presence of the mongolian fold in Orientals says nothing whatever about their intellectual capacities.) Some of the other physical components of Down's syndrome, including some that do not appear until after infancy, are short stature and slight build; a skull flattened in back; late-appearing, irregularly spaced teeth; a thick, protruding, stubby, fissured tongue; general motor retardation; and various physiological abnormalities including permanent sexual immaturity. Most mongoloids show severe mental deficiency, but the spread of intelligence reaches up to the normal level, so it is not safe to infer serious mental impairment on the basis of physical symptoms alone. Classically, mongoloid children are described as placid, cheerful, and easy to manage, although irresponsible. In point of fact, however, some mongoloids are mischievous and irritable, and many of them are inveterate show-offs.

Mongolism used to mean an early death, but medical progress has worked to the advantage of mongoloids as well as of other people, and a number of mongoloids live a long life. New techniques are being tried for the education of mongoloids with some degree of success, and there is hope that chemical therapies can be found to undo Down's syndrome as a somatic condition. Other conditions associated with chromosomal anomaly are intersex (incomplete differentiation into male or female), various deformities (whose origins cannot always be known for certain), and some forms of cancer. While these conditions are genetic, they are not inherited in the usual sense, and although they are in principle heritable, they are usually associated with inability to reproduce.

Other abnormal conditions detectable at birth are the product of environmental insults to the developing embryo. We have already mentioned in Chapter 1 such prenatally influenced conditions as the *thalidomide syndrome* and the blindness or deafness or deformity that can be caused by *rubella* in the mother early in pregnancy. (An interesting sidelight is that newborn babies whose mothers have had rubella during pregnancy are themselves highly infectious and need to be quarantined from the rest of the nursery.) Some conditions, such as *cretinism*, a pattern of stunted growth and mental retardation produced by inadequate functioning of the thyroid gland, have largely obscure origins. Fortunately, cretinism can be cured by continued treatment with thyroid extract. One other potential source of early abnormality, as pointed out in Chapter 1, is *incompatibility of blood type* between mother and child, as when an Rh-negative mother bears an Rh-positive baby.

The birth process itself contains such hazards as the risk of mechanical injury or of oxygen deficiency (*anoxia*) while the neonate is making the transition to independent breathing. Injury to the motor centers of the brain before birth or at birth can produce *cerebral palsy*. Characteristically, the victim's muscles are innervated in conflicting and uncoordinated patterns, so that he has great difficulty in walking, speaking, eating, and fine manipulations. His body may be racked into twisted attitudes by muscle tensions, he may involuntarily grimace a great deal, and he is likely to make a great many superfluous movements, sometimes in fixed, repetitive patterns. Because of their grotesque behavior and appearance, which to the ignorant often connoted insanity or feeble-mindedness, many cerebral palsied children used to be hidden away from public view. Cerebral palsy often has secondary effects beyond the primary one of motor impairment: perceptual disturbances, epilepsy, mental deficiency, and so forth. However, these secondary effects are by no means inevitable. Some victims of cerebral palsy reach a high level of achievement, and many lead a normal life including a job, marriage, and parenthood. The cerebral palsied child's poor motor control may make assessment of his intellectual abilities especially difficult, but special techniques for this purpose have been devised.[2] The physical and intellectual problems of cerebral palsy are often further complicated by emotional ones. Both the child and his parents may suffer considerable embarrassment and frustration, and in assessing the child's functioning it is not always possible to sort out the contributions of motor impairment, cognitive limitations, and emotional disturbances. Cerebral palsy, like other forms of brain damage, can produce either a generalized cognitive deficit or a special impairment such as difficulty with language. Nowadays, the cerebral palsied are no longer locked away from sight or relegated to the scrap heap: Educational and training procedures have been devised that show great promise of letting cerebral palsied people lead normal lives. We have not been able to find any research reports on the techniques known as "patterning," whereby brain-injured children are put through a series of intensive exercises, but accounts in the popular press suggest that these methods may have real value for cerebral palsied and other handicapped children.

Abnormal deliveries are said to produce a "continuum of reproductive casualty" ranging from cerebral palsy and epilepsy to elusive disturbances of functioning whose precise physical origins are hard to specify. A much-criticized but nevertheless intriguing study by Yacorzynski and Tucker[3] suggests that children who suffered anoxia at birth may, collectively, have a wider spread of intellectual functioning, both below and above average, than a group of normal-birth controls. Graham and associates[4] found that anoxic babies studied at age three showed, as a group, some impairment of functioning, but that a goodly number of individuals apparently escaped any serious consequences. A number of other investigators, notably Pasamanick and Knoblock,[5] conclude that minor birth injuries to the brain are responsible for subtle effects that do not show up until later in life. These effects include poor motor coordination, hyperactivity, and impairments of symbolic functioning. Studies of children with known birth abnormalities show a higher incidence of such difficulties later in life than is found in the children of normal births. Similarly, retrospective studies of children with various academic and behavior problems show a higher-than-expected frequency of difficult or traumatic births.[6] These two lines of evidence, prospective and retrospective, converge on the concept of *minimal brain damage,* discussed on page 537. The use of high forceps to speed delivery carries a risk of brain damage. Heavy sedation of the mother during labor produces sluggishness of some days' duration in the neonate, but little is known about whether there is any permanent damage.

Premature birth has its hazards, especially the threat of anoxia and also of excessive oxygen used to combat anoxia. Pure oxygen given in large quantities to premature babies can cause *retrolental fibroplasia*, changes in the internal structure of the eye which cause blindness. Since the discovery of the relationship between overgenerous use of oxygen and RLF, doctors are inclined to use oxygen sparingly with premature babies, and the incidence of RLF has declined following a brief (1940–1955) period of increase. However, the physician sometimes has to choose between the risk of RLF and the risk of the baby's dying, and a certain incidence of RLF is probably inevitable.

Blindness from other causes and deafness may also be present at birth. It should be remembered that there are many degrees of blindness and deafness, causing various degrees of disability and calling for different sorts of remedies. There is even some evidence to suggest that the use of hearing aids in early infancy can overcome some congenital deafness or partial deafness.[7] As we have said, the psychophysical techniques used to study neonatal perception may prove to be valuable diagnostic instruments for the early detection of sensory impairments (which also include color blindness and defective taste, smell, touch, pain sense, awareness of hot and cold, balance sense, and proprioception from the muscles and joints). There are, of course, various other physical disabilities that may be apparent at birth or shortly thereafter, some with psychological consequences: crippled limbs, heart malformations, harelip, cleft palate, and so forth. Fortunately, the total incidence of such conditions is quite low. Furthermore, surgery and the use of prosthetic devices, coupled with new educational techniques, are doing much to counteract even severe physical impairments.

Severe *mental retardation*, sometimes associated with demonstrable physical deficiencies and sometimes without known cause, may become apparent only during the course of infancy. Severely retarded infants are usually characterized by poor muscle tone and physical inactivity, emotional unresponsiveness, and greatly delayed development, so that they may still be lying helpless while their counterparts are scuttling about on all fours or even toddling. Moderate and mild degrees of mental retardation are extremely difficult to detect in infancy and may be reflected not at all in the baby's physical, motor, and emotional development. We must also bear in mind the wide range of normal development among infants, and parents should not rush to the conclusion that slower than average maturation means that their baby is mentally retarded. Many normal and even superior babies develop slowly early in life but, in their own good time, catch up.

Baby tests may indeed detect severe impairment, but otherwise are worthless for predicting later intellectual status. In general, if a baby is reasonably active and alert, responds emotionally to people and situations (and fear and rage are perfectly normal responses to some stimuli, including doting visitors who move in too fast), and if his pediatrician is satisfied with his progress, he is probably normal. Unvarying apathy seems to be the most important single danger sign. It is becoming evident, though, that the effects of emotional deprivation, stimulus deprivation, and cognitive deprivation take hold in infancy, and some unknown number of physically normal babies has almost certainly been made retarded by the lack of appropriate attention, vocal and verbal stimulation, play, and playthings. It used to be taken for granted that mentally defective babies should be whisked off to the nearest institution and forgotten. Nowadays, with the realization that putting a baby in an institution can be a premature entombment, and that much can be done to help flawed babies, there is a far greater tendency to keep them at home and to give them as nearly normal an upbringing as possible.

Pediatricians and child psychiatrists have come to recognize a condition called simply *failure to thrive*, marked by deficient physical development in the absence of any organic impairment.[8] Failure to thrive may be associated with a number of different specific symptoms: Feeding problems, chronic vomiting, diarrhea, constipation, distended bowels, sleep disturbances, and chronic crying and irritability are among the most common. Failure to thrive seems to be caused by disturbed relations between the baby and his parents, who show serious inadequacies in their personal functioning, as parents and otherwise. Another possible sign of infantile psychopathology is chronic and severe body-rocking, crib-rocking, or head-banging, analogous to the stereotyped, repetitive movements to be observed in some zoo animals. Less intense rocking or banging, however, may occur in perfectly sound babies. We have already mentioned, in Chapter 3, the *battered child syndrome* as one manifestation of disturbed parent-child relations.

Toddlerhood and the Preschool Years

By the end of infancy, any severe hereditary or congenital physical defects are likely to have come to light (a few rare inherited conditions like Huntington's chorea, a degenerative disease of the central nervous system, do not appear until maturity). By early childhood, more distinctly psychological problems sometimes appear. One such problem may be that of intermediate mental inadequacy, which may show up in greatly delayed language development or in failure to make normal progress from infantile speech to more mature forms. Mental inadequacy may, of course, have a physical basis, but we are often at a loss to account for it. In the absence of gross physical signs, however, special education of the kind pioneered by Samuel Kirk[9] can do a great deal to improve the intellectual functioning of seemingly retarded children, especially when begun early. In general, as the child gets older, he has to solve increasingly complex problems, and as life gets more complicated, lesser degrees of intellectual inadequacy become evident. Some, of course, show up only when the child goes to school and is faced with the special demands of school learning.

Some toddlers and preschool children—and even an occasional infant—live in a state of *chronic, diffuse emotional strain* which hampers their functioning and development and may foreshadow more serious disturbances to come. There are a number of signs which can tell parents or teachers when a child is suffering in this way. These are not signs for which adults need go looking, but to which they can be sensitive and recognize when they do occur. They are not signs of serious psychological disturbance, but of distress to be relieved. The reader should remember that no *single* sign need be cause for alarm; it is when they appear in combination that action may possibly be called for. One of the most sensitive barometers of a child's emotional state is the quality of his voice. A child whose voice is too consistently shrill, or harsh, or muffled, or flat and toneless, may—barring specific hearing defects—be having trouble with his emotions. He may be feeling emotions too strong for him to manage, he may be bottling up his feelings without any channels of direct discharge, or—even more serious—his capacity for emotional response may have been muted or deadened. Chronic emotional distress often shows up, too, in the psychosomatic evidences of autonomic imbalance of an acute or chronic nature, as on a child's skin, in the form of rapid and seemingly unprovoked flushing, paling, and sweating—and the fair-skinned reader should know that dark-skinned people also flush and go ashen, if not pale. Similarly, emotional strain can even provoke or contribute to the appearance of eczema. Chronic distress can sometimes be seen in the qualities of body movement, whether tense jerkiness or flaccid sluggishness. It may be revealed in constant sighing or yawning or swallowing. It can show up in digestive upsets such as frequent vomiting or urination without adequate physical cause. Sleep disturbances, including frequent nightmares and strong bedtime fears, may betray a more pervasive state of strain. The child who spends *long* periods doing nothing, the one who *constantly* plays with his genitals, or the child with *persistent* tics and twitches may be having emotional difficulties. In overall behavior, chronic stress may be expressed in either agitated restlessness or in dull listlessness—notice again that flattened or missing emotion is as much an indicator as emotional pyrotechnics. We should emphasize that emotional upset in children in this age range is directly and intimately tied to body functioning, an anticipation of the hysterical and psychosomatic manifestations we shall talk about later.

The distress signaled by symptoms of these kinds can often be relieved quite simply, by giving the child more overt affection or a little more freedom, by setting limits more definitely or by scaling down the standards he has to meet, by simplifying his environment or diversifying it, or, if he is old enough and if it can be done tactfully and sympathetically, by helping him talk about his feelings and by reassuring him about them. The important point is to try to understand the particular sources of the particular child's unhappiness and to rearrange things accordingly. Sometimes nothing can be done short of removing the child from his family, and since we are woefully short of good child care facilities, this is hardly a solution. Sometimes, too, we cannot unravel the causes of a child's distress, and sometimes, even when we can, his reaction patterns have so solidified that easy solutions are no longer possible. In some cases, adults may be completely unaware of how their own behavior affects the child—a mother who screams at her children wonders why the children scream so much, or the father who whips his children or constantly ridicules and belittles them cannot understand why they show him so little affection or respect, or parents of both sexes are puzzled when their attempts to breed self-sufficiency in the child make him cling harder than ever—and a certain number of parents seem incapable of learning that it is their behavior that produces in the child the very symptoms that they worry about. Various forms of psychotherapy may be helpful with young children, although more often it is the parents who need help in understanding themselves in relation to the child. The professional can sometimes help by explaining to parents what children are like (remember that people lived with children a long time before anybody began to notice their special characteristics), how differently they operate from adults, and how different their life spaces are.

More profound psychological disturbance may appear during this period in the form of *childhood schizophrenia,* an early form of the disorder which we shall discuss more fully under adolescence. In addition to the fairly classical, adultlike schizophrenia (which we, along with Szasz,[10] prefer to think of as a characteristic style of behaving rather than a disease entity) found in occasional young children, a special variety has been recognized, described, and studied within the last three decades. Kanner[11] has labeled this disorder *early infantile autism* and considers it a condition distinct from schizophrenia. We shall discuss autism in some detail because it is an easily recognizable pattern and, although uncommon, seems to be on the increase. The apparent increase may be simply a product of improved diagnosis which distinguishes autism from mental deficiency, although the picture has become obscured by the introduction of the concept of minimal brain dysfunction (see page 537) to account for some cases of what formerly would have been called autism. Certain features of autism are simply exaggerations of normal childhood behavior, but exaggerations so gross and so rigid that they become qualitatively different from the normal.

Autism may develop gradually, from early infancy onward, or it may appear almost abruptly, often between ages two and three, following a seemingly normal course of development. Parents report of the autistic infant that he does not call forth the ordinary parental sentiments, perhaps because he himself seems unresponsive to human stimulation. He may be described as "a very good baby," content to lie isolated in his crib without yelling constantly for attention. He may not smile, or he may smile at things rather than people, he may be indifferent to cuddling or even withdraw from it, he may never hold out his arms to ask to be picked up. Some—but not all—autistic children are hyperactive and hypermotile; some are expert escape artists and defy all parental efforts to confine them to crib, room, house, and yard, and some on the loose scale fire escapes and rooftops. They seem to have little sense of personal danger and repeatedly suffer severe injuries with no loss of the drive to keep going. Indifference to pain is thought by some psychiatrists to be one of the outstanding features of autism. Some autistic children show remarkable mechanical ingenuity, learning to operate latches, knobs, locks, and light switches, and to take things apart and put them back together at a very early age.

When autism appears after age two, parents may first be made aware that something is wrong by the child's failure to talk. Even more generally, autistic children fail to show the ordinary imitative behavior found in most babies. Quite commonly, the autistic child comes into professional hands initially as a case of suspected deafness. Some autistic children eventually learn to talk, in some cases very well, but their speech is likely to show certain abnormalities. One feature prominent in the speech of many autistic children is *echolalia,* a compulsive parroting of what they hear. Instead of answering a question, the child may simply repeat it, sometimes at great length. Such children appear to have unusual difficulty in making the transition to the use of the first person singular pronoun, simply referring to himself as he hears others do. Or the child may pick up a phrase, a name, a snatch of song, or even a long verse, and repeat it endlessly, sometimes as a reply to something addressed to him.

The most central and pervasive feature of autism is the lack of human contact, physical, visual, or verbal. The child may seem emotionally intense, but his emotions do not fit the usual qualitative categories of anger, fear, amusement, and so forth. His feelings seem to be bound up in inanimate—preferably mechanical or physically manipulable —things. The autistic child is fascinated by rhythmic, repetitive patterns. Not only does he memorize and repeat songs and verses, but he can spend protracted periods switching a light on and off, flushing a toilet, watching a record-player turntable spin, lighting matches, or operating a mechanical toy. Some psychiatrists have sought to capitalize therapeutically on the autistic child's mechanical preoccupations by having children communicate with a computer that asks the child questions (via tape) and then asks further questions depending on how the child replied to the one before. There is reason to wonder, of course, whether this approach may even further reinforce the child's attachment to machines to the neglect of people. The child himself may like to spin or twirl or roll, machinelike, or he may adopt ritualized, perseverative gestures or mannerisms. Like the fictionalized Jordi,[12] many autistic children carry with them at all times a "jiggler," typically a toy tied to the end of a string so that it can be taken out and jiggled in moments of tension. Autistic children show little interest in sex and rarely masturbate. They often do very well in unambiguous school subjects like mathematics, and some can perform prodigious feats of memory, analogous to those of the *idiot savant* (who may indeed have been, in some cases, an unrecognized autistic), such as being able to say on what day of the week any date over the past hundred years fell. The autistic child is not likely to have highly elaborate delusional ideas, although he may hate, for instance, to walk past an open garbage can for fear it will swallow him up. In general, it would seem that the autistic child has identified with the nonhuman world and treats other people—without hatred or malice—as though they are only another kind of thing. At the extreme, we may get the child who seems himself to have become a machine, as in Bettelheim's case of Joey the Mechanical Boy.[13]

Autistic boys outnumber autistic girls four to one. Typically, the autistic child is a firstborn, but some autistic boys have an older sister or brother. All reports agree that he is usually the child of intelligent but rigid and undemonstrative parents who may not comprehend the special needs of babies and who may even find it distasteful to minister to so messy a creature as a young baby—or perhaps only this particular baby. Rimland[14] has proposed that autism represents genetically high intelligence that has somehow been flawed, as by a disturbance in the gene system. A full-scale analysis of Rimland's arguments would require another book, and we must be content to say that we find more plausible the hypothesis that autism develops when the environment fails to provide the usual props for emotional development, leading to severely defective identification.

As in all nature-nurture discussions, of course, no absolute answer is possible simply because we cannot hold the variables constant, and most especially when we have to deal with retrospective data. Although it might appear from the autistic child's unresponsiveness that he is emotionally inert, close observation suggests that emotional responsiveness may simply have withered from lack of feedback, leaving him with emotions that are poorly differentiated as well as largely unexpressed. Away from home, the autistic child is prone to panic, indicating that he may have a stronger attachment to his family than we realize. Fear of strange situations might also account for his good behavior in school and for the fact that he seems never to get to know his classmates. Autistic behavior often seems to resemble an attempt to find refuge, order, control, predictability, meaning, and feeling in relations with things or with human beings reduced to the thing level. Ignorant of the meaning of human emotional relations, the child can find satisfaction in the play of empty sensory patterns. His adoption of rigid and repetitive behavior patterns can be seen as a way of preserving a fragile integrity and also as a defense against boredom.

About a third of autistic children are reported to grow into reasonably normal adulthood, although Kessler[15] questions whether the once-autistic child could ever hope to form true friendships and love relationships, or to establish meaningful communication beyond routine formulas and procedures; she also points out, however, that we have had no follow-up studies that would give us this information. According to Eisenberg and Kanner,[16] the best predictor of recovery is the acquisition of language by age five, and the most important factor in making recovery possible is acceptance by an understanding teacher at school—an understanding made difficult by the child's conspicuous abnormality and the sometimes disruptive effects of his occasionally tangential behavior. The usual therapies seem to be of little avail. There is some evidence that autism or at least some of its manifestations may be amenable to "behavior therapy," based on the principles of operant conditioning, in which desired forms of behavior (or approximations thereof) are promptly reinforced and undesirable forms ignored.[17] Behavior therapy seems to work quite well for many simple conditions, particularly those marked by a single symptom. It appears that a recent case of protracted sneezing was kept going partly by reinforcing effects of the attention it attracted; the sneezing stopped when sneezes met with mild punishment (electric shock to the finger) instead of concerned attention.[18]

A topic that is much debated is the existence or nonexistence of a condition called *minimal brain damage* or *minimal brain dysfunction*.[19] The abnormal behavior of some babies and young children is thought by some authorities to be caused by central nervous system pathology too slight to be detected by the usual diagnostic means. This explanation is invoked when there are no obvious inadequacies in the way parents deal with the child. It seems to us that the test of whether this explanation is meaningful and useful is whether people can devise accurate methods of differential diagnosis and distinctive treatment methods, medical or educational or both, specially suited to children who show the symptoms. Meanwhile, there is disagreement as to whether minimal brain damage actually exists and whether it is an adequate explanation, in and of itself, for the conditions to which it is applied.

Returning to more common types of disturbances in this developmental period, we saw in Chapter 6 that the self-awareness of the preschool years often brings with it a number of *fears*—of death and bogymen, of bodily mutilation, of terrors hidden in the darkness, of being orphaned, and so forth. Sometimes these are expressed openly, sometimes they are denied; sometimes a child forms a fear of some specifically threatening object, and sometimes he projects a nameless or unacknowledged dread upon some invented menace (such a projection is called a *phobia*). If the child's phantoms are pooh-poohed, or if they fail to take explicit shape, his fears may be more diffusely expressed, in a generalized shrinking timidity, in somatic symptoms, or in nightmares. When the child is basically secure, specific fears, especially if they can be formulated and dealt with sympathetically and realistically, come and go and do not constitute a major problem. It is only when the child becomes obsessed with some particular threat, amounting to a phobia, or when he is too pervasively and inexplicably anxious about everything, when his nightmares come too often and too terrifyingly, that his fears become symptomatic of real personality disturbance.

Late infancy, toddlerhood, and the preschool years are an especially unfavorable time for *hospitalization and surgery*. This is the period when children can least tolerate prolonged separation from their parents, and when body integrity, the focus of many fears, becomes a major issue. The best opinion seems to indicate that elective surgery should be deferred, wherever it is medically possible, at least until age three and preferably to age five or later. Very young infants seem to tolerate surgery well, especially if their mothers stay with them in the hospital. Past infancy, the important factor is being able to talk to the child about what is going to happen and prepare him for what might otherwise be a seriously disorienting experience. No matter at what age the child goes to the hospital, he should be told the truth; hospitalization is doubly traumatic if the child has been led to believe he was going to the circus, or to visit friends.[20]

Obviously, conditions arise which make it imperative to operate on or hospitalize young children. When this happens, special measures are needed to prevent secondary effects. In the matter of surgery, for instance, many doctors, recognizing the importance of emotional as well as surgical considerations, have learned to establish a relationship with the child, to let him cooperate in preliminary procedures, to avoid forcible handling, and to let him know as clearly and unthreateningly as possible what to expect. They have learned to give the child sedation in his own room before he is taken to the operating room. Preferably, a parent should be with the child both when he is put to sleep and when he comes out of the anesthetic. As for hospitalization itself, especially if it is prolonged, the main secondary effect to be feared is lassitude and apathy or sustained and generalized anxiety. One countermeasure is the hospital play program, where professionals and volunteers work to give pediatric patients the individual affection and stimulation necessary to normal functioning, and for which overworked doctors and nurses may not have time. A perhaps more radical measure, adopted by a few far-seeing hospitals, is to allow mothers to stay with their sick children, or to visit them at any hour or for as long as they wish. Not only does this work to the psychological benefit of young patients, but mothers can assume many routine nursing duties—trained nurses being in short supply—and lighten the hospital's administrative load.

In the preschool years, when language is being elaborated and consolidated, *speech defects* may be noted. Certain of these may have their origins in defects of the speech apparatus, making articulation difficult. The great majority of defects of articulation are due simply to immaturity, and the child straightens out his own pronunciation as he grows. Sometimes, though, these defects linger beyond their appointed time. When the child continues using baby talk long after his contemporaries have left it behind, it may be a sign that his parents are encouaging it by talking baby talk to him, or by overmothering and overprotecting him, or by making babyhood too attractive. When the child first begins to talk, of course, parental baby talk is almost inevitable. Once the child is well launched in speaking, however, it is time for the parents to resume using English. If the child reverts to baby talk after abandoning it, it may be a sign of regression due to some transient or permanent emotional strain. In such cases, baby talk is not something to be attacked directly. Indeed, nonorganic speech defects in general are cured not by direct attack but by providing the child with good speech models.

Probably the most frequent form of speech disorder in young children is *stuttering* (speech specialists today make no distinction between stuttering and stammering). Various theories to account for and various therapies to help stuttering have been advanced. Most theories, whether psychological (in terms of stuttering as a symptom of emotional disturbance) or physiological (in terms of short circuits in the brain), have not been able to withstand the facts, or else have been so abstract as to be untestable. A promising recent approach has placed stuttering partly under experimental control.[21] It is possible that in "natural" stuttering, as well as in stuttering induced artificially in the laboratory, the critical factor is a disturbance of feedback. Studies indicate that a smooth flow of speech is dependent on the speaker's listening to and monitoring, without any particular awareness of the process, his own speech output. Normally, the lag between speaking and hearing oneself speak is infinitesimal. Stuttering can be induced experimentally in anyone simply by producing a time lag of about one quarter of a second between the time a person speaks and the time his voice comes back to him. This is accomplished by having the person speak into a tape recorder which after the predetermined interval plays his voice back to him through headphones. (One can also, using videotape recorders, produce delayed visual feedback, with similar results.)[22]

Most therapies, it appears, at best can help the severe stutterer live more comfortably with his stuttering; few cures are claimed by responsible therapists. At worst, for reasons that will become clear in a moment, therapy—particularly if begun too early—may even exacerbate stuttering and make its removal more unlikely. For, along with Johnson,[23] the authors feel that the bulk of stuttering is created by adults who, reacting to normal speech hesitations and gropings, force the child to pay attention to his speech, generating a crippling self-consciousness about it, like that of the centipede who had gotten along perfectly well until an admiring ant asked him which leg he moved first, thereby rendering him unable to move.

All young children stumble and hesitate and make errors in speaking, but this only becomes a fixed pattern when parents hear the child's fumblings as stuttering and try to correct them. As with pronunciation, the child, left to himself, corrects his speech production and, with increasing practice, becomes more fluent. Once the child hears his own speech as stuttering, he becomes bound up in trying to control it, and then begins to stutter in earnest, exploding his words and writhing with the effort to keep his speech under control. Whatever other emotional or neurological factors may lie behind stuttering, there is ample evidence that it can be created; hence, it is a poor idea to tell a preschool child that he can talk better, that he should try to speak more slowly, or that he should repeat himself and "this time say it nicely"—which does not mean that parents should never correct those errors that have no special connection with stuttering.

Again in this section, let us emphasize that toddlerhood and the preschool years, too, have their normal "problems" calling for no special treatment whatever. Tantrums, negativism, destructiveness, toilet-training problems, thumb-sucking, masturbation, "selfishness," "cruelty," and so forth, at this age are not marks of derangement.

The Middle Years of Childhood

The most prominent difficulties of the middle years revolve around schooling and the child's ability to learn. *Learning difficulties* arise from many sources. First, there is *mental retardation,* intellectual disability not so severe as to incapacitate the child, but severe enough to interfere with school work. A number of children have intellectual abilities equal to their daily childhood pursuits—and even, later on, to simple jobs and having a family—but insufficient to master all the sometimes artificial and arbitrary tasks demanded by school. The limitations of such a child's intelligence may not be evident until he goes to school and is asked to deal with abstract symbols.

Once his limitations have been detected and verified by careful individual testing and evaluation, two courses of management are possible. The child can be written off as a lost cause and left to suffer out the years he is legally required to spend in school—there is special help available for almost all severely handicapped children, but the merely dull child may not be eligible for it. When such a course is followed, as it all too often is, the child can easily develop a sense of failure and worthlessness. Even his classmates are likely to take over the school's opinion of him and treat him as an outcast—except, of course, when he has some special socially redeeming quality such as athletic ability. He can react to his sense of inadequacy passively, sharing the world's contempt, or he can deny it and rebel against it in truancy or delinquency. In any case, he is not likely to derive much benefit from his incarceration in school.

The second course is to make allowances for his limitations, to find out what things he can do well, to encourage him to pursue such talents as he may have, and, patiently and sympathetically, to give him as much formal education as possible. If this second course is followed, he can have the sense of worth that everybody is entitled to, he can accept his limitations realistically because he also knows his capabilities, and he stands a good chance of enjoying life and of making his own valuable, if modest, contribution to society.

Not all learning difficulties, however, are due to organic limitations. A large variety of factors, including malnutrition and low socioeconomic status, can interfere with learning. A number of children of apparently poor endowment, for instance, have turned out to be suffering from some degree of *hearing loss,* short of deafness, or *impaired vision,* short of blindness. With these disabilities brought to light and corrected as much as possible, children can be put into classes (if necessary, with special facilities) where they can go on to normal achievements—always provided that they have not already been damaged by the experience of failure. For another common source of learning difficulty, which sometimes appears as a secondary effect of physical handicaps, is emotional interference.

Emotional interferences with learning are generally referred to as *learning blocks.* They most often appear in a context of parental over-ambition and pressure, which turn the child away from the learning process and make of it something extrinsic to his own wishes. Some children try hard to measure up to their parents' expectations, but the very effort that goes into trying produces anxiety that interferes with learning, each failure becomes more frustrating, generating new anxiety and confusion and making the next failure all the more probable. For other children, nonachievement becomes a weapon in an unconscious revolt against parental pressures. The child goes through all the motions of studying hard, applying all the learning devices he has been urged to use, but still, somehow, nothing seems to stay with him. He is consciously blameless, but he can still manage a sort of secret satisfaction at the distress his parents feel at his failure. At the same time, he neutralizes his parents, since he is already apparently doing everything possible, so that they cannot blame him either. Sarason and collaborators[24] have devoted a great deal of attention to the role of anxiety in school performance, to the relation between anxiety and intelligence test performance, and to the special kind of "test anxiety" that afflicts some children in the course of being evaluated. There seems to be little doubt that anxiety or lack of it plays an important part in how well a child does in school, but the data so far do not permit any broad generalizations.

In addition to difficulty with school work in general, there are a number of special disabilities centered about particular kinds of skills or materials, such as reading, spelling, or arithmetic. Possibly the most important of these, because it involves the most basic and general academic skill, is *reading disability.* Theorists have had a field day explaining reading disability in terms of brain function, sinistrality, mixed cerebral dominance, emotional blocks, lack of perceptual maturation to the point of "reading readiness," in happy disregard of contrary evidence. It now seems likely that ease in learning to read hinges almost entirely on prior experience—with shape discrimination, with shape naming, with learning the alphabet, with being read to, with drawing, and with language in general—to the point where it seems safe to say that for most children learning to read happens before they reach school, and that reading instruction simply crystallizes and organizes the ways of perceiving that the child has already acquired. Reading disability, then, is probably most often the result of impoverished perceptual and linguistic experience in the years before school, which would account for its high incidence in culturally deprived groups. There is every promise that the kinds of preschool experience offered under programs like Head Start will reduce materially the frequency of reading disability. *Arithmetic* or *number disability* used to be fairly common, but there is hope that the new approaches to teaching math starting in the early grades will help to eliminate this problem.

Lapouse[25] has investigated the frequency of psychiatric symptoms in a representative sample of 482 school-age children. The incidence of single severe symptoms was surprisingly high (40 per cent of the children had seven or more fears or worries and almost 20 per cent wet the bed at least occasionally), but these were only somewhat correlated with chronic maladjustment. Younger children showed more symptoms than older ones, but there were no differences between boys and girls.

A recent study by Achenbach[26] proposes a new classification for children's psychiatric conditions based on the clustering of symptoms. Achenbach's first classification is according to whether children show internalizing, self-directed symptoms, externalizing symptoms directed against the outside world, or less clearly directed symptoms (unclassified). The boys in Achenbach's sample tend to be externalizers at all ages except, for reasons unknown, eleven, twelve, and fifteen. Girls tend to be internalizers from age six onward, except at age twelve. Boys and girls show somewhat different symptom groupings. Both male and female externalizers show aggressive and delinquent behavior, but only the boys have sexual problems. Many more male than female externalizers show hyper-reactive (emotionally explosive) behavior. Males from all three groups show schizoid thinking and behavior, but only internalizing and unclassified girls do so. Internalizing boys and girls had obsessions, compulsions, and phobias (one cluster) and somatic complaints, but internalizing girls also had trouble with obesity, depression, and anxiety. The female unclassified group included a few subjects who had trouble with bed-wetting and other immaturities, which were not observed in the male subjects. Provocative though Achenbach's scheme is, it must be viewed as provisional until tested against an even larger sample of children.

DELINQUENCY

Delinquency often has its beginnings in the school years, although its most serious manifestations usually occur in adolescence. It is simple enough to define delinquent acts—stealing, vandalism, physical aggression, and so forth—in social terms, defined by consequences, but all these acts may have quite different psychological sources in the individual. Therefore, we are forced to draw a number of distinctions among the psychological origins of delinquent acts. First, we can recognize *normal* or casual delinquent behavior. Individually, probably every six- or seven-year-old does a certain amount of experimental stealing from his mother's pocketbook. This is not serious and will usually be outgrown without any special measures. In the gang, especially the boy gang, there is usually a certain amount of prankishness which often has a superficially delinquent character. In addition, boys are expected to do a certain amount of street fighting to prove their mettle. These manifestations again are not serious, and most children develop their own inhibitions and controls without any action by the authorities.

Second, there is what we may term *subcultural* (sometimes called *socialized*) delinquency. This is the second most common kind after normal delinquency. It is characteristic of the lower-class child who grows up into a ready-made delinquent culture within his own society, or turns to it when he finds himself blocked or rejected by the middle class. This is primarily gang delinquency, although it may be the breeding ground for later individual criminality. The important thing to recognize about subcultural delinquency is that, psychologically, it is not delinquency at all. It is only delinquency in terms of middle-class mores, which do not apply. The gang member is behaving in ways sanctioned by the culture he belongs to, and need feel absolutely no guilt. Indeed, to question the mores of the gang would be far more likely to make him feel guilty than almost any "delinquent" act he might perform. Subcultural delinquency, insofar as it is a gang enterprise, is more likely to be male than female. However, girl fighting gangs do exist. In addition, girls may be accepted into boy gangs, where they play the roll of queen bee or camp follower. Most female delinquency, though, including sexual delinquency, is likely to be of the neurotic or the acting-out type described below.

Third, there is *neurotic* delinquency. This often takes the form of stealing from his parents (or sometimes a teacher) by a child who feels isolated. Such stealing is often symbolic: The child is not interested in the money as such (he may even throw it away, or lose it, or simply forget what he did with it), but is, in effect, stealing the love he feels his parents will not give him. Or he may, unconsciously, steal as a way of punishing his parents for not loving him. He may steal in ways that seem to insure his being caught, as though seeking punishment to relieve some unconscious guilt. In some cases, children use the money they steal to buy favor with their peers, status they are otherwise denied. Obviously, neurotic delinquency does not call for punishment but for treatment. To avoid confusion, however, let us point out that neurotic delinquency is not a *neurosis,* a state of internal conflict which inhibits action and is expressed in particular symptoms such as diffuse anxiety, compulsive rituals or somatic complaints. We call this delinquency neurotic because it is an *indirect* expression of an unformulated need or wish.

The fourth type of delinquency, *acting-out* delinquency, where the individual freely expresses his impulses, particularly hostile ones, has something in common with all the others. Acting out refers to the free, deliberate, and often malicious indulgence of impulse, particularly in the sphere of aggression but also in other areas of delinquency such as vandalism. It is essentially a form of revolt. Like subcultural delinquency, it may be more or less consciously directed against the middle-class morality. Unlike subcultural delinquency, it may be more an individual matter requiring less sanction from group mores. Furthermore, the acting-out delinquent may himself come from the middle or upper classes; he may be motivated by hostility either against the adult world in general or against his parents in particular, or by simple boredom. Like neurotic delinquency, acting out may express unformulated needs that have nothing to do with the specific acts committed. In common with psychopathic behavior, to be described below, acting-out delinquency may betray a brutal disregard for other people's feelings. Unlike the psychopath, however, for whom other people's feelings simply do not count, the actor-out may quite consciously want to inflict pain, even though he may not know why or he may simply move trancelike through an orgy of destruction. He may well be a relatively gifted and forceful individual, caught up in a pattern of resentments and unstructured cravings and impulses, who needs help in finding ways to use his gifts in socially constructive ways.

Fifth and finally, there is *psychopathic* delinquency. Psychopathy certainly begins very early in life. Indeed, some authors still speak of *constitutional* (that is, hereditary or "built-in") *psychopathic personality*. The consensus seems now to be that psychopathy represents a failure of the basic identification process in the first five years of life, so that the individual becomes incapable of true feelings for others. This failure can in some cases be traced to a disruption of normal family relationships. However, it is worth noting that the psychopath has an essentially intact personality, but lacks strong emotional ties to reality. The psychopath is remarkable for his emotional blandness, particularly in regard to actions that would profoundly shock the normal individual. He is virtually lacking in conscience or superego, although he professes a recognition of and can speak smoothly in terms of devotion to accepted values. He makes glib promises and resolutions, but meanwhile may be picking the pocket of the person he is talking to. He is profoundly egocentric and can never quite see his own responsibility for anything that goes wrong. The psychopath's measured intelligence is within the normal range but his thinking is essentially superficial and external. In spite of ability to learn things, he does not profit by the lessons of his own experience, so that his behavior is out of keeping with what he abstractly knows. In fact, he not only seems indifferent to the consequences for other people of what he does, he does not seem concerned about the almost certainly unfortunate consequences for himself—he is incurably, unrealistically optimistic.

The psychopath steals even when he is sure to be caught. He lies even when there is no earthly reason for lying. He may be assaultive or even murderous—although many psychopaths are not at all physically aggressive—but even his violence or sadism has a shallow, unfeeling quality quite unlike that of the child who has a chip on his shoulder. He does physical harm as casually and unthinkingly as he lies or steals. Because he can learn the formulas to which other people respond, he can manipulate people, at least until they come to detect the meaninglessness of what he says. It is not that he specifically wishes people ill, but only that their needs and feelings have no immediacy for him. His own needs and wishes are paramount and absolute. Because he is normally intelligent, he can undertake elaborate plans for getting what he wants, but his thinking, which does not take full account of other people's views, is likely to go awry, and his schemes to collapse. Childhood psychopaths supply the bulk of the adult criminal population, but not all of them end up as criminals. Some simply become unpleasant characters who exploit and betray their friends and families but stay within the law. Some become drifters or marginal personalities. Some settle down to shallow respectability on a low socioeconomic level. A few, turning their talents into socially acceptable channels, become financial successes, but it is doubtful that they are able to establish satisfactory personal relationships. The political rabble-rouser, the lynch-mob leader, is likely to be a psychopath. Because of the psychopath's lack of strong feeling, punishment does not change his ways, he is extremely hard to deal with in psychotherapy, and we cannot be hopeful about those who are already among us. In terms of prevention, considering the apparent origins of pschopathy in a disturbance of early emotional relationships, we can only point to all the things we have said so far about sound emotional relationships in infancy and early childhood.

Adolescence

The excesses of normal adolescent behavior, like normal preschool behavior, often reach emotional extremes that might lead some people to conclude that adolescence itself may be a form of insanity. We hope we have made clear that such is not the case. Nevertheless, adolescence is a vulnerable period, in terms of both the painful problems the adolescent has to face and the reawakening of past developmental issues that were only partially resolved. (Psychiatrists speak of the disturbances of adolescence as *hebetic* or *heboid*.) It is during adolescence that a true *schizophrenic breakdown* may first occur; indeed, schizophrenia used to be known as *dementia praecox,* insanity of the young. Many normal adolescent traits in their extreme forms approximate schizophrenic behavior. Too persistent feelings of dislocation and estrangement, total docility or exaggerated rebelliousness, emotional volatility, feelings that everybody is against one, talk of suicide, and even idealism that seems to be a denial of reality may all have a schizophrenic flavor. Needless to say, most adolescents have developed a tough core of security and an anchorage in reality that permit them to withstand and thrive on the stresses of this period. Since, however, a few do break down, we should attempt to see the form that breakdowns are most likely to take.

Schizophrenia is actually a label that embraces several psychoses. All of these have in common a distortion of normal emotional responses and include ideas or feelings about reality which are incompatible with normal views. Ordinarily, the whole of reality is reshaped in keeping with a central conflict within the schizophrenic. This reshaping may take the form of *delusions,* unfounded but no less serious beliefs to the effect that people are trying to poison the individual, that they are accusing him of depraved practices or inviting him to engage in them, or that he has been endowed with special powers and dispensations. Schizophrenics may have delusions about their own bodies: that they are corrupted by strange diseases, that they are being controlled by malignant forces, that they are sensitive to radio waves, that their bodies contain various kinds of machines. Sometimes beliefs of this sort take the more concrete form of hallucinations, imaginary but nevertheless vivid experiences where the individual hears voices talking to him or about him, sees visions, or smells strange or foul odors. Notice that most sane people hallucinate occasionally, as when one hears his name called even though no one has spoken.

Schizophrenia does not always take such elaborate or explicit forms, however. Sometimes it is expressed in total apathy and inactivity, sometimes in grossly inappropriate emotional responses to standard reality: The individual may be quite unfeeling about something that is of vital importance to him, he may giggle foolishly in response to almost anything that happens, or he may fly into a rage over trifling setbacks. Some schizophrenics seem to be contented in their fantasy worlds, some seem to lack any emotion, while some are at constant war with their surroundings. They may feel harried by their enemies, they may be verbally abusive, they may take satisfaction in behaving outrageously, or they may be assaultive, self-destructive, or murderous.

Quite frequently, the central conflict of schizophrenia is a sexual one, although often heavily disguised. Conflicts over homosexual cravings, feelings of uncleanness, feelings of lack of control, a sense of being unwanted, a sense of vulnerability—all may enter into the schizophrenic pattern. We might also add that males are more prone than females to schizophrenia (as to most forms of emotional disturbance), but that some schizophrenic girls and women show this disorder in its most virulent forms. Most basically, the schizophrenic has a seriously disturbed self-image, and when he turns against the outside world it seems to be in an attempt to destroy the mirror in which he can see his own unbearably horrible image—or he may simply turn away from the world to deny the reality of his own feelings.

One hears schizophrenia spoken of as incurable. This is not necessarily the case. Some schizophrenics recover spontaneously from psychotic episodes, temporarily or permanently. Some can live comfortably as long as they remain in the sheltered environment of a hospital or even in a community that understands their weaknesses and needs. Some number show improvement in response to a number of treatments used singly or in combination: tranquilizing drugs, energizing drugs, shock therapies, and individual and group psychotherapy, among others. Some respond well to arrangements that permit them to live in the hospital but work in the community, or to live at home and spend their days in therapeutic programs in the clinic or hospital.

There is a great gulf between the legal and the practical view of what constitutes *sexual delinquency* in boys. For girls, the discrepancy is not so great, particularly if a girl incurs the biological penalty of becoming pregnant. For this reason, and because the adolescent girl may use sexual promiscuity as a weapon of revolt, sex offenses make up a very sizable proportion of delinquent behavior in girls. Psychologically, as we might expect from what was said in Chapter 11 about female sexuality, sexually delinquent behavior in girls often seems to have nonsexual origins. We have just pointed out that it may be an expression of adolescent revolt. It is rather often associated with simple-mindedness and a passive inclination to do what other people say. It may express a need for affection, for emotional contact and support in girls who lack warm attachments. In some cases, and under certain kinds of pressures, it appears to stem from a need to conform to group mores, from the threat of exile if one does not do as the others do. In general, sex delinquency in girls is often symptomatic of a deeper emotional disturbance or of personal inadequacy. Punitive measures are of little help and may only force a girl into a life of prostitution. Sympathetic case work, however, which can help the girl make practical adjustments, often accomplishes a rapid change. The second major kind of female delinquency is shop-lifting, sometimes for fun or profit but more often in response to neurotic needs.

Sexual deviations may appear in adolescence, although less commonly than the other phenomena we have been discussing. In girls, homosexuality as a fixed pattern, although less frequent than in boys, is probably the form which sexual deviation most often takes. There appear to be two main motivations behind female homosexuality. The first is deep-rooted hostility toward or fear of males. The second is psychological masculinity, a wish to assume the male role—this often extends beyond sexual practices to such matters as dress, mannerisms, speech, and so forth. In the latter case, men are viewed not as enemies but as competitors.

In boys, there are several forms of sexual deviation which may become serious problems during adolescence. It should be noted, however, that all these deviations may play a part in normal adolescent fantasies, and that some of them may actually be practiced experimentally, without their having any abnormal significance. Rape, which normal boys may fantasy but are extremely unlikely to execute, is ordinarily a part of subcultural delinquency, acting-out delinquency, or psychopathy, and does not require further discussion here. Closely allied to rape is sexual sadism. As we know, sex and violence do often become interwoven, and for certain unstable personalities may be interchangeable. Much of the pornographic literature addressed to late-school-age and adolescent boys (which they claim not to like but read avidly) is a compound of sex and sadism. For some normal children, such literature may serve a positive function by reassuring them that their fantasies are shared by other people. For a few near-psychotic or psychopathic children, however, such literature may possibly be pernicious, supplying a prototype for acting-out behavior. For yet others, likewise unstable but less inclined to act out, it can serve further to confuse their own feelings and attitudes.

A more common form of deviation in adolescent males is homosexuality. As in the case of female homosexuality, male homosexuality as a permanent life style often reflects fear or hatred of the opposite sex, or else a psychological identification with it. Negative feelings toward girls may be expressed as frank disgust or constant disparagement. Identification with the female role (which in many cases seems related to having an ineffectual father or to the father's being missing from the home) leads to conscious imitation of feminine ways. Homosexuality may also go along with a schizoid (schizophreniclike but still nonpsychotic) alienation from experience, so that the individual needs some extraordinary stimulus, perhaps with elements of revulsion, to arouse him sexually.

Yet another form of deviation is voyeurism, or Peeping Tom behavior. All youngsters, to satisfy their curiosity, do a certain amount of peeping and spying. However, when sexual spectacles become an end in themselves rather than a source of knowledge or stimulation, it is apparent that the individual's normal sexual orientation has been lost. Voyeurism (or exhibitionism) may be associated with feelings of sexual inadequacy, with a guilt about sexual feelings that can be appeased as long as sex is enjoyed only at a distance, or with more serious and generalized personality disturbances.

In practice, the adult homosexual or voyeur can often lead an outwardly normal life. Often, however, his personality organization is to some degree warped and his sex life unsatisfactory. In addition, he lives in constant danger of detection, which would lead, at best, to public shame and hostility, and, at worst, to imprisonment or mandatory hospitalization. Because such deviations are usually deeply embedded in the individual's character structure, they require prolonged psychotherapy aimed at a general revision of personality.

Although neurotic traits may appear earlier, it is ordinarily in adolescence or after, when the individual's ideal self has become differentiated from his other selves, that he is capable of full-blown *neurosis*, a state of conflict between antagonistic and often unformulated inner tendencies that drains his energies and hampers his functioning. As we mentioned previously, the neurotic individual's inner conflicts are seldom expressed directly. Basically, the neurotic person, unlike the psychotic or the psychopathic one, recognizes that he is blocked or ineffective by reason of characteristics within himself but beyond his voluntary control. The source of the neurosis is usually anxiety or guilt, against which the neurotic erects defenses which themselves impede his functioning. His tensions and defenses constitute the neurotic symptoms. Sometimes we find diffuse, "free-floating" anxiety ready to attach to any situation. However, the anxiety itself may be a defense against something else, such as pervasive but unacknowledged hostility. In some neurotics, the symptoms take more explicit, often symbolically meaningful forms, such as specific fears or phobias; ritualized, compulsive behavior; inability to make decisions (*abulia*); or a general sense of inadequacy, impotence, or worthlessness. These symptoms may affect only one sharply circumscribed area of functioning, or they may cripple the neurotic in all his activities.

One form of neurosis in adolescence is *hysteria,* inner conflict expressed usually through somatic symptoms. One form of hysterical behavior, now relatively rare (there are fashions in psychological disorders as in other things), is somatic dysfunction: hysterical blindness, deafness, paralysis, and so forth, where, although the affected organ is in good anatomical and physiological working order, the individual cannot use it. Such manifestations often seem to be a denial of the organ in an attempt to repudiate what it has experienced or done (a paralyzed hand, for instance, may serve to deny masturbation), to protect it from harm, to prevent its doing something in the future, or to justify the individual's helplessness—somatic dysfunctions are not uncommon among soldiers who would rather not fight, but they are wholly unconscious and so different from deliberate shirking.[27] Hysteria may take the form of hypochondria, a constant inventory of the body to see what has gone wrong, and a tendency to interpret normal and usually unnoticed body sensations as warnings of some dread disease process. We can see how adolescents, with their heightened body awareness, might be prone to hypochondriacal symptoms; almost all adolescents have spells of hypochondria and almost all outgrow it. Yet another hysterical manifestation, and a more serious one, is the unsuccessful suicide. This must be distinguished from the genuine suicide attempt, whether successful or not, which stems from a profound sense of despair or accompanies a psychotic breakdown. The hysterical gesture of suicide is usually an appeal for attention and affection and a means of reproaching an unsympathetic world. Even in cases where the danger of actual suicide is slight, suicidal gestures indicate emotional disturbance serious enough to call for professional help.

Hysteria often blends into *psychosomatic disorders,* where the body undergoes actual pathological changes as a result of corrosion by chronic conflicting emotions. On the borderline between hysteria and psychosomatic disorders, there are manifestations such as fainting, where the physical changes that go with emotion interfere with the blood supply to the brain. Another borderline phenomenon, usually beginning in adolescence, is *anorexia nervosa,* a condition in which the individual finds food, or most foods, inedible or revolting. Anorexia nervosa seems to occur most often in girls, and, according to one interpretation, seems to be an unconscious expression of fear of sexuality, where anything taken into the body connotes, symbolically, sexual penetration. Although anorexia nervosa does not lead directly to physiological disorders, its victims may become badly emaciated and suffer tissue damage due to malnutrition. They generally survive on small quantities of a few selected foods, but they may have to be hospitalized and fed intravenously.

At the opposite pole from anorexia stands the far more common condition of *bulimia,* or compulsive overeating. Bulimia may begin long before adolescence, and appears to be an infantile oral character trait. It often is a symbolic expression of a hunger for love and support. It has psychosomatic consequences in obesity and metabolic changes. Other more directly psychosomatic disorders, such as gastric ulcers, migraine, and so forth, can also be observed. It is worth mentioning that such somatic afflictions as eczema and asthma can be made worse or may even be triggered off by psychological upsets as early as infancy.

We might also say a word about individual differences in psychosomatic reactions. All strong emotions entail clearcut body changes. And, provided emotions are not so strong as to be disruptive, different emotions seem to entail different patterns of physiological change. But within this general framework, Lacey,[28] Wenger,[29] and others have demonstrated that individuals have their own characteristic ways of reacting to a variety of emotional situations. It can easily be observed that some people react predominantly (although other systems are also involved in varying degrees) with their pharyngeal mucous membranes, becoming all stuffed up; some with their tear ducts; some react with their skins, flushing or paling; in some, blood pressure goes up, in others down; some react with their muscles, tensing up; some with their digestive tracts, losing appetite or needing to eliminate. We are thus in a position to conjecture that the particular psychosomatic symptom that appears in individuals who live under prolonged emotional strains, and whose tissues break down before their personality organization, is a product of the particular chronic emotion which is at work within the person, of his idiosyncratic form of emotional response, and of tissue vulnerabilities such as a tendency to eczema or asthma. As we can see, the adolescent has moved into a stage of individualized complexity where, like most adults, he is a mixture of normal and abnormal, of strengths and weaknesses, of virtues and faults.

Help for Exceptional Children

Discussion of morbid conditions such as those described in this chapter may lead to certain anxieties, and we feel some obligation to try to put this discussion in its proper perspective. It is obvious that all the "abnormal" psychological symptoms we have described crop up in the most normal people. It is not necessarily the case that because a child shows some sign of psychological disturbance he is mentally ill. In the first place, his behavior may be a way of coping with essentially abnormal and stressful living conditions; in such cases, it is the environment that needs attention, and not the child. Furthermore, these symptoms by themselves do not indicate abnormal functioning. They express normal human potentialities shared by everybody. It is only when they begin to dominate the scene and interfere with effective living that they become abnormal and require special attention—which may occasionally consist of nothing more than the familiar prescription of a change of scene for a few weeks. At the other extreme, special attention may consist of prolonged psychotherapy. It should also be obvious that we are at a loss to explain in terms of situational influences many abnormalities thought to be psychological rather than organic, and we may need to give more consideration to constitutional strengths, weaknesses, capacities, and vulnerabilities. Some children survive objectively appalling childhoods without visible ill effects, while others seem to break down under apparently trifling stresses. Some break down or get off to a poor start and then recover with very little outside help, while others may spend a lifetime trying to find an identity they can call their own. Until the conditions of mental health and illness have been better defined, we can only offer the prescription that we have repeated throughout this book: love, emotional warmth, self-confidence and confidence in the child, solid but not overwhelming authority, enjoyment, opportunity for sound identifications, and encouragement—without coercion—to cognitive growth and to independence.

Meanwhile, some few children do have physical disabilities serious enough to affect their psychological functioning, and others do develop chronic psychological disorders. Fortunately, we live in an era when we can face such problems and try to deal with them realistically, instead of locking the child in a closet, castigating ourselves with guilt feelings, rattling family skeletons, and otherwise wasting valuable energies. It is hard for us to realize now that a generation ago people could not bring themselves to speak publicly of tuberculosis, cancer, or venereal disease, which, thanks largely to publicity by special interest groups, have been brought out into the open, where they can be dealt with. In the same way, we are now coming to acknowledge and attack such problems as emotional disturbance, schizophrenia, mental deficiency, epilepsy, cerebral palsy, and so forth. Possibly the most important effect of campaigns designed to focus public attention on these problems is that they have enabled parents to continue to be parents even when their children were severely disabled; they have made parents aware that children continue to be children in spite of disabilities, that they need the same basic emotional support that other children do.

Children with physical disabilities and severely disturbed children need outside professional help. Whether this kind of help is indicated for the child with emotional disturbances of slight or intermediate severity must be a matter for individual decision. Psychotherapy can help, but it cannot guarantee to do so. Furthermore it costs heavily, in terms both of money and psychic strain, and parents must weigh its possible benefits against its costs to them and to the child. And when they do elect psychotherapy—which often means psychotherapy for the entire family— they must be prepared to follow through wherever it leads. Sometimes, of course, less drastic measures than psychotherapy can be of therapeutic benefit. A good school or teacher, for instance, or participation in a recreation group, can often help a child immensely. Nevertheless, a professional opinion as to the most advisable measures is often helpful.

Unfortunately, for those who need and want professional help, there are not enough facilities to go around. The great middle classes are at a particular disadvantage when it comes to finding professional services. The well-to-do can pay for help, and there are many private and public agencies prepared to serve those with limited funds. However, for those readers who are seeking professional help, certain guidelines may be in order. Various professional specialties are licensed or certified by various accrediting agencies, but the individual's best assurance of qualified help is to obtain information from a reliable source. To find out where reputable psychiatric or psychological services can be obtained, the individual can apply to his pediatrician or family doctor, to the medical society of the county where he lives, to the nearest mental health clinic, to his county or local welfare agency, to the psychological association in his state, to the American Psychological Association, or to the psychology department or clinic of a college or university. For vocational guidance, a roster of qualified counselors is maintained by the National Vocational

Guidance Association. In the case of particular disabilities, parent or citizen groups have been set up to provide services or maintain a directory of where services are available. Among these are the United Cerebral Palsy Associations, the National Association for Retarded Children, the National Epilepsy League, the National Society for Crippled Children and Adults, the American Foundation for the Blind, the American Speech and Hearing Association, and the National Organization for Mentally Ill Children, plus, of course, many more. Many national foundation organizations have branch offices and clinics around the country, and application for help can be made directly to these. Otherwise, the national headquarters can direct applicants to the nearest facilities.

Pathology of the Environment

We have been talking thus far of problems which, regardless of their sources in the family or the social environment, are essentially problems of individual disturbance. These problems fall within the province of psychiatry and psychology. We should like to close our discussion of abnormalities of development with a discussion of the so-called sociopathies, pathologies of society, social organization, and family structure which may have deleterious effects on personality development. Obviously, we have taken some account of these throughout this book, and in the present chapter in references to mothering and to delinquency. We have implied earlier that intellectually sterile, unstimulating, and over-rigid patterns of schooling may well stifle or deform personal creativity and development. The even more damaging effects of the usual sorts of institutionalization have also been alluded to. We have even suggested that some whole cultures seem to represent lunacy made the norm. Now we should like to give more attention to problems which are the province of social work, the field of child welfare, and, in terms of academic disciplines, of sociology.

FAMILY PATHOLOGY

We should note that psychology and sociology are not exclusive disciplines. Their domains inevitably overlap a great deal. However, their emphases are quite different—so different, at times, that the same terms may have quite different meanings in the two disciplines. Sociologically, for instance, a "broken home" is one in which the parents are divorced or separated, or one or both parents dead, regardless of how successfully the remaining members live together as a family unit. Psychologically, on the other hand, a broken home is one in which life is made difficult either by the loss or absence of a parent or by interpersonal strife, even though all the family members are present to participate in it. We shall feel free to use this and other terms in a way biased toward psychology, simply because psychology is our business.

The most immediately important sociopathies, from the standpoint of child development, are those having to do with the family structure, particularly those disruptions which are called broken homes. Until thirty or forty years ago, most such homes were broken up as a result of the death of one or both parents. The efforts of those who attempted to help the survivors of broken homes were largely aimed at placing the children, usually in orphanages. The orphanage is now a vanishing institution, for two reasons. First of all, parents live longer—especially mothers, for whom childbirth is now rarely a hazard. Second, there has been a general recognition that the usual form of group care provided in orphanages leaves much to be desired. However, a contrary trend is generated by a need to provide facilities for illegitimate babies who, for one reason or another, cannot be adopted. As substitutes for orphanages there have now been developed programs to place children without parents in private homes, and to enable a surviving parent to keep his or her family together. Instead of going to institutions, many homeless children are placed in foster homes (temporary placements, with the child's keep paid for by the public or private agency in whose legal custody he remains) or adoptive homes (permanent placements, with the child becoming a legal member of the family). The second substitute for orphanages is the provision through various state agencies and the federal Social Security system of subsidies for widows and their dependent children, enabling them to keep their families together.

Certain flaws have appeared in the foster care and adoptive placement programs. One is that it is hard to find enough foster homes. Another shortcoming is apparent in the case of children who have to move repeatedly from one foster home to another, because of incompatibility or changed circumstances; such children develop a sense of repeated loss and rejection, and often become victims of psychopathology. Yet another flaw lies in the implicit assumption that any foster home is better than any institution. Some people have moved to improve institutional care instead of scrapping it. By raising the quality, psychological warmth, understanding, and training of personnel, by providing continuity of attachment between child and a particular person responsible for his care, and by organizing children into *small* groups on a family plan, a number of institutions are improving to the point where they may yet provide the best solution for children with special kinds of emotional disturbance that prevent their forming attachments to a foster family, and for children past the early school years.

Illegitimacy was at one time an unfavorable circumstance for child and mother alike. We have now come to realize that the child and his mother—often a confused adolescent—are people in need of help rather than punishment. It is not usually feasible for an unmarried mother to keep her child, but an adoptive home can often be found for him. Unfortunately, we have an overabundance of unwanted illegitimate Negro babies whom potential white parents are reluctant to adopt. Also, many states have laws that require the adoptive parents to be of the same religion as the baby's own mother, which often prevents adoptions that might otherwise have been arranged. Adoptive placement, too, at one time carried its risks—as it still may for babies adopted through extra-legal channels. Adoption agencies, however, have now set standards for adoptive families which help insure favorable environments for children. At times, indeed, these standards have been too inflexible, meaning that children have had to spend long waiting periods in the limbo of an agency, sometimes until they were too old to be good adoption risks. There has recently been an attempt to make standards more flexible and still insure a healthful home atmosphere. It has also become accepted practice to let adopted children know early that they are adopted, that they are, in fact, *chosen,* as a safeguard against their learning the fact accidentally and being overcome by the uncertainty and, perhaps, sense of rejection of not being with their own parents. On the other hand, too great an insistence on the child's adoptive status can raise a whole host of doubts and questions. Adoption agencies have also shown a greater willingness to place flawed babies with families who want them; such babies are often in demand by adoptive parents who would not otherwise be eligible or who are themselves handicapped in some way. A thorough study still needs to be made of how well adoption works, and what factors help and hinder the process.

Nowadays, of course, although children less often have to face the problems of being orphaned or branded as illegitimate, they still are confronted with the problems of homes broken by marital discord. In the lowest stratum of society there are many families where intermittent or changing or absent fathers are the rule, where the children's only tie, if any, is to the mother. Such families are particularly likely to breed feelings of isolation and rejection, hostility against society, delinquency, and a gang orientation. A number of writers have commented on the special identification problems of Negro males raised without fathers. Interestingly enough, a certain segment of upper-class society displays a similar pattern of multiple divorce (in the lowest-class families, of course, neither the marriage nor the divorce may be formalized), where there may be a tie with one parent but no clearcut, sustained family structure. For the children of such families, the boarding school may play the psychological role of orphanage and may be the only stable factor in the child's life.

In a sense even more disruptive is divorce in the middle-class family, founded as it is on a more definite assumption of permanence. Sometimes, of course, divorce seems to be the only answer. A family atmosphere of psychological divorce, permeated by coldness or open antagonism, may be even worse for the children. Divorce is simply an explicit acknowledgment that a marriage has failed, and, if anything, may have a stabilizing effect. Needless to say, even a badly spoiled marriage can sometimes be salvaged by putting it on a new footing where the parents' immaturities will not be in the forefront, and when this can be done—by family counseling, by psychotherapy, or otherwise—it is certainly preferable to divorce.

Divorce entails many secondary problems, of course, and these have to be met. Among the psychologically most important ones are those having to do with the children's divided loyalties and how their time is to be apportioned between the two parents. Some divorced parents work severe hardships on their children by trying to win their exclusive affection, by using them as a weapon against the other parent, by trying to justify their own point of view, and even by treating children as substitute spouses. Traumatic as divorce can be, there is general agreement that it is better than trying to maintain a pretense "for the children's sake." The children can more easily understand and accept a real break than deceptions which do not deceive but only baffle and disturb. One of the subtle and neglected aspects of divorce is the disruption of countless accumulated habit patterns, leading to disorientation, aimlessness, and often a loneliness that sends the divorced person rushing into a new liaison.

Home conditions of poverty and economic privation or uncertainty can expose the child to ills ranging from malnutrition to extremes of psychopathology. Although the acceptance of the principle of the welfare state has eliminated many of the conditions Dickens wrote about, we can still find nests of squalor on tenant farms, in migrant labor camps, and in the tenements of every city. Indeed, whole nations and, in the United

States, whole regions, such as Appalachia, suffer from economic blight. Economic poverty may remove the child from the culture at large and deprive him of all the stimulation to growth that is the lot of most children. Some families, of course, maintain their group and individual integrity in the face of the most grinding hardships. On the other hand, it may take more than economic relief to lift other families from a pattern of irresponsibility or depravity.

The social agencies in every community know certain families that can be counted on to produce more than their actuarial share of school failures, truancy, delinquency, sexual deviation, drunkenness and disorderliness, and disease, and of inadequate personalities who become the parents of other inadequate personalities in a recurring sequence that led early geneticists to talk of hereditary (rather than self-renewing) social incompetence. Social agencies have experimented with a cooperative total rehabilitation of such families, instead of the former piecemeal cleaning up of each problem as it arose. Such approaches have met with encouraging success, and may presage a wholly new concept in welfare work. Meanwhile, of course, government funds are going into antipoverty programs, and paid workers and volunteers are engaged in numerous remedial and preventive ventures.

Agencies and counselors, however, must take account of the possibly devastating effects of conflicts in cultural values. This danger is brought sharply to our attention in Hunt's study[30] of the ecology of mental disease. It came to Hunt's attention that a surprisingly large number of boys who had belonged to the same group in a depressed section of Washington developed some form of psychopathology. Investigating further, he found that those boys who had often taken part in the gang's sexual perversions *and* who had participated in neighborhood religious revivals were the ones who broke down. It was only when sexual perversion was joined to religion in the same individual, implying a state of severe conflict, that psychopathology resulted. Antipoverty and redevelopment programs can work only if we understand the phenomenon of "culture shock" and understand that we are engaged in cultural engineering—a realization that may cause us to reconsider some of our own middle-class assumptions.

We must make explicit that widespread prejudice against racial, ethnic, national, or religious groups is a form of social pathology. While the victims of prejudice may suffer immediate and obvious harm, the prejudiced are also the victims of culturally ordained unreason and suffer to the extent that their capacities for perceiving, feeling, and thinking are crippled by their misconceptions. It is obvious but often overlooked that prejudice generates reciprocal prejudice, so that minority groups may harbor irrational beliefs about and attitudes toward the prejudiced majority as well as crippling concepts of themselves.

DISASTER AND SOCIAL DISRUPTION

Finally, we should point out that in recent years social scientists have begun to gather and organize information about what happens to children in times of major social crisis due to man-made or natural disasters: war, flood, earthquake, windstorm, panic. It has always been obvious that children suffer from such crises, but now we are beginning to see more precisely what they suffer and how, and what sort of psychological safety precautions can be incorporated in disaster preparations. The growth of our civilization has produced two parallel trends. First, we are able to create disasters on a gigantic scale, in the form of nuclear bombing, biological warfare, concentration camps, forced migrations, and genocide. Second, we have become able to stand apart from our acts of mass destruction, assess them, and plan against the day when we turn our destructive forces against ourselves. Needless to say, we shall reach real social maturity only when such assessments and planning are no longer necessary.

Studies of adult morale have shown that panic is most likely to occur when the individual feels cut loose from his moorings in the group and does not have clearcut tasks to perform. For the child, at least up to age ten and probably beyond, the essential moorings are in family ties. As we have said previously, it was found that, in general, children evacuated to safety from the threat of aerial bombardment, but removed from their parents, suffered far greater psychological strain than those who remained with their parents even in the face of actual danger. At one time, disaster rescue and relief workers had as their first intuitive impulse the need to collect children and take them to a safe place where they could be cared for in groups. In the Dutch flood disasters of the early 1950's, by contrast, a deliberate attempt was made to take account of World War II experience and keep children with their families, or at least with their mothers and siblings—fathers, for the most part, being required to take part in emergency operations.[31]

American investigators, studying children's recovery from the psychological effects of such disasters as floods and tornadoes, have found that those children who had to step in and take over the functions and responsibilities of a dead or incapacitated parent or older sibling, and those who had the greatest opportunity to discuss and ventilate their experiences, were the first to recover. Ironically enough, "better-off" middle-class families, in which there was less likely to be a clearcut role for a child to assume, and which protectively tried to keep children from talking about the awful events they had witnessed, were likely to prevent children from discharging their accumulated feelings and thus helped perpetuate them. It should be noted, however, that adults are likely to misperceive the way children experience disaster; a superlative literary example of this is given in the novel *A High Wind in Jamaica*. Following a severe hurricane that demolished the family plantation, the mother observes:

> "That awful night!" said Mrs. Thornton, once, when discussing their plan of sending [the children] home to school: "Oh, my dear, what the poor little things must have suffered! Think how much more acute Fear is to a child! And they were so brave, so English. . . . You know, I am terribly afraid what permanent, *inward* effect a shock like that may have on them. Have you noticed they never so much as mention it? . . ."
>
> Meanwhile, the children, accepting the new life as a matter of course, were thoroughly enjoying it.[32]

We might mention in passing the nomadic societies of children that sprang up in southern and eastern Europe following World Wars I and II. Children separated from their parents formed roving, predatory bands which developed their own cultures of a highly psychopathic turn. Again there is a literary depiction of such behavior in *Lord of the Flies*,[33] which describes in harrowing detail the sociology of a group of castaway children (and which also teaches a Freud-like view of the intrinsic evil of human nature).

Studies on the effects of major social upheavals are, of course, only at the beginning, but their findings are important and dependable enough to make a vital difference in the thinking of those charged with planning for disaster relief. Meanwhile, we can see that we have our work cut out for us to provide a world fit for our children to grow up in.

REFERENCES / Chapter 13

[1] Kessler, J. W. *Psychopathology of Childhood*. Englewood Cliffs: Prentice-Hall, 1966.
[2] Haeusserman, E. *Developmental Potential of Preschool Children*. New York: Grune & Stratton, 1958.

³ Yacorzynski, G. K., and Tucker, B. E. What price intelligence? *American Psychologist*, 1960, 15, 201–203.

⁴ Graham, F. K., Ernhart, C. B., Thurston, D., and Craft, M. Development three years after perinatal anoxia and other potentially damaging newborn experiences. *Psychological Monographs*, 1962, 76, no. 3; see also Corah, N. L., Anthony, E. J., Painter, P., Stern, J. A., and Thurston, D. Effects of perinatal anoxia after seven years. *Psychological Monographs*, 1965, 79, no. 3.

⁵ Pasamanick, B., and Knobloch, H. Early feeding and birth difficulties in childhood schizophrenia: An explanatory note. *Journal of Psychology*, 1963, 56, 73–77.

⁶ Kawi, A. A., and Pasamanick, B. Prenatal and paranatal factors in the development of childhood reading disorders. *Monographs of the Society for Research in Child Development*, 1959, 24, no. 4.

⁷ Griffiths, C. *Hear*. New York: Exposition Press, 1966.

⁸ Leonard, M. F., Rhymes, J. P., and Solnit, A. J. Failure to thrive in infants. *American Journal of Diseases of Children*, 1966, 111, 600–612.

⁹ Kirk, S. A. *Early Education of the Mentally Retarded*. Urbana: University of Illinois, 1958; Kirk, S. A. *Educating Exceptional Children*. Boston: Houghton Mifflin, 1962.

¹⁰ Szasz, T. S. The uses of naming and the origin of the myth of mental illness. *American Psychologist*, 1961, 16, 59–65.

¹¹ Kanner, L. Early infantile autism. *Journal of Pediatrics*, 1944, 25, 211–217.

¹² Rubin, T. I. *Jordi*. New York: Macmillan, 1960.

¹³ Bettelheim, B. Joey: A "mechanical boy." *Scientific American*, March, 1959. See also the same author's *The Empty Fortress: Infantile Autism and the Birth of Self*. New York: Free Press, 1967. An interesting case of pseudo-autism is described in Axline, V. *DIBS: In Search of Self*. Boston: Houghton, Mifflin, 1964.

¹⁴ Rimland, B. *Infantile Autism*. New York: Appleton-Century-Crofts, 1964. See especially Part II.

¹⁵ Kessler, *op. cit.*, Chapter 11.

¹⁶ Eisenberg, L., and Kanner, L. Early infantile autism, 1943–55. *American Journal of Orthopsychiatry*, 1956, 27, 556–566.

¹⁷ Wolf, M. M., Risley, T., and Mees, H. Application of operant conditioning procedures to the behavior problems of an autistic child. *Behavior Research and Therapy*, 1964, 1, 305–312; Hewett, F. M. Teaching speech to an autistic child through operant conditioning. *American Journal of Ortho-psychiatry*, 1965, 35, 927–936; Grossberg, J. M. Behavior therapy: A review. *Psychological Bulletin*, 1964, 62, 73–88.

¹⁸ Still sneezing. *Time*, April 22, 1966, p. 52.

¹⁹ U. S. Department of Health, Education, and Welfare. *Minimal Brain Dysfunction in Children*. Washington: U. S. Government Printing Office, National Institute of Neurological Diseases and Blindness Monograph no. 3, 1966; Work, H. H., and Haldane, J. E. Cerebral dysfunction in children. *American Journal of Diseases of Children*, 1966, 111, 573–580; in Something wrong with his brain, II, *ibid.*, 571–572, Work cautions that a diagnosis of brain damage, unless coupled with a discussion of psychological needs, can

induce in parents attitudes of hopelessness, hostility, or rejection, making the problem worse than ever. Prechtl (Prechtl, H. F. R. In Foss, B. M. (ed.) *Determinants of Infant Behavior II.* New York: Wiley, 1963, pp. 53–66) believes that signs of minimal brain damage may be detectable even in the neonate.

[20] Levy, D. M. Psychic trauma of operations in children. *American Journal of Diseases of Children,* 1945, 69, 7–25; Robertson, J. *Young Children in Hospitals.* New York: Basic Books, 1958.

[21] Fillenbaum, S. Impairment in performance with delayed auditory feedback as related to task characteristics. *Journal of Verbal Learning and Verbal Behavior,* 1963, 2, 136–141.

[22] Smith, W. M., McCrary, J. W., and Smith, K. U. Delayed visual feedback and behavior. *Science,* 1960, 132, 1013–1014.

[23] Johnson, W., *et al.* A study of the onset and development of stuttering. *Journal of Speech and Hearing Disorders,* 1942, 7, 251–257.

[24] Sarason, S. B., Hill, K. T., and Zimbardo, P. G. A longitudinal study of the relation of test anxiety to performance on intelligence and achievement tests. *Monographs of the Society for Research in Child Development,* 1964, 29, no. 7.

[25] Lapouse, R. The epidemiology of behavior disorders in children. *American Journal of Diseases of Children,* 1966, 111, 594–599.

[26] Achenbach, T. M. The classification of children's psychiatric symptoms: A factor analytic study. *Psychological Monographs,* 1966, 80, no. 6.

[27] Arluck, E. W. *Hypnoanalysis: A Case Study.* New York: Random House, 1964. PP 26.

[28] Lacey, J. I. The evaluation of autonomic responses: Toward a general solution. *Annals of the New York Academy of Sciences,* 1956, 67, 123–164.

[29] Wenger, M. A. The measurement of individual differences in autonomic balance. *Psychosomatic Medicine,* 1941, 3, 427–434.

[30] Hunt, J. McV. An instance of the social origin of conflict resulting in psychoses. *American Journal of Orthopsychiatry,* 1938, 8, 158–164.

[31] Querido, A., and Mead, M. Mental health and the floods in Holland. *World Mental Health,* 1953, 5, 34–38.

[32] Hughes, R. *A High Wind in Jamaica* (also published as *The Innocent Voyage*). New York: New American Library, 1965 (originally published in 1929), p. 41.

[33] Golding, W. *Lord of the Flies.* New York: Coward-McCann, 1954. (Also available in paperback.)

APPENDIX

A Brief Note
on Films

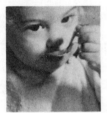

In their teaching, the authors find it profitable to make generous use of films on infant and child behavior. Even when students have access to real live children, films serve a number of important functions. They provide common, repeatable situations for practice in observing, recording, and interpreting behavior. They can demonstrate particular kinds and aspects of behavior that students might spend precious and fruitless hours waiting to catch. They permit an acquaintance with children of an age (notably early infancy), of types (emotionally disturbed children, for instance), or in situations (such as faraway lands, institutions, and so forth) that are not ordinarily available to students. However, we have found it necessary to relate films closely to issues being discussed in class, lest they form merely an interlude between discussions. And because students readily fall into the passive set that goes with watching pictures in a darkened room, merely allowing entertainment to flow over them, it is important to help them see a film as an opportunity for critical observation, and to urge them to question its assumptions just as they would those of a written article.

The Vassar series, *Studies of Normal Personality Development,* distributed, for rental and sale, by the New York University Film Library, 26 Washington Place, New York, N.Y. 10003, comprises a group of films with much the same systematic approach to childhood as this book:

A Long Time to Grow:

> PART I. *Two- and Three-Year-Olds in Nursery School* (Camera follows activities and learning behavior of nursery-school children throughout the day and various seasons of the year. 35 min.)

PART II. *Four- and Five-Year-Olds in School* (Fours seen in familiar world of activities and interests; fives begin to enter more formalized, enlarging world. 40 min.)

PART III. *Six-, Seven- and Eight-Year-Olds—Society of Children* (Entrance of children into world of tradition, magic, and customs handed down from one generation to the next and resistant to change. 30 min.)

Preschool Incidents

(A series of films designed to stimulate discussion. The problems raised are left unanswered. The solutions are to come about through discussion within the group. The incidents are shown twice):

When Should Grownups Help?—(Four episodes in which adult may or may not have needed to assist child. For discussion or use as an observation exercise. 14 min.)

When Should Grownups Stop Fights?—(Four episodes involving conflicts among two- to five-year-olds, without showing resolution. For discussion or use as an observation exercise. 15 min.)

. . . And Then Ice Cream—(Two episodes: One in a school where dessert is a reward for eating the first course and the second in one where intake is up to the child. For discussion or use as an observation exercise. 11 min.)

This Is Robert

(Case study of a child with normal emotional problems, particularly of aggression. Focuses on the preschool years, with supplementary material on prior and subsequent development. Projective play methods are used extensively. 80 min.)

Meeting Emotional Needs in Childhood: The Groundwork of Democracy

(How parents and schools contribute to mental health, with special attention to the middle years of childhood. An older film, partly replaced by Part III of *A Long Time to Grow*. 32 min.)

Understanding Children's Play

(Produced by the Caroline Zachry Institute of Human Development; now distributed as part of the Vassar series. The values of an array of preschool play materials for children and for adults who wish to observe them. 11 min.)

Pay Attention

(Problems and education of deaf and hard-of-hearing children. 27 min.)

Learning Is Searching: A Third Grade Studies Man's Early Tools

(An example of liberal education in the primary grades. 30 min.)

The use of projective techniques in the study of normal personality development:

Finger Painting
> (Although not usually thought of as a projective method, finger painting gives the child wide scope for behavior expressive of personality. Shows personal styles of nine different children. 22 min., color, silent.)

Balloons: Aggression and Destruction Games
> (L. J. Stone. Two children between ages of four and five from similar backgrounds photographed through one-way screen while reacting to test situations. Differences in response to a graduated series of opportunities and invitations to break balloons. 17 min.)

Frustration Play Techniques
> (Eugene Lerner, 35 min.):

> PART I. *Blocking Games* (Shows test situations in which the experimenter, in dealing with several children individually, presents obstructions to the children's play in order to observe their characteristic variations in behavior response. Thus the series of games serves to indicate how each child responds to intrusions, prohibitions, and competitions.)

> PART II. *Frustration and Hostility Games* (Reveals how the child responds to a series of frustrations. He is given a series of attractive toys but can play uninterruptedly with each for only a short time. After each toy is taken away, an uninteresting stick is substituted, thus providing, on the play level, a parallel to the boring and interfering routines of life.)

Abby, a Backward Look
> (Development of a child during the first two years, shown in chronologically reversed sequence. 30 min.)

Starting Nursery School: Patterns of Beginning
> (An approach to the issue of separation—of "leaving home and mother" to start school. 23 min.)

Incitement to Reading
> (The latest in the Vassar series. How the combined first and second grades of a liberal private school learned to read. 37 min.)

In addition, the Vassar Film Program has made films for Project Head Start. These are available free of charge from the nearest office of Modern Talking Pictures Services, Inc., or inquire of Project Head Start, Office of Economic Opportunity, 1100 Eighteenth Street, N.W., Washington, D.C. 20506:

Vassar College Nursery School—A Camera Visit

(Shows a two-days-a-week program, using the facilities of the regular nursery school; provides opportunity for seeing a well-equipped nursery school. 35 min.)

A Pre-Kindergarten Program—A Camera Visit to New Haven

(Presents, in the gymnasium of the neighborhood recreation center, one of the sixteen pre-kindergartens of this city's public schools and some of its special problems. 30 min.)

Los Nietos Kindergarten—A Camera Visit

(In a predominantly Mexican-American neighborhood, this public school kindergarten was held in a summer program not unlike those of Head Start. 25 min.)

The following three training films for Head Start teachers were produced by Vassar in 1967:

Organizing Free Play

Head Start to Confidence

Discipline and Self-Control

We have also used to good advantage a number of films not of our own making. The following selection is not exhaustive: it consists of some of the films we have found most applicable to our own teaching and which are therefore relevant to teaching based on this text. Various film libraries have these films. The best sources generally are the New York University Film Library (see above) and the Psychological Cinema Register, Pennsylvania State University, University Park, Pennsylvania 16802.

And So They Grow

(Produced by the Play Schools Association. 28 min.)

Angry Boy

(A dramatization of the problem of hidden hostility in a child. 35 min.)

Baboon Behavior

(Irven DeVore, University of California. Film record of the results of a year's field study of baboons in the Royal Nairobi National Park in Kenya; a comparison between pertinent aspects of baboon behavior and their counterparts in human development and behavior. 31 min.)

A Balinese Family

(One of a series produced by Gregory Bateson and Margaret Mead. A study of a Balinese family and their three youngest children. 17 min.)

Bathing Babies in Three Cultures
(Gregory Bateson and Margaret Mead. A comparative series of sequences showing the interplay between mother and child in three different settings. 9 min.)

Behavior of Animals and Human Infants in Response to a Visual Cliff
(R. D. Walk and E. J. Gibson. A comparative study of depth discrimination by young animals and human infants. 15 min.)

Birth and the First Fifteen Minutes of Life
(René A. Spitz. Shows second and third stages of labor and early behavior. 10 min., silent.)

A Chance at the Beginning
(Anti-Defamation League for Martin Deutsch and Channel 13, New York. Demonstrates how preschool training for culturally deprived children can provide a sound foundation for the development of each child's abilities. 26 min.)

A Chance for Change
(Produced by Adam and Ellen Giffard, Scientific Film Services. A sensitive and brilliant recording on film of an imaginative program of compensatory education in rural Mississippi, making use of "indigenous personnel" supervised by trained nursery-school educators. 40 min.)

A Child Went Forth
(Losey and Ferno, Brandon Films. An intimate, affectionate picture of two- to seven-year-olds in a "progressive" nursery camp; still valuable though made in the 1940's. 20 min.)

Childhood Rivalry in Bali and New Guinea
(Gregory Bateson and Margaret Mead. A series of scenes in which children of the same age in the two cultures respond to various situations. 17 min.)

Children in the Hospital
(Produced by Dr. Edward Mason of Harvard University. Illustrates types of emotional responses of four- to eight-year-olds to the stress of hospitalization, illness, and separation. 44 min.)

Children Without
(NEA. A commentary on the current problem in education involving the disadvantaged child. 29 min.)

Clinical Aspects of Childhood Psychosis
(Produced by the Institute of Psychiatry, London, England. An attempt to summarize the clinical findings in seventy cases of childhood psychosis. 55 min., silent.)

Constitutional and Environmental Interactions in Rearing Four Breeds of Dogs

(D. G. Freedman. Illustrates procedures and findings of experiment in which different breeds of dogs are raised in either "indulged" or "disciplined" fashion following weaning at three weeks of age. 19 min.)

Development of Behavior in the Duck Embryo

(Gilbert Gottlieb and Zing-Yang Kuo. A Peking duck egg is opened, its inner membrane made transparent, and embryonic activity observed throughout the twenty-seven-day development period. 21 min.)

Development of the Smile and Fear of Strangers in the First Year of Life

(D. G. Freedman. Development of smile and fear of strangers during the first year of life in identical and fraternal twins. 22 min.)

Diagnosis of Childhood Schizophrenia

(Produced by the Brooklyn Juvenile Guidance Center, Inc. Traces the step-by-step procedure of screening clinical data in order to establish the diagnosis of childhood schizophrenia. 35 min.)

Eternal Children

(National Film Board of Canada. Presents an intimate study of the special problems of retarded children and their parents. 30 min.)

First Days in the Life of a New Guinea Baby

(Gregory Bateson and Margaret Mead. A series of scenes beginning immediately after birth with special emphasis on the infant's readiness to respond. 19 min.)

First Steps

(United Nations Film Board. Shows how the proper care of crippled children and the understanding of their emotional conditions may help them to become useful citizens. 11 min.)

Focus on Behavior: A World to Perceive

(National Educational Television. Describes the research of Witkin and of Gibson and Walk. 30 min.)

Focus on Behavior: The Conscience of a Child

(National Educational Television. Describes Sears' research at Stanford. 30 min.)

Food and Maternal Deprivation

(Jenny Aubry for l'Association pour la Santé Mentale de l'Enfance. Part of the record collected by the French research unit studying the effects of maternal deprivation on child development. See MATERNAL DEPRIVATION IN YOUNG CHILDREN. 20 min.)

Four Families:

PART I. (Margaret Mead. Comparison of family life in India and France. 30 min.)

PART II. (Margaret Mead. Comparison of family life in Japan and Canada. 31 min.)

Going to Hospital with Mother

(James Robertson. How the staff of a British hospital has improvised a method of routinely admitting the mothers of patients under school age. See A TWO-YEAR-OLD GOES TO HOSPITAL. 45 min.)

Grief

(Part of the series produced by Spitz. Shows drastic effects of separation from the mother and general deprivation during infancy. 30 min., silent.)

He Acts His Age

(Crawley Films, Ltd., for the National Film Board of Canada. Describes the activities of children at different age levels and suggests that such activities are a gauge of emotional and mental development. 13 min.)

How Babies Learn

(Bettye M. Caldwell and Julius B. Richmond. Describes some of the important developmental advances made by babies during the first year of life. 35 min.)

Imitation in a Home-Raised Chimpanzee

(K. J. Hayes and C. Hayes. Viki, home-raised chimpanzee, shown at twenty to thirty-six months in variety of imitative activities. 17 min., silent.)

Incident on Wilson Street

(NBC News Production. A positive approach to problems affecting children in the learning process. 54 min.)

Karba's First Years

(Gregory Bateson and Margaret Mead. One of a series on Character Formation in Different Cultures. Development in a Balinese child; valuable in teaching about cultural differences in child-rearing. 19 min.)

Maternal Deprivation in Young Children

(Jenny Aubry and Genevieve Appell. One of a series sponsored by the Centre Internationale de l'Enfance. Effects of psychotherapeutic treatment on mother-deprived children. 30 min.)

Mechanical Interest and Ability in a Home-Raised Chimpanzee:

PART I. (K. J. Hayes and C. Hayes. Follows from age eight months to age six years, development of Viki's manual dexterity. 17 min., silent.)

PART II. (K. J. Hayes and C. Hayes. Shows Viki's behavior in response to water, over ages nine months to six years; and behavior in connection with fire, over ages three to five years. 18 min., silent.)

Michael: A Mongoloid Child

(Produced by the British Film Institute. An intimate study of a mongoloid teen-ager living on a farm in rural England. 14 min.)

Mother Love

(From TV program *Conquest*. Dr. Harry F. Harlow studies the effect of substitution of wire- and cloth-mothers for real ones on young rhesus monkeys. 26 min.)

My Own Yard to Play In

(Edward Harrison Productions. Received citation at Venice Festival. Brief and simple film showing resourcefulness of children playing in a large city. 9 min.)

Nature and Development of Affection

(H. F. Harlow and R. Zimmerman. Illustrates a series of observations and experiments analyzing the variables underlying nature and development of affection in primates. See MOTHER LOVE. 19 min., silent.)

Operation Head Start

(Paul Burnford Film Productions. The home and classroom experiences of a child in the Head Start program. 16 min.)

Passion for Life

(Sponsored by the Film Board of the United Nations. The main theme of the charmingly told story is the struggles and triumphs of progressive education in a French village community. 80 min.)

Portrait of a Disadvantaged Child: Tommy Knight

(McGraw-Hill. A day in the life of a slum child. 16 min.)

The Quiet One

(McGraw-Hill. The story of an only child and victim of a disrupted Harlem home, and of the work of the Wiltwyck School in psychological rehabilitation. 67 min.)

The Search for the Lost Self

(Murray Lerner, MPO. Sensitive, *cinéma vérité* description of a day-school program for seriously disturbed children. 58 min.)

The Smiling Response

(Part of the Spitz series. The development of the smile in infancy. 20 min.)

Some Basic Differences in Newborn Infants During the Lying-In Period
> (One of a series produced by Margaret E. Fries and Paul J. Woolf. Old, silent film, with some poor sections photographically; nonetheless valuable in suggesting early temperamental differences. 23 min., silent.)

That the Deaf May Speak
> (Produced for the Lexington School for the Deaf in New York City. The problems of deaf children and the methods of teaching employed in overcoming this handicap. 42 min.)

Thursday's Children
> (Produced at the Royal School for the Deaf, Margate, England. The story of how a group of deaf children from four to seven are led out of their world of silence. Methods used differ from those in P A Y A T - T E N T I O N, the Vassar film. Remarkable photography of children's faces and expressions. 19 min.)

Trance and Dance in Bali
> (Gregory Bateson and Margaret Mead. May be combined usefully with K A R B A ' S F I R S T Y E A R S. 20 min.)

A Two-Year-Old Goes to Hospital
> (James Robertson. Part of a research project on "The Effects of Personality Development of Separation from the Mother in Early Childhood." Describes the behavior of a twenty-nine-month-old child during eight days in a hospital ward. See G O I N G T O H O S P I T A L W I T H M O T H E R. 50 min.)

Uzgiris and Hunt Scales of Infant Psychological Development
> (A series of six films to be released in 1968 on: Object Permanence, Development of Means, Imitation, Operational Causality, Object Relations in Space, and Development of Schemas; all based on Piaget's work, produced by Psychological Development Laboratory, University of Illinois, Urbana, Ill., 61801. Each approx. 35 min.)

BIBLIOGRAPHY

This list contains, in addition to titles cited in the text and at the end of each chapter, certain references of general interest.

ACHENBACH, T. M. The classification of children's psychiatric symptoms: A factor analytic study. *Psychological Monographs,* 1966, 80, no. 6.

ADER, R. F. Social factors affecting emotionality and resistance to disease in animals: III. Early weaning and susceptibility to gastric ulcers in the rat. A control for nutritional factors. *Journal of Comparative and Physiological Psychology,* 1962, 55, 600–602.

ADLER, A. *The Practice and Theory of Individual Psychology.* New York: Harcourt, Brace, 1923.

ADLER, R. Onward and upward with the arts: The new sound. *New Yorker,* February 20, 1965, pp. 63–105.

ADORNO, T. W., FRENKEL–BRUNSWIK, E., LEVINSON, D. J., and SANFORD, R. N. *The Authoritarian Personality.* New York: Harper, 1950.

AINSWORTH, M. D. S. The effects of maternal deprivation. *Public Health Papers,* no. 14. Geneva: World Health Organization, 1962.

———. *Infancy in Uganda.* Baltimore: Johns Hopkins University, 1967.

ALAIN–FOURNIER, H. *The Wanderer.* New York: New Directions, 1946 (originally *Le Grand Meaulnes,* 1913).

ALLEN, K. E., HART, B., BUELL, J. S., HARRIS, F. R., and WOLF, M. M. Effects of social reinforcement on isolate behavior of a nursery school child. *Child Development,* 1964, 35, 511–518.

ALLPORT, G. W. Eidetic imagery. *British Journal of Psychology,* 1924, 15, 99–120.

———. *The Use of Personal Documents in Psychological Science.* New York: Social Science Research Council, 1942.

———. *Becoming.* New Haven: Yale, 1955.

———. The fruits of eclecticism—bitter or sweet? *Psychologia,* 1964, 7, 1–14.

———, and VERNON, P. E. *Studies in Expressive Movement.* New York: Macmillan, 1933.

ALTMANN, S. A. Primate behavior in review. *Science,* 1965, 150, 1440–1442. (Reviews of Schrier, Harlow, and Stollnitz's *Behavior of Non-human Primates* and DeVore's *Primate Behavior.*)

———. (ed.) *Social Communication among Primates.* Chicago: University of Chicago, 1966.

ALTUS, W. D. First born and last born children in a child development clinic. *Journal of Individual Psychology,* 1964, 20, 179–182.

———. Birth order and its sequelae. *Science,* 1966, 151, 44–49.

AMERICAN PSYCHOLOGICAL ASSOCIATION. Education for research in psychology. *American Psychologist,* 1960, 15, 158–159.

AMES, L. B. The development of the sense of time in the young child. *Journal of Genetic Psychology,* 1946, 68, 97–125.

———. The sense of self of nursery school children as manifested by their verbal behavior. *Journal of Genetic Psychology,* 1952, 81, 193–232.

———, and LEARNED, J. Imaginary companions and related phenomena. *Journal of Genetic Psychology,* 1946, 69, 147–167.

ANASTASI, A. Heredity, environment, and the question "How?" *Psychological Review,* 1958, 65, 197–208.

ANDERSON, J. E. Child development: An historical perspective. *Child Development,* 1956, 27, 181–196.

ANSBACHER, H. L. and R. R. *The Individual Psychology of Alfred Adler.* New York: Basic Books, 1956.

APGAR, V. Perinatal problems and the central nervous system. In U.S. Dept. of Health, Education, and Welfare, Welfare Administration, Children's Bureau. *The Child with Central Nervous System Deficit.* Washington: U.S. Government Printing Office, 1965, pp. 75–76.

ARDREY, R. *The Territorial Imperative.* New York: Atheneum, 1966.

ARLUCK, E. W. *Hypnoanalysis: A Case Study.* New York: Random House, PP. 26, 1964.

ASCH, S. E. Studies in the principles of judgments and attitudes: II. Determination of judgments by group and ego standards. *Journal of Social Psychology,* 1940, 12, 433–465.

———, and NERLOVE, H. The development of double function terms in children: An exploratory investigation. In Kaplan, B., and Wapner, S. (eds.) *Perspectives in Psychological Theory.* New York: International Universities, 1960, pp. 47–60.

ASHBY, H. *Health in the Nursery.* London: Longmans, Green, 1898.

ASHTON-WARNER, S. *Teacher.* New York: Simon & Schuster, 1963.

AXLINE, V. *DIBS: In Search of Self.* Boston: Houghton Mifflin, 1964.

BALTIMORE CITY PUBLIC SCHOOLS. *An Early School Admission Project: Progress Report 1963–64.* Baltimore: Baltimore City Public Schools, 1964.

BARKER, R. G., DEMBO, T., and LEWIN, K. Frustration and regression: An experiment with children. *University of Iowa Studies in Child Welfare,* 1941, 18, no. 1.

———, WRIGHT, B. A., MEYERSON, L., and GONICK, M. R. *Adjustment to Physical Handicap and Illness: A Survey of the Social Psychology of Physique and Disability.* New York: Social Science Research Council, 1953.

BARTH, L. G. *Embryology.* New York: Holt, Rinehart, & Winston, 1953.

BARTOSHUK, A. K. Human neonatal cardiac responses to sound: a power function. *Psychonomic Science,* 1964, 1, 151–152.

BATESON, G., JACKSON, D., HALEY, J., and WEAKLAND, J. Toward a theory of schizophrenia. *Behavioral Science,* 1956, 1, 251–264.

———, and MEAD, M. *Balinese Character.* New York: New York Academy of Sciences, 1942.

BAYER, L. M., and BAYLEY, N. *Growth Diagnosis.* Chicago: University of Chicago, 1959.

BAYLEY, N. Consistency and variability in the growth of intelligence from birth to eighteen years. *Journal of Genetic Psychology,* 1949, 75, 165–196.

———. On the growth of intelligence. *American Psychologist,* 1955, 10, 805–818.

BEACH, F. A., and JAYNES, J. Effects of early experience upon the behavior of animals. *Psychological Bulletin,* 1954, 51, 239–263.

BENDER, L., and VOGEL, F. Imaginary companions of children. *American Journal of Orthopsychiatry,* 1941, 11, 56–66.

BENEDICT, R. Continuities and discontinuities in cultural conditioning. *Psychiatry,* 1938, 1, 161–167.

BENNETT, E. L., DIAMOND, M. C., KRECH, D., and ROSENZWEIG, M. R. Chemical and anatomical plasticity of brain. *Science,* 1964, 146, 610–619.

BENNETT, R., and NAHEMOV, L. Institutional totality and criteria of social adjustment in residences for the aged. *Journal of Social Issues,* 1965, 21, 44–78.

BEREITER, C., and ENGELMANN, S. *Teaching Disadvantaged Children in the Preschool.* Englewood Cliffs: Prentice-Hall, 1966.

BERENDA, R. W. *The Influence of the Group on the Judgments of Children.* New York: King's Crown Press, 1950.

BERNSTEIN, B. Elaborated and restricted codes: Their social origins and some consequences. *American Anthropologist,* 1964. no. 6, part 2, 55–69.

BETTELHEIM, B. Joey: A "mechanical boy." *Scientific American,* March, 1959.

———. *The Empty Fortress.* New York: Free Press, 1967.

BEXTON, W. H., HERON, W., and SCOTT, T. H. Effects of decreased variation in the sensory environment. *Canadian Journal of Psychology,* 1954, 8, 70–76.

BIBER, B. Premature structuring as a deterrent to creativity. *Bank Street College of Education Publications,* n.d., no. 67 (originally *American Journal of Orthopsychiatry,* 1959, 29, no. 2.)

BIRCH, H. G., and LEFFORD, A. Intersensory development in children. *Monographs of the Society for Research in Child Development,* 1963, 28, no. 5.

BIRNS, B., BLANK, M., BRIDGER, W. H., and ESCALONA, S. B. Behavioral inhibition in neonates produced by auditory stimuli. *Child Development,* 1965, 36, 639–645.

BITTERMAN, M. E., WODINSKY, J., and CANDLAND, D. K. Some comparative psychology. *American Journal of Psychology,* 1958, 71, 94–110.

BLANK, M., and BRIDGER, W. H. Cross-modal transfer in nursery-school children. *Journal of Comparative and Physiological Psychology,* 1964, 58, 277–282.

BLAUVELT, H. Dynamics of the mother-newborn relationship in goats. In Schaffner, B. (ed.) *Group Processes: Transactions of the First Conference.* New York: Macy Foundation, 1955, pp. 221–258.

———, and McKENNA, J. Mother-neonate interaction: Capacity of the human newborn for orientation. In Foss, B. M. (ed.) *Determinants of Infant Behavior* (q. v.) pp. 3–29.

BLISS, E. D. (ed.) *Roots of Behavior.* New York: Harper, 1962.

BORING, E. G. *A History of Experimental Psychology.* New York: Appleton-Century-Crofts, second edition, 1950.

BOUSFIELD, W. A. The occurrence of clustering in the recall of randomly arranged associates. *Journal of General Psychology,* 1953, 49, 229–240.

BOWER, T. G. R. Stimulus variables determining space perception in infants. *Science,* 1965, 149, 88–89.

———. Slant perception and shape constancy in infants. *Science,* 1966, 151, 832–834.

BOWLBY, J. *Child Care and the Growth of Love.* London: Pelican, second edition, 1965.

BRACKBILL, Y., and THOMPSON, G. G. (eds.) *Behavior in Infancy and Early Childhood.* New York: Free Press, 1967, pp. 259–274.

BRADLEY, N. C. The growth of the knowledge of time in children of school-age. *British Journal of Psychology,* 1947, 38, 67–78.

BRIDGES, K. M. B. Emotional development in early infancy. *Child Development,* 1932, 3, 324–341.

BROWN, F. A. Living clocks. *Science,* 1959, 130, 1535–1544.

BRUCE, H. M. A block to pregnancy in the mouse caused by the proximity of strange males. *Journal of Reproductive Fertility,* 1960, 1, 96.

BRUNER, J. S. *The Process of Education.* Cambridge: Harvard, 1960.

———. After John Dewey, what? *Bank Street College of Education Publications,* 1961, no. 54 (originally published in *Saturday Review,* June 17, 1961).

———. *On Knowing.* Cambridge: Harvard-Belknap, 1962.

BÜHLER, C. *The First Year of Life.* New York: John Day, 1930.

BURGHARDT, G. M. and HESS, E. H. Food imprinting in the snapping turtle, Chelydra serpentina. *Science,* 1966, 151, 108–109.

BURNET, F. M. Immunological recognition of self. *Science,* 1961, 133, 307–311.

CALDWELL, B. M. Mother-infant interaction in monomatric and polymatric families. *American Journal of Orthopsychiatry,* 1963, 33, 653–664.

———. The effects of infant care. In HOFFMAN, M. L., and HOFFMAN, L. W. (eds.) *Review of Child Development Research* (q.v.), vol. I.

———. *Preschool Inventory Manual.* The author, 1965.

CALHOUN, J. G. Population density and social pathology. *Scientific American,* February, 1962, pp. 139–148.

CAMPBELL, D. T. Social attitudes and other acquired behavioral dispositions. In KOCH, S. (ed.) *Psychology: A Study of a Science* (q.v.).

CANNON, W. B. *Bodily Changes in Pain, Hunger, Fear, and Rage.* New York: Appleton-Century, second edition, 1929.

———. *Wisdom of the Body.* New York: Norton, 1939.

CARMICHAEL, L. (ed.) *Manual of Child Psychology.* New York: Wiley, second edition, 1954.

CARPENTER, E., VARLEY, F., and FLAHERTY, R. *Eskimo.* Toronto: University of Toronto, 1959.

CARR, H. A., and WATSON, J. B. Orientation in the white rat. *Journal of Comparative Neurology,* 1908, 18, 27–44.

CARSON, R. *The Silent Spring.* Boston: Houghton Mifflin, 1962.

CARY, J. *A House of Children.* New York: Harper, 1955.

CASLER, L. The effects of supplementary verbal stimulation on a group of institutionalized infants. *American Psychologist,* 1965, 20, 476 (abstract).

CASSIRER, E. Le langage et la construction du monde des objets. *Journal de Psychologie Normale et Pathologique,* 1933, 30, 18–44.

———. *An Essay on Man.* New York: Doubleday, Anchor Books, 1954.

CAUDILL, W., and WEINSTEIN, H. Maternal care and infant behavior in Japanese and American urban middle class families. In König, R., and Hill, R. (eds.) *Yearbook of the International Sociological Association,* 1966.

CAVINESS, J. A., and GIBSON, J. J. The equivalence of visual and tactual stimulation for the perception of solid forms. Paper read at meetings of Eastern Psychological Association, 1962.

CHASTAING, M. Premiers sourires enfantins. In *Rencontre/Encounter/Begegnung.* Utrecht and Antwerp: Spectrum, 1957, pp. 80–87.

CHESLER, M. A. Ethnocentrism and attitudes toward the physically disabled. *Journal of Personality and Social Psychology,* 1965, 2, 877–882.

CHILD STUDY ASSOCIATION OF AMERICA. *Parents' Guide to Facts of Life for Children.* New York: Maco, 1965.

CHODOFF, P. A critique of Freud's theory of infantile sexuality. *American Journal of Psychiatry,* 1966, 123, 507–518.

CHOMSKY, N. Review of *Verbal Behavior,* by B. F. Skinner. *Language,* 1959, 35, 26–58.

CHURCH, J. *Language and the Discovery of Reality: A Developmental Psychology of Cognition.* New York: Random House, 1961.

————. Innovations, excellence, and children's learning. *Bank Street College of Education Publications,* 1962 (originally published in *School and Society,* 1962, 90, 401–404).

————. (ed.) *Three Babies.* New York: Random House, 1966.

————, and INSKO, C. A. Ethnic and sex differences in sexual values. *Psychologia,* 1965, 8, 153–157.

CLEMENS, S. L. *The Adventures of Huckleberry Finn,* 1884.

CLOCK, R. O. *Our Baby.* New York and London: Appleton, 1912.

COHEN, W. Spatial and textural characteristics of the *Ganzfeld. American Journal of Psychology,* 1957, 70, 403–410.

COMALLI, P. E., WAPNER, S., and WERNER, H. Interference effects of Stroop color-word test in children, adults, and aged. Paper read at meeting of Eastern Psychological Association, 1960.

COMMAGER, H. S. (ed.) *America in Perspective.* New York: New American Library, 1947.

CONN, J. H., and KANNER, L. Children's awareness of sex differences. *Journal of Child Psychiatry,* 1947, 1, 3–57.

CORAH, N. L., ANTHONY, E. J., PAINTER, P., STERN, J. A., and THURSTON, D. Effects of perinatal anoxia after seven years. *Psychological Monographs,* 1965, 79, no. 3.

CRABTREE, C. A. Effects of structuring on productiveness of children's thinking. *Dissertation Abstracts,* 1962, 23, 161. Reprinted in Gordon, I. J. (ed.), *Human Development.* Chicago: Scott, Foresman, 1965, pp. 249–250.

CRONBACH, L. J. A validation design for qualitative studies in personality. *Journal of Consulting Psychology,* 1948, 12, 365–374.

CROWELL, D. C., SHIRO, L. K., CADE, T. M., LANDAU, B., and BENNETT, H. L. Progress report: Preschool readiness project. Honolulu: University of Hawaii, 1966 (mimeographed).

CROWELL, D. H., DAVIS, C. M., CHUN, B. J., and SPELLACY, F. J. Galvanic skin reflex in newborn humans. *Science,* 1965, 148, 1108–1111.

CRUICKSHANK, W. M. *Psychology of Exceptional Children and Youth.* Englewood Cliffs: Prentice-Hall, second edition, 1963.

DANIELSSON, B. *Love in the South Seas.* London: George Allen & Unwin, 1956.

DARBY, C. L., and RIOPELLE, A. J. Observational learning in the rhesus monkey. *Journal of Comparative and Physiological Psychology,* 1959, 52, 94–98.

DARWIN, C. A biographical sketch of an infant. *Mind,* 1877, 2, 285–294.

DAVIS, C. M. Results of the self-selection of diets by young children. *Canadian Medical Association Journal,* 1939, 41, 257–261.

DAVIS, H. V., SEARS, R. R., MILLER, H. C., and BRODBECK, A. J. Effects of cup, bottle, and breast feeding on oral activities of newborn infants. *Pediatrics,* 1948, 2, 549–558.

DAVIS, R. C., BUCHWALD, A. M., and FRANKMAN, R. W. Autonomic and muscular responses, and their relation to simple stimuli. *Psychological Monographs,* 1955, 69, no. 405.

————, GARAFALO, L., and KVEIM, K. Conditions associated with gastrointestinal activity. *Journal of Comparative and Physiological Psychology,* 1959, 52, 466–475.

DAWE, H. C. An analysis of two hundred quarrels of preschool children. *Child Development,* 1934, 5, 139–157.

DENENBERG, V. H., HUDGENS, G. A., and ZARROW, M. X. Mice reared with rats: Modification of behavior by early experience with another species. *Science,* 1963, 143, 380–381.

———, and WHIMBEY, A. E. Infantile stimulation and animal husbandry: A methodological study. *Journal of Comparative and Physiological Psychology,* 1963, 56, 877–878.

DENNIS, W. Piaget's questions applied to a child of known environment. *Journal of Genetic Psychology,* 1942, 60, 307–320.

———. Historical beginnings of child psychology. *Psychological Bulletin,* 1949, 46, 224–235.

———. Animistic thinking among college and university students. *Scientific Monthly,* 1953, 76, 247–250.

———, and NAJARIAN, P. Infant development under environmental handicap. *Psychological Monographs,* 1957, 71, no. 7.

DEUTSCHE, J. M. *The Development of Children's Concepts of Causal Relations.* Minneapolis: University of Minnesota, 1937.

DILLON, M. S. Attitudes of children toward their own bodies and those of other children. *Child Development,* 1935, 5, 165–176.

DOBZHANSKY, T. *Mankind Evolving.* New Haven: Yale, 1962.

DOLLARD, J., DOOB, L. W., MILLER, N. E., MOWRER, O. H., SEARS, R. R., *et al. Frustration and Aggression.* New Haven: Yale, 1939.

DOUVAN, E., and ADELSON, J. *The Adolescent Experience.* New York: Wiley, 1966.

DOXIADIS, S., VALAES, T., KARAKLIS, A., and STAVRAKAKIS, D. Risk of severe jaundice in glucose-6-phosphate-dehydrogenase deficiency of the newborn. *The Lancet,* Dec. 5, 1964, pp. 1210–1212.

DRILLIÉN, C. M. *The Growth and Development of the Prematurely Born Infant.* Baltimore: Williams & Wilkins, 1964.

DuBois, C. The dominant value profile of American culture. *American Anthropologist,* 1955, 57, 1232–1239.

DUKES, W. F. N = 1. *Psychological Bulletin,* 1965, 64, 74–79.

DUMAS, G. *Traité de Psychologie.* Paris: Alcan, 1923.

DUNN, L. C., and DOBZHANSKY, T. *Heredity, Race and Society.* New York: Mentor, revised edition, 1952.

EASTMAN, N. J. *Expectant Motherhood.* Boston: Little, Brown, second edition, 1956.

EISENBERG, L., and KANNER, L. Early infantile autism, 1943–55. *American Journal of Orthopsychiatry,* 1956, 27, 556–566.

ELEFTHERIOU, B., BRONSON, F. H., and ZARROW, M. X. Interaction of olfactory and other environmental stimuli on implantation in the deer mouse. *Science,* 1962, 137, 764.

ENDLER, N. S., and BOULTER, L. R. *Contemporary Issues in Developmental Psychology.* New York: Holt, Rinehart, & Winston, 1967.

ENGEN, T., LIPSITT, L. P., and KAYE, H. Olfactory responses and adaptation in the human neonate. *Journal of Comparative and Physiological Psychology,* 1963, 56, 73–77.

ERIKSON, E. H. *Childhood and Society.* New York: Norton, 1951.

ESCALONA, S., and HEIDER, G. M. *Prediction and Outcome.* New York: Basic Books, 1959.

EVANS, B. *The Natural History of Nonsense.* New York: Vintage, 1958 (originally published in 1946).

FANTZ, R. L. Pattern vision in newborn infants. *Science,* 1963, 140, 296–297.

———. Visual perception from birth as shown by pattern sensitivity. In Caldwell, B. M., Fantz, R. L., Greenberg, N. H., Stone, L. J., and Wolff, P. H. New issues in infant development. *Annals of the New York Academy of Science,* 1965, 118, 783–866.

FAUST, M. S. Developmental maturity as a determinant in prestige of adolescent girls. *Child Development,* 1960, 31, 173–184.

FIEDLER, M. F. *Deaf Children in a Hearing World.* New York: Ronald, 1952.

———, and STONE, L. J. The Rorschachs of selected groups of children in comparison with published norms: II. The effects of socio-economic status on Rorschach performance. *Journal of Projective Techniques,* 1956, 20, 276–279.

FILLENBAUM, S. Impairment in performance with delayed auditory feedback as related to task characteristics. *Journal of Verbal Learning and Verbal Behavior,* 1963, 2, 136–141.

FISCHBERG, M., and BLACKLER, A. W. How cells specialize. *Scientific American,* September, 1961, pp. 121–140.

FISHER, C., GROSS, J., and ZUCH, J. A cycle of penile erections synchronous with dreaming (REM) sleep. *Archives of General Psychiatry,* 1965, 12, 29–45.

FISKE, D. W., and MADDI, S. R. (eds.) *Functions of Varied Experience.* Homewood, Ill.: Dorsey, 1961.

FLORY, C. D. Osseous development in the hand as an index of skeletal development. *Monographs of the Society for Research in Child Development,* 1936, 1, no. 3.

FORGAYS, D. G., and FORGAYS, J. W. The nature of the effect of free environmental experience in the rat. *Journal of Comparative and Physiological Psychology,* 1952, 45, 322–328.

FOSS, B. M. (ed.) *Determinants of Infant Behavior.* New York: Wiley, 1961.

———. *Determinants of Infant Behavior II.* New York: Wiley, 1963.

FOWLER, W. Cognitive learning in infancy and early childhood. *Psychological Bulletin,* 1962, 59, 116–152.

FRANK, L. K. The fundamental needs of the child. *Mental Hygiene,* July, 1938, pp. 353–379.

———. *Projective Methods.* Springfield, Ill.: Thomas, 1948.

———. *On the Importance of Infancy.* New York: Random House, 1966, PP 32.

FREEDMAN, D. G. Constitutional and environmental interactions in rearing of four breeds of dogs. *Science,* 1958, 127, 585–586.

———. The differentiation of identical and fraternal infant twins on the basis of filmed behavior. Paper read at *Second International Congress of Human Genetics,* 1961.

———, KING, J. A., and ELLIOT, O. Critical period in the social development of dogs. *Science,* 1961. 133, 1016.

FREEDMAN, M. B. As older sexual codes crumble on campus, a newer honesty takes their place. In Time, Inc., *The Young Americans.* New York: Time-Life Books, 1966, pp. 98–99.

FREUD, S. *Collected Papers.* London: Hogarth, 1950.

———. *A General Introduction to Psychoanalysis.* New York: Liveright, 1935.

FRIEDAN, B. *The Feminine Mystique.* New York: Norton, 1963.

FRIEDENBERG, E. Z. *The Vanishing Adolescent.* Boston: Beacon, 1959.

———. *Coming of Age in America.* New York: Random House, 1966.

GARDNER, E. J. *Principles of Genetics.* New York: Wiley, 1960.

GARRATY, J. A. The interrelations of psychology and biography. *Psychological Bulletin,* 1954, 51, 569–582.

GELLERT, E. Children's conceptions of the content and functions of the human body. *Genetic Psychology Monographs,* 1962, 65, 293–405.

GESELL, A., and ILG, F. L. *Infant and Child in the Culture of Today.* New York: Harper, 1943.

————, and THOMPSON, H. Twins T and C from infancy to adolescence: A biogenetic study of individual differences by the method of co-twin control. *Genetic Psychology Monographs*, 1941, 24, 3–121.

————, ————, and AMATRUDA, C. S. *The Psychology of Early Growth*. New York: Macmillan, 1938.

GHENT, L. Form and its orientation: A child's-eye view. *American Journal of Psychology*, 1961, 74, 177–190.

GOETHE, J. W. v. *Leiden des jungen Werthers*, 1795.

GOLDFARB, W. Psychological privation in infancy and subsequent adjustment. *American Journal of Orthopsychiatry*, 1945, 15, 247–255.

GOLDING, W. *Lord of the Flies*. New York: Coward-McCann, 1954. (Also available in paperback.)

GOLDSTEIN, K. *The Organism*. New York: American Book Company, 1939.

————, and SCHEERER, M. Abstract and concrete behavior. *Psychological Monographs*, 1941, 53, no. 2.

GOODENOUGH, F. L., and ANDERSON, J. E. Psychology and anthropology: Some problems of joint import for the two fields. *Southwestern Journal of Anthropology*, 1947, 3, 5–14.

GOODMAN, M. E. Child's-eye view of the world of people. *Wheelock Alumnae Quarterly*, Winter, 1965, pp. 7–10.

GOODMAN, P. *Growing Up Absurd*. New York: Random House, 1960.

————. Moral youth in an immoral society. In Time, Inc., *The Young Americans*. New York: Time-Life Books, 1966, pp. 18–19, 110–111.

GRAHAM, F. K. Behavioral differences between normal and traumatized new borns. I. The test procedures. *Psychological Monographs*, 1956, 70, no. 20.

————, ERNHART, C. B., THURSTON, D., and CRAFT, M. Development three years after perinatal anoxia and other potentially damaging newborn experiences. *Psychological Monographs*, 1962, 76, no. 3.

————, MATARAZZO, R. G., and CALDWELL, B. M. II. Standardization, reliability, and validity. *Psychological Monographs*, 1956, 70, no. 21.

GRAY, S. W., and KLAUS, R. A. An experimental preschool program for culturally deprived children. *Child Development*, 1965, 36, 887–898.

GRIFFITHS, C. *Hear*. New York: Exposition Press, 1966.

GRIFFITHS, R. *A Study of Imagination in Early Childhood*. London: Kegan Paul, 1935.

————. *The Abilities of Babies*. New York: McGraw-Hill, 1954.

GROSE, R. F., and BIRNEY, R. C. (eds.) *Transfer of Learning*. Princeton: Van Nostrand, 1963.

GROSSBERG, J. M. Behavior therapy: A review. *Psychological Bulletin*, 1964, 62, 73–88.

GUILFORD, J. P. *The Nature of Human Intelligence*. New York: McGraw-Hill, 1967.

GUILLAUME, P. Les débuts de la phrase dans le langage de l'enfant. *Journal de Psychologie Normale et Pathologique*, 1927, 24, 203–229.

GUNTHER, M. Infant behavior at the breast. In Foss, B. M. (ed.) *Determinants of Infant Behavior*. New York: Wiley, 1961, pp. 37–44.

GYORGY, P., DHANAMITTA, S., and STEERS, E. Protective effects of human milk in experimental staphylococcus infection. *Science*, 1962, 137, 338–340.

HABER, W. B. Reactions to loss of limb: Physiological and psychological aspects. *Annals of the New York Academy of Sciences*, 1958, 74, 14–24.

HAEUSSERMAN, E. *Developmental Potential of Preschool Children*. New York: Grune & Stratton, 1958.

HAGGARD, E. A., BREKSTAD, A., and SKARD, Å. G. On the reliability of the anamnestic interview. *Journal of Abnormal and Social Psychology*, 1960, 61, 311–318.

HALL, C. S. The inheritance of emotionality. *Sigma Xi Quarterly*, 1938, 26, 17–27, 37.

HALL, E. T. *The Silent Language*. Garden City: Doubleday, 1959. (Also available in paperback.)

HALL, G. S. *Adolescence*. New York: Appleton: 1904, 2 vols.

HALPERN, E. The effects of incompatibility between perception and logic in Piaget's stage of concrete operations. *Child Development*, 1965, 36, 491–497.

HARLOW, H. F. The nature of love. *American Psychologist*, 1958, 13, 673–685.

―――. The heterosexual affectional system in monkeys. *American Psychologist*, 1962, 17, 1–9.

―――, and HARLOW, M. K. Social deprivation in monkeys. *Scientific American*, 1962, 207, 136–146.

―――, and KUENNE, M. Learning to think. *Scientific American*, 1949, 181, 36–39.

HARTLEY, R. E. *Growing Through Play*. New York: Columbia University, 1952.

―――, FRANK, L. K., and GOLDENSON, R. M. *Understanding Children's Play*. New York: Columbia University, 1952.

HARVEY, O. J., and CONSALVI, C. Status and conformity to pressures in informal groups. *Journal of Abnormal and Social Psychology*, 1960, 60, 182–187.

HATCH, A., BALAZS, T., WIBERG, G. S., and GRICE, H. C. Long-term isolation stress in rats. *Science*, 1963, 142, 507.

HAYES, C. *The Ape in Our House*. New York: Harper, 1951.

HAYNES, H., WHITE, B. L., and HELD, R. Visual accommodation in human infants. *Science*, 1965, 148, 528–530.

HAZLITT, V. Children's thinking. *British Journal of Psychology*, 1930, 20, 354–361.

HEBB, D. O. Heredity and environment in mammalian behaviour. *British Journal of Animal Behaviour*, 1953, 1, 43–47.

HECHINGER, G., and HECHINGER, F. M. *Teen-age Tyranny*. New York: Morrow, 1963.

HEIDBREDER, E. (Studies in concept formation and thinking; for complete bibliography, see D. H. RUSSELL, *Children's Thinking*.)

HEIDER, F., and SIMMEL, M. An experimental study of apparent behavior. *American Journal of Psychology*, 1944, 57, 243–259.

HELD, R., and HEIN, A. Movement-produced stimulation in the development of visually-guided behavior. *Journal of Comparative and Physiological Psychology*, 1963, 56, 872–876.

HENDRY, C. E., LIPPITT, R., and ZANDER, A. *Reality Practice as Educational Method*. New York: Beacon House, 1944.

HERON, W., DOANE, B. K., and SCOTT, T. H. Visual disturbances after prolonged perceptual isolation. *Canadian Journal of Psychology*, 1956, 10, 13–18.

HESS, E. H. Imprinting in birds. *Science* , 1964, 146, 1128–1139.

HESS, R. D., and SHIPMAN, V. C. Early experience and the socialization of cognitive modes in children. *Child Development*, 1965, 36, 869–886.

HEWETT, F. M. Teaching speech to an autistic child through operant conditioning. *American Journal of Orthopsychiatry*, 1965, 35, 927–936.

HILGARD, E. R., and BOWER, G. H. *Theories of Learning*. New York: Appleton-Century-Crofts, third edition, 1966.

HIRSCH, J. Behavior genetics and individuality understood. *Science*, 1963, 142, 1436–1442.

HOCHBERG, J., and BROOKS, V. Pictorial recognition as an unlearned ability: A study of one child's performance. *American Journal of Psychology*, 1962, 75, 624–628.

HOFFMAN, M. L., and HOFFMAN, L. W. (eds.) *Review of Child Development Research*. New York: Russell Sage, Vol. I, 1964; Vol. II, 1967.

HOLLINGSHEAD, A. B. *Elmtown's Youth*. New York: Wiley, 1949.

HONZIK, M. P., MACFARLANE, J. W., and ALLEN, L. The stability of mental test performance between two and eighteen years. *Journal of Experimental Education*, December, 1948, pp. 309–324.

HOUSE, B. J., and ZEAMAN, D. Reward and nonreward in the discrimination learning of imbeciles. *Journal of Comparative and Physiological Psychology*, 1958, 51, 614–618.

HSU, C. Y. Influence of temperature on rat embryos. *Anatomical Research*, 1948, 100, 79–90.

HUANG, I. Children's conception of physical causality: A critical summary. *Journal of Genetic Psychology*, 1943, 63, 71–121.

HUGHES, R. *A High Wind in Jamaica* (also published as *The Innocent Voyage*). New York: New American Library, 1965 (originally published in 1929).

HUNT, J. McV. An instance of the social origin of conflict resulting in psychoses. *American Journal of Orthopsychiatry*, 1938, 8, 158–164.

———. *Intelligence and Experience.* New York: Ronald, 1961.

HUNTER, W. S. The delayed reaction in animals and children. *Behavior Monographs*, 1913, 2, no. 1.

HUNTON, V. C. The recognition of inverted pictures by children. *Journal of Genetic Psychology*, 1955, 86, 281–288.

IGEL, G. J., and CALVIN, A. D. The development of affectional responses in infant dogs. *Journal of Comparative and Physiological Psychology*, 1960, 53, 302–305.

INHELDER, B. Criteria of the stages of mental development. In Tanner, J. M., and Inhelder, B. *Discussions on Child Development.* New York: International Universities, 1953, I, 75–107.

———, and PIAGET, J. *The Early Growth of Logic in the Child.* New York: Harper & Row, 1964.

IRWIN, O. C., and WEISS, A. P. A note on mass activity in newborn infants. *Journal of Genetic Psychology*, 1930, 38, 20–30.

ISAACS, S. *Intellectual Growth in Young Children.* London: Routledge, 1930.

———. *Social Development in Young Children.* London: Routledge, 1933.

JENKINS, J. J., and PALERMO, D. S. Further changes in word association norms. *Journal of Personality and Social Psychology*, 1965, 1, 303–309.

———, and RUSSELL, W. A. Systematic changes in word association norms: 1910–1952. *Journal of Abnormal and Social Psychology*, 1960, 60, 293–304.

JERSILD, A. T., and HOLMES, F. B. *Children's Fears.* New York: Bureau of Publications, Teachers College, Columbia University, 1935.

JOHNSON, R. C. Similarity in IQ of separated identical twins as related to length of time spent in same environment. *Child Development*, 1963, 34, 745–749.

JOHNSON, W., *et al.* A study of the onset and development of stuttering. *Journal of Speech and Hearing Disorders*, 1942, 7, 251–257.

JONES, M. C. Psychological correlates of somatic development. *Child Development*, 1965, 36, 899–911.

———, and BAYLEY, N. Physical maturing among boys as related to behavior. *Journal of Educational Psychology*, 1950, 41, 129–148.

JOYCE, J. *A Portrait of the Artist as a Young Man.* New York: Modern Library, 1928 (originally published in 1917, also available in paperback).

KAGAN, J., and MOSS, H. A. *Birth to Maturity.* New York: Wiley, 1962.

KALISH, R. A. The aged and the dying process: The inevitable decisions. *Journal of Social Issues*, 1965, 21, 87–96.

KAMII, C. K., RADIN, N. L., and WEIKART, D. P. A. A two-year preschool program for culturally disadvantaged children. Paper read at meetings of American Psychological Association, 1966.

KANNER, L. Early infantile autism. *Journal of Pediatrics*, 1944, 25, 211–217.

KAPLAN, B., and WAPNER, S. (eds.) *Perspectives in Psychological Theory.* New York: International Universities, 1960.

KARDINER, A., and associates. *The Psychological Frontiers of Society.* New York: Columbia University, 1945.

KATCHER, A. The discrimination of sex differences by young children. *Journal of Genetic Psychology,* 1955, 87, 131–143.

KAWI, A. A., and PASAMANICK, B. Prenatal and paranatal factors in the development of childhood reading disorders. *Monographs of the Society for Research in Child Development,* 1959, 24, no. 4.

KAWIN, E. Parenthood in a free nation. Volume II: *Early and Middle Childhood.* New York: Macmillan, 1961.

KELLER, L., COLE, M., BURKE, C. J., and ESTES, W. K. Reward and information values of trial outcomes in paired-associate learning. *Psychological Monographs,* 1965, 79, no. 12.

KENDLER, T. S., and KENDLER, H. H. Reversal and nonreversal shifts in kindergarten children. *Journal of Experimental Psychology,* 1959, 58, 56–60.

KESSLER, J. W. *Psychopathology of Childhood.* Englewood Cliffs: Prentice-Hall, 1966.

KIMBLE, D. P. (ed.) *The Anatomy of Memory.* Palo Alto: Science and Behavior Books, 1965.

KINSEY, A. C., and associates. *Sexual Behavior in the Human Male.* Philadelphia: Saunders, 1948.

————. *Sexual Behavior in the Human Female.* Philadelphia: Saunders, 1953.

KIRK, S. A. *Early Education of the Mentally Retarded.* Urbana: University of Illinois, 1958.

————. *Educating Exceptional Children.* Boston: Houghton Mifflin, 1962.

KIRKENDALL, L. A., and LIBBY, R. W. Interpersonal relationships—crux of the sexual renaissance. *Journal of Social Issues,* 1966, 22, 45–59.

KLATSKIN, E. H., JACKSON, E. B., and WILKIN, L. C. The influence of degree of flexibility in maternal child care practices on early child behavior. *American Journal of Orthopsychiatry,* 1956, 26, 79–93.

KLÜVER, H. Eidetic imagery. In Murchison, C. *Handbook of Child Psychology.* Worcester: Clark University, second edition, 1933, pp. 699–722.

————. The study of personality and the method of equivalent and non-equivalent stimuli. *Character and Personality,* 1936, 5, 91–112.

KOCH, S. (ed.) *Psychology: A Study of a Science.* New York: McGraw-Hill, vol. 6, 1963.

KOFF, R. H. Systematic changes in children's word-association norms 1916–63. *Child Development,* 1965, 36, 299–305.

KOFFKA, K. *Principles of Gestalt Psychology.* New York: Harcourt, Brace, 1935.

KOHLBERG, L. Development of moral character and moral ideology. In HOFFMAN, M. L., and HOFFMAN, L. W. (eds.) *Review of Child Development Research* (q.v.), I, 383–431.

KOHLER, I. On the Structuring and Transformation of the Perceptual World. New York: International Universities, 1964.

KRASNER, L. Studies of the conditioning of verbal behavior. *Psychological Bulletin,* 1958, 55, 148–170.

KREEZER, G., and DALLENBACH, K. M. Learning the relation of opposition. *American Journal of Psychology,* 1929, 41, 432–441.

KREUTTER, M. The teacher in the brown paper bag. *Urban Review,* May, 1966.

KROGMAN, W. M. Trend in the study of physical growth in children. *Child Development,* 1940, 11, 279–284.

————. The physical growth of children. *Monographs of the Society for Research in Child Development,* 1955, 20, no. 1.

KRON, R. E., STEIN, M., and GODDARD, K. E. A method of measuring sucking behavior of newborn infants. *Psychosomatic Medicine*, 1963, 25, 181–191.

KUENNE, M. R. Experimental investigation of the relation of language to transposition behavior in young children. *Journal of Experimental Psychology*, 1946, 36, 371–490.

KUO, Z.-Y. *The Dynamics of Behavior Development: An Epigenetic View.* New York: Random House, PP 34, 1967.

LACEY, J. I. The evaluation of autonomic responses: Toward a general solution. *Annals of the New York Academy of Sciences*, 1956, 67, art. 5, 123–164.

———, and DALLENBACH, K. M. Acquisition by children of the cause-effect relationship. *American Journal of Psychology*, 1939, 52, 103–110.

LANGNESS, L. L. *The Life History in Anthropological Science.* New York: Holt, Rinehart, & Winston, 1965.

LAPOUSE, R. The epidemiology of behavior disorders in children. *American Journal of Diseases of Children*, 1966, 111, 594–599.

LENNOX, B. Chromosomes for beginners. *The Lancet*, 1961, i, no. 7185, 1046–1051.

LEONARD, M. F., RHYMES, J. P., and SOLNIT, A. J. Failure to thrive in infants. *American Journal of Diseases of Children*, 1966, 111, 600–612.

LEOPOLD, W. F. *Speech Development of a Bilingual Child.* Evanston-Chicago: Northwestern University Studies in the Humanities, 6, 1939–1949, 4 vols.

———. *Bibliography of Child Language.* Evanston: Northwestern University, 1952.

LEVINE, J., FISHMAN, C., and KAGAN, J. Social class and sex as determinants of maternal behavior. Paper read at meetings of American Orthopsychiatric Association, 1967.

LEVINE, S. The psychophysiological effects of early stimulation. In BLISS, E. L. (ed.) *Roots of Behavior* (q.v.).

———, and MULLINS, R. F. Hormonal influences on brain organization in infant rats. *Science*, 1966, 152, 1585–1592.

LEVY, D. M. Experiments on the sucking reflex and social behavior in dogs. *American Journal of Orthopsychiatry*, 1934, 4, 203–224.

———. Studies in sibling rivalry. *Research Monographs of the American Orthopsychiatric Association*, 1937, 2.

———. On instinct-satiation: An experiment on the pecking behavior of chickens. *Journal of Genetic Psychology*, 1938, 18, 327–348.

———. *Maternal Overprotection.* New York: Columbia University, 1943.

———. Psychic trauma of operations in children. *American Journal of Diseases of Children*, 1945, 69, 7–25.

———. Advice and reassurance. *American Journal of Public Health*, 1954, 44, 1113–1118.

———. The relation of animal psychology to psychiatry. *Medicine and Science*, 1954, 16, 44–75.

———. The infant's earliest memory of inoculation: A contribution to public health procedures. *Journal of Genetic Psychology*, 1960, 96, 3–46.

LEWIN, K. *A Dynamic Theory of Personality.* New York: McGraw-Hill, 1935.

———. Behavior and development as a function of the total situation. In CARMICHAEL, L. *Manual of Child Psychology* (q.v.), pp. 918–970.

———, LIPPITT, R., and WHITE, R. Patterns of aggressive behavior in experimentally created "social climates." *Journal of Social Psychology*, 1939, 10, 271–299.

LEWIS, M. M. *How Children Learn to Speak.* New York: Basic Books, 1959.

LIPPITT, R., and WHITE, R. The "social climate" of children's groups. In Barker, R., Kounin, J. S., and Wright, H. F. (eds.) *Child Behavior and Development.* New York: McGraw-Hill, 1943, pp. 485–508.

LIPSITT, L. P., ENGEN, T., and KAYE, H. Developmental changes in the olfactory threshold of the neonate. *Child Development,* 1963, 34, 371–376.

———, and LEVY, N. Electrotactual thresholds in the neonate. *Child Development,* 1959, 30, 547–554.

LIPTON, E. L., STEINSCHNEIDER, A., and RICHMOND, J. B. Swaddling, a child care practice. *Pediatrics,* 1965, 35, 521–567.

LOBB, H. Vision *versus* touch in form discrimination. *Canadian Journal of Psychology,* 1965, 19, 175–187.

LONG, L., and WELCH, L. (Studies in concept formation; for complete bibliography, see RUSSELL, D. H. *Children's Thinking.*)

LORENZ, K. Z. *King Solomon's Ring.* New York: Crowell, 1952.

LOWIE, R. H. Review of Gusinde, M. *Die Feuerlander Indianer.* Mödling bei Wien: Anthropos, 1937. *American Anthropologist,* 1938, 40, 495–503.

LYND, H. M. *On Shame and the Search for Identity.* New York: Harcourt Brace, 1958.

———. Some questions raised by experiences of shame. Paper read at meetings of the American Psychological Association, 1966.

LYND, R. S. and H. M. *Middletown in Transition.* New York: Harcourt Brace, 1937.

LYNES, R. *A Surfeit of Honey.* New York: Harper, 1957.

MACCOBY, E. E., and BEE, H. L. Some speculations concerning the lag between perceiving and performing. *Child Development,* 1965, 36, 368–377.

MacDONALD, D. Profile of Eugene Gilbert. *The New Yorker,* November 22, 1958, pp. 57 ff., and November 29, 1958, pp. 57 ff.

MACFARLANE, J., ALLEN, L., and HONZIK, M. P. *A Developmental Study of the Behavior Problems of Normal Children between Twenty-one Months and Fourteen Years.* Berkeley: University of California, 1954.

MACHOTKA, P. The development of esthetic criteria in childhood: I. Justifications of preference. *Child Development,* 1966, 37, 877–885.

MacRAE, D. A test of Piaget's theories of moral development. *Journal of Abnormal and Social Psychology,* 1954, 49, 14–18.

MAIER, N. R. F. Reasoning in children. *Journal of Comparative Psychology,* 1936, 21, 357–366.

———. Maier's law. *American Psychologist,* 1960, 15, 208–212.

MALTZ, H. E. Ontogenetic changes in the meaning of concepts as measured by the semantic differential. *Child Development,* 1963, 34, 667–674.

MANN, T. *Stories of Three Decades.* New York: Knopf, 1936.

MARETZKI, T. W., and MARETZKI, H. *Taira: An Okinawan Village.* New York: Wiley, 1966.

MASLOW, A. H. Self-actualizing people: A study of psychological health. *Personality Symposia,* 1950, 1, 11–34.

McCANDLESS, B. Environment and intelligence. *American Journal of Mental Deficiency,* 1952, 56, 596–597.

McCARTHY, D. Language development in children. In CARMICHAEL, L. *Manual of Child Psychology* (q.v.), pp. 492–630.

McCLELLAND, D. C. *The Achieving Society.* Princeton: Van Nostrand, 1961.

McGINLEY, P. *The Love Letters of Phyllis McGinley.* New York: Viking, 1954.

MEAD, M. *And Keep Your Powder Dry.* New York: Morrow, 1942.

———. *Male and Female.* New York: Morrow, 1949.

———, and MACGREGOR, F. C. *Growth and Culture: A Photographic Study of Balinese Childhood.* New York: Putnam, 1951.

———, and WOLFENSTEIN, M. (eds.) *Childhood in Contemporary Cultures.* Chicago: University of Chicago, 1955.

587

MEDAWAR, P. H. *The Future of Man.* New York: Basic Books, 1959.

MEIER, G. W. Other data on the effects of social isolation during rearing upon adult reproductive behaviour in the rhesus monkey (Macaca-Mulatta). *Animal Behaviour,* 1965, 13, 228–231.

MELZACK, R., PENICK, E., and BECKETT, A. The problem of "innate fear" of the hawk shape. *Journal of Comparative and Physiological Psychology,* 1959, 52, 694–698.

MERLEAU–PONTY, M. *Phénoménologie de la Perception.* Paris: NRF, 1945.

MERRILL PALMER QUARTERLY, 1964, 10, no. 3. Selected papers from the Institute for Developmental Studies, Arden House Conference on pre-school enrichment of socially disadvantaged children.

MERTON, R. K. *On the Shoulders of Giants.* New York: Free Press, 1965.

MEYER, EDITH. Comprehension of spatial relations in preschool children. *Journal of Genetic Psychology,* 1940, 57, 119–151.

MEYERSON, L. Somatopsychology of physical disability. In CRUICKSHANK, W. M., *Psychology of Exceptional Children and Youth* (q.v.).

MICHOTTE, A. *La Perception de la Causalité.* Louvain: Institut Supérieur de Philosophie, 1946.

MILLER, G. A., GALANTER, E., and PRIBRAM, K. H. *Plans and the Structure of Behavior.* New York: Holt, 1960.

MILLER, L. Children and money. *Redbook,* November, 1959, 39–41, 66, 68.

MILLER, N. E. The perception of children. *Journal of Genetic Psychology,* 1934, 44, 321–339.

MILLER, R. R., and SCHULTZ, R. J. All-female strains of the teleost fishes of the genus Poeciliopsis. *Science,* 1959, 130, 1656–1657.

MILLER, W., and ERVIN, S. The development of grammar in child language. In Bellugi, U., and Brown, R. (eds.) The acquisition of language. *Monographs of the Society for Research in Child Development,* 1964, 29, no. 1.

MILLS, D., and BISHOP, M. Onward and upward with the arts: Songs of innocence. *The New Yorker,* November 13, 1937, pp. 32–42.

MINTZ, B. (ed.) *Environmental Influences on Prenatal Development.* Chicago: University of Chicago, 1958.

MINUCHIN, P., and BIBER, B. A child development approach to language in the preschool disadvantaged child. Paper read at meetings of the Society for Research in Child Development, 1967.

MISCHEL, W., and METZNER, R. Preference for delayed reward as a function of age, intelligence and length of delay interval. *Journal of Abnormal and Social Psychology,* 1962, 64, 425–431.

MITTWOCH, U. Sex differences in cells. *Scientific American,* July, 1963, pp. 54–62.

MOLTZ, H., and STETTNER, L. J. The influence of patterned-light deprivation on the critical period for imprinting. *Journal of Comparative and Physiological Psychology,* 1961, 54, 279–283.

MONTAGU, M. F. A. Adolescent sterility. *Quarterly Review of Biology,* 1939, 14, 13–34 and 192–219.

———. *The Direction of Human Development.* New York: Harper, 1955.

———. *Prenatal Influences.* Springfield, Ill.: Thomas, 1962.

MOORE, A. U. Studies on the formation of the mother-neonate bond in sheep and goat. Paper read at meetings of the American Psychological Association, 1960.

MOORE, T., and UCKO, L. E. Night waking in early infancy. *Archives of Disease in Childhood,* 1957, 32, 333–342.

MOWRER, O. H. *Learning Theory and the Symbolic Processes.* New York: Wiley, 1960.

————, and Mowrer, W. M. Enuresis—A method for its study and treatment. *American Journal of Orthopsychiatry*, 1938, 3, 436–459.

Munn, N. L. *The Evolution and Growth of Human Behavior*. Boston: Houghton Mifflin, second edition, 1965.

Murphy, G. *Personality: A Biosocial Approach to Origins and Structures*. New York: Harper, 1947.

————. *Historical Introduction to Modern Psychology*. New York: Harcourt, Brace, revised edition, 1949.

————. *Human Potentialities*. New York: Basic Books, 1958.

————, Murphy, L. B., and Newcomb, T. M. *Experimental Social Psychology*. New York: Harper, revised edition, 1937.

Murphy, L. B. *Social Behavior and Child Personality*. New York: Columbia University, 1937.

————. *The Widening World of Childhood*. New York: Basic Books, 1962.

————, and associates. *Personality in Young Children*. New York: Basic Books, 1956.

Mussen, P. H. (ed.) *Handbook of Research Methods in Child Development*. New York: Wiley, 1960.

Nash, O. *The Ogden Nash Pocket Book*. New York: Pocket Books, 1944.

Neilon, P. Shirley's babies after fifteen years: A personality study. *Journal of Genetic Psychology*, 1948, 73, 175–186.

Nelson, T. H. The Hypertext. *International Federation for Documentation: Abstracts, 1965 Congress*, p. 80.

Newman, H. H., Freeman, F. N., and Holzinger, K. J. *Twins*. Chicago: University of Chicago, 1937.

Nicolson, A. B., and Hanley, C. Indices of physiological maturity: derivation and interrelationships. *Child Development*, 1953, 24, 3–38.

Nixon, R. E. *The Art of Growing*. New York: Random House, 1962.

Ogburn, W. F., and Bose, N. K. On the trail of the wolf-children. *Genetic Psychology Monographs*, 1959, 60, 117–193.

Olson, W. C., and Hughes, B. O. The concept of organismic age. *Journal of Educational Research*, 1942, 36, 525–527.

Olum, V. Developmental differences in the perception of causality. *American Journal of Psychology*, 1956, 69, 417–423.

Opie, I., and Opie, P. *The Lore and Language of School Children*. Oxford: Clarendon, 1959.

Ortar, G. R. Classification of speech directed at children by mothers of different level of education and cultural background. Paper read at 18th International Congress of Psychology, 1966.

Osgood, C. E. On understanding and creating sentences. *American Psychologist*, 1963, 18, 735–751.

Palermo, D. S., and Jenkins, J. J. Changes in word associations of fourth- and fifth-grade children from 1916 to 1961. *Journal of Verbal Learning and Verbal Behavior*, 1965, 4, 180–187.

Papoušek, H. Conditioning during early postnatal development. In Brackbill, Y., and Thompson, G. G. (eds.) *Behavior in Infancy and Early Childhood*. New York: Free Press, 1967, pp. 259–274.

Pasamanick, B., and Knoblock, H. Early feeding and birth difficulties in childhood schizophrenia: An explanatory note. *Journal of Psychology*, 1963, 56, 73–77.

Patel, A. S., and Gordon, J. E. Some personal and situational determinants of yielding to influence. *Journal of Abnormal and Social Psychology*, 1960, 61, 411–418.

PESTALOZZI, J. *How Father Pestalozzi Educated and Observed His Three-and-a-Half-Year-Old Son,* 1774.

PIAGET, J. *Judgment and Reasoning in the Child.* New York: Harcourt, Brace, 1928.

———. *The Child's Conception of the World.* New York: Harcourt, Brace, 1929.

———. Das Umdrehen des Gegenstandes beim Kind unter einem Jahr. *Psychologishe Rundschau,* 1932, 4, 110–115.

———. *The Moral Judgment of the Child.* Glencoe: Free Press, 1948 (originally published in 1932).

———. How children form mathematical concepts. *Scientific American,* November, 1953, pp. 74–79.

———. *The Construction of Reality in the Child.* New York: Basic Books, 1954.

PINCUS, G. The breeding of some rabbits produced by artificially activated ova. *Proceedings of the National Academy of Sciences,* 1939, 25, 557–559.

PINNEAU, S. R. The infantile disorders of hospitalism and anaclitic depression. *Psychological Bulletin,* 1955, 52, 429–452.

PINTNER, R., and LEV, J. Worries of school children. *Journal of Genetic Psychology,* 1940, 56, 67–76.

PLATT, J. R. The step to man. *Science,* 1965, 149, 607–613.

POLANYI, M. *Personal Knowledge.* Chicago: University of Chicago, 1958.

PRATT, K. C. The neonate. In CARMICHAEL, L. (ed.) *Manual of Child Psychology* (q.v.), pp. 215–291.

———, NELSON, A. K., and SUN, K. H. The behavior of the newborn infant. *Ohio State University Studies, Contributions to Psychology,* 1930, 10.

PREYER, W. *Die Seele des Kindes,* 1882.

PROVENCE, S., and LIPTON, R. *Children in Institutions.* New York: International Universities, 1962.

PYLES, M. K., STOLZ, H. R., and MACFARLANE, J. S. The accuracy of mothers' reports on birth and developmental data. *Child Development,* 1935, 6, 165–176.

QUERIDO, A., and MEAD, M. Mental health and the floods in Holland. *World Mental Health,* 1953, 5, 34–38.

RABBAN, M. Sex-role identification in young children in two diverse social groups. *Genetic Psychology Monographs,* 1950, 42, 81–158.

RADKE, M. J., and TRAGER, H. G. Children's perceptions of the social roles of Negroes and whites. *Journal of Psychology,* 1950, 29, 3–33.

———, ———, and DAVIS, H. Social perceptions and attitudes of children. *Genetic Psychology Monographs,* 1949, 40, 327–447.

RAINWATER, L. Some aspects of lower class sexual behavior. *Journal of Social Issues,* 1966, 22, 96–108.

RAPAPORT, D. (ed.) *Organization and Pathology of Thought.* New York: Columbia University, 1951.

READ, K. *The Nursery School.* Philadelphia: Saunders, fourth edition, 1966.

REYNOLDS, M. M. *Negativism of Preschool Children.* New York: Bureau of Publications, Teachers College, Columbia University, 1928.

———, and MALLAY, H. Sleep of young children. *Journal of Genetic Psychology,* 1933, 43, 322–351.

RHEINGOLD, H. L. The modification of social responsiveness in institutionalized babies. *Monographs of the Society for Research in Child Development,* 1956, 21, no. 2.

RIBBLE, M. A. *The Rights of Infants.* New York: Columbia University, revised edition, 1965.

RICHARDSON, C., and CHURCH, J. A developmental analysis of proverb interpretations. *Journal of Genetic Psychology,* 1959, 94, 169–179.

RICHMOND, J. B., LIPTON, E., and STEINSCHNEIDER, A. Observations on differences in autonomic nervous system function between and within individuals during early infancy. *Journal of the American Academy of Child Psychiatry,* 1962, 1, 83.

RICHTER, C. P. Total self-regulatory functions in animals and human beings. *Harvey Lectures,* 1942–43, 38, 63–103.

RIESEN, A. H. The development of visual perception in man and chimpanzee. *Science,* 1947, 106, 107–108.

RIESMAN, D., in collaboration with Reuel Denny and Nathan Glazer. *The Lonely Crowd.* New Haven: Yale, 1950.

RIMLAND, B. *Infantile Autism.* New York: Appleton–Century–Crofts, 1964.

RING, K., LIPINSKI, C. E., and BRAGINSKY, D. The relationship of birth order to self-evaluation, anxiety reduction, and susceptibility to emotional contagion. *Psychological Monographs.* 1965, 79, no. 10.

RIOPELLE, A. J. Observational learning of a position habit by monkeys. *Journal of Comparative and Physiological Psychology,* 1960, 53, 426–428.

ROBERTS, E. Thumb and finger sucking in relation to feeding in early infancy. *American Journal of Diseases of Children,* 1944, 68, 7–8.

ROBERTS, K. E., and SCHOELLKOPF, J. A. Eating, sleeping, and elimination practices of a group of two-and-one-half-year-old children. *American Journal of Diseases of Children,* 1951, 82, 121–152.

ROBERTSON, J. *Young Children in Hospitals.* New York: Basic Books, 1958.

ROBINOWITZ, R. Learning the relation of opposition as related to scores on the Wechsler Intelligence Scale for Children. *Journal of Genetic Psychology,* 1956, 88, 25–30.

ROBINSON, H. B. An experimental examination of the size-weight illusion in young children. *Child Development,* 1964, 35, 91–107.

ROFFWARG, H. P., MUZIO, J. N., and DEMENT, W. C. Ontogenetic development of the human sleep-dream cycle. *Science,* 1966, 152, 604–619.

ROSENBLATT, J. S., TURKEVITZ, G., and SCHNEIRLA, T. C. Early socialization in the domestic cat as based on feeding and other relationships between female and young. In Foss, B. M. (ed.) *Determinants of Infant Behavior* (q.v.).

ROSENBLITH, J. F., and ALLINSMITH, W. (eds.) *The Causes of Behavior.* Boston: Allyn and Bacon, second edition, 1966.

ROSENTHAL, R. *Pygmalion in the Classroom.* New York: Holt, Rinehart & Winston, in press.

ROSENZWEIG, M. R. Environmental complexity, cerebral change, and behavior. *American Psychologist,* 1966, 21, 321–332.

———, KRECH, D., BENNETT, E. L., and ZOLMAN, J. F. Variation in environmental complexity and brain measures. *Journal of Comparative and Physiological Psychology,* 1962, 55, 1092–1095.

ROSENZWEIG, S., and KOGAN, K. L. *Psychodiagnostics.* New York: Grune & Stratton, 1949.

ROSS, J. B., and MCLAUGHLIN, M. M. (eds.) *A Portable Medieval Reader.* New York: Viking, 1949.

ROSSI, E. L., and ROSSI, S. I. Concept utilization, serial order and recall in nursery-school children. *Child Development,* 1965, 36, 771–778.

ROTH, P. *Letting Go.* New York: Random House, 1962.

ROTHBART, M. K., and MACCOBY, E. E. Parents' differential reactions to sons and daughters. *Journal of Personality and Social Psychology,* 1966, 4, 237–243.

RUBIN, T. I. *Jordi.* New York: Macmillan, 1960.

RUSSELL, D. H. *Children's Thinking.* Boston: Ginn and Co., 1956.

SACKETT, G. P. Effect of rearing conditions upon the behavior of rhesus monkeys. *Child Development,* 1965, 36, 855–868.

SALINGER, J. D. *The Catcher in the Rye.* Boston: Little, Brown, 1951.

SAMPSON, E. E. The study of ordinal position: Antecedents and outcomes (1964, mimeographed).

SANGER, M. D. Language learning in infancy: A review of the autistic hypothesis and an observational study of infants. Unpublished Ed. D. Thesis, Harvard University, 1955.

SARASON, S. B., and GLADWIN, T. Psychological and cultural problems in mental subnormality: A review of research. *Genetic Psychology Monographs,* 1958, 57, 3–290.

———, HILL, K. T., and ZIMBARDO, P. G. A longitudinal study of the relation of test anxiety to performance on intelligence and achievement tests. *Monographs of the Society for Research in Child Development,* 1964, 29, no. 7.

SAYEGH, Y., and DENNIS, W. The effects of supplementary experiences upon the behavioral development of infants in institutions. *Child Development,* 1965, 36, 81–90.

SCHAEFER, E. S. A circumplex model for maternal behavior. *Journal of Abnormal and Social Psychology,* 1959, 59, 226–235.

SCHEERER, M. Cognitive theory. In Lindzey, G. (ed.) *Handbook of Social Psychology.* Cambridge: Addison–Wesley, 1954, I, 91–142.

SCHEIN, M. W., and HALE, E. B. The effect of early social experience on male sexual behavior of androgen-injected turkeys. *Animal Behavior,* 1959, 7, 189–200.

SCHIFF, W. Perception of impending collision. *Psychological Monographs,* 1965, 79, no. 11.

SCOTT, J. P. *Animal Behavior.* Chicago: University of Chicago, 1958. (Also available in paperback.)

———. Critical periods in behavioral development. *Science,* 1962, 138, 949–958.

———, and FULLER, J. L. *Genetics and the Social Behavior of the Dog.* Chicago: University of Chicago, 1965.

SCUPIN, E. and G. *Bubis erste Kindheit.* Leipzig: Grieben, 1907.

SEARLE, L. V. The organization of hereditary maze-brightness and maze-dullness. *Genetic Psychology Monographs,* 1949, 39, 279–325.

SEARS, R. R. *Survey of Objective Studies of Psychoanalytic Concepts.* New York: Social Science Research Council, 1943.

———, MACCOBY, E. E., and LEVIN, H. *Patterns of Child Rearing.* Evanston: Row, Peterson, 1957.

———, and WISE, G. W. Relation of cup feeding in infancy to thumb-sucking and the oral drive. *American Journal of Orthopsychiatry,* 1950, 20, 123–138.

SHERIF, M., HARVEY, O. J., WHITE, B. J., HOOD, W. R., and SHERIF, C. W. *Intergroup Conflict and Cooperation: The Robbers Cave Experiment.* Norman, Okla: University Book Exchange, 1961.

SHERMAN, M. The differentiation of emotional responses. *Journal of Comparative Psychology,* 1927, 7, 265–284.

———. The differentiation of emotional responses in infants: II. The ability of observers to judge the emotional characteristics of the crying of infants and of the voice of the adult. *Journal of Comparative Psychology,* 1927, 7, 335–351.

SHERWIN, R. V. The law and sexual relationships. *Journal of Social Issues,* 1966, 22, 109–122.

SHESH, D. B. Measurement of aesthetic sense of children. *Psychologia,* 1966, 9, 236–238.

SHINN, M. W. *Biography of a Baby.* Boston: Houghton Mifflin, 1900.

SHIRLEY, M. M. *The First Two Years, A Study of Twenty-Five Babies,* Minneapolis: University of Minnesota, 1931–1933, 3 vols.

SHUTTLEWORTH, F. K. The physical and mental growth of girls and boys age six to nineteen in relation to age at maximum growth. *Monographs of the Society for Research in Child Development,* 1939, 4, 3.

————. The adolescent period: A graphic atlas. *Monographs of the Society for Research in Child Development,* 1949, 14, 1.

————. The adolescent period: A pictorial atlas. *Monographs of the Society for Research in Child Development,* 1949, 14, 2.

SIGEL, I. E. How intelligence tests limit understanding of intelligence. *Merrill-Palmer Quarterly of Behavior and Development,* 1963, 9, 39–56.

SIMMEL, M. L. The absence of phantoms for congenitally missing limbs. *American Journal of Psychology,* 1961, 74, 467–470.

SIMPSON, G. G. The biological nature of man. *Science,* 1966, 152, 472–478.

SINGER, J. L. *Daydreaming.* New York: Random House, 1966.

SIQUELAND, E. R., and LIPSITT, L. P. Conditioned headturning in human newborns. *Journal of Experimental Child Psychology,* 1966, 3, 356–376.

SKEELS, H. M. Adult status of children with contrasting early life experiences. *Monographs of the Society for Research in Child Development,* 1966, 31, no. 3.

SKINNER, B. F. *Walden Two.* New York: Macmillan, 1948.

————. Behaviorism at fifty. *Science,* 1963, 140, 951–958.

SMITH, C. J. Mass action and early environment in the rat. *Journal of Comparative and Physiological Psychology,* 1959, 52, 154–156.

SMITH, H. T. Report on nurse-infant interactions. Unpublished.

SMITH, M. B. Socialization for competence. *Social Science Research Council Items,* 1965, 19, 17–23.

SMITH, R. P. *"Where Did You Go?" "Out." "What Did You Do?" "Nothing."* New York: Norton, 1957. (Also available in paperback).

————. *How to Do Nothing with Nobody, All Alone by Yourself.* New York: Norton, 1958.

SMITH, S. M., BROWN, H. O., TOMAN, J. E. P., and GOODMAN, L. S. The lack of cerebral effects of D-Tubocurarine. *Anesthesiology,* 1947, 8, 1–14.

SMITH, W. M., McCRARY, J. W., and SMITH, K. U. Delayed visual feedback and behavior. *Science,* 1960, 132, 1013–1014.

SOLLENBERGER, R. T. Some relationships between the urinary excretion of male homone by maturing boys and their expressed interests and attitudes. *Journal of Psychology,* 1940, 9, 179–189.

SOLOMON, R. L. Punishment. *American Psychologist,* 1963, 18, 239–253.

SONTAG, L. W. The significance of fetal environmental differences. *American Journal of Obstetrics and Gynecology,* 1941, 42, 996–1003.

————. Differences in modifiability of fetal behavior and physiology. *Psychosomatic Medicine,* 1944, 6, 151–154.

————, and REYNOLDS, E. L. The Fels composite sheet: I. A practical method for analyzing growth progress. *Journal of Pediatrics,* 1945, 26, 327–335.

SPEARMAN, C. E. *The Creative Mind.* New York: Appleton, 1931.

SPEARS, W. C. Assessment of visual preference and discrimination in the four-month-old infant. *Journal of Comparative and Physiological Psychology,* 1964, 57, 381–386.

SPENCE, K. W. Cognitive factors in the extinction of the conditioned eyelid response in humans. *Science,* 1963, 140, 1224–1225.

SPERRY, R. W. Summation. In KIMBLE, D. P. (ed.) *The Anatomy of Memory* (q.v.), pp. 140–177.

SPIKER, C. C., and McCANDLESS, B. R. The concept of intelligence and the philosophy of science. *Psychological Review,* 1954, 61, 255–266.

SPIRO, M. E. *Children of the Kibbutz.* Cambridge: Harvard, 1958.

SPITZ, R. A. Hospitalism. An inquiry into the genesis of psychiatric conditions in early childhood. *Psychoanalytic Study of the Child,* 1945, 1, 53–74.

———. Hospitalism: A follow-up report. *Psychoanalytic Study of the Child,* 1946, 2, 113–117.

———. The smiling response: A contribution to the ontogenesis of social relations. *Genetic Psychology Monographs,* 1946, 34, 57–125.

———. The psychogenic diseases in infancy: An attempt at their etiologic classification. *Psychoanalytic Study of the Child,* 1951, 6, 255–275.

———. *The First Year of Life.* New York: International Universities, 1965.

SPOCK, B. *Baby and Child Care.* New York: Pocket Books, 1957.

SPRINGER, D. Development in young children of an understanding of time and the clock. *Journal of Genetic Psychology,* 1952, 80, 83–96.

STAPLES, R. The responses of infants to color. *Journal of Experimental Psychology,* 1932, 15, 119–141.

STECHLER, G. Newborn attention as affected by medication during labor. *Science,* 1964, 144, 315–317.

STERNGLASS, E. J. Cancer: Relation of prenatal radiation to development of the disease in childhood. *Science,* 1963, 140, 1102–1104.

STEVENSON, H. W., and McBEE, G. The learning of object and pattern discrimination by children. *Journal of Comparative and Physiological Psychology,* 1958, 51, 752–754.

STODDARD, G. D. *The Meaning of Intelligence.* New York: Macmillan, 1943.

STOLZ, H. R., and STOLZ, L. M. *Somatic Development of Adolescent Boys.* New York: Macmillan, 1951.

STOLZ L. M. Youth: The Gesell Institute and its latest study. *Contemporary Psychology,* 1958, 3, 10–15.

———, and collaborators. *Father Relations of War-Born Children.* Stanford: Stanford University, 1954.

STONE, L. J. Experiments in group play and readiness for destruction. In Lerner and Murphy (eds.), Methods for the study of personality in young children. *Monographs of the Society for Research in Child Development,* 1941, pp. 101–155.

———. *Finger Painting: Children's Use of Plastic Materials.* A Guide to the Film. New York: New York University Film Library, 1944.

———. Some problems of filming children's behavior: A discussion based on experience in the production of "Studies of Normal Personality Development." *Child Development,* 1952, 23, 227–233.

———. A critique of studies of infant isolation. *Child Development,* 1954, 25, 9–20.

———. He still learns through his play. In *Childcraft.* Chicago: Field Enterprises, 1954, 13, 151–161.

———, FIEDLER, M. F., and FINE, C. G. Preschool education of deaf children. *Journal of Speech and Hearing Disorders,* 1961, 26, 45–60.

STOTLAND, E., and DUNN, R. E. Identification, "oppositeness," authoritarianism, self-esteem, and birth order. *Psychological Monographs,* 1962, 76, no. 9.

STOTT, L. H., and BALL, R. S. Infant and preschool mental tests. *Monographs of the Society for Research in Child Development,* 1965, 30, no. 3.

STRAUSS, A. L. The development of conceptions of rules in children. *Child Development,* 1954, 25, 193–208.

Swan, C. Rubella in pregnancy as an aetiological factor in congenital malformation, stillbirth, miscarriage, and abortion. *Journal of Obstetrics and Gynaecology of the British Empire*, 1949, 56, 341–363 and 591–605.

Szasz, T. S. The uses of naming and the origin of the myth of mental illness. *American Psychologist*, 1961, 16, 59–65.

Tanner, J. M. *Education and Physical Growth*. London: University of London, 1961.

Tauber, E. S., and Koffler, S. Optomotor response in human infants to apparent motion: Evidence of innateness. *Science*, 1966, 152, 382–383.

Taussig, H. B. The thalidomide syndrome. *Scientific American*, August, 1962, 29–35.

Terman, L. M., *et al. Genetic Studies of Genius*. Stanford: Stanford University, vol. I, 1925.

———, and Tyler, L. E. Psychological sex differences. In L. Carmichael, *Manual of Child Psychology* (q.v.), pp. 1064–1114.

Thiessen, D. D., and Rodgers, D. A. Population density and endocrine function. *Psychological Bulletin*, 1961, 58, 441–451.

———, Zolman, J. F., and Rodgers, D. A. Relation between adrenal rate, brain cholinesterase activity, and hole-in-wall behavior of mice under different living conditions. *Journal of Comparative and Physiological Psychology*, 1962, 55, 186–190.

Thomas, A. S., Birch, H. G., Hertzog, M. E., and Korn, S. *Behavioral Individuality in Early Childhood*. New York: New York University, 1963.

Thompson, W. R., and Heron, W. The effects of restricting early experience on the problem-solving capacity of dogs. *Canadian Journal of Psychology*, 1954, 8, 17–31.

———, and Schaefer, T. Early environmental stimulation. In Fiske, D. W., and Maddi, S. R. (eds.) *Functions of Varied Experience*. Homewood, Ill.: Dorsey, 1961.

Tiedemann, D. *Beobachtung über die Entwicklung der Seelenfähigkeiten bei Kindern*, 1787.

Tighe, T. J. Reversal and nonreversal shifts in monkeys. *Journal of Comparative and Physiological Psychology*, 1964, 58, 324–326.

Todd, T. W. The roentgenographic appraisement of skeletal differentiation. *Child Development*, 1930, 1, 298–310.

Tryon, R. C. Genetic differences in maze-learning ability in rats. *Thirty-ninth Yearbook of the National Society for the Study of Education*, 1940, 111–119.

Tyler, L. E. *Tests and Measurements*. Englewood Cliffs: Prentice-Hall, 1963.

———. *The Psychology of Human Differences*. New York: Appleton-Century-Crofts, 1965.

U. S. Bureau of the Census. *Statistical Abstract of the United States*. Washington: U. S. Government Printing Office, 1957 and 1962.

U. S. Dept. of Health, Education, and Welfare. *Minimal Brain Dysfunction in Children*. Washington: U. S. Government Printing Office, National Institute of Neurological Disease and Blindness Monograph no. 3, 1966.

U. S. Dept. of Health, Education, and Welfare, Children's Bureau. *Bibliography on the Battered Child*. Washington: U. S. Government Printing Office, 1961 (mimeographed).

———. *Infant Care*. Washington: U. S. Government Printing Office (periodically revised).

———. *Prenatal Care*. Washington: U. S. Government Printing Office (periodically revised).

————. *Your Child From One to Six*. Washington: U. S. Government Printing Office (periodically revised).

————. *Your Child From Six to Twelve*. Washington: U. S. Government Printing Office (periodically revised).

————. *The Adolescent in Your Family*. Washington: U. S. Government Printing Office (periodically revised).

VALENTINE, C. W. The colour perception and colour preference of an infant during its fourth and eighth months. *British Journal of Psychology*, 1913–14, 6, 363–386.

————. *The Normal Child: And Some of His Abnormalities*. Baltimore: Penguin, 1956.

VAN DEN BERG, J. H. *The Changing Nature of Man*. New York: Dell, 1964.

VERPLANCK, W. S. A glossary of some terms used in the objective science of behavior. *Psychological Review*, 1957, 64, Supplement 8, 42 pp.

WALK, R. D., and GIBSON, E. J. A comparative and analytical study of visual depth perception. *Psychological Monographs*, 1961, 75, no. 15.

WALTERS, R. H., MARSHALL, W. E., and SHOOTER, J. R. Anxiety, isolation, and susceptibility to social influence. *Journal of Personality*, 1960, 28, 518–529.

WANN, K., DORN, M., and LIDDLE, E. *Fostering Intellectual Development in Young Children*. New York: Columbia University, 1962.

WARFIELD, F. *Cotton in My Ears*. New York: Viking, 1948.

WARKANY, J. Etiology of mongolism. *Journal of Pediatrics*, 1960, 56, 412–419.

WATSON, J. B. *Psychology from the Standpoint of a Behaviorist*. Philadelphia: Lippincott, 1919.

————. *Psychological Care of Infant and Child*. New York: Norton, 1928.

WEATHERLY, D. Self-perceived rate of physical maturation and personality in late adolescence. *Child Development*, 1964, 35, 1197–1210.

WEININGER, O. Mortality of albino rats under stress as a function of early handling. *Canadian Journal of Psychology*, 1953, 7, 111–114.

WEINREICH, U. Travels through semantic space. *Word*, 1958, 14, 346–366.

————. On the semantic structure of language. In Greenberg, J. H. (ed.) *Universals of Language*. Cambridge: M.I.T., 1963.

WEIR, R. H. *Language in the Crib*. The Hague: Mouton, 1962.

WELCH, L., and LONG, L. (Studies in concept formation; for complete bibliography, see RUSSELL, *Children's Thinking*.)

WENGER, M. A. The measurement of individual differences in autonomic balance. *Psychosomatic Medicine*, 1941, 3, 427–434.

WERNER, H. *Comparative Psychology of Mental Development*. Chicago: Follett, revised edition, 1948.

————, FREUD, A., SEARS, R. R., and FRANK, L. K. *Symposium on Genetic Psychology*. Worcester: Department of Psychology, Clark University, 1950.

————, and KAPLAN, B. *Symbol Formation*. New York: Wiley, 1963.

————, and KAPLAN, E. The acquisition of word meanings. *Monographs of the Society for Research in Child Development*, 1950, 25, no. 1.

WERTHEIMER, M. Psychomotor coordination of auditory and visual space at birth. *Science*, 1961, 134, 1692.

WHITE, B. L. The development of perception during the first six months of life. Paper read at meetings of the American Association for the Advancement of Science, 1963.

————, and HELD, R. Plasticity of sensori-motor development in the human infant. In ROSENBLITH, J. F., and ALLINSMITH, W. (eds.) *The Causes of Behavior*. Boston: Allyn & Bacon, second edition, 1966.

WHITE, R. K., and LIPPITT, R. O. *Autocracy and Democracy*. New York: Harper, 1960.

WHITE, R. W. Motivation reconsidered: The concept of competence. *Psychological Review*, 1959, 66, 297–333.

———. Ego and reality in psychoanalytic theory. *Psychological Issues*, 1963, Monograph No. 11.

———. *Lives in Progress*. New York: Holt, Rinehart, & Winston, second edition, 1966.

WHITING, J. S. M., and CHILD, I. L. *Child Training and Personality*. New Haven: Yale, 1953.

WHORF, B. L. *Language, Thought, and Reality*. Edited by J. B. Carroll. New York and Cambridge: Wiley and M.I.T., 1956.

WILKINSON, F. R., and CARGILL, D. W. Repression elicited by story material based on the Oedipus complex. *Journal of Social Psychology*, 1955, 42, 209–214.

WILLIAMS, C. D. The elimination of tantrum behavior by extinction procedures. *Journal of Abnormal and Social Psychology*, 1959, 59, 269.

WILLIAMS, R. J. The biological approach to the study of personality. Paper given at the Berkeley Conference on Personality Development in Childhood, 1960.

WILSON, J. J., WILSON, B. C., and SWINYARD, C. A. Two-point discrimination in congenital amputees. *Journal of Comparative and Physiological Psychology*, 1962, 55, 482–485.

WILSON, R. S. Personality patterns, source attractiveness, and conformity. *Journal of Personality*, 1960, 28, 186–199.

WINDLE, W. F. Neuropathology of certain forms of mental retardation. *Science*, 1963, 140, 1186–1191.

WITHERS, C. *A Rocket in My Pocket*. New York: Holt, 1948.

WITKIN, H. A. and associates. *Personality through Perception*. New York: Harper, 1954.

WOHLWILL, J. F. The perception of size and distance relationships in perspective drawings. Paper read at meetings of Eastern Psychological Association, 1962.

———, and WIENER, M. Discrimination of form orientation in young children. *Child Development*, 1964, 35, 1113–1125.

WOLF, M. M., RISLEY, T., and MEES, H. Application of operant conditioning procedures to the behavior problems of an autistic child. *Behavior Research and Therapy*, 1964, 1, 305–312.

WOLFENSTEIN, M. The emergence of fun morality. *Journal of Social Issues*, 1951, 7, 15–25.

WOLFF, P. H. Observations on the early development of smiling. In Foss, B. M. (ed.) *Determinants of Infant Behavior* II, pp. 113–138. New York: Wiley, 1963.

———. Observations on newborn infants. *Psychosomatic Medicine*, 1959, 21, 110–118.

WOLFF, W. *The Expression of Personality*. New York: Harper, 1943.

———. *The Personality of the Preschool Child*. New York: Grune & Stratton, 1946.

WOODCOCK, L. P. *Life and Ways of the Two-Year-Old*. New York: Dutton, 1941.

WOODWORTH, R. S. *Contemporary Schools of Psychology*. New York: Ronald, revised edition, 1948.

WORK, H. H., and HALDANE, J. E. Cerebral dysfunction in children. *American Journal of Diseases of Children*, 1966, 111, 573–580.

WRIGHT, H. F. *Recording and Analyzing Child Behavior*. New York: Harper & Row, 1967.

YACORZYNSKI, G. K., and TUCKER, B. E. What price intelligence? *American Psychologist*, 1960, 15, 201–203.

YARROW, L. J. Separation from parents during early childhood. In HOFFMAN, M. L., and HOFFMAN, L. W. (eds.) *Review of Child Development Research* (q.v.), vol. I.

ZAMENHOF, S. MOSLEY, J., and SCHULLER, E. Stimulation of the proliferation of cortical neurons by prenatal treatment with growth hormone. *Science,* 1966, 152, 1396–1397.

ZAZZO, R. Le problème de l'imitation chez le nouveau-né. *Enfance,* 1957, 2, 135–142.

PHOTO SOURCES

*The authors are grateful for permission to use photographs
from the following sources:*

Eve Arnold for the photo on p. 2

Irene Bayer/Monkmeyer Press Photo Service for the photo on p. 333

Gregory Bateson and Margaret Mead for the photo on p. 2 (from FIRST DAYS IN THE LIFE OF A NEW GUINEA BABY, Film, New York University Film Library) and the photos on pp. 106, 114, 145, 151, 274, and 301 (from *Balinese Character: A Photographic Analysis,* New York: The New York Academy of Sciences, Special Publications, Vol. II, 1942; Reissued 1962)

Marc and Evelyne Bernheim/Rapho Guillumette Pictures for the photo on p. 363

Esther Bubley for the photo on p. 30

Bettye Caldwell, Director, Children's Center, Syracuse, N.Y., for the photos on pp. 99, 309, 335

Alexandria Church for the photos on pp. 248, 361, 368

W. L. Faust for the photos on pp. 362, 368

The Ford Foundation for the photo on p. 151

Rita Freed for the photo on p. 460

P. W. Freeland/The Franklin Institute for the photos on pp. 403, 411

Louis Georgianna, Upstate Medical Center, Syracuse, N.Y., for the photo on p. 99

Harry F. Harlow for the photos on p. 111

Ken Heyman for the photos on pp. 149, 365

Dorothy Levens, Director of the Vassar College Nursery School, for the photos on pp. 332, 333, 338, 341–343, 347–348

Leviton-Atlanta for the photos on pp. 497, 501

Fred W. McDarrah for the photos on pp. 469, 473

The McGraw Hill Book Company for the photos on the title page and pp. 3, 24–25 (from Edith L. Potter, *Fundamentals of Human Reproduction,* McGraw-Hill Book Co., 1948)

Wayne Miller for the photos on the title page and pp. 65, 83, 133, 363, 390–391

Theodor H. Nelson for the photo on p. 419

The Office of Economic Opportunity for the photos on pp. 148, 340, 334, 525

Ruth Orkin for the photo on p. 406

Myron Papiz for the photos on pp. 335, 343

Fred Schnell for the photos on pp. 434, 461

Ray Shaw for the photos on p. 365

The Society of Brothers for the photos on the title page and pp. 332, 348 (from *Children in Community 1963,* edited by the Society of Brothers and published by The Plough Publishing House, Rifton, New York)

Time/Life for the photos on pp. 114, 362, 418, 419

Burk Uzzle for the photo on p. 335

The Vassar Film Program for the photos on pp. 83, 86–87, 92, 248, 256 (from ABBY'S FIRST TWO YEARS); the photo on p. 93 (from INCITEMENT TO READING); and the photos on p. 333 (from STARTING NURSERY SCHOOL)

INDEX

A NOTE ON THE TYPE

The text of this book is set in Caledonia, a typeface designed by W(illiam) A(ddison) Dwiggins for the Mergenthaler Linotype Company in 1939. Dwiggins chose to call his new typeface Caledonia, the Roman name for a Scotland, because it was inspired by the Scotch types cast about 1833 by Alexander Wilson & Son, Glasgow type founders. However, there is a calligraphic quality about this face that is totally lacking in the Wilson types. Dwiggins referred to an even earlier typeface for this "liveliness of action"—one cut around 1790 by William Martin for the printer William Bulmer. Caledonia has more weight than the Martin letters, and the bottom finishing strokes (serifs) of the letters are cut straight across, without brackets, to make sharp angles with the upright stems, thus giving a "modern face" appearance.

W. A. DWIGGINS (1880–1956) was born in Martinsville, Ohio, and studied art in Chicago. In 1904 he moved to Hingham, Massachusetts, where he built a solid reputation as a designer of advertisements and as a calligrapher. He began an association with the Mergenthaler Linotype Company in 1929, and over the next twenty-seven years designed a number of book types for that firm. Of especial interest are the Metro series, Electra, Caledonia, Eldorado, and Falcon. In 1930, Dwiggins first became interested in marionettes, and through the years made many important contributions to the art of puppetry and the design of marionettes.

Manufactured in the United States of America by American Book–Stratford Press, Inc. Design by Leon Bolognese.